Integrated Clinical Orthodontics

Integrated Clinical Orthodontics

Edited by

Vinod Krishnan, BDS, MDS, MOrth, RCS Ed

Professor, Department of Orthodontics, Sri Sankara Dental College, Trivandrum, Kerala, India

Ze'ev Davidovitch, DMD, Cert Ortho

Professor of Orthodontics, Emeritus, Harvard University, Boston, Massachusetts, USA

Clinical Professor, Department of Orthodontics, Case Western Reserve University, Cleveland, Ohio, USA

WILEY-BLACKWELL

A John Wiley & Sons, Ltd., Publication

This edition first published 2012
© 2012 by Blackwell Publishing Ltd

Blackwell Publishing was acquired by John Wiley & Sons in February 2007. Blackwell's publishing program has been merged with Wiley's global Scientific, Technical and Medical business to form Wiley-Blackwell.

Registered office: John Wiley & Sons, Ltd, The Atrium, Southern Gate, Chichester, West Sussex, PO19 8SQ, UK

Editorial offices: 9600 Garsington Road, Oxford, OX4 2DQ, UK
  The Atrium, Southern Gate, Chichester, West Sussex, PO19 8SQ, UK
  2121 State Avenue, Ames, Iowa 50014-8300, USA

For details of our global editorial offices, for customer services and for information about how to apply for permission to reuse the copyright material in this book please see our website at www.wiley.com/wiley-blackwell.

Library of Congress Cataloging-in-Publication Data
Integrated clinical orthodontics / edited by Vinod Krishnan, Ze'ev Davidovitch.
   p. ; cm.
  Includes bibliographical references and index.
   ISBN 978-1-4443-3597-2 (hardback)
  I. Krishnan, Vinod.   II. Davidovitch, Zeev.
  [DNLM: 1. Orthodontics–methods.   WU 400]
  LC classification not assigned
  617.6'43–dc23

                                        2011034246

A catalogue record for this book is available from the British Library.

Wiley also publishes its books in a variety of electronic formats. Some content that appears in print may not be available in electronic books.

Set in 10/12 pt Minion by Toppan Best-set Premedia Limited, Hong Kong
Printed and bound in Singapore by Markono Print Media Pte Ltd

1   2012

Dedicated to

My ever-inspiring family, who supported me throughout this project
My children, Jithu and Malu

My mentors, Dr Jyothindra Kumar (orthodontist) and the late Dr Ponnuswamy (anatomist),
who changed the way I looked at my profession

and

All those who would love to see advancement in the 'Science of Orthodontics'

Vinod Krishnan

My wife, for her continuous support and advice; my children, for their compassion and constructive suggestions;
and my grandchildren, for their excellence in computer science

Ze'ev Davidovitch

Dedication

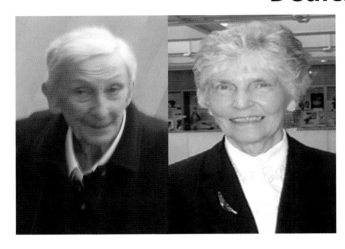

Laure Lebret and Anna-Marie Grøn: for lives committed to integrated orthodontic education

It is fitting to dedicate a book titled *Integrated Clinical Orthodontics* to two teachers whose lives were committed to interactive and integrated education: Laure Lebret and Anna-Marie Grøn. Both were full-time faculty members in the Departments of Orthodontics at the Forsyth Dental Center (initially The Forsyth Infirmary for Children and now The Forsyth Institute) and the Harvard School of Dental Medicine. The two affiliated institutions co-sponsored the orthodontic postgraduate program in an unparalleled combination until 1990. Together with Dr Coenrad F A Moorrees, the Chairman of both departments for over 40 years, they were the pillars of a unique educational program. The fact that the three of them originated from three different countries stands as an important detail in the history of a program whose graduates have spread worldwide, carrying with them the notion that professional excellence requires constant curiosity, and a search for contributing factors derived from any reasonable source. Coenrad Moorrees was born in Holland, Laure Lebret in France, and Anna-Marie Grøn in Denmark. Each was touched with difficult experiences during the Second World War.

To many generations of Harvard/Forsyth orthodontic graduates, our education was nurtured with the indelible impact of these three teachers, who were role models of civility, collegiality, scientific thinking, and productivity. Dr Moorrees departed in 2003, Dr Lebret in 2009, and one year later, Dr Grøn joined them, leaving behind a legacy of goodness, along with the hard and patient work of educating hundreds of orthodontists, many of whom became academicians, among them an unconventional number of chairpersons or program directors.

Laure Lebret and Anna-Marie Grøn were pioneer women, as dentists, orthodontists, and postgraduate teachers. Known as the important cornerstones in Coenrad Moorrees'

team, both had solid and independent cores with sharp minds and caring dispositions. They were involved with Dr Moorrees in seminal studies on the dentition and various aspects of facial growth, the most important of which was a long-term study of over 400 sets of twins, investigating the relation of facial and dental development.

In addition to co-authoring papers with Dr Moorrees and other workers on dental development, natural head position, and the mesh diagram analysis, Laure Lebret worked and published on the growth of the human palate, the reproducibility of rating stages of tooth movement, and physiological tooth migration. While tackling with Dr Moorrees the principles of diagnosis and also dental development, Anna-Marie Grøn's role was cut in the equally demanding and meticulous research of reproducibility of rating stages of osseous development, and the prediction of the timing of tooth emergence. The research that both women engaged in was not easy, for they mastered the intricacies of, and fully understood the variations in, clinical research, let alone longitudinal investigations with thousands of collected measurements per child. Their inquiry was clean, responsible, and painfully detailed. Their publications are, currently some 40 and 50 years later, having an impact on clinical decisions for thousands of children worldwide. One particular summary of much of the combined efforts of Lebret, Grøn, and Moorrees is embedded in a paper entitled 'Growth studies of the dentition: a review' (Moorrees CF, Grøn AM, Lebret LM, Yen PK, Fröhlich FJ, *American Journal of Orthodontics* 1969; 55: 600–16). Rarely is it not referenced in a paper or chapter on dental development.

Beyond the research and organized, clear didactics, the clinical teaching of Grøn and Lebret was in line with what today is labeled evidence-based practice and critical appraisal. 'Justify the plan', was their modus operandi, and 'consider the alternatives', before you decide. They were not necessarily unique in these requests. They simply transferred their research experience into daily clinical practice. They translated the central tendencies developed by research into the individual environment, to choose and deliver sound individualized treatment. That was the educational culture they helped us go through, and later propagate on our own as we became educators.

For all the gifts of knowledge and humanity they bestowed on their students worldwide, we dedicate this book to Laure Lebret and Anna-Marie Grøn. They deserve recognition in a book built around the idea of integrated sciences in the ever-expanding world of clinical orthodontics. By honouring their memory, we acknowledge that the explorations are going on, extending from theirs, for the benefit of mankind.

Joseph G Ghafari, DMD
Ze'ev Davidovitch, DMD

Contents

List of Contributors

Nina K Anderson PhD
Clinical Instructor
Department of Developmental Biology
Harvard School of Dental Medicine
Boston, Massachusetts
USA

Neslihan Arhun DDS, PhD, MSc
Associate Professor
Department of Conservative Dentistry
Baskent University, Faculty of Dentistry
Ankara
Turkey

Ayca Arman-Ozcirpici DDS, PhD
Associate Professor
Department of Orthodontics
Baskent University, Faculty of Dentistry
Bahcelievler, Ankara
Turkey

Adrian Becker BDS, LDS, DDO
Clinical Associate Professor Emeritus
Department of Orthodontics and Center for the Treatment of
Craniofacial Disorders in Special Needs Individuals
The Hebrew University-Hadassah School of Dental Medicine
Jerusalem
Israel

Nabil F Bissada DDS, MSD
Professor and Chair
Department of Periodontics
Case Western Reserve University
School of Dental Medicine
Cleveland, Ohio
USA

William A Brantley PhD
Professor and Director
Graduate Program in Dental Materials Science
Division of Restorative and Prosthetic Dentistry, College of
Dentistry
and
Department of Biomedical Engineering, College of Engineering
Ohio State University
Columbus, Ohio
USA

Stella Chaushu DMD, MSc
Associate Professor and Chair
Department of Orthodontics and Center for the Treatment of
Craniofacial Disorders in Special Needs Individuals
The Hebrew University-Hadassah School of Dental Medicine
Jerusalem
Israel

George J Cisneros DMD, MMSc
Professor and Chair
Department of Orthodontics
New York University College of Dentistry
New York
USA

Adriana Da Silveira DDS, MS, PhD
Chief of Orthodontics
Dell Children's Craniofacial & Reconstructive Plastic Surgery Center
and
Adjunct Assistant Professor
Department of Biomedical Engineering
University of Texas at Austin
Austin, Texas
USA

Gunnar Dahlén BSc, DDS, PhD (Dr Odont)
Professor and Chairman
Department of Oral Microbiology
Institute of Odontology
Sahlgrenska Academy at University of Gothenburg
Gothenburg
Sweden

Ze'ev Davidovitch DMD, Cert Ortho
Professor of Orthodontics, Emeritus
Harvard University, Boston
Massachusetts
USA
and
Clinical Professor
Department of Orthodontics
Case Western Reserve University
Cleveland, Ohio
USA

Linda A DiMeglio MD, MPH
Associate Professor
Section of Pediatric Endocrinology and Diabetology
Riley Hospital for Children
Indiana University School of Medicine
Indianapolis, Indiana
USA

Theodore Eliades DDS, MS, Dr Med, PhD
Professor and Director
Graduate Program in Dental Materials Science
Center of Dental Medicine, University of Zurich
Zurich
Switzerland

Kaj Fried DDS, PhD
Professor of Neuroscience
Karolinska Institutet
Department of Dental Medicine
Huddinge
Sweden

Joseph G Ghafari DMD
Professor and Head
Division of Orthodontics and Dentofacial Orthopedics
American University of Beirut Medical Center
Beirut
Lebanon

Donald B Giddon MA, DMD, PhD, FACD
Associate Professor of Clinical Pediatrics
Department of Developmental Biology
Harvard School of Dental Medicine
Boston, Massachusetts
USA

Nadine G Haddad MD, FAAP
Associate Professor of Clinical Pediatrics
Indiana University School of Medicine
Riley Hospital for Children
Section of Endocrinology and Diabetology
Indianapolis, Indiana
USA

James K Hartsfield Jr DMD, MS, MMSc, PhD, FACMG, CDABO
Adjunct Professor
Department of Orthodontics and Oral Facial Genetics
Indiana University School of Dentistry
and
Department of Medical and Molecular Genetics
Indiana University School of Medicine
and
Department of Orthodontics
University of Illinois at Chicago College of Dentistry
Chicago, Illinois
USA

Mark S Hochberg DMD
Program Director
Emeritus, Pediatric Dentistry, Interfaith Medical Center
and
Attending, New York Presbyterian Hospital
New York
USA

Julie Holloway DDS, MS
Program Director
Graduate Prosthodontics Program
Ohio State University College of Dentistry
Columbus, Ohio
Ohio
USA

Sarandeep Huja DDS, PhD
Program Director
Graduate Orthodontics Program
Ohio State University College of Dentistry
Columbus, Ohio
USA

Sanjivan Kandasamy BDSc, BScDent, DocClinDent, MOrthRCS, MRACDS
Clinical Associate Professor
Dental School
University of Western Australia
and
Centre for Advanced Dental Education
St Louis University
St Louis, Missouri
USA

Nina Kaukua DDS
Post Doctoral Fellow
Columbia University Medical Center
Craniofacial Regeneration Center, College of Dental Medicine
New York
USA

O P Kharbanda BDS, MDS, MOrth RCS Ed, MMEd
Professor and Head
Department of Orthodontics and Dentofacial Deformities
Centre for Dental Education and Research
All India Institute of Medical Sciences
New Delhi
India

Neal D Kravitz DMD, MS
Faculty, Washington Hospital Center
Washington, DC
and
Baltimore College of Dental Surgery
Dean's Faculty, University of Maryland
Baltimore, Maryland
USA

Vinod Krishnan BDS, MDS, MOrth RCS (Edin)
Professor
Department of Orthodontics
Sri Sankara Dental College
Trivandrum, Kerala
India

Simone Kucska BDS, MSD
Kucska Facial Orthopedics
Sao Paulo, Brazil
and
Post-Doctoral Scholar
Los Angeles, California
USA

Anne Marie Kuijpers-Jagtman DDS, PhD
Professor of Orthodontics
Head of Department of Orthodontics and Craniofacial Biology
Head of Cleft Palate Craniofacial Unit
Radboud University Nijmegen Medical Center
Nijmegen
The Netherlands

Maria J Kuriakose BDS, PhD, Cert Ortho
Associate Professor
Department of Cleft and Craniomaxillofacial Surgery
Amrita Institute of Medical Sciences
Kochi, Kerala
India

Anthony T Macari DDS, MS
Instructor/Clinical Director
Division of Orthodontics and Dentofacial Orthopedics
American University of Beirut Medical Center
Riad El Solh
Beirut
Lebanon

Jeremy J Mao DDS, PhD
Professor and Zegarelli Endowed Chair
Columbia University
Director, Center for Craniofacial Regeneration
Senior Associate Dean for Research
Columbia University College of Dental Medicine
New York
USA

Birte Melsen DDS, Dr Odont
Professor and Chairman
Department of Orthodontics, School of Dentistry
Faculty of Health Sciences, Aarhus University
Aarhus
Denmark

Elliott M Moskowitz DDS, MSd, CDE
Clinical Professor
Department of Orthodontics
New York University College of Dentistry
New York
USA

Neal C Murphy DDS, MS
Clinical Associate Professor
Departments of Orthodontics & Periodontics
Case Western Reserve University
School of Dental Medicine
Cleveland, Ohio USA

David R Musich DDS, MS
Clinical Professor of Orthodontics
University of Pennsylvania School of Dental Medicine
Philadelphia, Pennsylvania
and
Lecturer
Department of Orthodontics
University of Illinois, School of Dentistry
Chicago, Illinois
Private practice
Schaumburg, Illinois
USA

Omur Polat Ozsoy DDS, PhD
Associate Professor
Department of Orthodontics
Baskent University, Faculty of Dentistry
Ankara
Turkey

Carole A Palmer EdD, RD, LDN
Professor
Division of Nutrition and Oral Health Promotion
Department of Public Health and Community Service
Tufts University School of Dental Medicine
Boston, Massachusetts
USA

Hyo-Sang Park DDS, MSD, PhD
Professor and Chair
Department of Orthodontics, School of Dentistry
Kyungpook National University
and
Director, Orthodontic Research Center, Kyungpook National
University Hospital
Daegu
Korea

Sherry Peter BDS, MDS, FRCS
Clinical Professor
Department of Cleft and Craniomaxillofacial Surgery
Amrita Institute of Medical Sciences
Kochi, Kerala
India

Ameet V Revankar BDS, MDS
Assistant Professor
Department of Orthodontics and Dentofacial Orthopedics
SDM College of Dental Sciences and Hospital
Dharwad, Karnataka
India

Donald J Rinchuse DMD, MS, MDS, PhD
Professor and Graduate Orthodontic Program Director
Seton Hill University
Greensburg, Pennsylvania
USA

Lauren Schindler MS, RD
Senior Bariatric Dietitian
St Alexius Hospital NewStart
St Louis, MO
USA

Joseph Shapira DMD
Professor and Chair
Department of Pediatric Dentistry
The Hebrew University-Hadassah School of Dental Medicine
Jerusalem
Israel

Mete Ungor DDS, PhD
Professor
Head of Department of Endodontics
Baskent University, Faculty of Dentistry
Ankara
Turkey

Meade C Van Putten Jr, DDS, MS
Director of Maxillofacial Prosthodontics
The AG James Cancer Hospital and Solove Research Institute
Ohio State University
Columbus, Ohio
USA

Carlalberta Verna DDS, PhD
Associate Professor
Department of Orthodontics, School of Dentistry
Faculty of Health Sciences, Aarhus University
Aarhus
Denmark

Neeraj Wadhawan BDS, MDS
Research Officer
Department of Orthodontics and Dentofacial Deformities
Centre for Dental Education and Research
All India Institute of Medical Sciences
New Delhi
India

Eric Lye Kok Weng BDS, MDS, FRA CDS, FAMS
Consultant
Department of Oral and Maxillofacial Surgery Singapore
and
Assistant Director
Integrated Sleep Service
Changi General Hospital
Singapore

Mimi Yow BDS, FDS RCS, MSc (Orthodontics), FAMS
Senior Consultant
Department of Orthodontics
National Dental Centre
Singapore
and
Clinical Associate Professor
Faculty of Dentistry
National University of Singapore
Singapore

Preface

The subject of this book, integrated clinical orthodontics, seemed initially to be a straightforward topic. After all, we know that we depend on each other, in all walks of life, not excluding orthodontics. Therefore, we thought that it would be helpful to try to compose a publication that would reflect clearly each area where orthodontists interact with experts in other medical specialties, in an effort to upgrade their services to their patients.

Each individual who needs, seeks, or receives orthodontic care, differs from every other individual, molecularly, functionally, and esthetically. This natural variability is reflected in the orthodontic clinic, defining the identity of the specialty whose experts could be beneficial to the orthodontist and the patient alike. Our goal has been to learn from people engaged in clinical research in different medical fields, about their experience and advice on interactions with orthodontists. These interactions stem from the simple fact that none of us knows everything, and whether we like it or not, we depend on the professional opinions of our colleagues in other specialties, whose knowledge can remedy the voids in our own.

In planning the contents of this book, we immediately realized that there are many fields of knowledge that can augment the diagnostic and therapeutic capabilities of the orthodontist. In fact, we were amazed at the large number of these specialties, clearly reflected in the number of chapters in this book, 25, each dedicated to a specialty whose members interact with orthodontists. This increasingly widening scope of orthodontics is enabled by the availability and relative ease of electronic communication, and the expanding new findings in medicine and dentistry. It becomes increasingly difficult to command all relevant information about emerging new and exciting fields, such as tissue engineering and stem cells, and becoming aware of ongoing progress in seemingly traditional fields, such as genetics, psychology, and material science. Interaction with others seems to offer the means to clarify and confirm the identity of clinical findings in the diagnostic phase, and elucidate the road ahead, in terms of treatment plans and the choice of the most suitable mechanotherapy for the individual patient.

The concept emerging from this book is that orthodontics is not merely an exercise in wire bending, but rather a specialty leaning on many others. Interactions, whenever indicated, between the orthodontist and other medical specialists are a powerful tool on the way to excellence. In short, we would like to see each and every reader of this book to think like a healthcare professional and as a conscientious member of the dental profession who wishes to bring credit upon a high calling that has lifted itself from a questionable mechanical art to a most respected and esteemed health service to humankind.

We would like to extend our heartfelt thanks to all our contributing authors, who have generously shared their valuable knowledge and wisdom for the benefit of all those who are eager to learn about the advancements in 'science of orthodontics'. We were excited to read the manuscripts and are hopeful that the response of our esteemed readers will be the same too. Although the chapters are based on the contributors' own work and experiences, all the information can be applied to similar settings across the world.

We would also like to express our sincere gratitude to all the staff at Wiley-Blackwell, Oxford, UK, especially Sophia Joyce, Nick Morgan, Catriona Cooper, Lucy Nash, and James Benefield, as well as Lotika Singha (copyeditor), and Anne Bassett (project manager) whose relentless efforts helped us to accomplish this laborious, but fulfilling, task.

Vinod Krishnan
Ze'ev Davidovitch
Editors

1

The Increased Stature of Orthodontics

Ze'ev Davidovitch, Vinod Krishnan

Summary

Orthodontists treat patients with orofacial anomalies, including malocclusions, by applying mechanical forces to the crowns of teeth. These forces are transmitted to the tissues surrounding the roots of the teeth, enticing their cells to remodel these tissues, thereby enabling the teeth to move to new, preferred positions. Like any other tissues and organs in the human body, dental tissues and cells are controlled by the nervous, immune, vascular, and endocrine systems, as well as by factors such as psychological stress, nutrition, medications, and local and systemic diseases. Since the jaws are integral parts of the body as a whole, orthodontic diagnosis must include detailed information on any deviation from general health norms, and these data should be reflected in the treatment plan. Therefore, when specific pathologies are identified, an interaction with the appropriate healthcare provider who is treating the patient should occur, or a referral made to another specialist. The advice obtained from these experts can have a substantial impact on the orthodontic diagnosis and treatment plan. Continuing advances in medicine and dentistry increase the scope, importance, and value of these interactions. This introductory chapter discusses the need and rationale for interactions in specific situations, and this book includes details of conditions that require advice from specific specialists. The focus on this expanding scope is derived from the notion that biology plays a pivotal role in orthodontics, and that pertinent information regarding the health status of individual candidates for orthodontic treatment might have long-lasting effects on the course and outcomes of orthodontic treatment.

Introduction

Facial esthetics, balance, and harmony, and/or their absence, have attracted attention from time immemorial, by artist and art viewer alike. Facial expressions can readily reflect various moods, emotions, and feelings, thereby conveying unspoken messages from person to person. The mouth is an essential component of this anatomical–physiological–emotional complex, by virtue of its ability to participate actively in these functions, involving its soft (cheeks, lips, and tongue) and hard (jaws and teeth) tissues. Painters, sculptors, and photographers have noted these features, and frequently, when creating images of human faces, included the rest of the body, or at least the torso, in their art work, demonstrating acceptance of the principle that the face and the rest of the body are one unit. The specialty of orthodontics is taught predominantly as a field of endeavor dedicated to the improvement of orofacial esthetics and function. Consideration of biological principles and constraints is shadowed by the desire of both the patient and his/her orthodontist to achieve noticeable improvement in the position and location of the malpositioned crown(s), ignoring the fact that the crowns are anchored in the jaws by their roots, which are surrounded by tissues that act and react like any other organ to any local or systemic factor that comes their way. This situation is similar to an iceberg, visible partially above the water surface, but invisible under it.

Malocclusions are situations where individual teeth or entire dental arches are positioned in undesirable locations, either esthetically or functionally. The goal of orthodontics is to correct or minimize deviations from accepted normal characteristics of dental occlusion, orofacial function, and esthetics. We tend to focus on these deviations from normalcy as the main target of our specialty, while keeping other health-related issues far in the background, sometimes behind the horizon, as if a malocclusion exists in a vacuum, detached from the rest of the body. Maintenance of this outlook may, however, jeopardize the quality of orthodontic diagnosis, treatment plan, outcome, and long-term maintenance of the corrected malocclusion. What is

Integrated Clinical Orthodontics, First Edition. Edited by Vinod Krishnan, Ze'ev Davidovitch.
© 2012 Blackwell Publishing Ltd. Published 2012 by Blackwell Publishing Ltd.

required for attainment of optimal results in orthodontics is broadening of its scope, to include other specialties, dental and medical, that may expose etiological factors, and biological processes that could determine the nature of the cellular/tissue response to mechanotherapy. In short, we should not treat a malocclusion, but rather *a person* with a malocclusion (McCoy, 1941; Kiyak, 2008).

Presently, orthodontics is viewed by the general population as a field occupied mainly by concerns about facial esthetics, and limited to the application of 'braces' to crooked teeth. This image has been cultivated and nurtured by many members of the orthodontic specialty, because it simplifies their lives by highlighting the known fact that teeth move when subjected to mechanical forces. This outlook is deeply embedded in the curricula of the majority of the orthodontic educational/training programs around the world. Orthodontic residents are made to believe, at least subconsciously, that correcting a malocclusion in a human being is just as easy as moving metallic teeth through the warm, soft wax of a typodont (Davidovitch and Krishnan, 2009). Furthermore, this attitude has encouraged general dentists to engage in the practice of orthodontics without obtaining proper education that would qualify them for this task. An example of a poor outcome of such treatment is seen in Figure 1.1. However, orthodontics, which had been viewed until recently as being mainly a technique-oriented profession, has actually evolved into a comprehensive specialty, with a rapidly expanding scope, increasingly interacting with experts in biology, medicine, dentistry, engineering, and computer science. These interactions can provide the orthodontist with important information pertaining to individual patients that may lead to modifications in the diagnosis and treatment plans.

Voluminous expansion of the scientific and clinical bases of orthodontics is occurring in various directions, biological and technical. The role of biology in the diagnosis, treatment planning, and treatment of individual patients is becoming increasingly clear (Cartwright, 1941; Davidovitch and Krishnan, 2009). An orthodontist may be an expert in mechanics, but he/she is not a nutritionist, psychologist, pediatrician, endocrinologist, primary care physician, oral and maxillofacial surgeon, endodontist, prosthodontist, or any other medical and/or dental specialist. Therefore, it seems only prudent to request advice from other specialists whenever a condition is recognized in a person seeking orthodontic treatment, or in a patient who is already being treated.

The reality is that people who possess malocclusions may also have pathological conditions that could significantly impact the course and outcome of orthodontic treatment. This probability creates a need to consult and interact with other specialists familiar with an individual patient, or with the health problem afflicting this individual. Moreover, some people may have communicable diseases that may endanger the well-being of others who are in their environ-ment. The existence of rapid communication systems enables an orthodontist to easily seek advice from other specialists, leading to the crafting of diagnoses and treatment plans tailored specifically for each individual patient. These systems are also very useful in fostering strong doctor–patient trust, increasing cooperation and improving outcomes.

Likewise, recent advances in material science, metallurgy and biomedical engineering have introduced an increasing array of alloys, capable of generating a wide spectrum of mechanical forces. A continuous interaction between the orthodontist and these engineers has already produced major changes in the design of orthodontic brackets, and the composition of the metallic and nonmetallic wires that generate the proper orthodontic forces, while controlling factors such as friction and strain. This interaction is a fertile ground for the development of new appliances capable of engendering optimal tooth movement, biologically and mechanically, for each patient. Moreover, these engineers are crucial participants in the design and manufacturing of the multiple prototypes of metallic implants and mini-implants, which are used for the creation of intraoral anchorage, thereby taking away this responsibility from teeth and thus avoiding altogether any undesirable tooth movement.

The pioneers of modern orthodontics were pathfinders in a field full of challenges and obstacles. Those leaders utilized the best therapeutic tools available for eliminating malocclusions, paving the way for greater achievements by their successors. Edward H Angle, the 'father of modern orthodontics', advocated at the end of the nineteenth century the inclusion of basic medical sciences, such as anatomy, physiology, and pathology, in the curriculum designed for educating dentists as specialists in orthodontics. He apparently saw clearly the functional connection between the head and the rest of the body. Three decades on, one of his students, Albert Ketcham (1929), in attempting to elucidate the reasons for dental root resorption (a major undesirable side effect of tooth movement), concluded that the etiology is associated with the patient's metabolism. In the following years, resorption of roots was attributed to factors such as nutritional deficiencies, hormonal fluctuations, genetic predisposition, and psychological stress. All these factors point to the notion that tissue remodeling that facilitates tooth movement is dependent, at least in part, on the unique pathophysiological profile of the individual patient. Detailed information on this biological profile may be obtained from a number of different healthcare providers familiar with individual patients.

However, despite the recognition of the importance of life sciences in orthodontic education and practice, considerable emphasis is still being placed on the mechanical aspect of this specialty. Consequently, conditions such as excessive root resorption are labeled as idiopathic, unpre-

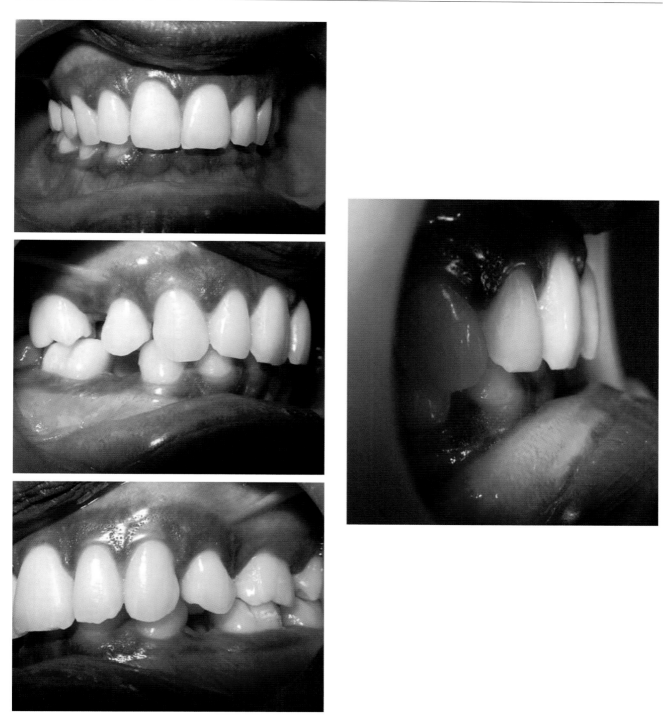

Figure 1.1 Poorly executed orthodontic treatment by a general practitioner. Ignoring the absence of mandibular central incisors, the practitioner extracted all the second premolars but was then unable to close the spaces entirely, ending with excessive overjet and a very deep bite.

dictable and an 'act of God'. These explanations fly in the face of the long-recognized principle of the intimate union between biology and mechanics in orthodontic therapy. This proximity was first suggested by Farrar (1888), who speculated that tooth movement is facilitated by either

resorption or bending of the alveolar bone, or by both processes. Farrar's comment was surprisingly correct, although it was based on empirical evidence. Experimental evidence supporting Farrar's hypothesis was provided by Sandstedt (1904–5), and by Baumrind (1969). While Sandstedt used histological sections to demonstrate that paradental cells are responsible for the force-induced tissue remodeling, Baumrind confirmed in experiments on rats that orthodontic forces indeed bend the alveolar bone.

The broadening scope of orthodontics

The chief purpose of orthodontic treatment is to assist nature in the proper development of the orofacial system in growing children, and correct malocclusions in young and adult patients. Ideally, orthodontics should be practiced in a facility that houses all other medical specialists, such as a hospital, or a large group practice. In such an environment, reaching various experts and obtaining their advice about health-related problems of individual orthodontic patients may be accomplished with relative ease. Specialists such as primary care/family physicians, orthopedists, surgeons, psychologists and nutritionists may be within walking distance from the orthodontic clinic. However, the widespread network of electronic communications today has enabled an orthodontist to refer a patient for consultation and receive the specialist's opinion in a timely fashion, without dependence on geographical proximity or venue location.

Contemporary orthodontics is a fusion of biology and mechanics, starting with the process of diagnosis, which is based on estimating and documenting the extent of malocclusion, as well as asking: 'Who is the patient, biologically?' This question must be answered before any plans of tooth movement can be contemplated. The presence of any systemic or local pathological condition may cause significant alterations in the orthodontic therapeutic plans for any and every individual patient, regardless of age or gender. A comprehensive orthodontic diagnosis should start with a detailed presentation of the patient's biological profile, including all conditions that may impact on mechanotherapy. This segment of the diagnosis is followed by a detailed description of the malocclusion. The biological segment is the part where interaction with specialists in various medical fields is expressed, and is later reflected in the crafting of an individual treatment plan. A brief example of such a diagnosis is as follows: 'AZ is a 34-year-old female nurse, mother of a two children, with multiple sclerosis that started 5 years ago, with a history of familial neuropathies. She has a Class II Division 1 malocclusion, with a steep mandibular plane, an 8° ANB angle, and a 12 mm overjet'. This diagnosis is a presentation of the main systemic and orofacial findings, which pave the way, together, to a proper treatment plan. For the sake of providing the best treatment plan for AZ, it would be beneficial to seek the advice of the other specialists who take care of her, such as her personal physician, neurologist, and nutritionist. Their opinions may turn out to be valuable in guiding the orthodontist toward a treatment plan that would be optimal and practical for this individual patient.

A similar malocclusion in a different patient may read as follows: 'RM is a 14-year-old boy, entering the pubertal growth spurt, who has type 1 diabetes, allergies, and asthma, with a Class II Division 1 malocclusion, a steep mandibular plane, and an 8 mm overjet.' This concise but detailed diagnosis implies that the patient is growing and has health-related issues that may overshadow the orthodontic problem and its treatment outcome. Systemic issues of this nature, involving the immune, endocrine, and vascular systems, may alter the response of cells surrounding teeth to applied mechanical stress, modify the velocity of tooth movement and contribute to the creation of undesirable side effects to orthodontic treatment, such as irreversible loss of alveolar bone and shortening of dental roots. Moreover, if medical and/or socioeconomic problems are ignored, and are allowed to persist, maintenance of the corrected malocclusion may be jeopardized. Therefore, in the case of RM, it may be advisable for the orthodontist to communicate with the patient's pediatrician, endocrinologist, and nutritionist prior to solidifying the diagnosis and treatment plan.

The orthodontic patient as a human being

Orthodontists not only see young individuals, who are ready to face the world with a lot of enthusiasm and confidence, but also adult patients with various needs and expectations. In some instances, patients may be having psychosocial issues, and may seek orthodontic therapy in an attempt to alleviate their personality deficits, improve their social status and find solutions to problems in their professional and personal life. It is extremely important to realize that every patient considered for treatment is an individual with a metabolic profile and physiological traits unique to him/her (Bartley et al., 1997) even though all humans share similar genetic, anatomical, physiological, and biochemical bases. The interindividual differences may arise from physical, social, ethnic, psychological, and metabolic variations, among other factors. It is important to realize that orthodontic treatment is provided to vital tissues that respond in a similar fashion in all patients. However, the extent, duration, and outcome of this response are frequently dependent on biological factors only remotely related to the malocclusion at hand.

The pattern and timing of craniofacial growth and development events are intimately associated with somatic growth-related functions, controlled and regulated by a myriad of chemical and physical factors, of internal and external origin, interacting with target cells in many or all organs and systems. This complex reality faces every orthodontist, as well as any other healthcare provider. It is rather unrealistic to expect that any one individual, in any medical specialty, would be able to comprehend, manage, and memorize all this voluminous knowledge. Hence the need for the orthodontist to keep abreast of new developments in the entire field of medicine, and to interact with members of other specialties whenever a situation arises that requires input from other experts.

One fundamental interaction in this formula is between orthodontists, who move teeth with mechanical forces, and the experts who create the means to generate these forces: biomedical and metallurgical engineers. The requirement for a perpetual interaction between experts in these entities is because orthodontic tooth movement requires close interaction between the biological and the mechanical environments (Krishnan and Davidovitch, 2006a; Meikle, 2006) and, even in a healthy patient, the response to orthodontic forces can vary from time to time, because the duration of treatment is often measured in years. In addition, the presence of an underlying ailment that affects the physiological condition may alter the nature of the acute and chronic inflammation that are core events in tooth movement, and modify craniofacial growth and development (Alvear et al., 1986). Cellular signaling molecules generated either in the vicinity of the periodontal ligament or in distant sites have the potential to disrupt tooth movement by altering the levels of biomolecules in the local biological environment of the periodontal ligament (Krishnan and Davidovitch, 2006b).

The patient's biological status – does it influence orthodontic treatment?

Due to the uniqueness of every individual patient's biology, it is imperative for the orthodontist to create and maintain open communication channels with practitioners in every medical field. Patients may be referred for consultation to their personal physician, or to experts in specific areas, such as endocrinology, neurology, immunology, genetics, metabolism, pulmonology, nutrition, psychology, and infectious diseases. Each organ or tissue system in a pathological state may have profound effects on paradental cells and tissues, by transferring signal molecules through the vascular system to any tooth being moved, and all the cells surrounding it.

Inflammation is a central coordinator of orthodontic tooth movement, and as such, it ushers leukocytes and plasma out of the mechanically stressed capillaries, which become hyperpermeable in reaction to the release of vasoactive neurotransmitters from the strained nerve terminals. In this fashion, leukocytes that had become primed in remote diseased organs can enter strained dental and paradental tissues, and interact with cells carrying receptors for signaling molecules synthesized by the migratory immune cells. Experiments with human periodontal ligament (PDL) fibroblasts *in vitro,* revealed that these cells respond readily to cytokines, growth factors, colony stimulating factors and chemo-attractant signals, all of which are produced and released by the newly arrived leukocytes (Saito et al., 1990a,b). This intimate correlation between tooth movement and pathological conditions that happen elsewhere in the body is the main reason for interacting with physicians, nutritionists, psychologists or other experts in healthcare provision.

Many individuals seeking orthodontic care have systemic ailments, such as asthma, and are usually already under treatment for these conditions at the time of their orthodontic diagnosis appointment(s). This treatment often entails the use of various prescription and/or over-the-counter medications. Some of these medications may have insignificant effects on the process of tissue remodeling evoked by the orthodontic forces, but others, such as steroidal and nonsteroidal anti-inflammatory drugs, anti-cancer medications, immune suppressors, statins, and anti-osteoporotic medications, may reach the cells in and around moving teeth by exiting, in the plasma, through capillaries that have become hyperpermeable by the applied stress (Krishnan and Davidovitch, 2006b). It is, therefore, important to record all the medications taken regularly by a patient before the onset of orthodontic treatment, as well as during the course of therapy. Once a complete list of medications taken regularly by a patient is obtained, it is essential to search for information about their desirable and undesirable effects. This information can be readily found on the internet and in current pharmacopeias. An example of a profound effect of a nonsteroidal anti-inflammatory drug on cells involved in orthodontic tissue remodeling is demonstrated in Figure 1.2, showing the mesially-located, stretched PDL and alveolar bone surface lining cells of a maxillary cat canine that had been moved distally for 24h, with a force of 80 g. The tissue sections were stained immunohistochemically for prostaglandin E2, a ubiquitous inflammatory mediator. A section taken from a control cat untreated by the nonsteroidal anti-inflammatory drug, indomethacin, shows cells intensely stained for PGE2, while a section obtained from an indomethacin-treated cat demonstrates a marked reduction of staining intensity, suggesting that this drug may have a profound effect on tooth movement.

Nutrition may play an important role in determining the pattern and course of tooth movement (Palmer, 2007). A modern diet consists of proper amounts of proteins, carbohydrates, lipids, vitamins, and trace elements. However, within the same community, marked differences between individuals may be found in the relative proportion of each dietary component, and even greater differences are known to exist between members of diverse communities, despite their geographical proximity. Some items in the diet may be essential for eliciting a vigorous cellular response to mechanical forces. For example, vitamin C is an essential co-factor in the synthesis of collagen by fibroblasts, and vitamin D_3 is a key regulator of the mobilization of calcium into and out of the intestine, kidney, and skeleton. Proteins provide the amino acids needed for building and remodeling tissues surrounding moving teeth; carbohydrates supply the energy required for all cellular

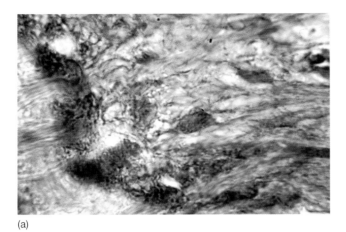
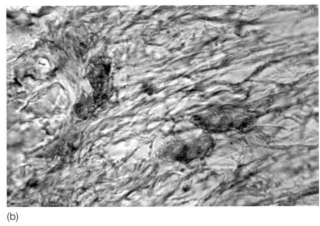

(a)   (b)

Figure 1.2 Immunohistochemical staining for prostaglandin (PG) E2 in sagittal sections, 5 μm thick, of maxillary canines of 1-year-old cats, after 24 hours of distal movement by an 80 g translatory force. (a) Periodontal ligament (PDL) tension site of control cat, showing distinct staining in alveolar bone osteoblasts. (b) PDL tension site of a cat injected subcutaneously with indomethacin, 5 mg/kg, at the time of appliance activation. The staining intensity for PGE2 in osteoblasts and PDL cells is light.

activities, and lipids are a critical part of every cell's plasma membrane.

Some dietary components may be detrimental to the patient's health and well-being, and have a negative effect on dental and paradental tissues. In the case of alcohol, its chronic excessive consumption may cause dental root resorption in orthodontic patients, by causing liver cirrhosis, disrupting the hydroxylation of vitamin D_3 in the liver, thereby evoking increased production of parathyroid hormone (PTH), necessary for the maintenance of calcium homeostasis (Ghafari, 1997). This hormone is implicated in the resorption of mineralized tissues, including dental roots. For these reasons it may be helpful to obtain detailed information about the dietary habits of every patient prior to the onset of orthodontic treatment. An evaluation of individual daily diets by a qualified nutritionist may supply the orthodontist with important clues regarding expectations of individual tissue responses to orthodontic mechanotherapy.

Regulation of mammalian body functions is dominated to a large extent by three systems: the nervous, immune, and endocrine systems. Persons seeking orthodontic care sometimes have ailments that affect one or more of these systems. Treating such patients orthodontically with little consideration for their systemic abnormalities may result in some unpleasant surprises for the patients, as well as for their orthodontists. For example, a patient with an existing condition such as multiple sclerosis may develop trigeminal neuralgia early in the course of orthodontic treatment, because of the acute pain generated every time the orthodontic appliance is activated. The pain may even be amplified because of the direct contact between the denuded, unmyelinated trigeminal nerve fibers. In cases such as this, and in patients with other neurological diseases, either

central or peripheral, administration of orthodontic forces may exacerbate the neurological condition, and/or be affected by it. Moreover, medications taken by these patients may also alter the pattern of tissue response to orthodontic forces (Krishnan and Davidovitch, 2006b). Therefore, it may be prudent to seek the advice of the neurologists treating such patients.

The immune system is a network of biological structures and processes within an organism that protects against disease by identifying and killing pathogens and tumor cells. It detects a wide variety of agents, from viruses to parasitic worms, and needs to distinguish them from the organism's own healthy cells and tissues in order to function properly. Detection is complicated as pathogens can evolve rapidly, producing adaptations that avoid the immune system and allow the pathogens to successfully infect their hosts (Abergerth and Gudmundsson, 2006). The immune system provides the leukocytes required for the induction and maintenance of inflammation, which is the mechanism whereby tissue remodeling facilitates tooth movement. Disorders of the immune system, such as immunodeficiency that occurs when the immune system is less active than normal, result in recurring and life-threatening infections. Immunodeficiency can either be the result of a genetic disease, such as severe combined immunodeficiency, or secondary to pharmaceutical therapy or an infection (such as the acquired immune deficiency syndrome (AIDS), which is caused by the retrovirus human immunodeficiency virus (HIV)). In contrast, autoimmune diseases result from a hyperactive immune system attacking normal tissues, as if they were foreign organisms. Common autoimmune diseases include Hashimoto thyroiditis, rheumatoid arthritis, diabetes mellitus type 1 and lupus erythematosus. Figure 1.3 shows intraoral views in a 39-year-old

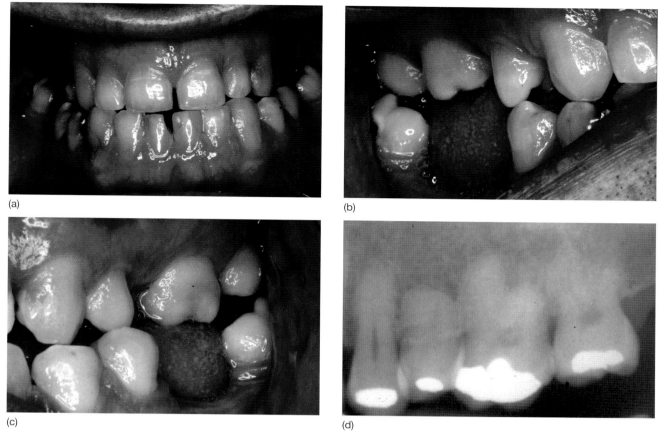

Figure 1.3 A malocclusion in a 39-year-old man with a number of systemic diseases. (a) Frontal view of the dentition, demonstrating a midline shift and bilateral posterior crossbite. (b, c) Left and right views of the dentition, showing spaces resulting from prior tooth extractions. Tipping of teeth into the extraction sites is visible in both dental arches. (d) The maxillary periapical radiograph reveals severe shortening of the premolar and molar roots.

man with a history of diabetes mellitus type 1, Hashimoto thyroiditis and depression. He had an obvious malocclusion and his systemic diseases were being treated by a variety of medications. In view of the multiplicity of diseases and the numerous medications taken by this patient, the patient's physician recommendation was to refrain from orthodontic treatment. The decision to not consider orthodontics was reached on the basis of input from the patient's physician, dentist, and a prosthodontist.

The endocrine system is a system of glands, each of which secretes a specific type of hormone to regulate the body and act as an information signal system, much like the nervous system. A hormone is a chemical transmitter released from specialized cells into the bloodstream, which transports it to specialized organ-receptor cells that respond to it. Hormones regulate many functions of an organism, including mood, growth and development, tissue function and metabolism. Together with the nervous system, the endocrine system regulates and integrates the body's metabolic activities. The endocrine system meets the nervous system at the hypothalamus. The hypothalamus, the main

integrative center for the endocrine and autonomic nervous systems, controls the function of endocrine organs by neural and hormonal pathways.

Application of orthodontic forces increases the blood flow into the tooth and the paradental tissues (Kvinnsland et al., 1989; Ikawa et al., 2001) and their capillaries become hyperpermeable, fostering plasma extravasation. This local alteration in the vascular system can cause an increase in the tissue concentration of hormones, of which some, like parathyroid hormone, calcitonin and thyroxin are known to regulate bone metabolism (Copp and Cheney, 1962; Mundy et al., 1976; Parfitt, 2003; Martin, 2004; Poole and Reeve, 2005). Figure 1.4 presents photomicrographs of the alveolar bone and PDL, as seen in sections stained immunohistochemically for 3′, 5′-adenosine monophosphate (cyclic AMP or cAMP). The sections were obtained from three young adult cats. Figure 1.4a is from an untreated (control) cat and shows mild cellular staining intensity for cAMP near a maxillary canine. Figure 1.4b is from a cat whose maxillary canine was subjected to 24 hours of distal movement. This figure is from the zone of tension in the

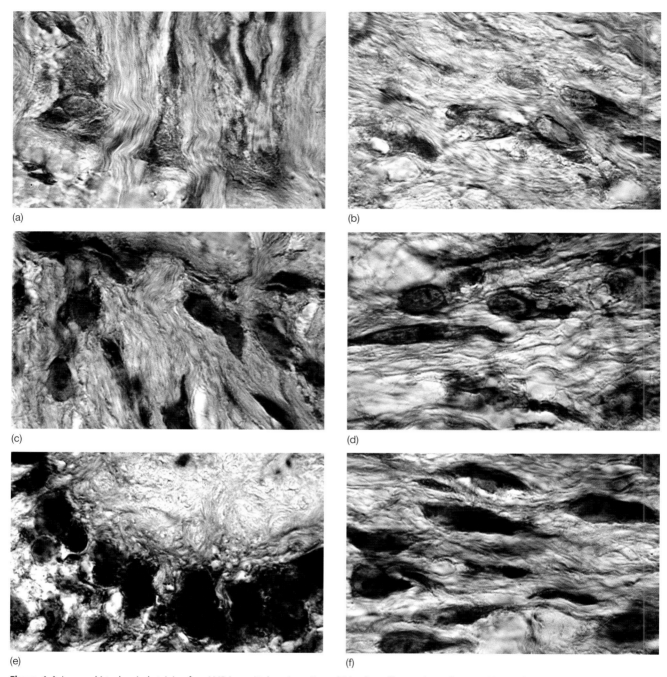

Figure 1.4 Immunohistochemical staining for cAMP in sagittal sections, 5 μm thick, of maxillary canines of 1-year-old cats after 24 hours of distal movement by an 80 g translatory force. (a) Osteoblasts and (b) periodontal ligament (PDL) fibroblasts from a control cat (no orthodontic force). (c) Osteoblasts and (d) fibroblasts in PDL tension site (cat received orthodontic force, but no parathyroid hormone (PTH)). (e) Osteoblasts and (f) fibroblasts in PDL tension site. This cat received orthodontic force, and a subcutaneous injection of PTH, 30 IU/kg, at the time of the appliance activation. The intensity of staining for cAMP is light in the untreated control animal, pronounced in the animal that was treated by force alone, and was very intense in the animal treated by force and PTH.

PDL, demonstrating intense staining for cAMP, resulting from the orthodontic force. Figure 1.4c was derived from a cat that had been treated in the same manner as the one shown in Figure 1.4b, and in addition received a subcutaneous injection of PTH, 30 IU/kg, 2h before euthanasia. In this figure, the cells are stained extremely dark, reflecting a high concentration of cellular cAMP. Since this cyclic nucleotide represents cellular activation by extracellular signals, it is reasonable to conclude that the biological response to orthodontic forces may be sensitive to hormonal concentrations in the blood. These concentrations are modified significantly by pathological conditions that develop in specific endocrine glands, suggesting that an opinion of an endocrinologist about the patient's hormonal profile could be very helpful in crafting a proper orthodontic diagnosis and treatment plan.

Orthodontists treat human beings, who sometimes are unable or unwilling to acknowledge and comply with their share of responsibility and effort dictated by the treatment regimen. Frequently, such behavioral patterns stem from psychological stresses, rooted in genetic, developmental, and/or environmental etiologic factors. Hence, psychology is apparently a crucial element in determining and forecasting the degree of success or failure of orthodontic treatment. Psychology is a field that focuses on studying the mind. Psychologists attempt to understand the role of mental functions in individual and social behavior, while also exploring underlying physiological and neurological processes. Psychologists study such topics as perception, cognition, attention, emotion, motivation, brain functioning (neuropsychology), personality, behavior, and interpersonal relationships. Deviation from the norm in any of these areas may harbor the seed of failure of orthodontic treatment. A review of records of about 1100 patients who had completed orthodontic treatment revealed that those who had been diagnosed before the onset of treatment as having had psychological problems, such as mood swings and anxiety, displayed a high risk of developing excessive root resorption during the course of treatment (Davidovitch et al., 2000). This undesirable outcome could have been the result of alterations in the hypothalamic–pituitary–adrenal axis, caused by the psychological problems. Another unexpected side effect of orthodontic treatment in a psychologically stressed patient is alopecia totalis (Davidovitch and Krishnan, 2008) (Figure 1.5a–g). Apparently, the mind is an important determinant of the degree of success of orthodontic treatment. Therefore, it seems advantageous to interact with a psychologist whenever a psychological issue is diagnosed, both before and during treatment.

Interactions between dentists who practice one or more specialties are almost axiomatic. Patients with malocclusions are frequently being referred to an orthodontist for an initial examination and assessment of the degree of need for orthodontic care. The referring person may be a general dentist who controls the dental health of the patient and his/her family, a periodontist, a pedodontist or another dental specialist. After examining the patient, the orthodontist informs the referring dentist about his/her findings and recommendation, and whenever necessary, they coordinate the timing of various treatment phases. However, sometimes elimination of a complex malocclusion, which involves the teeth, their surrounding tissues, as well as the facial muscles and skeleton, requires the construction of a comprehensive treatment plan by a number of specialists.

Such is the case in caring for patients with orofacial clefts and other craniofacial anomalies, where teams of experts convene to discuss each patient's individual needs in a detailed and carefully coordinated sequence. These teams include experts in pediatrics, plastic surgery, psychology, social work, nutrition, dentistry, and orthodontics. A similar team approach is adopted for the treatment of adults who require reconstructive treatment. The team in this case may include a general dentist and specialists in periodontics, endodontics, maxillofacial surgery, prosthodontics, and orthodontics.

The orthodontist's professional wish-list includes a comfortable, painless experience for all patients, efficient treatment of short duration, avoidance of iatrogenic damage, and a guarantee that the teeth have been moved to their best position, from where there is no relapse. The duration of tooth movement may be shortened significantly by decortication of the alveolar bone, leading to release of stem cells from the bone marrow, and the engineering of new tissues (Wilcko et al., 2009).

Conclusions

Treatment of a malocclusion requires high technical skills and a thorough comprehension of biological sciences, because teeth transfer the applied orthodontic force to their surrounding tissues, where strained cells remodel the PDL and alveolar bone, allowing the teeth to move to new positions. The biological component reflects the nature of the anticipated clinical response, and highlights the plethora of differences between all patients. These physiological and pathological differences may have profound effects on the outcomes of treatment. Detailed descriptions of these conditions may be found in the library or on the internet, but in addition it is advisable to communicate effectively with each patient, and with all experts who have examined and treated the patient previously. These specialists can share invaluable information about their own observations of the patient's biological and therapeutic profile. Such details should be included in the diagnosis, and reflected in the treatment plan, that may differ from a plan that addresses only the morphological features of a malocclusion.

The continuous evolution in material and biological sciences will strengthen further the interactions between orthodontists and other healthcare specialists, leading the way toward sustainable corrections of malocclusions and craniofacial anomalies. These unfolding advances will continue to reduce the distance to the elusive target of optimal orthodontics. The common thread that unifies specialists in various disciplines is the desire to share, contribute to and participate in efforts to improve everybody's body and spirit, a universal goal that knows no boundaries.

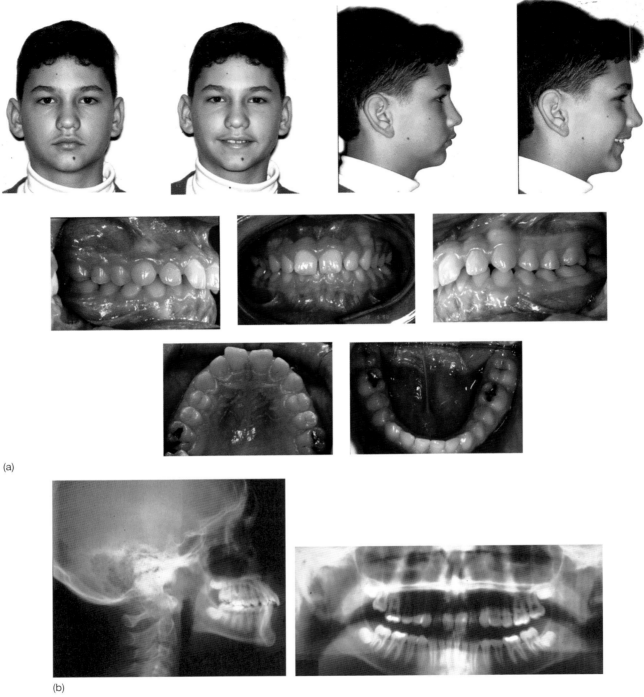

(a)

(b)

Figure 1.5 (a) Pre-treatment extra- and intraoral photograph of MV, at age 12 years and 10 months. Note good symmetry, smiling picture revealing maxillary midline is shifted 3.5 mm, a convex profile. Teeth in occlusion show a deep anterior overbite (80–90%) and spaces between the maxillary incisors. The maxillary midline is shifted 3.5 mm to the right. On the right side, the buccal occlusion is neutral and spaces are seen between the maxillary incisors and mesial to the canine. Left side shows a Class II Division 1 molar relationship as well as spaces between the maxillary incisors and mesial to the canine. Occlusal view of maxillary dental arch shows a parabolic shape, spaces between the anterior teeth from canine to canine, and distolabial rotations of both central incisors. Mandibular dental arch shows a U-shape, without any spacing or crowding of teeth. (From Davidovitch Z, Krishnan V (2008), courtesy of Quintessence Publishing Co Inc, Chicago.) (b) Pre-treatment lateral cephalogram demonstrating normal anteroposterior and vertical relationships between the jaws, a favorable inclination of the anterior cranial base and the palatal and mandibular planes, and a deep overbite in the incisor region. The panoramic radiograph reveals all teeth to be present and normal dental development. (From Davidovitch Z, Krishnan V (2008), courtesy of Quintessence Publishing Co Inc, Chicago.)

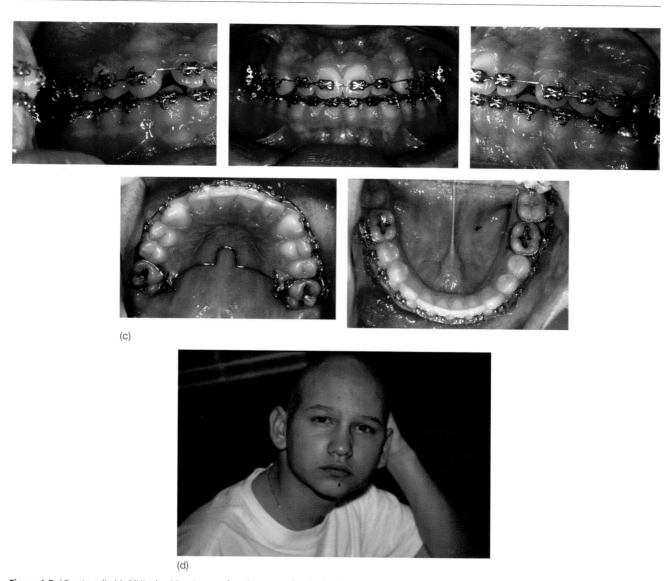

(c)

(d)

Figure 1.5 (*Continued*) (c) MV's dentition 1 year after the onset of orthodontic treatment. Frontal view and both left and right lateral views demonstrated accumulation of dental plaque and food debris in the canine and premolar regions between the brackets and the gingival margin. Occlusal view shows spaces between the maxillary canines and lateral incisors. (From Davidovitch Z, Krishnan V (2008), courtesy of Quintessence Publishing Co Inc, Chicago.) (d) Photograph of MV in October 1991, 9 months after the beginning of orthodontic treatment, 1 month after he lost all his scalp hair (alopecia totalis). (From Davidovitch Z, Krishnan V (2008), courtesy of Quintessence Publishing Co Inc, Chicago.)

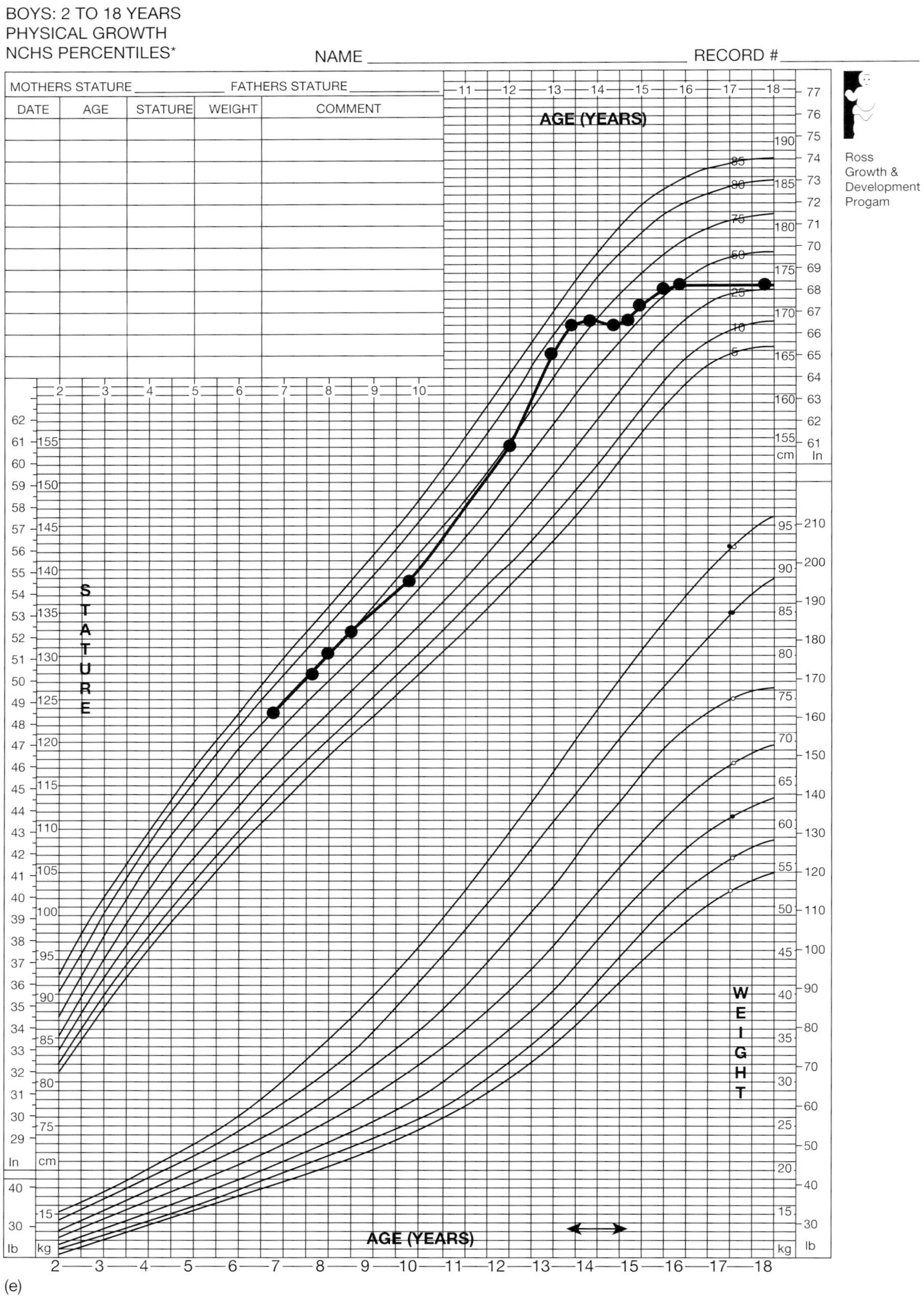

BOYS: 2 TO 18 YEARS
PHYSICAL GROWTH
NCHS PERCENTILES*

(e)

Figure 1.5 (*Continued*) (e) Physical growth (stature) curve of MV, revealing the somatic growth inhibitory effects of the corticosteroid treatment that was implemented in an attempt to restart new hair growth. The hormonal treatment failed to stimulate hair growth. (From Davidovitch Z, Krishnan V (2008), courtesy of Quintessence Publishing Co Inc, Chicago.)

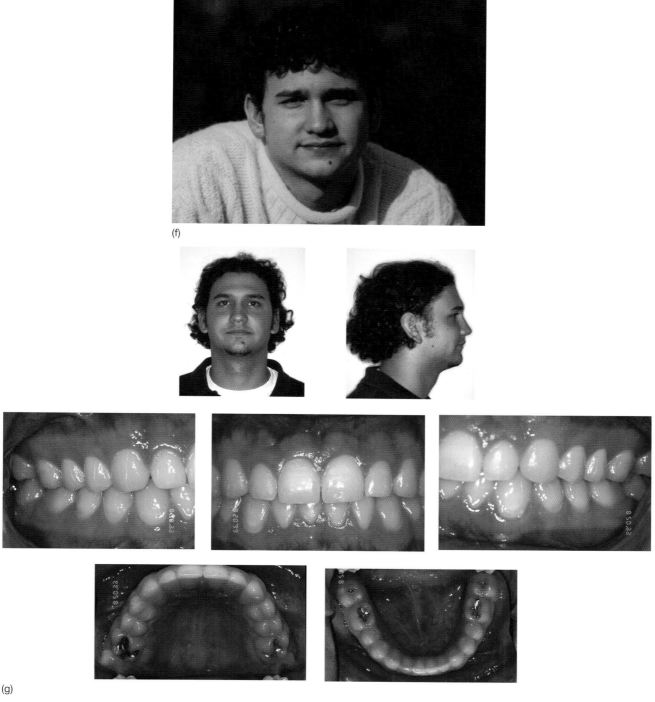

(f)

(g)

Figure 1.5 (*Continued*) (f) Photograph of MV taken in December 1993, 11 months after the completion of his orthodontic treatment and 1.5 years of treatment with vitamin D_3. Apparently, this treatment mode was successful in restoring hair growth. (From Davidovitch Z, Krishnan V (2008), courtesy of Quintessence Publishing Co Inc, Chicago.) (g) Extra- and intraoral photographs of MV taken in August 1999. His hair remained intact. (From Davidovitch Z, Krishnan V (2008), courtesy of Quintessence Publishing Co Inc, Chicago.)

References

Agerberth B, Gudmundsson GH (2006) Host antimicrobial defence peptides in human disease. *Current Topics in Microbiology and Immunology* 306: 67–90.

Alvear J, Artaza C, Vial M, Guerrero S, et al. (1986) Physical growth and bone age of survivors of protein-energy malnutrition. *Archives of Disease in Childhood* 61: 257–62.

Bartley AJ, Jones DW, Weinberger DR (1997) Genetic variability of human brain size and cortical gyral patterns. *Brain* 120(Pt 2): 257–69.

Baumrind S (1969) A reconsideration of the property of the pressure tension hypothesis. *American Journal of Orthodontics* 55: 12–22.

Cartwright FS (1941) Extending the scope of orthodontics. *American Journal of Orthodontics and Oral Surgery* 27: 394–8.

Copp DH, Cheney B (1962) Calcitonin – a hormone from the parathyroid which lowers the calcium-level of the blood. *Nature* 193: 381–2.

Davidovitch Z, Krishnan V (2008) Adverse effects of orthodontics. A report of two cases. *World Journal of Orthodontics* 9: 268.

Davidovitch Z, Krishnan V (2009) Role of basic biological sciences in clinical orthodontics: a case series. *American Journal of Orthodontics and Dentofacial Orthopedics* 135: 222–31.

Davidovitch Z, Lee YJ, Counts AL, et al. (2000) The immune system possibly modulates orthodontic root resorption. In: Z Davidovitch, J Mah (eds) *Biological Mechanisms of Tooth Movement and Craniofacial Adaptation*. Boston, MA: Harvard Society for the Advancement of Orthodontics, pp. 207–17.

Farrar JN (1888) *Irregularities of the Teeth and their Correction*, vol 1. New York, NY: DeVinne Press, p. 658.

Ghafari JG (1997) Emerging paradigms in orthodontics – an essay. *American Journal of Orthodontics and Dentofacial Orthopedics* 111: 573–80.

Ikawa M, Fujiwara M, Horiuchi H, et al. (2001) The effect of short-term tooth intrusion on human pulpal blood flow measured by laser Doppler flowmetry. *Archives of Oral Biology* 46: 781–7.

Ketcham AH (1929) A progress report of an investigation of apical root resorption of vital permanent teeth. *International Journal of Orthodontics, Oral Surgery and Radiology* 15: 310–28.

Kiyak HA (2008) Does orthodontic treatment affect patients' quality of life? *Journal of Dental Education* 72: 886–94.

Krishnan V, Davidovitch Z (2006a) Cellular, molecular, and tissue-level reactions to orthodontic force. *American Journal of Orthodontics and Dentofacial Orthopedics* 129: 469, e1–32.

Krishnan V, Davidovitch Z (2006b) The effect of drugs on orthodontic tooth movement. *Orthodontics and Craniofacial Research* 9: 163–71.

Kvinnsland S, Heyeraas K, Ofjord ES (1989) Effect of experimental tooth movement on periodontal and pulpal blood flow. *European Journal of Orthodontics* 11: 200–5.

Martin TJ (2004) Does bone resorption inhibition affect the anabolic response to parathyroid hormone? *Trends in Endocrinology and Metabolism* 15: 49–50.

McCoy JD (1941) The general health benefits of orthodontic treatment. *American Journal of Orthodontics and Oral Surgery* 27: 369–78.

Meikle MC (2006) The tissue, cellular, and molecular regulation of orthodontic tooth movement: 100 years after Carl Sandstedt. *European Journal of Orthodontics* 28: 221–40.

Mundy GR, Shapiro JL, Bandelin JG, et al. (1976) Direct stimulation of bone resorption by thyroid hormones. *Journal of Clinical Investigatoins* 58: 529–34.

Palmer CA (2007) Effective communication in dental practice. In: *Diet, Nutrition and Oral Health*, 2nd edn. Upper Saddle River, NJ: Pearson, pp 409–52.

Parfitt AM (2003) Parathyroid hormone and periosteal bone expansion. *Journal of Bone and Mineral Research* 17: 1741–3.

Poole K, Reeve J (2005) Parathyroid hormone–a bone anabolic and catabolic agent. *Current Opinion in Pharmacology* 5: 612–17.

Saito S, Ngan P, Saito M, et al. (1990a) Effects of cytokines on prostaglandin E and cAMP levels in human periodontal ligament fibroblasts in vitro. *Archives of Oral Biology* 35: 387–95.

Saito S, Ngan P, Saito M, et al. (1990b) Interactive effects between cytokines on PGE production by human periodontal ligament fibroblasts in vitro. *Journal of Dental Research* 69: 1456–62.

Sandstedt C (1904) Einige beiträge zur theorie der zahnregulierung. *Nord Tandlaeg Tidskr* 5: 236–56.

Wilcko MT, Wilcko WM, Pulver JJ, et al. (2009) Accelerated osteogenic orthodontics technique: a 1-stage surgically facilitated rapid orthodontic technique with alveolar augmentation. *Journal of Oral and Maxillofacial Surgery* 67: 2149–59.

2

Effective Data Management and Communication for the Contemporary Orthodontist

Ameet V Revankar

Summary

In this modern competitive era, technology offers all of us modalities we can use to stand above the rest. Health information technology has the potential to greatly improve healthcare alongside yielding huge savings. Over the past several decades, computer systems and information technology have pervaded all aspects of dentistry, successfully bridging the divide between the clinical setting and research. However, this transformative technology demands learning of new skills to understand, maintain and use it effectively, and to deliver what it promises to deliver. The role of communication processes, verbal/nonverbal, oral/written, in human interactions needs no emphasis, as it forms the core basis of all successful relationships across humanity beyond creed, race, and ethnicity. One such relationship is the doctor–patient relationship, which is constantly evolving. Having moved from paternalistic to 'equal partners', it is now more likely progressing towards a 'service provider–consumer' format. Moreover, in the new 'cyber age' reliance on electronic communication is constantly on the rise, far superseding interpersonal contacts. This chapter discusses the integration of information technology systems in orthodontics, to improve work flow and efficiency, as well as for the management and protection of electronic data from theft and corruption. It also discusses the various methods of electronic communication in patient management per se, as well as electronic communication with other specialists and peers, and its increasing role in orthodontic education.

Introduction

Information technology refers to the use of computers and software to produce, manipulate, store, communicate, and/or disseminate information. Computerized data management systems are becoming an integral part of any healthcare system and transforming it through integration of all clinical disciplines. Although encoding clinical data into a computer is a positive step, it is not enough. A continuity-of-care record is needed in order to document, measure, support and coordinate within and between specialties. The challenges in this task include the threat of information overload, the need to provide for data-sharing between specialists, the appropriate use of the data for the delivery of healthcare, and prevent misuse and loss of data. All of these challenges need to be considered before installation of health information technology (Boyd et al., 2010).

Effective communication is defined as the exchange of information and a person's beliefs to provide feedback and communicate one's message. When translated to the doctor–patient scenario, communication entails the ability of the doctor to comprehend fully the patient's concern and medical information, diagnose the problem, and advocate a treatment plan, to the satisfaction of both parties. In this communication process, the doctor and the patient assume the roles of the communicator and the receiver, alternately, until a common consensus is arrived at. The ultimate goal of an effective communication process is to foster a strong doctor–patient relationship, linked to important outcomes of care–treatment compliance (Francis et al., 1969; DiMatteo, 1995), clinical outcomes (Greenfield et al., 1988; Kaplan et al., 1989), malpractice claims (Beckman et al., 1994), and transfer of patients between doctors (Marquis et al., 1983). Evidence indicates that good doctor–patient relationships are on the decline, due to consumer-centric attitudes, decrease in professionalism, and commercialization of healthcare delivery systems (Chaitin et al., 2003). The path to a better doctor–patient relationship demands better communication, aimed at the patient's perspective of treatment and includes the patient as a collaborative partner with his or her doctor (Roter, 2000;

Integrated Clinical Orthodontics, First Edition. Edited by Vinod Krishnan, Ze'ev Davidovitch.
© 2012 Blackwell Publishing Ltd. Published 2012 by Blackwell Publishing Ltd.

Murphy et al., 2001), beginning with scheduling the patient's initial visit, progressing through diagnostic records, scheduling diagnosis, treatment planning, finances, finally culminating in the execution of the treatment plan. All the aforementioned tasks are aided by use of software programs that can enhance the doctor–patient experience, taking it to previously inconceivable heights.

The role of information technology in the orthodontic practice

Practice management systems

Practice management software (PMS) is a computer program/s that performs and organizes the administrative and clinical areas of an orthodontic practice. Traditionally PMS was limited to administrative tasks, and the electronic medical record (EMR) system was meant for maintaining patient medical records. However, the current versions of PMS available for orthodontic use have integrated EMRs and track appointments, billing, clinical information, and aids in patient communication, helping orthodontists to manage everyday tasks more efficiently than ever. A PMS also tracks referrals with generation of new referral reports, while managing incoming referrals from other specialists.

Patient demographic documentation by the assistant

Patient demographic documentation often starts when a new patient fills out a detailed information chart, which includes the patient's name, address, contact information, birth date, employer, and insurance information. Office staff manually enter this information into the software. The software can automatically interact with the relevant insurance company server in real time when connected over the internet, to verify the patient's credentials.

Scheduling patient visits

Patient appointment scheduling programs, the most important among administrative tasks, should consider proper management of the practitioner's time, cost-effectiveness, flexibility, which can reduce overheads and increase patient satisfaction. Various software programs are available for scheduling patient visits – integrated

through an interactive voice-based system (IVRS), which can be phone based or integrated into the office website (web based). The web module IVRS may be integrated into a single program that is also amenable to manual entries by the office staff. Such administrative applications deployed over the internet, enable patients to interact with the organizational aspects of the orthodontic practice. Online appointment scheduling, pre-registration, pre-visit preparations, and out-of-pocket treatment cost estimates all enhance communication and convenience. By having more control and a sense of participation in the administrative processes of the orthodontic office, patients may develop greater trust in the practice as a whole and potentially a better relationship with the doctor (Anderson et al., 2003).

Payment/financial record maintenance

It is paramount to document financial details for each appointment, to ensure transparency and ease of insurance claims, if applicable. Each charge usually corresponds to a particular service performed during a particular appointment, and most of the time multiple treatment procedures are performed by the operator. The settlement of the insurance claim, if applicable, may be performed as an automated process by the software, using proprietary electronic data interchange with the insurance company's server. This process is termed electronic claims submission (ECS). Electronic fund transfer (EFT) is the process whereby patients can pay a fee by electronic means, such as credit/debit card. Online banking can be automatically drafted by the software, enabling automatic debit from the payer's account, and deposit it into the practice's account on due dates (Lewis, 2006). The aforementioned steps of appointment scheduling, capturing patient demographics, and performing billing tasks are usually integrated into one module – the PMS (Table 2.1).

Advantages of using PMS

A PMS:

- Enables easy identification of new patients and round-the-clock appointment scheduling

Table 2.1 Comparison of patient management software systems

Software	Website	Special features
Dentimax	www.dentimax.com/	IVRS, e-module
SaralDent Dental	www.saralindia.com/	Manual SMS and email reminders
Medipac Dental	www.e2ilabs.com/	Automated SMS and email reminders
Curve Hero	www.curvedental.com/	Web-based interface; anytime/anywhere access

All are shareware. Free demo copies can be downloaded from the company websites.
IVRS, interactive voice-based system.

- Enhances ability to manage multiple appointment schedules
- Helps locate patient records easily by name or date
- Makes easy the process of call-backs, rescheduling, and referring of patients to different offices
- Minimizes recalls, missed and overlapping appointments
- Makes possible cross-scheduling among multiple clinics and medical offices
- Reduces staffing and administrative overhead, thus enhancing revenue
- Has built-in reports that help save time and reduce paper clutter
- Prompts sending reminder letters/phone calls/SMS to patients in what are known as patient communication systems
- Reduces stress for the patients and staff
- Eliminates the need to physically transfer patient information from one place to another
- Enables transparency in financial transactions with the use of EFT and ECS.

Although an electronic patient record (EPR) offers several advantages over conventional paper records, it suffers the risk of tampering. Attorney Arthur Pearson points out that in case of litigation, the prosecution could easily argue that the patient's electronic record has been tampered with, and this would put the defendant in an indefensible position (Scholz, 1989). Methods to overcome this issue include creating monthly duplicates of datasets, which are placed in an offsite data server 'escrow', or having printed records, as well. The former option is expensive and, the latter defeats the very purpose of having a 'paperless' electronic record. Current PMS/EMR program databases have features discouraging/preventing tampering. They usually require two digital signatures for every entry completed. Any changes/additional entries are added as a separate addendum entry. Tampering is quite an arduous task, even for experienced programmers. In the unlikely event that data have been tampered with, the electronic trail is traceable in case of litigation (Starke and Starke, 2006).

The deployment of PMS or other solutions for a 'paperless office' requires the setting up of a local area network (LAN) with a server and client system architecture (Haeger, 2005). Alternatives include internet program delivery (IPD)- or application service provider (ASP)-based solutions, which are basically outsourced hosting and delivery of management software, including data backup and archiving, and therefore do not require extensive hardware setup in the office.

Advantages of ASP solutions over office installed/maintained programs include (Lewis, 2006):

- No need to enforce local data management and protection systems

- EPRs are recorded/stored in the ASP server and thus available from any geographical location in the internet-connected world
- The patient data access system is easily integrated on the office website, providing patients, insurance agencies, and referring doctors with easy access
- Customer support is rapid in case of the unforeseen event, because the servers are offsite, in the custody of the ASP provider.

Although safety of patient data is of major concern as the data is stored on 'out of office' servers, these ASP servers are managed by professionals, and are compliant with privacy norms and data protection policies.

Computer-aided diagnosis and treatment planning to enhance communication

Case documentation

The majority of available software for orthodontic offices includes case documentation modules for routine dental complaints, and special modules for all dental specialties (Figure 2.1). These programs allow the practitioner to make accurate diagnoses and create compelling treatment plans. Some software vendors offer case sheet customization based on the practitioner's needs. The integrated functions and features enable the practitioner to present recommendations to patients in a way that they can understand, making communication easier.

Diagnostic record taking

Digital photographs

Digital photography has replaced film-based cameras due to its unparalleled advantages in routine clinical practice over conventional film images, for example immediate visualization of the captured image, possibility of image enhancement, indefinite 'shelf life' of the 'soft copy', ease of printing and duplication, absence of film, processing costs, and ease of electronic transmission around the world (Sandler et al., 2002; Revankar et al., 2009a). Further, the immediate availability of images enables the doctor to demonstrate the current status of the patient's dentition and extraoral features to them. Digital photography experience has been enhanced by availability of programs that can perform wireless transfer of photographs from the camera to the computer (Revankar et al., 2010), ability to automatically tag photographs with DICOM (digital imaging and communication in medicine)-compatible data, automatic parsing of duplicate photographs, and colour/hue matching (Halazonetis, 2004). It is now possible to integrate cone-beam computed tomography (CBCT) data in DICOM format with standard extraoral frontal photographs of the patient to generate three-dimensional (3D) facial photographs without the need for 3D facial camera

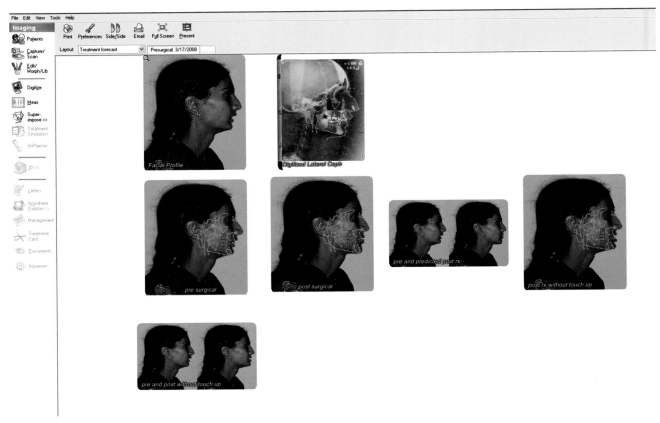

Figure 2.1 Example of an orthodontic case documentation module.

systems (Mah, 2007). This is sometimes referred to as 2D facial photo wrap (Dolphin Imaging and Management Solutions, Chatsworth, CA) (Figure 2.2) and is definitely a giant step ahead in rendering a visual identity to the patient's 3D volume.

E-models
The transition from physical study models to 3D images is progressing slowly due to the expensive nature of the 3D model scanners. Desktop-based model scanners are available both in the LASER (light amplification by stimulated emission of radiation) and optical/white structured light variety (Table 2.2). However, outsourcing options are available, whereby the physical models or impressions can be sent to the 3D modeling company and the 3D models generated from it are downloaded through the internet (Table 2.3). The orthodontist has to log on to the company website with his or her unique case ID enabling round-the-clock access to the digital models (Figure 2.3). These 3D models have proved to be viable alternatives to plaster models, in terms of measurements, diagnosis of malocclusion, and treatment planning (Tomassetti et al., 2001; Stevens et al., 2006).

An alternative to standard impression techniques is intraoral scanning, termed 'dedicated impression scanning

systems' and capable of generating 3D models. The first dedicated impression scanning system in orthodontics is the Orascanner (Suresmile, OraMatrix, Richardson, Texas, USA), a light-based imaging device that projects a precisely patterned grid onto the teeth. The orthodontist can make a diagnosis and plan treatment on the computer, using software tools to measure tooth and arch dimensions (Mah and Sachdeva, 2001). The virtual models also act as a valuable tool for patient education (Figure 2.4).

Digital radiography
Radiographic imaging has now progressed from 2D to 3D with the increasing use of CBCT. 3D CBCT scans are also being used as alternatives to standard plaster models (Figure 2.5) and 3D-based dental measurement (3DD) programs (El-Zanaty et al., 2010). The advantages of 3D CBCT models over conventional plaster and other forms of digital models are (Chenin et al., 2009):

- Include not only the tooth crown, but also the roots
- Impactions/developing teeth and alveolar bone can be visualized
- Dynamic virtual setup simulation and generation of stereolithographic models using computer-aided manufacturing (CAM) is possible.

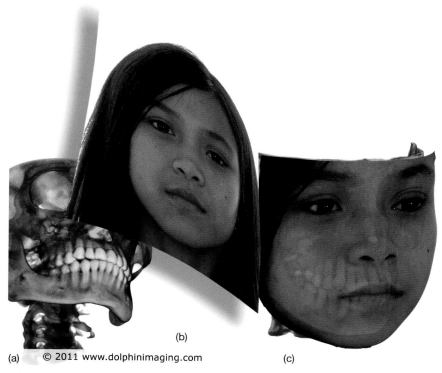

(a)   © 2011 www.dolphinimaging.com   (b)   (c)

Figure 2.2 2D facial wrap. (a) 3D craniofacial skeleton rendering from cone-beam computed tomography data. (b) Standard 2D digital photograph of the patient. (c) Facial photo wrap. (Image courtesy of Dolphin Imaging and Management Solutions, Chatsworth, CA; www.dolphinimaging.com.)

Table 2.2 Commercially available desktop model scanners

Name of the scanner	Type of scanner	Output format	Website
3Shape R700 Orthodontic 3D scanner	LASER	STL, DICOM	www.cadbluedental.com
Maestro 3D dental scanner	Structured light	STL, PLY, OBJ, ASC, VRML	www.maestro3d.com
ShapeGrabber Ai210D 3D dental scanner	LASER	STL	www.dentalscanner.com

STL, stereolithography; ASC, Autodesk, Inc 3D file; DICOM, digital imaging and communications in medicine; OBJ, wavefront technologies format; PLY, polygon file format; VRML, virtual reality modeling language.

Table 2.3 Commercial outsourcing-based digital modeling and archiving solutions

Solution	Company	Website
Orthocad	Cadent, Carlstadt, NJ, USA	www.cadentinc.com
e-model	GeoDigm, Chanhassen, MI, USA	www.geodigmcorp.com
Orthoplex	Dentsply GAC International Bohemia, NY, USA	www.gacintl.com/orthoplex
Ortholoine	Objet Geometries Inc Billerica, MA, USA	www.objet.com/Pages/Case_Studies/Medical/Ortholine
Anadent 3D	Sinthanayothin C, Thailand	www.anadent3d.com
Orthomodel	Tarcan B, Istanbul, Turkey	www.orthomodel.com/eng

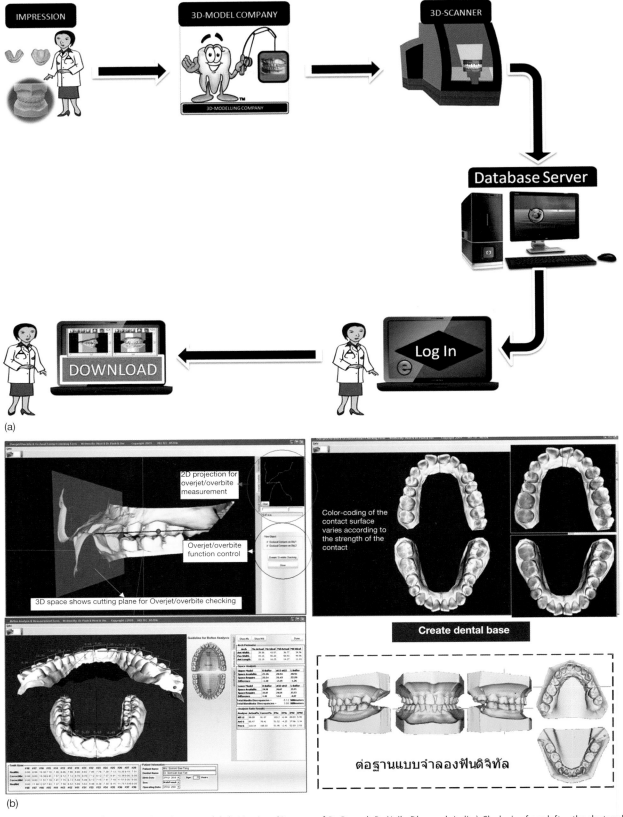

Figure 2.3 (a) Flow chart for outsourcing plaster model digitization. (Courtesy of Dr Roopak D. Naik, Dharwad, India.) Clockwise from left – the doctor ships the rubber base impressions or plaster casts to the 3D model company and 3D scanning is accomplished in the company's scanner. Following this the digital models are available on the company's secure login webpage where the doctor logs in to see the models or download them. (b) Visualization and manipulation of digital models in Anadent 3D software. (Image courtesy Dr Sinthanayothin C, NECETC, Thailand.)

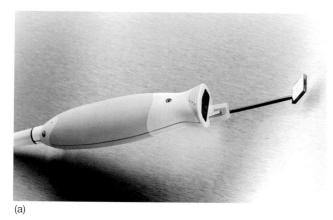

(a)

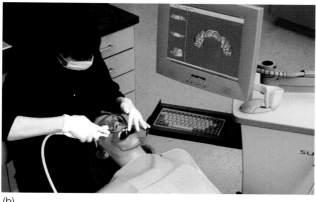

(b)

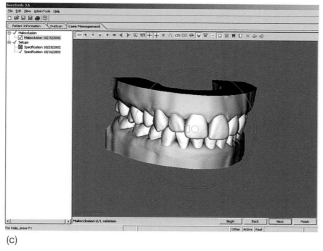

(c)

Figure 2.4 (a) The Orascanner apparatus. (b) Intraoral scanning with the Orascanner. (c) 3D digital model generated from the scan. (Image courtesy Dr Rohit Sachdeva, OraMetrix, Inc., Richardson, TX.)

Two-dimensional cephalometry

There have been tremendous advancements in the field of lateral cephalometric radiograph digitization, tracing, analyses, and treatment prediction, and a horde of cephalometric software is available for this mundane task. Online cephalometric analysis alternatives (Abraham, 2007) are also available (per case charge) that do not require the

purchase and instalation of software (Table 2.4). Either digital or film radiographs, scanned or photographed on a viewer, can be used with a scale adjacent to the film that enables software calibration. At the time of writing, digitization of the film prior to automatic analysis is on the brink of change from manual to automatic landmark identification, using the 'neural-associative-processor-based' hardware recognition systems (Yagi and Shibata, 2003). These systems have been demonstrated successfully to identify landmarks automatically, with high accuracy without human input in both adults and adolescents (Tanikawa et al., 2010).

Three-dimensional cephalometry

Since the inception of the cephalostat, Broadbent tried advocating a 3D stereoscopic analysis, and suggested combined use of the lateral cephalogram, postero-anterior radiograph, and a submental vertex view (Broadbent, 1931). However, the essence of Broadbent's cephalostat was lost over the decades, when orthodontists worldwide used the lateral cephalogram, which is a 2D representation of a 3D object, as the primary diagnostic head film with its inherent disadvantages. As pointed out earlier, 3D cephalometry with the newer CBCT machines is as close as it can get to craniometry in the intact human (Gribel et al., 2011a,b). The biggest problem with 3D cephalometry is the absence of population norms for the 3D measurements, and this was recently addressed by Gribel et al. (2011a,b). Assessment of changes due to growth or treatment as well as evaluation of internal structures can be done using 3D volumetric superimposition technology (Dolphin 3D, Dolphin Imaging and Management Solutions, Chatsworth, California, USA).

Discussing treatment with the patient

A motivated patient who understands and undertakes responsibility for his or her treatment is an asset to any practitioner. To inspire treatment compliance, a patient needs to understand the treatment procedure he or she might undergo, which is graphically possible with the aid of interactive motivational software (Table 2.5). The graphical simulation of a treatment procedure to be undertaken can aid eliciting truly informed consent (Figure 2.7). Commensurate with the fact that the human brain registers and recalls more of what is seen in comparison with inputs received through the other senses, there is evidence suggesting that these computer-based visual patient education programs enable better recall and hence positive feedback from the patient, in comparison with traditional means of patient education alone (Patel et al., 2008). Post-treatment, predicted profiles of the patient can also help in this endeavor. In fact, it is mandatory in some countries to show the software-generated post-treatment composites of varied treatment options to the patient before treatment (Figure 2.8). Previously, only 2D profile predictions were possible. However, with 'dynamic CBCT' technology it is now

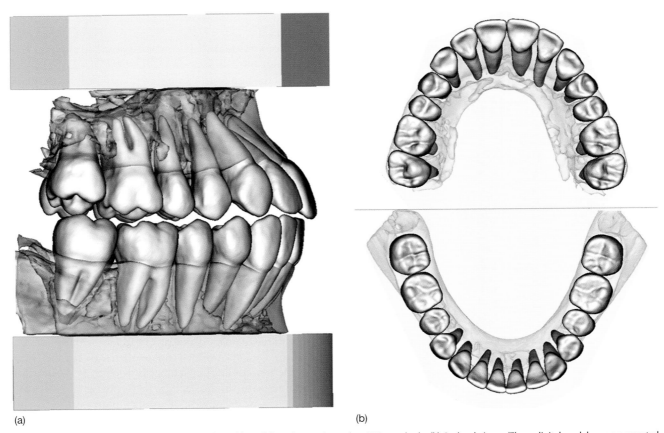

(a)   (b)

Figure 2.5 Dental models generated from CBCT data. (a) Models on bases trimmed to ABO standards. (b) Occlusal views. (These digital models were generated with Anatomodel software. Anatomage Inc., San Jose CA www.anatomage.com; reproduced with permission from German and German, JCO April 2010).

Table 2.4 Comparison of various 2D and 3D cephalometric software

Software	Website	Special features
Viewbox	www.dhal.com	3D module for CBCT data
Onyxceph	http://2i.webworld.org/	Model analysis from photographs
Ceph Basic	www.image-instruments.de/ceph-basic/en/index_us.htm	Includes patient education module
Dolphin Imaging	www.dolphinimaging.com	3D module for CBCT data
Vistadent	www.gactechnocenter.com/V3D.htm	3D module for CBCT data
Anatomage 3D	www.anatomage.com	Automatic digitization
Cephanalysis.com	www.cephanalysis.com	Outsourcing; per case

CBCT, cone-beam computed tomography.

possible to generate 3D composites of predicted treatment outcomes (Figure 2.9).

Other arenas of communication

Communication using the internet

The internet is probably the biggest invention of the millennium and among mankind's best, comparable with the invention of the integer zero by Indian mathematicians of yore. The internet has made communicating between geographically distant locations and time zones incredibly easy. In orthodontics, this means easy and reliable dissemination of information, electronic patient communication and appointment scheduling, patient referral to colleagues, transfer of patient records, online diagnostic aids, backup and retrieval, journal manuscript submissions, distant learning through webinars, real time interaction without physical presence of faculty, and much more (Engilman

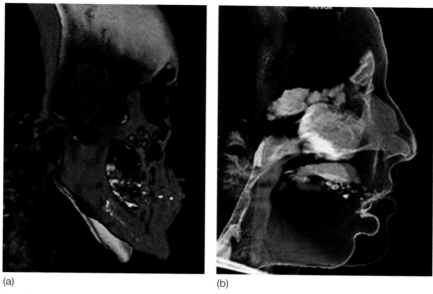

Figure 2.6 Pre- and post-3D volumetric superimpositions of mandibular advancement surgery. (a) Hard tissue superimposition: blue is post surgical. (b) Soft tissue superimposition. (Image courtesy of Dolphin Imaging and Management Solutions, Chatsworth, CA; www.dolphinimaging.com.)

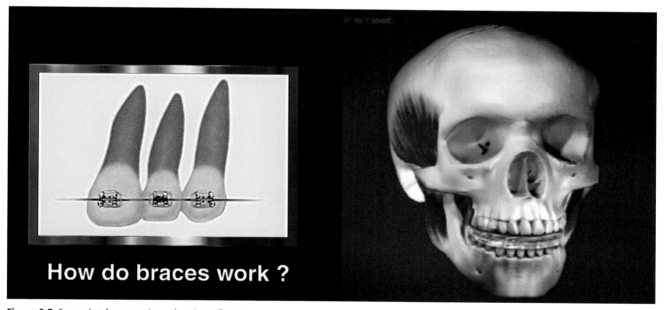

Figure 2.7 Screenshot from a patient education software.

Table 2.5 Patient education software

Software	Website
Caesy	www.caesy.com/
Optio	www.optiopublishing.com/
Orasphere	www.orasphere.com/
Consult Pro	www.consult-pro.com/
Dolphin Aquarium	www.dolphinimaging.com
Orthomation	www.gactechnocenter.com

et al., 2007). Modes of communication using the internet include (Revankar and Gandedkar, 2010):

- Email (electronic mail)
- File transfer protocol (FTP)
- Hyper text transfer protocol (HTTP) file transfer
- RFB (remote frame buffer) protocol and VNC (virtual network computing)
- VoIP (voice over internet protocol)
- Video teleconferencing/videoconferencing (tele-orthodontics) (Figure 2.10).

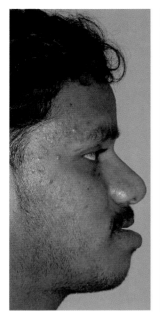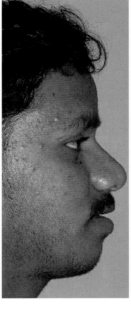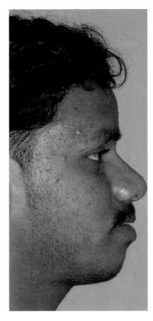

Figure 2.8 Predicted post-treatment profiles for varied treatment plans in an orthognathic patient, generated with Dolphin Imaging 10. (Image courtesy of Dolphin Imaging and Management Solutions, Chatsworth, CA; www.dolphinimaging.com.)

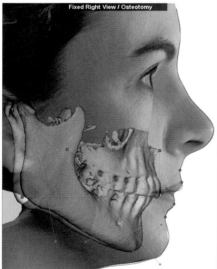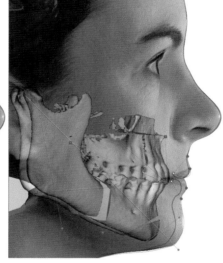

(a)

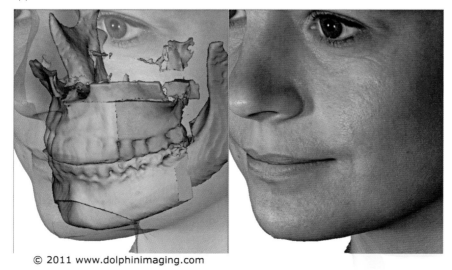

(b)

Figure 2.9 3D soft tissue prediction of orthognathic surgery. (a) Mandibular osteotomy on cone-beam computed tomography (CBCT) dataset – right view. (b) Mandibular osteotomy on CBCT dataset – 45° view. (Image courtesy of Dolphin Imaging and Management Solutions, Chatsworth, CA; www.dolphinimaging.com.)

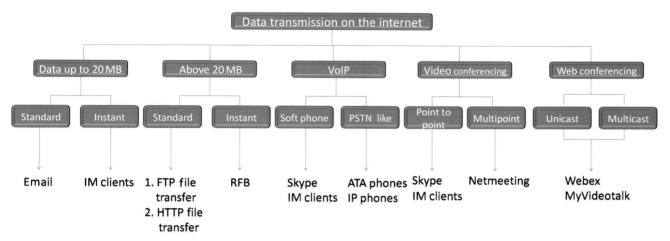

Figure 2.10 Schematic representation showing the various methods of data transmission over the internet and their associated protocols.

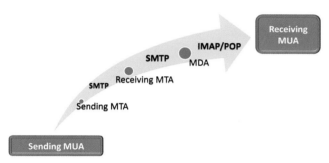

Figure 2.11 Email transmission and the underlying protocol. Email servers/MTAs/MDAs use SMTP to send and receive email messages; user-level client mail applications typically only use SMTP for sending messages to a mail server for relaying to other MUAs. For receiving messages, MUAs usually use either POP or IMAP to access their mail box accounts on a mail server following authentication. MUA, mail user agent; MTA, mail transfer agent; SMTP, simple mail transfer protocol; MDA, mail delivery agent; IMAP, internet message access protocol; POP, post office protocol.

Email

Email has become the standard form of mail, with land mail being dubbed as 'snail mail' in this fast-paced world. Instant data transmission is now a necessity in every field, including orthodontics. The internet serves as an effective platform, transcending all dimensions – space, time, and matter – for exchanging information with patients, peers, consultants, manuscript transactions, leisure, etc., to name a few. The amount of content a typical email can hold ranges from 10 megabytes (MB) to a maximum of 20 MB, depending on the service provider. Simple mail transfer protocol (SMTP) is the current internet standard for email transmission across internet protocol (IP) networks (Figure 2.11).

Email communication pertaining to appointment reminders, payment receipts and birthday/festival wishes enhance the doctor–patient relationship (Anderson et al., 2003) by providing the patient with a 'sense of importance'. Email appointment reminders can save the reception staff

time on confirming appointments using phone calls, effectively reducing the 'number of no shows' (Povolny, 2002). Dedicated online patient communication (OPC) programs are available and automate the emailing chore; they can integrate with the office PMS, extracting data pertaining to payments, insurance claims, and appointment schedules (Ortho Sesame software, PT Interactive Tukwila, Wash; TeleVox Software, Mobile, Ala; www.televox.com). These OPC suites can be integrated onto the office website, enabling patients to enter their email addresses in the database as well as access their information online from the office website as described below. However, some clinicians are of the opinion that email communication has a negative impact on doctor–patient relations because of the lack of the nonverbal component (body language) that is vital to a successful interpersonal contact (Baur, 2000).

File transfer protocol

FTP allows transmission of much larger files. The process typically involves the acquisition of an 'user account' on an FTP server, either free or paid, following which the user uploads files onto the server. Once a file is uploaded, it is available for download worldwide, provided the downloader has the user account details for the uploaded file. Some FTP servers such as Drive HQ (www.drivehq.com/FTP) provide 1 gigabyte (GB) of free space and upload of a maximum file size of 100 MB/file for free users. FTP was a popular protocol a decade ago but is no longer in vogue today, except for special applications such as webpage/content uploads for uploading content on the office website.

Hyper text transfer protocol file transfer

HTTP is similar to FTP, the difference being that this protocol is browser based (Internet Explorer/Mozilla Firefox) and runs on the World Wide Web platform, the predominant

Table 2.6 Comparison of various HTTP file servers

HTTP file server	Maximum file size[a] allowed	Password[a] file protection	Searchable data base
www.rapidshare.com	200 MB/file unlimited storage	No	No
www.mediafire.com	100 MB/file unlimited storage	Yes	Yes
www.adrive.com	Up to 50 GB both file size and storage	No	Yes
www.sendthisfile.com	100 MB/file	Yes	No

[a]For free users. Generally subscription services allow uploading of large files of ranging from 2 GB/file to 10 GB/file depending upon the file server.

platform on the 'WEB' as of this date, because of its user-friendliness and graphical user interface. Many websites provide simple-to-use data upload service, both free and paid. The user can choose to password protect a file or keep it open to access. Once uploaded, the file is available for download all over the internet, any number of times, and can serve multiple downloads at the same instance as well. The standard procedure requires the uploader to distribute the link to download the file via email, message boards, websites or any other form of communication. Some file servers allow the user to place their file in a searchable database (Table 2.6). Large file transfers up to 2 terabytes (TB)/session are now feasible, thus making the transfer of large patient image files/radiographs, procedure videos, and lectures possible. Most manuscript submission systems for international orthodontic journals also follow this protocol for electronic manuscript submission.

Remote frame buffer protocol

RFB protocol enables remote access to graphical interfaces. Along with virtual network computing (VNC), it forms the heart of applications such as TeamViewer and Dynagate (TeamViewerGmbH, Göppingen, Germany), which enables real-time file transfer. TeamViewer establishes true virtual private network (VPN)-encrypted connection, enabling direct high-speed file transmission from one user end to the other (point to point) without an intervening file server. Files can also be transferred through popular instant messaging clients, such as Yahoo messenger, Google Talk, and Skype, using the same protocol. These applications can be used for real-time textual 'chat' between practitioners, student/faculty instructions, and online patient support via 'chat rooms' embedded on the office website. Offsite information systems management, which involves 'out-of-office' management of 'in-office computer systems' that is operating any computer system on an internet-connected network as though the remote operator is physically present on the local computer, is possible with applications such as TeamViewer. 'Chat room' discussions for interactive learning have been implemented, but have not been very successful, probably because this form of education is not 'taken seriously' unless accompanied by a video feed (Proffit, 2005).

Voice over internet protocol

VoIP or IP telephony as it is popularly known, is based on a simple method of converting analog signals (for instance sound waves) into digital packets before being transmitted over the internet. Soft phones (VoIP software running on a computer) are free to use for computer-to-computer calling anywhere in the internet-connected world. They can also be used to call conventional phones (landlines and cell phones) at nominal prices. Other endpoints for using the VoIP protocol may be the analog telephone adapter (ATA) and IP phones (Mupparapu, 2008). These phones do not require an intervening computer to process the voice call and can be used like standard public switched telephone network land phones. Wi-Fi phones that use VoIP when located in a Wi-Fi hotspot are also available. Applications such as Fring (www.fring.com) enable Symbian/Windows smart cell phones to do the same, when connected to a Wi-Fi network, enabling cross platform connectivity with other VoIP and instant messaging clients. This technology can be used for cheap voice calling in comparison with the traditional telephone system, especially when call volumes are high and office overheads are to be kept low (Mupparapu, 2008).

Video teleconferencing/video conferencing

This is a set of interactive telecommunication technologies that allow two or more locations to interact via two-way video and audio transmissions simultaneously. The simplest video conferencing system – point to point – and suitable for individual use at home or private orthodontic office, consists of inexpensive equipment, namely a PC, a web camera, software and a high-speed internet connection (Engilman et al., 2007). This technology is shaping the future, enabling interaction among colleagues, for case discussions – interactive seminar instruction in orthodontic residency programs (Bednar et al., 2007; Engilman et al., 2007; Miller et al., 2007).

Traditional computer-assisted learning (CAL), the multimedia approach to learning, is a form of self-instruction in which material can be presented via text, visual, sound, and motion digital files (Rosenberg et al., 2005). CAL is not a novel method of learning, having been in existence for as long as computers have been around. It is a necessary tool in the current educational system (Rosenberg et al., 2010) and offers several advantages (Rosenberg et al., 2003).

- It motivates and generates interest in the student towards the subject.
- Students can learn at their own pace and review the lesson any number of times.
- Students can access the system in a convenient, distraction-free environment.
- Multimedia and interactive animations can enhance self-communication and understanding.
- They can reduce the need for educators.

Meta-analyses have found that CAL increased student examination scores by 0.3 standard deviations, decreased instructor-based learning schedules (Kulik and Kulik, 1991), and led to a small to moderate improvement in student scholastic achievement (Dacanay and Cohen, 1992). Controlled trials in orthodontics, comparing CAL with conventional teaching methods, are split between no difference (Clark et al., 1997), significant advantage of CAL over conventional teaching (Luffingham, 1984; Irvine and Moore, 1986; Al-Jewair et al., 2009), and significant advantage of conventional methods over CAL (Hobson et al., 1998). Current evidence suggests that CAL is definitely useful as an adjunct to conventional teaching but cannot be used as the only teaching modality (Rosenberg et al., 2010).

Web conferencing

This is a conglomeration of various protocols delivering simultaneous multicast video, audio conferencing, real-time file transfer, and screen sharing, used to conduct live meetings, training, or presentations via the internet. In a web conference, each participant sits at his or her own computer and is connected to other participants via the internet. This arrangement can be either a downloaded application on each attendee's computer or a web-based application, where all attendees access the meeting by clicking on a link distributed by email (meeting invitation) to enter the conference.

Multicenter web conferencing, with high-speed internet networks, forms the back bone of high-quality interactive, long-distance seminar instructions (Bednar et al., 2007). The convergence of two major forces – evolving technology and orthodontic educator shortage – is leading to further development of virtual classrooms for interactive learning (Scholz, 2005). However, technology is still evolving and some disadvantages exist in interactive web conferencing.

- Active participation of each and every participant cannot be ensured, especially so in a large group because of the

difficulties in installing multiple tracking cameras and locating microphones to ensure voice clarity throughout the room.
- There are inherent problems with the reliability of the high-speed internet connections.
- Supplemental electronic teaching materials are not inbuilt within the system and need to be distributed by other means before the session.

Web conferencing also forms the basis of futuristic tele-orthodontics. Telemedicine currently offers real-time 'live' and 'store and forward' videoconferencing and consultations (Miller, 2003). At present, tele-orthodontics is the delivery of some aspect of orthodontic care where the patient and doctor are geographically separated. According to Favero et al. (2009) minor orthodontic emergencies can be resolved easily at home, reassuring patient and parents, and limiting visits to the orthodontic office to cases of real need.

Internet-based applications will neither replace 'hands-on' care and treatment from the doctor, nor the social quality of a personal interview. However, this new technology is affecting the quantity and quality of health information that patients can obtain, the number of aspects of care being provided, and the nature of the doctor–patient relationship (Hollander and Lanier, 2001). The World Wide Web is a sea of knowledge, full of readily available information. Many patients confront their doctor with information they have gleaned from the internet. Some doctors are alarmed by this, while others embrace the role of the internet with their patients and provide health information and links to preferred sources of health information on their own websites. It is the responsibility of the doctor to guide the patients toward credible resources because knowledge resources on the internet are a mixed bag with variable contents, quality, and readability (Antonarakis and Kiliaridis, 2009). With level access to information about the full range of treatment options, patients are actively participating in deciding on a course of treatment and other aspects of their healthcare.

Evidence on the internet

The internet is a great resource for readily accessible evidence. Various scientific literature databases such as PubMed, MEDLINE, Cochrane, EMBASE, DARE, ERIC, and Google scholar, can be searched for pertinent information. In 2006, the Council on Scientific Affairs (COSA), a division of the American Association of Orthodontists (AAO), developed a website for evidence-based orthodontic literature, linked to the AAO members' area. The data on pertinent topics listed on these 'organization endorsed' websites should be held with high regard as it usually presents chimeric data synthesized from the best available evidence.

The office website

The internet is a significant consumer research resource center in the current era. Hence, building up a practice website, and maintaining and making web presence noticeable are critical. Web presence can be enhanced by search engine optimization and pay per click advertisements on other popular websites using Google Ads. Even broadcasting yourself through the popular social networking websites – Facebook (www.facebook.com), Orkut (www.orkut.com), Twitter (www.twitter.com) and YouTube (www.youtube.com) – to expand your reach is now possible.

Apart from advertising, the office website is an important cornerstone for a successful doctor–patient relationship. Being the face of the doctor's practice, the website typically includes information about the doctor, office staff, equipment, office policies, and values. A prospective patient can relate these values to him or herself. This 'initial communication' may lay the groundwork for a good doctor–patient relationship by providing a sense of trust and shared values. There is evidence to prove that incorporation of certain design characteristics and content on the office website are important for attracting prospective new patients. The following content is deemed to be critical to attract new patients (Wallin, 2009):

- Doctor's photograph – a color photo in 'usual clothing' with a child or their family
- Patient-focused content throughout the website
- Warm doctor's statement – demonstrating care and concern for patients
- Doctor's credentials and experience listing, including information about continuing education, to show that the doctor is abreast with the latest technologies and techniques
- Individual staff photographs, with information about each staff member, showing their friendliness towards patients
- First visit page – a compelling page as to why patients should choose this particular practice, what happens at the first visit and consultation fees
- Happy people's photographs – emotionally impactful smiling faces (which look as if they could be faces of patients) throughout the website
- Warm and friendly design theme without pop-ups, splash pages, and auto music or advertisements.
- Before and after treatment page – with three to six compelling, full-face photographs of the doctor's patients.

When consulting a professional agency to design a website for your office, remember that most of them churn out 'template-based' websites, which ultimately result in all 'orthodontic office websites' designed by the same agency looking similar to each other (Turpin, 2008). Creating individuality for your practice is very important; hence the doctor's inputs to the web designer on the design, textual content, photographs, and videos for the office website cannot be underplayed. The website should be an interactive hub where patients, both old and new, can find answers to their questions. New patient registration can be done through the website, as mentioned earlier. Further, a health history form can be provided online so that the prospective patient can fill in the necessary details before arriving at the office. Patients already into treatment can be provided with secure access to their own personal orthodontic health record through the website.

Electronic data management

From the preliminary step of patient communication, diagnostic record making, and treatment planning, to the future follow-up regimen, digital technology delivers unparalleled and unique services to orthodontics. With the advent of this technology, orthodontists around the globe have embraced the 'techno-wave' in various forms. Data storage has also seen a change from paper to disk drives and photographic film to flash cards. Changes in the method of storage, have led to new challenges in data protection, from termites to computer viruses (Revankar et al., 2009b). The Wikipedia online encyclopedia defines computer malware, also called malicious software, as 'software designed to infiltrate or damage a computer system without the owner's informed consent' (Malware, 2010). The expression is a general term used by computer professionals to refer to a variety of forms of hostile, intrusive, or annoying software or program codes, which can often be destructive, if appropriate and timely action is not undertaken.

Most people are unaware of the term malware and use the term computer virus incorrectly to describe all sorts of malware, as not all malware are viruses but all viruses are malware. The legal codes of several American states, including California and West Virginia refer to malware as a *computer contaminant* (National Conference of State Legislatures, 2008). Of late, the majority of computer code being released is malicious. Preliminary results from Symantec (Symantec Internet Security Threat Report, 2007) sensors published in 2008, suggested that 'the release rate of malicious code and other unwanted programs may be far exceeding that of legitimate software applications'. According to F-Secure, 'As much malware was produced in 2007 as in the previous 20 years altogether' (F-Secure Corporation, 2007) Malware's most common pathway from criminals to users is through the internet, by email and the World Wide Web. In a setup like a dental office, malware can spread rapidly to even standalone systems through the pervasive use of thumb/flash drives for data transfer.

Protection against malware

Most systems contain *bugs* (vulnerabilities), which may be exploited by malware. Typical examples are *buffer over-*

runs, in which an interface designed to store data in a small area of memory allows the caller to supply too much, and then overwrites its internal structures. This function may be used by malware to force the system to execute its code. Hence, the first line of defense against malware is to fix the vulnerabilities in software platforms, especially in the operating system. The most effective and easiest method of doing this in Microsoft's Windows operating system is to turn on *automatic updates*. This allows the operating system to download and apply critical updates to software regularly, thus patching the loopholes as much as possible.

An integrated anti-malware suite, comprising an antivirus, antispyware, anti-root kit and a firewall forms the second line of defense. Availability of these integrated solutions is widespread, but it is imperative that your security suite does not lend false positives as much as it is important that it detects true positives. Another prime consideration is that the anti-malware suite is light on system memory. There are both freeware and subscription security suites available. Independent antivirus testing websites such as AV comparatives (Box 2.1) can guide decisions and you can

always use Google to find more testers. However, these testers are effective only if they are frequently updated for virus *signature database*, given the fact that it is the malware that is written first and then the *definition updates* for the anti-malware suite. However, no battery of security software can provide total immunity, which means that one can still get infected even though one stays updated. The best way to protect oneself in a high-risk environment such as the World Wide Web is to reduce system vulnerability by not using a full privileges account, such as the *administrator* but to use a *restricted/limited/standard* user account with a software restriction policy in force.

It is of utmost importance to configure the firewall to *interactive mode* rather than *automatic mode* to be fully aware of the established connections and to be able to block illegitimate ones. This is quite difficult for the novice user, but can be learnt with a little practice. It is presumed here that practicing 'safe internet behavior', is of utmost importance. The top eight cyber security practices are as follows.

- *Protect your personal information* – includes information such as credit card numbers, social security number, user names and passwords and other sensitive information. Never store this information on your computer or allow password remember/auto complete in the web browser.
- *Know who you are dealing with online* – includes issues such as not disclosing one's identity/sensitive information to strangers as well as to unsecure websites.
- Use a security suite with up-to-date *virus definitions*.
- Use updated versions of operating system and browser software.
- Regularly back up your important files. One can use offline/online backup solutions.
- Do not download and install software from unverified sources. It should be noted that there are many fake free anti-malware suites floating on the internet which are in fact Trojan droppers – do not fall for the bait!
- Do not install pirated software, or play with cracks, patches and keygens to convert trial software into a full version. It is illegal as well as very risky in terms of system security.
- Do not visit websites that claim to provide illegal downloads of movies, software (warez), etc.

More details on safe internet practices can be found at Stay Safe Online, a website of the National Cyber Security Alliance (see Box 2.1).

For more security, in the scenario of thumb/flash drive infections, software that restricts auto-launching of all codes from removable drives may be installed (Box 2.1). These software provide the required protection for stand alone/non-networked computer systems in the office, from 'wild threats' and form the basis of the 'prevention is better than cure' policy.

Box 2.1 Products and programs for data protection and recovery

- Acronis true image, Acronis Inc., Woburn Massachusetts, USA: www.acronis.com/
- AV-Comparatives, Innsbruck, Austria: www.av-comparatives.org
- CCleaner, Piriform, London, England: www.ccleaner.com
- ComputerHope.com, West Jordan, Utah, USA: www.computerhope.com/issues/chsafe.htm
- Data Recovery Doctor, Pro Data Doctor: www.datadoctor.in
- ESET 5.NOD32 Antivirus for MS-DOS, ESET, San Diego, California, USA: www.eset.com
- HijackThis, Trend Micro, Cupertino, California, USA: www.trendsecure.com/portal/en-US/tools/security_tools/hijackthis
- Ice Sword, XFocus: www.antirootkit.com/software/IceSword.htm
- Knoppix, Knopper.net, Schmalenberg, Germany: www.knoppix.com
- Norton Ghost, Symantec, Cupertino, California, USA: http://us.norton.com/ghost
- Recover My Files, GetData Software Development Company, Hurstville, New South Wales, Australia: www.recovermyfiles.com
- Stay Safe Online, National Cyber Security Alliance, Washington DC, USA: www.staysafeonline.info
- Stinger, McAfee, Santa Clara, California, USA: http://vil.nai.com/vil/stinger
- Symantec, Cupertino, California, USA: http://security.symantec.com/sscv6/default.asp?langid=ie&venid=sym
- The Live CD List, FrozenTech, Santa Barbara, California, USA: www.livecdlist.com
- Ubuntu, registered trademark of Canonical, London, UK: www.ubuntu.com
- USB FireWall, Net Studio: www.net-studio.org/application/usb_firewall.php
- USBAntiVirus International Inc.: www.usbantivirus.net.
- Windows CleanUp!, Steven Gould, Dallas, Texas, USA: www.stevengould.org
- Windows, Microsoft Corporation: www.microsoft.com

Combating a malware infection

Despite all safety measures, a malware infection may still occur. The steps to be followed if the inevitable happens to the Microsoft Windows operating system (the most widely used operating system), is as follows:

- Reboot/restart the machine and enter the safe mode
- Turn off system restore
- Do a full system anti-malware scan in safe mode (with updated definitions)

- Install and run a temporary file cleaner and standalone malware shredders.

Reboot/restart the machine and enter the safe mode

For entering the *safe mode* on most systems running Microsoft Windows, hit the F8 key repeatedly when the system is booting (Figure 2.12a,b). Additional details on entering the *safe mode* in all Microsoft Windows versions can be found at Computer Hope (see Box 2.1). In this mode, the system loads only the most *critical drivers* and in

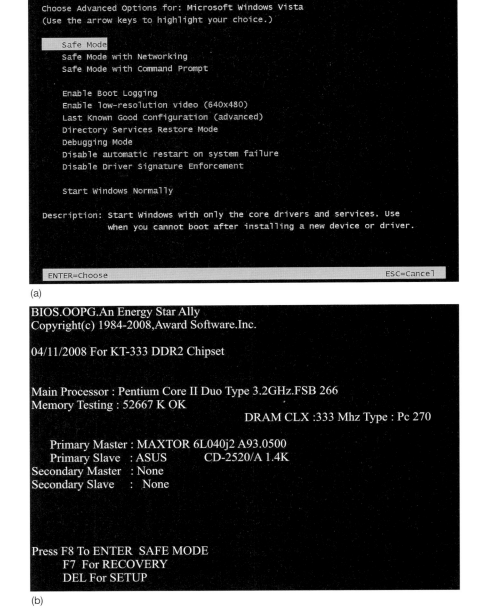

(a)

(b)

Figure 2.12 (a) Entering 'safe mode' from 'Advanced Boot Options' after rebooting computer. (b) The prompt to press F8 key to enter safe mode.

case one of your other drivers is infected, it can still be disinfected. This action cannot be performed in the normal mode, when these drivers may also be loaded.

Turn off system restore

In the Microsoft Windows operating environment, the system restore feature is found under the 'performance' section of the 'control panel'. It should be turned off before running a malware scan, because after the system is disinfected, it restores partition, and if left intact, it might inadvertently *restore* the malware back, like the proverbial phoenix.

Do a full system anti-malware scan in safe mode (with updated definitions)

Once you have entered the safe mode and turned off system restore, run a full system anti-malware scan with updated definitions. Alternatively, run a *DOS* based antimalware scanner such as ESET NOD32 antivirus (see Box 2.1). The advantage of DOS-based scanners is that one does not need to load the operating system. These scanners make it possible to scan from the DOS mode, thus making all system files (even the critical ones) available for the scan. This method is similar to physically connecting the system disk to a different computer and doing a 'scan from the outside'.

Install and run a temporary file cleaner and standalone malware shredders

This step can be done before or after running the antimalware scan. These utilities remove the unnecessary files called temporary files that Windows generates in the course of operation. Several freeware, such as Windows Clean Up and Piriform cleaner, are available (see Box 2.1). In addition to these, it is prudent to run standalone malware shredders such as Stinger, browser hijackers such as Hijack This, and rootkit revealers such as Ice Sword (Box 2.1). This function ensures disinfection of malware that goes undetected in the standard malware scan. One could also run an online scan at major antivirus provider websites such as ESET and Symantec, among others.

Some PMS and EMR solutions have integrated intrusion detection software, which runs in the background scanning for security breaches that might compromise patient data privacy such as a Trojan horse. On detection, the PMS/EMR will refuse to run, and will notify the user that the system is compromised. Privacy compliance for electronic patient data is paramount in laws such as the HIPAA (Health Insurance Portability and Accountability Act) and HITECH Act (Health Information Technology for Economic and Clinical Health Act) in the USA and patient data intrusion may have serious implications. A particular example that is often cited with regard to breached security involved a bank officer who used a database of cancer patients to call in loans (Sweeney, 1997).

What are the measures to safeguard data in the event of a system boot failure?

The prime method to save one's data is to always store it in a local hard disk drive partition other than that used by your operating system. For example, you could install the operating system in drive C, and store the data in drive D. This plan ensures that data is always safe, even in case you need to format the operating system residing in drive C.

What if one has not foreseen this problem or, for example, you have valuable data on the desktop, which by default is part of drive C and the system refuses to boot. Formatting in such circumstances would lead to irrecoverable data loss. In this scenario, boot the system from a compact disk drive using a bootable operating system disk (live compact disk) such as Linux Ubuntu or Knoppix. A list of bootable operating systems is available at The Live CD List (see Box 2.1). Booting from the live disk may require changing the boot order in the BIOS (Basic Input/Output settings). The primary function of the BIOS is to identify and initialize system component hardware (such as the video display card, hard disk, and floppy disk), when the computer is powered on. A specific boot order is followed when the BIOS searches for the operating system. For example: (1) Local hard disk, (2) CD drive, and (3) floppy drive. Booting from a live CD requires that the CD drive is designated as the first boot option in the BIOS. To change the BIOS settings, press the key designated for BIOS setup at the startup screen; in Figure 2.12b, this is the 'Del' key. Once you have logged in, you can access the local hard disk drives and after successfully doing so, it becomes a matter of common sense to transfer the data to portable media such as an external hard disk drive.

Data backup and recovery

Backup

Electronic data loss is an ever-present risk associated with newer technology owing to malware infection, and software or hardware failure. The best way to ensure safety is to conduct routine backups of important data onto physical media (onsite) or over the internet into a secure web server (offsite). Backing up direct data (such as images or standard files) onto a physical medium such as a hard disk drive or a compact disk is a simple matter of copying the files. However, copying programs or the status of an entire system (along with the operating system and installed programs) requires full system screenshot or a ghost image of the system, so that in the event of a system failure there is no need to reinstall program files. To generate a ghost image, special programs such as Norton Ghost or Acronis true image (see Box 2.1) are required. The ghost images generated by these programs may be used to restore the entire state of an operating system, along with the associated programs and data, at the time the ghost image was created. These ghost backup files can be stored on- or offsite. Websites such as Oaktreestorage.com and offsite backup solutions.com (see Box 2.1) provide an algorithm wherein each large file is divided into 100 or more parts and each part carries a 'marker' indicating whether anything within that 1/100 has been modified since the last time. Therefore, only portions that have been modified are reuploaded. This process is termed incremental backup (Redmond, 2008).

Recovery of lost data

Some programs enable the user to recover deleted data or data from formatted disks, such as Recover my files or Data recovery doctor (see Box 2.1). However, the disk should be physically intact to attempt recovery. Especially important is image recovery from memory cards used in digital cameras, lost due to accidental deletion/corruption/formatting. The following are certain circumstances, which can lead to such a situation.

- *Failure to 'safely remove' the memory card.* Corruption of the files usually occurs when there is a physical separation of the card when a transaction is in progress, especially during image transfer. However, this error might no longer pose a problem when 'hot swap' device standards become more widely available. This problem is also not an issue with wireless transfer of images.
- *Accidental deletion of the images.* This mistake usually occurs in large setups, where the same digital camera is shared by many operators. This problem can be overcome by enabling *autotransfer* in a wireless image transfer setup (Revankar et al., 2010), which transfers the images wirelessly to the *paired* computer, as and when they are shot. However, this corrective move does not eliminate the possibility of images being inadvertently deleted on the computer. Better still, if the images do not require editing (which is unlikely in our scenario), wirelessly print your images through a *paired* printer, using PictBridge, without the need for an intermediate computer.
- *Accidental formatting of the card.*
- *Physical damage to the card.*

Several commercial software programs are available for recovering lost images from deleted/corrupted/formatted memory cards. Most of these programs are shareware, requiring their purchase. Some freeware for computers running Microsoft Windows operating system are shown in Table 2.7.

Virtual patient record for integration of specialties

Over the years, electronic medical records/EPRs have evolved to help healthcare providers with structured and helpful information. However, most electronic record systems associated with a specific specialty are independent and isolated and do not communicate with other specialties, thus effectively addressing the specificities of that specialty alone, rather than the patient as a whole. Patients receive services which are provided by numerous specialists and institutions, including healthcare professionals, hospitals, outpatient care services, drug stores, and interdisciplinary healthcare workers such as nurses and laboratory support personnel. For the benefit of the patient, these heterogeneous working groups need to be monitored for coordinated activities with an excellent, workable, user-friendly communication system.

Integration of healthcare information systems is essential to improve communication and data use for healthcare delivery, research and management. Integrating data from heterogeneous sources is an uphill task, because the individual feeder systems usually differ in several aspects, such as functionality, presentation, terminology, data representation, and semantics (Lenz and Kuhn, 2003). The vision of seamless healthcare is based on integrated healthcare processes enabled by seamless information technology IT support. Realizing the vision of seamless healthcare requires the establishment of basic communication infrastructure. Once this network infrastructure is set up, the interoperability is based on the adoption of standard data formats at each feeder level. Syntactical standards are meant for the correct transmission of medical and administrative data between heterogeneous and distributed medical information systems. These standards are mainly HL7/CDA (Health Level Seven/Clinical Document Architecture), DICOM, and UN/EDIFACT (United Nations/Electronic Data Interchange For Administration, Commerce and Transport).

Semantic standards, on the other hand, ensure correct interpretation of the content of the electronically exchanged data. Established standards are LOINC (Logical Observation

Table 2.7 Comparison of three image recovery software programs

Software	Supported file formats	Supported operating systems	Recovery from formatted cards	Recovery from damaged cards
Picajet photo recovery	JPEG, TIF	Windows NT, 2000, XP	Yes	No
Artplus digital photorecovery	JPEG, TIF, DNG	Windows Vista, XP, 2000, 98, Me, NT	Yes	Yes
Photoextractor	JPEG	Windows NT, 2000, 2003 XP	Yes	No

Identifiers Names and Codes), SNOMED (Systematized Nomenclature of Medicine), and MeSH (Medical Subject Heading). Following data standards when implementing healthcare information technology networks will ensure seamless integration of EPR, from diverse systems into a single centralised repository, thus providing a holistic approach to healthcare. The central database may be accessed by patients, various healthcare providers, insurance agencies, and government regulators. Protection of patient confidentiality in such an environment requires the enforcement of certain technical constraints. These include authentication (ensuring that the user is indeed an authorized user), access control (allowing users access only to information that they need to know), and auditing (keeping a record of who has accessed what). For example, insurance agencies are allowed access to only the treatment procedures carried out and the fee for each procedure.

HIPAA compliance for electronic protected health information (EPHI)

Health information transmission via email is a standard mode of communication between orthodontists and other colleagues, as well as with healthcare companies. HIPAA was enacted in 1996 to regulate the availability, confidentiality, integrity and usage of patient electronic protected health information (EPHI). Standard emails result in transmission of unsecured PHI. An email message bound to a particular destination may cross anywhere between three and 10 or more internet service provider ISPs or mail relay systems before it reaches its final destination, providing ample opportunity for interception and tampering. Transmitting unsecured PHI poses a legal risk to the orthodontist, and to any other involved party, by endangering the patient's privacy.

Email encryption is a mathematical exercise that hides information in plain sight. Encryption applies mathematical formula/manipulation to the email message (including attachments), so that the message contents are hidden from everyone except the recipient. The fact that we are transmitting email messages without any encryption means that we are transmitting unsecured EPHI (HIPAA, 2009a).

HIPAA is a set of federal regulations that requires healthcare organizations and businesses that handle confidential patient health information to simplify and standardize data exchange, in an effort to protect the security, privacy, and confidentiality of that information (HIPAA, 2009b). HIPAA established a set of uniform standards for the privacy of PHI, which encompass electronic, oral and printed data or exchange of individually identifiable health information. On violation of the guidelines, HIPAA imposed penalties ranging from '[US]$100 per violation, up to $25 000 per year for each requirement violated'. Criminal violations can result in penalties 'from $50 000 in fines and one year in prison, up to $250 000 in fines and 10 years in prison' (Weil

2) (HIPAA Law, 2009). There are two possible methods for encrypting emails:

- Use of web-based encrypted mail providers – ASP
- Use of desktop-based email encryption.

Web-based encrypted mail providers

Many web-based email providers offer encrypted email services (ASP). The following providers are sufficiently competent to handle EPHI and its transmission (basic service is free to use):

- www.hushmail.com
- www.imedicor.com.

This model utilizes a third-party hosted mail client for secure delivery of email. The message is transmitted via secure transmission protocols, between the client web browsers and delivered to the ASP-hosted mail server, while a notification message is forwarded to the intended recipient. The intended recipient then actively requests delivery of the message at the secured ASP-hosted mail site. The advantage of this method is that confidential and authenticated exchanges can start immediately by any internet user worldwide, since there is no requirement for installation of any software, nor to obtain or to distribute cryptographic keys beforehand.

Desktop-based email encryption

There are several dedicated clients available for desktop-based email encryption, with their own dedicated email servers, as well as those which provide encryption add-ons for existing desktop email applications such as Outlook Express and Mozilla Thunderbird (Table 2.8). This method is based on the public key encryption architecture. In public key encryption, two keys are generated by every user – one is the public key and the other is a corresponding private key (Rubin, 1995). The public key is to be distributed, whereas the private key is kept confidential. In this method of encryption, you can send encrypted emails to anyone who has sent you their public key. Similarly, anyone who has your public key can send you encrypted messages. Only the owner of the private key corresponding to the public key will be able to decrypt and read the messages, thus providing 'confidentiality'. One can also attach digital signatures to emails using the private key, and the recipient can ascertain that the email was indeed sent by the person who he or she claims to be, using the sender's corresponding public key, thus providing 'assurance' against 'social engineering'. Digital signatures help prevent impostors from sending emails that appear to have come from you (Figure 2.13).

Privacy protection on non-internet-connected computers

When patient data are stored on a standalone computer or when communications occur within one's own local area

Table 2.8 Desktop-based HIPAA-compliant email clients

Software	License	Standalone	Website
Private Mail	Freeware	Yes – works with Hotmail	www.trusttone.com/
Mirracrypt	Shareware	No – plugin for Outlook 2003 and 2007	www.mirrasoft.com/
Mirramail	Shareware	Yes – works with any email service provider	www.mirrasoft.com/
Stealth	Freeware	No – plugin for Outlook 2003 and 2007	www.trusttone.com/

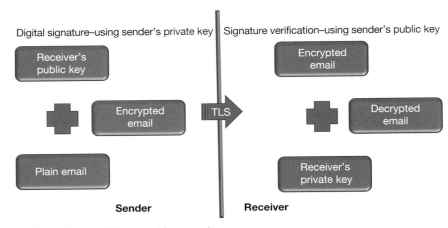

Figure 2.13 Public key encryption architecture. TLS, transport layer security.

network (LAN), it does not necessarily require encryption. However, these computers should be secure enough by allowing authorized password access to maintain HIPPA compliance. These systems should have 30-day password changing policies in force. To ensure total privacy compliance, all computer systems should enforce authentication, access control, and auditing (as discussed earlier). These three features should be integrated in any software that handles EPHI, including PMS and EMR solutions, to be HIPAA compliant.

Workstations used for storage and transmission of EPHI must contain an updated virus scan, updated operating system patches, and an anti-spyware product with appropriate firewalls. When a workstation is no longer used for EPHI storage or is decommissioned, the data on that system should be completely erased by special procedures such as low-level disk formatting to ensure data are completely removed from all sectors of the hard disk. All workstations should have antitheft measures in place. In case of theft, the concerned government agency should be notified along with all patients whose EPHI is stolen if the data were not encrypted. Therefore, it is wise to encrypt all EPHI even though HIPAA does not specify this for standalone workstations. However, all EPHI on removable and portable media such as laptops, tablets, handhelds, thumbdrives, floppy disks, and compact disks should be encrypted. Encrypting large folders or entire drives requires dedicated

encryption utilities. A simple to use freeware is AxCrypt (Axantum Software AB, Järfälla, Sweden). AxCrypt is driven by 128-bit AES (advanced encryption standard), secure enough for all nonclassified data as well as classified data up to the 'secret level' (AES, 2010).

Conclusion

Technology is complementing traditional communication methods in all aspects of orthodontics, but the enunciated role of technology is to enhance, not substitute, the role of personal interaction. Information technology applications and data management systems for orthodontics continue to evolve rapidly. The goal of wise implementation of these systems in orthodontics is to amplify the effectiveness of the system as a whole.

In the orthodontic team, all of the participants need to be informed and engaged for smooth running of the system. Most of the applications described in this chapter are required for the smooth functioning of today's orthodontic offices. Practitioners should develop a comprehensive plan for implementing or updating the IT infrastructure in their offices. Issues to be considered in technology purchasing decisions include usability, integration, work flow support, cost–benefit analysis, and compliance with acts such as the HIPAA and HITECH. An all-in-one solution, probably ASP-driven (no maintenance), for practice management, electronic orthodontic records, imaging and other diagnostics, and interactive patient electronic communication, which is secure, backs up automatically, is tamper proof, provides authentication, access control and auditing, is the way to go in the future. Intelligent face and patient input recognizing systems, recognizing the personality types and thus providing customized questionnaires and patient education systems to maximize understanding and thus compliance resulting in near to ideal treatment results, are possible areas of research in health information technology. A nationwide unitary patient secure electronic medical data database may be maintained and constantly updated through a network of data collection satellite/feeder units in each specialty. This database could be called upon to provide data requested by the user depending on the user access level.

Tele-orthodontics is another promising area of development, offering the possibility of being able to provide comprehensive diagnosis and advice from geographically distant areas, thus carrying healthcare to remote and inaccessible areas. This evolution is what health information technology promises to deliver by enhancing communication between doctors and their patients, colleagues and specialists, educators and students, as well as each and everyone in the specialty.

References

Abraham Z (2007) Photo archiving, cephalometric analyses, and information sharing on the Internet. *American Journal of Orthodontics and Dentofacial Orthopedics* 131: 98–100.

AES (2010) *Advanced Encryption Standard*. Available at: http://en.wikipedia.org/wiki/Advanced_Encryption_Standard (accessed July 2010).

Al-Jewair TS, Suri S, Shah PS (2009) Computer-assisted learning in orthodontic education: a systematic review and meta-analysis. *Journal of Dental Education* 73: 730–9.

Anderson JG, Rainey MR, Eysenbach G (2003) The impact of CyberHealthcare on the physician-patient relationship. *Journal of Medical Systems* 27: 67–84.

Antonarakis GS, Kiliaridis S (2009) Internet-derived information on cleft lip and palate for families with affected children. *Cleft Palate Craniofacial Journal* 46: 75–80.

Baur C (2000) Limiting factors on the transformative powers of email in patient-physician relationships: a critical analysis. *Health Communications* 12: 239–59.

Beckman HB, Markakis KM, Suchman AL, et al. (1994) The doctor-patient relationship and malpractice. Lessons from plaintiff depositions. *Archives of Internal Medicine* 154: 1365–70.

Bednar ED, Hannum WM, Firestone A, et al. (2007) Application of distance learning to interactive seminar instruction in orthodontic residency programs. *American Journal of Orthodontics and Dentofacial Orthopedics* 132: 586–94.

Boyd AD, Funk EA, Schwartz SM, et al. (2010) Top EHR challenges in light of the stimulus. Enabling effective interdisciplinary, intradisciplinary and cross-setting communication. *Journal of Healthcare Informatics and Management* 24: 18–24.

Broadbent BH (1931) A new x-ray technique and its application to orthodontia. *Angle Orthodontist* 1: 45–66.

Chaitin E, Stiller R, Jacobs S, et al. (2003) Physician-patient relationship in the intensive care unit: erosion of the sacred trust? *Critical Care Medicine* 31: S367–72.

Chenin DL, Chennin DA, Chennin ST, et al. (2009) Dynamic cone-beam computed tomography in orthodontic treatment. *Journal of Clinical Orthodontics* 43: 507–12.

Clark RD, Weerakone S, Rock WP (1997) A hypertext tutorial for teaching cephalometrics. *British Journal of Orthodontics* 24: 325–8.

Dacanay LS, Cohen PA (1992) A meta-analysis of self-instruction in dental education. *Journal of Dental Education* 56: 183–9.

DiMatteo MR (1995) Patient adherence to pharmacotherapy: the importance of effective communication. *Formulary* 30: 596–8, 601–2, 605.

El-Zanaty HM, El-Beialy AR, Abou El-Ezz AM, et al. (2010) Three-dimensional dental measurements: An alternative to plaster models. *American Journal of Orthodontics and Dentofacial Orthopedics*, 137, 259–65.

Engilman WD, Cox TH, Bednar ED, et al. (2007) Equipping orthodontic residency programs for interactive distance learning. *American Journal of Orthodontics and Dentofacial Orthopedics* 131: 651–5.

Favero L, Pavan L, Arreghini A (2009) Communication through telemedicine: home teleassistance in orthodontics. *European Journal of Paediatric Dentistry* 10: 163–7.

Francis V, Korsch BM, Morris MJ (1969) Gaps in doctor-patient communication. Patients' response to medical advice. *New England Journal of Medicine* 280: 535–40.

F-Secure Corporation (2007) F-Secure reports amount of malware grew by 100% during 2007. Press release. Available at: www.f-secure.com/f-secure/pressroom/news/fs_news_20071204_1_eng.html (accessed July 2010).

Greenfield S, Kaplan SH, Ware JE Jr, et al. (1988) Patients' participation in medical care: effects on blood sugar control and quality of life in diabetes. *Journal of General Internal Medicine* 3: 448–57.

Gribel BF, Gribel MN, Manzi FR, et al. (2011a) From 2D to 3D: an algorithm to derive normal values for 3-dimensional computerized assessment. *Angle Orthodontist* 81: 5–12.

Gribel BF, Gribel MN, Frazao DC, et al. (2011b) Accuracy and reliability of craniometric measurements on lateral cephalometry and 3D measurements on CBCT scans. *Angle Orthodontist* 81: 28–37.

Haeger RS (2005) Establishing an all-digital office. *Journal of Clinical Orthodontics* 39: 81–95.

Halazonetis DJ (2004) How can I match the color on 2 intraoral digital images? *American Journal of Orthodontics and Dentofacial Orthopedics* 126: 518–19.

HIPAA (2009a) *Health Insurance Portability and Accountability Act*. Available at: http://en.wikipedia.org/wiki/Health_Insurance_Portability_and_Accountability_Act (accessed August 2010).

HIPAA (2009b) *General Information Overview*. Available at: www.cms.hhs.gov/hipaaGenInfo/ (accessed August 2010).

HIPAA Law (2009) Available at: www.cms.hhs.gov/HIPAAGenInfo/Downloads/HIPAALaw.pdf (accessed August 2010).

Hobson RS, Carter NE, Hall FM, et al. (1998) study into the effectiveness of a text-based computer-assisted learning program in comparison with seminar teaching of orthodontics. *European Journal of Dental Education* 2: 154–9.

Hollander S, Lanier D (2001) The physician-patient relationship in an electronic environment: a regional snapshot. *Bulletin of the Medical Library Association* 89: 397–9.

Irvine NR, Moore RN (1986) Computer-assisted instruction in mixed dentition analysis. *Journal of Dental Education* 50: 312–15.

Kaplan SH, Greenfield S, Ware JE Jr (1989) Assessing the effects of physician-patient interactions on the outcomes of chronic disease. *Medical Care* 27: S110–27.

Kulik CC, Kulik JA (1991) Effectiveness of computer-based instruction: an updated analysis. *Computers in Human Behaviour* 7: 75–94.

Lenz R, Kuhn KA (2003) Towards a continuous evolution and adaptation of information systems in healthcare. *International Journal of Medical Informatics* 73: 75–89.

Lewis CA (2006) The advantages of paperless option. *Journal of Clinical Orthodontics* 40: 299–305.

Luffingham JK (1984) An assessment of computer-assisted learning in orthodontics. *British Journal of Orthodontics* 11: 205–8.

Mah J (2007) The evolution of digital study models. *Journal of Clinical Orthodontics* 41: 557–61.

Mah J, Sachdeva R (2001) Computer-assisted orthodontic treatment: the SureSmile process. *American Journal of Orthodontics and Dentofacial Orthopedics* 120: 85–7.

Malware (2010) Available at: http://en.wikipedia.org/wiki/Malware (accessed September 2010).

Marquis MS, Davies AR, Ware JE Jr (1983) Patient satisfaction and change in medical care provider: a longitudinal study. *Medical Care* 21: 821–9.

Miller EA (2003) The technical and interpersonal aspects of telemedicine: effects on doctor-patient communication. *Journal of Telemedicine and Telecare* 9: 1–7.

Miller KT, Hannum WM, Morley T, et al. (2007) Use of recorded interactive seminars in orthodontic distance education. *American Journal of Orthodontics and Dentofacial Orthopedics* 132: 408–14.

Mupparapu M (2008) Voice over internet protocol for the orthodontic practice: A sensible switch from plain old telephone service. *American Journal of Orthodontics and Dentofacial Orthopedics* 133: 470–5.

Murphy J, Chang H, Montgomery JE, et al. (2001) The quality of physician-patient relationships. Patients' experiences 1996–1999. *Journal of Family Practice* 50: 123–9.

National Conference of State Legislatures (2008) *Virus/Contaminant/Destructive Transmission Statutes by State.* Available at: www.ncsl.org/programs/lis/cip/viruslaws.htm (accessed September 2010).

Patel JH, Moles DR, Cunningham SJ (2008) Factors affecting information retention in orthodontic patients. *American Journal of Orthodontics and Dentofacial Orthopedics* 133: S61–7.

Povolny B (2002) Online patient communications. *American Journal of Orthodontics and Dentofacial Orthopedics* 121: 655–8.

Proffit WR (2005) Multicenter, internet-based orthodontic education: A research proposal. *American Journal of Orthodontics and Dentofacial Orthopedics* 127: 164–7.

Redmond RW (2008) The advantages of offsite backups. *Journal of Clinical Orthodontics* 42: 457–60.

Revankar AV, Gandedkar NH (2010) Effective communication for the cyberage. *American Journal of Orthodontics and Dentofacial Orthopedics* 137: 712–14.

Revankar AV, Gandedkar NH, Ganeshkar SV (2009a) 'Oops i deleted it' – A solution for recovering deleted or reformatted digital images from memory cards. *American Journal of Orthodontics and Dentofacial Orthopedics* 135: 820–22.

Revankar AV, Gandedkar NH, Ganeshkar SV (2009b) Securing your digital data against computer threats. *Journal of Clinical Orthodontics* 43: 393–9.

Revankar AV, Gandedkar NH, Ganeshkar SV (2010) WI-PICS -Wireless and beyond. *American Journal of Orthodontics and Dentofacial Orthopedics* 137: 147–9.

Rosenberg H, Grad HA, Matear DW (2003) The effectiveness of computer-aided, self-instructional programs in dental education: a systematic review of the literature. *Journal of Dental Education* 67: 524–32.

Rosenberg H, Sander M, Posluns J (2005) The effectiveness of computer-aided learning in teaching orthodontics: A review of the literature. *American Journal of Orthodontics and Dentofacial Orthopedics* 127, 599–605.

Rosenberg H, Posluns J, Tenenbaum HC, et al. (2010) Evaluation of computer-aided learning in orthodontics. *American Journal of Orthodontics and Dentofacial Orthopedics* 138: 410–19.

Roter D (2000) The enduring and evolving nature of the patient-physician relationship. *Patient Education and Counseling* 39: 5–15.

Rubin AD (1995) Secure distribution of electronic documents in a hostile environment. *Computer Communications* 18: 429–34.

Sandler PJ, Murray AM, Bearn D (2002) Digital records in orthodontics. *Dental Update* 29: 18–24.

Scholz RP (1989) Computerized patient records – A potential risk. *American Journal of Orthodontics and Dentofacial Orthopedics* 95: A42.

Scholz RP (2005) Commentary. *American Journal of Orthodontics and Dentofacial Orthopedics* 127: 167.

Starke KM, Starke GT (2006) Office-based medical records. In: PW Iyer, JB Lewin, MA Shea (eds) *Medical Legal Aspects of Medical Records.* Tucson, AZ: Lawyers and Judges Publishing Company Inc, p. 314.

Stevens DR, Flores-Mir C, Nebbe B, et al. (2006) Validity, reliability, and reproducibility of plaster vs digital study models: Comparison of peer assessment rating and Bolton analysis and their constituent measurements. *American Journal of Orthodontics and Dentofacial Orthopedics* 129: 794–803.

Sweeney L (1997) Weaving technology and policy together to maintain confidentiality. *Journal of Law, Medicine and Ethics* 25: 98–110.

Symantec Internet Security Threat Report (2007) *Trends for July-December 2007 (Executive Summary).* Available at: http://eval.symantec.com/mktginfo/enterprise/white_papers/bwhitepaper_exec_summary_Internet_security_threat_report_xiii_04–2008.en-us.pdf (accessed September 2010).

Tanikawa C, Yamamoto T, Yagi M, et al. (2010) Automatic recognition of anatomic features on cephalograms of preadolescent children. *Angle Orthodontist* 80: 812–20.

Tomassetti JJ, Taloumis LJ, Denny JM, et al. (2001) A comparison of 3 computerized Bolton tooth-size analyses with a commonly used method. *Angle Orthodontist* 71: 351–7.

Turpin DL (2008) Create and update your office web site. *American Journal of Orthodontics and Dentofacial Orthopedics* 133: 779.

Wallin WS (2009) Does your website draw new patients? *American Journal of Orthodontics and Dentofacial Orthopedics* 136: 746–51.

Yagi M, Shibata T (2003) An image representation algorithm compatible with neural-associative-processor-based hardware recognition systems. *IEEE Transactions on Neural Networks* 14: 1144–61.

3

Orthodontic Diagnosis and Treatment Planning: Collaborating with Medical and Other Dental Specialists

Om P Kharbanda, Neeraj Wadhawan

Summary

Orthodontists – as specialists – are expected to be proficient in diagnosing anomalies of the face, teeth, and jaws, as well as identifying any coexisting deviations in physiological functions and systemic pathologies. As a member of the healthcare provider system, an orthodontist should have sufficient knowledge to recognize and record the etiology of a presenting malocclusion, which may be the result of a variety of systemic or local aberrations. This means any anomalies of anatomy, physiology, and the various medical conditions that may directly or indirectly influence the orthodontic diagnosis, treatment plan, mechanotherapy, or the prognosis of the case should be taken note of. In addition, the existing oral health conditions and problems with the dentition, ranging from quality and quantity of dentition, morbidity associated with childhood trauma, dental caries, and/or periodontal diseases, which might require close collaboration with a variety of dental specialists, should be recorded. This chapter aims to deal with these issues and provide a framework for interaction and collaboration with medical and dental specialists, based on a holisitic approach to orthodontic diagnosis and treatment planning. The goal is to help the reader develop an aptitude to communicate with a variety of healthcare specialists to undertake, reconsider, stop, or reschedule orthodontic treatment with due precaution.

Introduction

Success in any healthcare profession depends largely on accurate diagnosis, formulation of appropriate treatment goals, and their precise implementation. Currently, patients with orthodontic needs span across a wide range of age groups, personalities, social strata, and ethnic backgrounds, with varying levels of expectations (Abu Alhaija et al., 2010). Additionally, the increasing number of adult patients means that the present-day orthodontist is faced with an array of systemic (van Venrooy and Proffit, 1985; Patel et al., 2009) as well as local conditions (Basdra et al., 2001; Altug-Atac and Erdem, 2007) that may affect both the general as well as oral health status of the individual. It is now accepted that 'It is no longer appropriate to deny elective dental or medical care to patients with diagnoses that have historically been associated with poor outcomes' (Sonis, 2004). The recent medical and dental advances have made it possible for many patients with significant medical and dental disorders to be successfully managed in the orthodontic office (Lux et al., 2005), provided the orthodontist has a sound knowledge base and is keen to interact with other medical and dental professionals (Patel et al., 2009).

An orthodontic graduate first needs to be a good oral diagnostician and a good physician, before becoming a good orthodontist. We, as orthodontists, often make a diagnosis after taking a short medical history, complemented by a physical examination concentrating only on facial appearance (in general) and occlusion (local) alone. This approach, which is more appropriately termed 'regional diagnosis', reveals the existing malocclusion but lacks an overall perspective, and, in this process, the bigger picture of the medical, psychological, and pathological processes occurring elsewhere in the body gets ignored. This approach makes proper recognition of existing systemic conditions, and their effects on orthodontic treatment, difficult, if not impossible to comprehend. In our 'play safe' approach, many of us end up refusing treatment to patients who could be treated successfully with suitable precautions and professional interaction with the other medical/dental specialists. To rectify this approach, it is recommended to include a module on diagnosis and management of medical conditions in orthodontic training programs, with sufficient exposure in clinical settings in multispecialty hospitals. This will allow development of an attitude that encourages a more professional approach when interacting with our medical and surgical colleagues, while recognizing and realizing our responsibilities and limitations. Up-to-date knowledge of medical problems should be aimed for, so that proper communication protocols can be followed while referring patients to other medical and dental colleagues.

The other side of the story

Since oral health can have a significant impact on the general health, dental health is often a great concern for the medical fraternity (George et al., 2010; Yasny, 2010). Mutual referral systems are useful in these situations, with medical personnel – including specialists – referring patients with dental and oral health-related problems to the dental specialists with greater zeal, provided the specialists on both sides are confident about and comfortable while interacting with each other. We should recognize that none of us can possibly treat all the diseases of the human body. Thus, a 'two-way interaction' is important for providing a better level of healthcare.

Orthodontic diagnosis from a broad perspective

From a mere tooth-moving specialty, orthodontics has emerged to become a branch of dentistry with deep scientific and evidence-based perspectives of its biomechanical principles. Often, clinicians remain preoccupied with the mechanotherapeutic features of various appliances and philosophies, ignoring the fact that teeth are a part of larger, intricately linked biological systems of the body which influence the response of teeth to mechanical stimuli.

Every patient is unique, with metabolic traits that are individually specific to him or her (Sidell and Kaminskis, 1975; Morrison et al., 1992; Bartley et al., 1997) even though all humans have similar basic anatomical, physiological, and biochemical features. It must be appreciated that treatment is being delivered not to an artificial set of typodont teeth, but rather to vital tissues – which have the capacity to respond differently to the same treatment protocol under the same physiological conditions in different individuals (Ren et al., 2003; McConkey, 2004; Williams, 2008), altered physiological conditions in the same individual (Brambilla et al., 1981), and in various pathological conditions (Salerno et al., 1982; Verna et al., 2000).

The craniofacial complex can be considered as an organization of many small organ systems and components, such as the dentoalveolar structures, the nervous system, the muscular system, the soft tissue matrix, and the air passages. These structures are so intricately interlinked that disturbances in the physiology, anatomy, or function of any one component structure are bound to cause an imbalance in the whole of the craniofacial complex. This understanding should be clearly reflected in orthodontic diagnosis and treatment planning.

Concurrently, a thorough knowledge of subjects such as anthropology, genetics, growth and development, nutrition, psychology, endocrinology, and kinesiology can help us gather critically important data regarding the various aspects of general health and disease. Along with this knowledge, the use of advanced biochemical, microbiologic, and radiologic investigative procedures can help to optimally diagnose a malocclusion, thus reducing the chances of treatment failure. In brief, a comprehensive approach toward diagnosis and treatment planning helps in categorizing patients according to their general health status and biological limitations, and increases the probability of a successful treatment outcome.

The first interaction with the patient

The initial examination is the most overlooked step as far as orthodontic diagnosis is concerned. Planning for an orthodontic examination should begin even before the patient visits the orthodontic office, through careful screening via telephonic conversation with trained office personnel, or alternatively, through electronic mailing of the patient's knowledge of their medical history to the orthodontic office prior to the scheduled appointment. This preliminary review will often highlight important medical conditions such as endocrine, hematological, cardiac, renal, hepatic, pulmonary, and allergic disorders, as well as dental health-related conditions. Such information is important for the orthodontist to prepare for the appointment, and plan various investigative procedures and anticipated referrals in advance, which can translate into increased efficiency and reduced time required for the screening and risk assessment of the patient. This strategy should ultimately lead to increased patient satisfaction and higher confidence levels, and lesser chances of complications later during therapy.

Comprehensive diagnosis and treatment planning should start at the time of the first interaction with the prospective patient (Kharbanda, 2009). The very short 'look-see' examination is no longer considered adequate with the increasing number of patients with medical problems seeking orthodontic treatment. At the first visit, the orthodontist should enquire about the problems and the expectations of the patient and parents from orthodontic treatment (Figure 3.1), and concurrently perform an appraisal of the patient's psy-

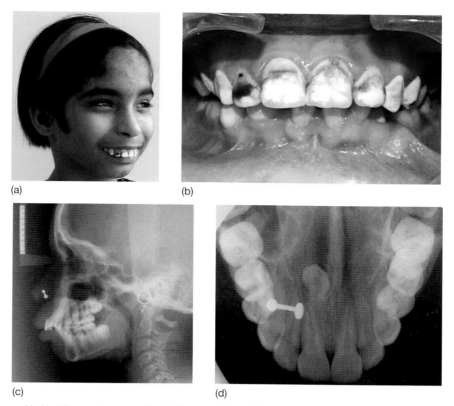

(a)   (b)

(c)   (d)

Figure 3.1 (a–d) A 12-year-old girl with severely compromised vision attended with her parents for protrusion of her upper teeth and poor dental esthetics. She had a Class II malocclusion with bimaxillary protrusion and severe discoloration of the dentition due to fluorosis. Radiographic examination also revealed an inverted and unerupted mesiodens. The diagnosis and treatment plan in such a case must include evaluation of expectations of patient and parents in view of the reduced vision of the girl, who may not fully appreciate the benefits of the improved esthetics following orthodontic treatment and correction of the discolored anterior teeth. It is also pertinent to elicit the intensity of concern in the patient and parents towards the discoloration and protrusion as well as the motivational factors with regard to treatment.

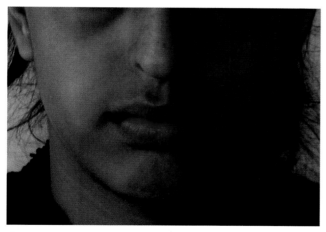

Figure 3.2 A 12-year-old girl with congenital strawberry angioma on the left side of her face reported for orthodontic consultation. A strawberry angioma of the face may be associated with disorders such as encephalotrigeminal angiomatosis (which is associated with epilepsy of the contralateral cerebral hemisphere). Hence, presence of such a lesion warrants further investigations to rule out such disorders. Angiomas of the face may extend into the oral cavity as well or they may occur as an isolated lesion within the oral cavity. These lesions are known to bleed excessively following episodes of trauma associated with extraction, injection of local anesthesia and even trauma from orthodontic appliances.

chological profile, as treating patients with unrealistic expectations or with extreme mood fluctuations may result in an unhappy ending (Al-Omiri and Alhaija, 2006). Following this initial scrutiny, a systematic procedure of examination should be followed, starting with the craniofacial region. If the examination or the previous medical history indicates the presence of an underlying pathology or abnormality, further investigations in the form of referrals and advanced diagnostic tests should be undertaken (Figure 3.2).

The importance of the medical history in the orthodontic diagnosis and treatment planning

Many patients today would already be taking short-or long-term medications, which may influence paradental tissue remodeling (Krishnan and Davidovitch, 2006) and consequently, tooth movement. Drugs such as steroids, when taken for long periods, as in chronic asthma or for immunosuppression, may predispose teeth to iatrogenic root resorption following application of a mechanical stimulus (McNab et al., 1999). In certain instances, for example, in the presence of sexually transmitted diseases such as human immunodeficiency virus (HIV) infection or syphilis, the patient may hesitate to give a complete and realistic history. Thus, it becomes the prerogative of the treating doctor to sufficiently evaluate the patient, both prospectively and retrospectively, to obtain a detailed health history during the first visit and/or the subsequent visits. In this regard, the orthodontist and office personnel should be able to judge from the mannerisms, attitude, and the current health condition of the patient whether further investigations and/ or precautions are warranted before and/or during treatment.

A detailed medical history is an extremely useful tool for evaluating the existing health status of an individual, and identifying any medical disorders that he/she may have. Diseases of chronic duration, those of severe intensity, those affecting bone metabolism, and those altering the inflammatory pathways have a particularly important bearing on the orthodontic treatment plan (Sonis, 2004; Patel et al., 2009). Besides nutritional imbalances, developmental disorders, and skeletal malformations, chronic diseases, liver dysfunctions, renal impairments, cardiac and pulmonary anomalies, and erosive joint diseases can all impact physiological growth, and thus, orthodontic treatment (Table 3.1).

Chromosomal aberrations and embryologic defects including deformities of the orofacial complex – where do orthodontists stand in their diagnostic approach?

Development of craniofacial structures is largely determined by the cells of the neural crest, which give rise to the branchial arches during embryonic development. In the 4th week of intrauterine life, the mandibular arch (also the hyoid and glossopharyngeal arches) forms discrete processes, which form the future maxilla and mandible. While the paired mandibular processes merge with each other in the midline by the 4th week, the maxillary process continues to contribute to the formation of the secondary palate, the upper jaw and lateral portions of the upper lip (Sperber et al., 2001). The period between the 6th and 12th week of intrauterine life is considered to be critical for craniofacial development (Finkelstein, 2001), and anomalies during this period result in a variety of craniofacial defects (these are covered in greater detail in Chapters 7–9). Most of the congenital disorders result from unknown causes. However, in the light of newer research, many of the unknown causes have been identified, and now multifactorial etiology is considered the commonest cause of congenital defects, whereas isolated genetic defects have been described in 10–30% of cases (Kumar, 2008). Genetic inheritance can follow a variety of patterns, from simple mendelian inheritance to complex polygenic traits with variable penetrance and expression across generations. In order to accurately diagnose the etiology of the condition and the inheritance pattern, the orthodontist has to identify the role of genetics and delineate it from the environmental influences. Familial comparisons, pedigree analysis, and sometimes, simple cephalometric analysis, may be valuable tools in identifying and differentiating the role of genetic aberrations in the causation of these conditions.

Orthodontists often encounter conditions resulting from embryonic developmental defects, such as cleft of lip and palate, hemifacial microsomia, maxillofacial dysplasias, vertical facial clefts, and micro/macrognathia. Being an active member of the craniofacial team, it is the responsibility of the orthodontist to be able to recognize the basic features of a congenital growth anomaly or a genetically linked syndrome. A thorough extraoral and intraoral examination can reveal vital information of an underlying syndrome/ congenital deformity, (Table 3.2 and Figure 3.3). Facial features such as sparse hair on the head, frontal bossing, depression of the nasal bridge, telecanthus, low-set ears, typical epicanthal folds, coloboma, defects of the external ear, and facial clefts are characteristic features seen in many craniofacial syndromes. It is important to note that many craniofacial deviations may be associated with systemic alterations, such as osteogenesis imperfecta with dentinogenesis imperfecta, or craniofacial clefts, in association with velocardiofacial and Aperts syndrome.

In sum, an orthodontist should be able to identify severe conditions, and make appropriate referrals to medical specialists and/or the craniofacial and genetic centers, while managing the lesser severe ones themselves, without inflicting further trauma on the psychological status of the already burdened patient.

Acute and chronic infections (systemic and local)

Various systemic diseases, and those locally affecting the craniofacial complex, have the propensity to contribute to the etiology of malocclusion, directly or indirectly, in both the prenatal and postnatal stages. Chronic systemic infections such as tuberculosis, hepatitis, nephritis, and HIV may indirectly contribute to a malocclusion by causing disruption in systemic growth during childhood. Acute perinatal infections such as the TORCH complex (Toxoplasmosis, Other infections, Rubella, Cytomegalovirus, Herpes simplex) can lead to congenital deformities in the offspring, including craniofacial clefts. Diseases such as congenital syphilis, apart from systemic alterations, can lead to an array of orofacial malformations such as saddle nose, depressed nasal bridge, and hypoplasia of the molars and incisors.

Late natal or acute childhood infections can cause temporary cessation of tooth development, which may be evident as enamel hypoplasia. In other instances, infections from distant foci, acute or chronic, may disseminate via blood, and lodge into one of the jaw bones, leading to osteomyelitis (Fabe, 1950; Carek et al., 2001), and consequent destruction of the bone architecture and/or growth disturbance. Involvement of the temporomandibular joint (TMJ), due to similar reasons, or from local spread of infections from adjacent structures, as in mastoiditis (Hadlock

Table 3.1 Common causes of short stature

1. Intrauterine growth retardation (low birth weight):
   a) Sporadic
   b) Syndromic

2. Chronic diseases and disturbances of organ systems:
   a) Diseases/abnormalities of organ systems like cardiac, renal, hepatic, hematologic and pulmonary systems.
   b) Diseases/ afflictions of the GIT causing malabsorption:
      (i) Inflammatory bowel disease
      (ii) Celiac disease
      (iii) Enteropathies
   c) Chronic infections causing failure to thrive like AIDS, tuberculosis.

3. Nutritional disturbances:
   a) Decreased caloric intake
   b) Protein energy malnutrition (PEM)
   c) Micronutrient deficiency like zinc and iron

4. Endocrinologic disorders:
   a) Growth hormone deficiency: Familial, primary, secondary, idiopathic.
   b) Glucocorticoid excess: Cushing's syndrome
   c) GH (growth hormone) insensitivity: deficiency of IGF-1 (Insulin-like Growth Factor)
   d) Hypothyroidism
   e) Poorly controlled diabetes mellitus
   f) Pseudohypoparathyroidism

5. Chromosomal aberrations:
   a) Turners syndrome
   b) Down syndrome

6. Skeletal disorders:
   a) Achondrodysplasia
   b) Chondrodystrophy

7. Inborn errors of metabolism:
   a) Mucopolysaccharidosis
   b) Various metabolic storage diseases like Hurler's disease, Niemann Pick's disease.

8. Psychosocial dwarfism (functional)

9. Chronic drug intake:
   a) Corticosteroids
   b) Methylphenidate and other amphetamines

10. Normal variation of growth:
    a) Familial tendency for short stature/Genetic
    b) Constitutional delay in growth

Table adapted from: Lifshitz (2007); Crocetti, Barone (2004); Fujieda, Tanaka (2007); Matfin (2009).

Table 3.2 Syndromes affecting face and jaws associated with Class II/Class III malocclusion

Condition	Features	Etiology
Class II Hemifacial microsomia (Goldenhar syndrome)	Unilateral dysplasia of the ear, hypoplasia of mandibular ramus, cardiac and renal abnormalities	Most cases sporadic; few familial instances; pedigrees compatible with autosomal dominant and recessive transmissions
Pierre Robin complex	Micrognathia; cleft palate and glossoptosis. This condition may occur as an isolated malformation complex or part of a broader pattern of abnormalities	Heterogeneous
Treacher Collins syndrome	Dysplastic low-set ears; downslanting palpebral fissures; micrognathia	Genetic/autosomal dominant
Class III Apert syndrome	Craniosynostosis proptosis hypertelorism; downslanting palpebral fissures; symmetric syndactyly of hands and feet	Genetic/autosomal dominant
Crouzon syndrome	Craniosynostosis; maxillary hypoplasia accompanied by relative mandibular prognathism; shallow orbits; proptosis	Genetic/autosomal dominant
Achondroplasia	Short-limbed dwarfism; enlarged head; depressed nasal bridge; lordosis; high palate	Genetic/autosomal dominant
Syndromes associated with mandibular prognathism Basal cell nevus (Gorlin syndrome)	Macrocephaly; frontal and parietal bossing; prognathism; multiple jaw cysts; multiple basal cell carcinomas; bifid ribs	Genetic/autosomal dominant
Klinefelter syndrome	Mandibular prognathism; skeletal disproportion; gynecomastia; small testicles	Commonly 47, XXY karyotype XXXY and XXXXY also occur
Osteogenesis imperfecta	Fragile bones; blue sclera; deafness; mandibular prognathism	Autosomal dominant (common type)

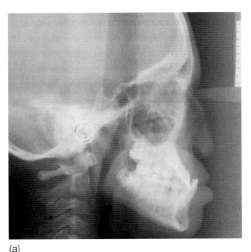
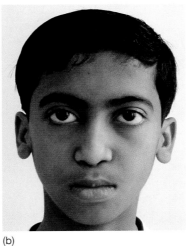
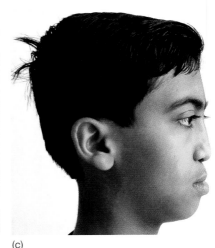

(a) (b) (c)

Figure 3.3 a-c Binder syndrome. This 11-year-old boy, who attended the orthodontic clinic for fixed appliance treatment, had a flat midface due to a retrognathic maxilla, broad flat nose, horizontal nostrils, short columella, and an apparent lack of nasal bridge. The radiograph confirmed a short anterior cranial base, small cranial base angle, reduced sagittal depth of nasopharynx, hypoplasia of the anterior nasal spine, downward inclination of the nasal bones and extremely reduced sagittal maxillary length. The patient was diagnosed as having Binder syndrome after consulting with the oral medicine department, the differential diagnosis of which includes acrodysostosis and Stickler syndrome. Additional investigations may be required for differential diagnosis of the case from other similar conditions.

et al., 2001) or otitis media (Semlali et al., 2004; Prasad et al., 2007), can lead to arthrosis, adhesions, and regressive changes within the joint, which may affect growth and function of the mandible, resulting in malocclusion. The role of tonsillitis and rhinitis in the etiology of mouth breathing and development of adenoid facies, cannot be overemphasized.

Many infectious bacterial, fungal, parasitic, and viral diseases require utmost consideration to prevent nosocomial transmission of the disease. Minor problems, such as aphthous ulcerations, aerobic and anaerobic infections of the oral cavity, may be effectively managed by the well-trained orthodontist. However, since many systemic infectious diseases, such as infectious mononucleosis, mumps, measles, tuberculosis, HIV, and leukemia may also have similar oral manifestations, it becomes extremely important to differentiate local lesions from lesions that are signs of major systemic conditions to allow timely intervention and management by trained personnel. In such situations, the orthodontist should collaborate with the physician to avoid the risks associated with spread of disease and complications that may arise during orthodontic treatment.

Deficiency states and malnutrition

Craniofacial and dental development is profoundly influenced by the availability of essential nutrients. Malnourished children tend to become disabled, incapable of resisting a disease or withstanding its onset and progress. Animal studies have demonstrated that in rats fed on a low-calcium and vitamin D-deficient diet, increase in body weight is impaired and the craniofacial dimensions are reduced (Engström et al., 1982a,b). There is no general agreement whether growth retardation during early infancy in humans is reversible in later years. Research findings on children surviving protein calorie malnutrition (PCM) have shown that severe malnutrition early in life affects their post-malnutrition growth, with reduced height and head size (Krueger 1969; Alvear et al., 1986). Other epidemiological studies have shown that catch-up growth subsequent to malnutrition compensates for previous growth retardation, and results in normal stature of previously malnourished children (Garrow and Pike, 1967; Graham and Adrianzen, 1972). Dreizen et al. (1967) stated that chronic undernutrition in the presence of nutritional or metabolic disease slows down the rate of skeletal maturation, delays the onset of menarche, and retards the epiphyseal fusion period.

These research findings may have diagnostic implications, wherein children with Class II malocclusion with nutritional deficiency, in general, could present with smaller physical and craniofacial dimensions. Those with unusual smaller dimensions may need to be discussed with a pediatrician and a nutritionist for their nutritional requirements, which might have a bearing on the quality of the response to functional appliance treatment as well as on the tissue response during orthodontic tooth movement. Similarly, vitamin deficiency, such as vitamin C (Litton, 1974) or D (Collins and Sinclair, 1988) deficiency, may affect the remodeling response of the periodontal ligament and the alveolar bone to orthodontic forces. For a detailed description on how nutritional factors influence orthodontic diagnosis and treatment planning, and how an orthodontist should obtain nutrition data from patients, see Chapter 5.

Endocrinological and metabolic anomalies in the etiology of malocclusion

The endocrine system is an intricate network that is regulated at various levels by human physiological processes. This system is responsible for regulation of the metabolic processes throughout the body, controlling the growth and differentiation of various parts of the skeleton. Hence, disruption of any part of this system may lead to widespread alterations of the human physiology, resulting in metabolic, anatomical, and/or growth-related disturbances. Although a disturbance in virtually any part of the endocrine system would be expected to have orthodontic implications, disorders of the pituitary, thyroid, parathyroid, and pancreas are of particular interest to the orthodontist. In many instances, an alert dental professional may be the first person to suspect a systemic anomaly (Cohen and Wilcox, 1993; Vitral et al., 2006; Gosau et al., 2009), leading to the diagnosis of an underlying endocrinological disorder.

The pituitary gland

The physical and mental development of a child is controlled to a great extent, apart from other genetic and nutritional factors, by the pituitary and the thyroid glands (Setian, 2007). Pituitary hormones control the functioning of various other endocrine glands, as well as the linear growth of the skeleton. Consequently, disturbances of the pituitary function (and that of hypothalamus) are associated with alteration of function of most other endocrine glands. Deficiency of growth hormone, one of the many hormones produced by the pituitary, is associated with reduced stature and reduced growth and development of the craniofacial complex (manifesting as a retrognathic maxilla and mandible) and shortened cranial base length (Cantu et al., 1997; Van Erum et al., 1998). Interestingly, it has been reported that dental age may not be retarded in growth hormone deficiency states (Van Erum et al., 1998). The use of hormone replacement therapy, in conjunction with orthodontic treatment for growth modulation highlights the importance of interactive care (Davies and Rayner, 1995; Hwang and Cha, 2004). On the other hand, growth hormone excess, which usually occurs secondary to a somatotrophic pituitary adenoma (Matfin 2009), causes gigantism in childhood and acromegaly in adults. Any child or an adult who presents with unexplained gain in height and/or mandibular prominence should be suspected for gigantism (Yagi et al., 2004), and should be referred to an endocrinologist for further investigations and management. It is important to know that although gigantism/acromegaly typically occurs in isolation, it may be associated with other pathological endocrine conditions such as multiple endocrine neoplasia (MEN) (Yagi et al., 2004; Accurso and Allem, 2010), McCune–Albright syndrome (MAS), neurofibromatosis and the Carney complex (Eugster and Pescovitz, 1999). See Chapter 11 for a detailed description of these conditions.

The thyroid gland

Euthyroid state is essential for normal mental and skeletal development and maturation, and adult bone maintenance (Harvey et al., 2002; Murphy and Williams, 2004). A hypothyroid state during pregnancy and early childhood results in various developmental disturbances and defects, including neurological deficits. Hypothyroidism (Figure 3.4) during pregnancy and in early childhood causes mental retardation, growth arrest, delayed bone maturation, and epiphyseal dysgenesis (Rivkees et al., 1988; Bassett et al., 2007). In older children and adolescents, however, mental deficits may not be marked, but the delay in skeletal maturation is evident. Orofacial alterations include enlargement of the tongue (Wittmann, 1977), delayed tooth eruption, tendency for mouth breathing, Class II malocclusion due to a retruded mandible, short posterior facial height, and anterior open bite (Shirazi et al., 1999), all of which contribute to the development of malocclusion.

In contrast, juvenile thyrotoxicosis leads to accelerated growth and advanced bone age, but it also induces short stature due to premature fusion of the growth plates as well as craniosynostosis (Bassett et al., 2007). In adults, thyrotoxicosis accelerates bone loss, causing osteoporosis (Murphy and Williams, 2004), and even minor disturbances of thyroid status increase the risk of fractures (Bassett et al., 2007).

At the present time, owing to early recognition of thyroid deficiency states, the classic manifestations of thyroid disease may not be evident in all individuals with thyroid disorders. Also, subclinical thyroid disease is being diagnosed more frequently in clinical practice in young and middle-aged people, as well as in the elderly, with a reported prevalence of 4–10% in the adult population (Canaris et al., 2000; Hollowell et al., 2002). Subclinical hyper- and hypothyroidism may have repercussions on the cardiovascular system and bone, as well as on other organs and systems (Biondi and Cooper, 2008). Hence, the clinician has to be vigilant and informed to be able to suspect or diagnose an underlying thyroid disease. For example, a lack of response to functional appliance treatment in a case of skeletal Class II malocclusion after a reasonable period of time and excellent patient cooperation

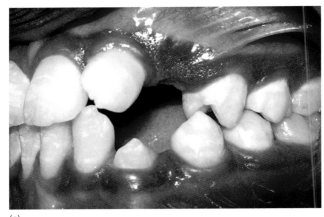

(a)

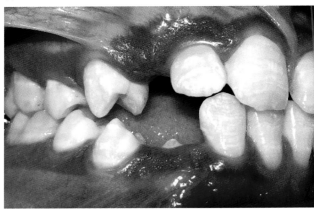

(b)

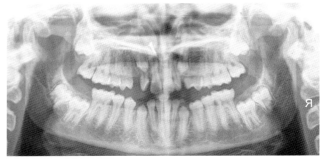

(c)

Figure 3.4 Intraoral views and radiographs of an 18-year-old girl diagnosed with hypothyroidism show delayed eruption of multiple teeth.

may be because of an underlying growth hormone or thyroid disorder. The literature supports the view that thyroid hormone replacement therapy results in rapid catch-up growth (Rivkees et al., 1988; Teng et al., 2004). It has been suggested that orthodontic treatment should be combined with hormone replacement therapy for optimum results (Verna et al., 2000).

Pancreas

Diabetes mellitus, a disorder of carbohydrate, protein, and fat metabolism due to absolute or relative deficiency of insulin, is one of the commonest metabolic disorders. The disorder, especially when poorly controlled, leads to widespread changes such as nephropathy, neuropathy, retinopathy, and vascular disease, as well as cardiovascular and cerebrovascular complications, among other possibilities (Vernillo, 2001). Uncontrolled diabetes predisposes to severe and rapidly progressive periodontal disease, osteoporosis, and increased propensity to infections, all of which can be factors in the etiology of malocclusion. It can also lead to alteration in the timing of tooth eruption, causing accelerated development until about 10–11 years of age, and delayed development after that (Adler et al., 1973; Orbak et al., 2008). In addition, diabetes is also associated with an exaggerated inflammatory response during normal tooth eruption (Orbak et al., 2008), xerostomia, burning mouth syndrome, candidiasis, delayed and abnormal wound healing, diminished salivary flow, and salivary gland enlargement. A child or adult with symptoms of dry mouth/burning sensation, ketone smell from the mouth, unusual intensity of periodontal breakdown, inflamed gingivae with pockets should raise the suspicion of underlying diabetes mellitus (Lamster et al., 2008).

Neuromuscular disorders in the etiology of orthodontic problems

The influence of neuromuscular harmony on dental development, occlusion, and functions such as mastication, deglutition, speech, and respiration is well established. Animal studies have confirmed alteration in the craniofacial skeletal structures secondary to loss of muscle tone (Babuccu et al., 2009; Tsai et al., 2010). Consequently, any degenerative or inflammatory disorder affecting the neuromuscular system can have significant influence on growth and remodeling of the dentofacial structures. Disorders such as chronic seizures, hemiparesis, and cerebral and cranial nerve palsies can cause alterations in the muscle tone, leading to imbalance of forces and consequent adaptation of the skeletal structures (Fong et al., 2003), including the craniofacial skeleton, with subsequent development of a malocclusion (Cascino et al., 1993; Trujillo et al., 2002; Portelli et al., 2009).

Seizure disorders, which are one of the most common neurological disorders with an incidence of 1–3% (depending on age) (Annegers, 1997), can result in orofacial trauma (Sheller, 2004) and asphyxiation because of appliance aspiration during an episode of seizures. Patients with chronic seizures may manifest body asymmetry (Fong et al., 2003), including forehead and facial structures (Tinuper et al., 1992), altered mental status and poor oral hygiene, while patients on long-term drug therapy may show gingival hyperplasia (Sheller, 2004) and bone mineral loss (Sheth, 2004). Moreover, hypercementosis, root shortening, anomalous tooth development, delayed eruption, and cervical lymphadenopathy have also been documented in patients with seizure disorders (Johnstone et al., 1999). Since orthodontic appliances often consist of a variety of metal fixtures, they have the ability to alter or distort the signals produced by magnetic resonance (MR) and computed tomography (CT) machines (Sadowsky et al., 1988; Sheller, 2004). Hence, in patients with suspected organic lesions causing seizures who may require MR imaging or CT scanning, the presence of an orthodontic appliance may act as an impediment in the imaging process, which needs to be considered while planning the treatment.

An overview of systemic disturbances in relation to orthodontic treatment planning

Although the discussion of each disease or organ system is beyond the scope of this chapter, this section will briefly highlight the diseases affecting major organ systems and their implications for orthodontic diagnosis and treatment planning.

Psychiatric disorders

A majority of patients attending an orthodontic clinic are children and young adults at various stages of maturation, with rapid and drastic changes taking place, both in their minds and bodies. These patients are prone to the development of psychological/psychiatric disorders. It is reported that up to 14–20% of American children and adolescents may develop psychiatric disorders (Cassidy and Jellinek, 1998). In addition, adults going through difficult phases of life may also develop psychiatric problems. It is, therefore, imperative that the orthodontist be well conversant with psychology as well as any abnormal behavior which might point towards a psychiatric disorder or substance misuse.

The psychiatric disorders most commonly encountered by the orthodontist are either major depressive disorder (MDD) or attention deficit hyperactivity disorder (ADHD) (Neeley et al., 2006a). Any history, sign, or symptom that points toward a psychiatric disorder or a sudden or unusual change in a patient's behavior during treatment requires discussion with the parents and the family physician, who may consider consultation with a clinical psychologist/psychiatrist. In addition, patients with ADHD may be under treatment with amphetamines such as methylphenidate, which predisposes them to xerostomia, dysphagia, sialoadenitis, stomatitis, bruxism, and growth disturbances (Elia et al., 1999). These possibilities have important orthodontic implications as non-compliance with maintenance of oral hygiene, instructions in placement of elastics at home, difficult behavior during orthodontic procedures, and missed appointments can lead to treatment failure. Therefore, pretreatment evaluation of the patient must include questions about prior or current illness and medication. Any treatment plan should include a discussion with the treating psychiatrist, as discussed in Chapter 4.

Substance misuse is also a significant problem among adolescents with a reported prevalence of up to 40% among tenth graders in the USA (Neeley et al., 2006b). Intravenous drug users may have diseases that are transmitted through blood, such as HIV infection (Leukefeld et al., 1990) and Hepatitis B (Gillchrist, 1999). A suspected case may need to be referred to a medical specialist after consultation with a psychologist.

Diseases of the respiratory system

Diseases of the respiratory system can be broadly divided into those affecting the upper and the lower airways. Diseases of the upper airway can be an outcome of anatomical, physiological, or pathological restrictions of airway space in the nose, pharynx, and the larynx. Chronic restriction of the nasal airway due to sinusitis, tonsillitis, adenoiditis, and allergic rhinitis leads to mouth breathing, and further to the classic adenoid facies as well as a change in the craniofacial flexure. Disorders of the lower airway, such as asthma, chronic bronchitis and other chronic pulmonary diseases increase the breathing effort and affected cases may display orofacial changes similar to those seen with mouth breathing, apart from consequences related to impaired general health due to low oxygenation of the blood. Moreover, children with severe asthma may be using oral or inhaled steroids, which may cause a reduction in the salivary flow (Laurikainen and Kuusisto, 1998), predispose to oral candidiasis, and increase risk of root resorption (Davidovitch and Krishnan, 2009). A proper consultation with a pulmonologist is deemed essential while treating these patients, so that any complications that may develop in due course during orthodontic treatment can be effectively managed.

Diseases of the cardiovascular system

Patients with congenital heart disease and valvular defects often have poor general health, retarded physical growth, increased susceptibility to infections, such as infective endocarditis, and are at a high risk of bleeding (if on anticoagulants). In general, patients with mild valvular dysfunction are able to tolerate dental procedures well, but patients with mitral regurgitation are particularly susceptible to exacerbation of pulmonary edema and acute shortness of breath (Warburton and Caccamese, 2006).

Infective endocarditis

This is a serious condition with an incidence of 1.6–6.2 per 100,000 patients (Prendergast, 2006) and a high annual mortality approaching 40% (Cabell et al., 2002). Various dental and orthodontic procedures predispose the patient to systemic bacteremia, which, in the presence of predisposing cardiac defects may lead to episodes of infective endocarditis. Any patient prone to infective endocarditis should be considered for treatment only after consultation with the treating physician. Although the need for routine use of

antibiotic prophylaxis against infective endocarditis in dental procedures remains controversial (Gould et al., 2006), the use of prophylactic antibiotics in high-risk cases (Task Force on Infective Endocarditis, 2004) is still advisable whenever a procedure likely to cause bacteremia is carried out. If a patient develops symptoms of infective endocarditis during treatment, immediate referral to a cardiologist is advisable.

Coronary artery disease and hypertension

Patients with angina or uncontrolled hypertension will be poor orthodontic patients because they are prone to cardiovascular accidents and stroke. In addition, many of these patients are taking antiplatelet and anticoagulant drugs, making them prone to bleeding. It must be kept in mind that patients with a history of hypertension are prone to episodes of hypertensive emergencies leading to cardiovascular or cerebrovascular accidents (Marik and Varon, 2007), and that certain conditions, such as adrenal tumors, Grave's disease, chronic renal disorders and vascular disorders, are known to trigger hypertensive crises (Lip and Beevers, 2005). Hence, a complete medical evaluation as well as consultation with the patient's cardiologist is imperative during diagnosis and treatment planning.

Diseases of the gastrointestinal tract

The liver is the principal metabolic storehouse of the body and carries out many important functions such as synthesis of plasma proteins and clotting factors, bile formation, drug elimination and detoxification of many substances, and formation of urea. Liver dysfunction leads to multiple, widespread alterations in the body. Patients with chronic liver disease may have malnutrition and growth failure, edema due to loss of plasma proteins, portal hypertension, variceal bleeding, hypersplenism, coagulopathy, and susceptibility to infections, as well as renal, pulmonary, and neurological complications. Patients with a liver transplant may be under immunosuppressive therapy, side effects of which include osteoporosis and susceptibility to infections (Patel et al., 2009). Consequently, in view of their compromised health status, a gastroenterologist's opinion must be sought before considering the patient for orthodontic treatment.

Viral hepatitis

This is perhaps the most common cause of hepatitis worldwide caused by six distinct viruses: HAV, HBV, HCV, HDV, HEV and HGV (Gillchrist, 1999). In the developed world, the major contributors are the viral vectors, which spread via blood or person-to-person contact, while in developing countries water-borne transmission and orofecal transmission also play a significant role. The disease burden of viral hepatitis is considerable. Person-to-person transmission of viral agents, especially bloodborne ones such as HBV, HCV, and HDV, is a worldwide concern. Healthcare-related transmission is an important source of new HBV infections worldwide (Centers for Disease Control and Prevention, 1989; Shepard et al., 2006). An orthodontist should be aware of the risks associated with transmission of viral agents in the symptomatic, as well as in the carrier stage. Moreover, patients with viral hepatitis may be under treatment with antiviral agents such as ribavirin, lamivudine, adefovir, and tenofovir, which have side effects such as renal tubular injury and hemolytic anemia. Similarly, therapeutic use of biological agents such as interferon 2α may be associated with flu-like symptoms, leukopenia, thrombocytopenia, psychiatric disturbances, hearing loss, and alopecia (Sonneveld and Janssen, 2010).

Gastric pathologies

Gastric pathologies such as acute and chronic gastritis and gastroesophageal reflux may present with halitosis, which may or may not be accentuated by poor oral hygiene. Moreover, gastric upset leads to a variety of oral changes, such as excessively coated tongue and enamel erosions secondary to acid regurgitation. Enamel erosions are particularly common in conditions such as gastroesophageal reflux disease (Daley and Armstrong, 2007), hiatus hernia, chronic alcoholism, and bulimia (Little, 2002).

Intestinal pathologies

Intestinal pathologies such as inflammatory bowel disease (ulcerative colitis, Crohn's disease) cause malabsorption and deficiency of important vitamins and minerals, e.g. iron and vitamin B_{12} (Field et al., 1995). In addition, patients with inflammatory bowel disease may present with oral mucosal ulceration (which may be confused with aphthous stomatitis) (Ruiz-Roca et al., 2005), denudation of the mucosa, and papillary/polypoid growths. It is estimated that approximately 10% of patients with inflammatory bowel disease may develop TMJ arthritis (Ruiz-Roca et al., 2005).

Renal diseases

The incidence of chronic renal disease is increasing worldwide (Ansell et al., 2002). Renal disease often results in a wide array of endocrine and metabolic anomalies, altered serum ionic balance, edema, uremia, hypertension, hyperactivity of the renin–angiotensin system, reduced erythropoietin levels, anemia, malnutrition, bleeding disorders, reduced immunocompetence, and osteodystrophy (Jaffe et al., 1990; Nadimi et al., 1993; Proctor et al., 2005). The oral findings in azotemia include stomatitis, candidiasis, xerostomia, gingivitis, and the classic uremic fetor (Kho et al., 1999).

Dental alterations also include localized radiolucent jaw lesions with or without 'ground glass' appearance, the classic 'brown tumors' of hyperparathyroidism (Okada et al., 2000), and enlargement of the skeletal bases (Nadimi et al., 1993). Pathological mobility of the teeth (Carmichael et al., 1995), loss of lamina dura, delayed tooth eruption (Jaffe et al., 1990), and an increased incidence of noncarious tooth loss (Proctor et al., 2005) Additionally, enamel hypoplasia of the primary and permanent teeth (Kho et al., 1999; Al Nowaiser et al., 2003) and narrowing or calcification of the pulp chamber of teeth in adults with chronic renal disease has also been reported (Nasstrom et al., 1985; Galili et al., 1991; Nasstrom, 1996). Patients with end-stage renal disease or transplants are usually on corticosteroid or immunosuppressant therapy, which makes them prone to systemic infections, gingival hypertrophy, and steroid-related iatrogenic root resorption (Colvard et al., 1986; Kennedy and Linden 2000). All these pathological conditions, especially osteodystrophy, have profound effects on the orthodontic treatment plan, and should be taken into consideration while formulating a treatment plan for the individual patient. Successful treatment in such compromised cases has been reported (Walker et al., 2007).

Allergic disorders

Allergic reactions to natural rubber latex (NRL), metals such as nickel and chromium, acrylics and composites, and disinfectants are not rare in orthodontic offices. Two types of immunological reactions, type I (acute reactions, anaphylaxis), and type IV (delayed hypersensitivity) (contact dermatitis) reactions, are especially important to the orthodontist. NRL, used in manufacturing of gloves and oral elastics, induces allergic reactions in less than 1% of the general population, 5–15% of healthcare workers, and 24–60% of patients with spina bifida (Poley and Slater, 2000). NRL allergy can manifest as both type I and type IV reactions while metal allergies, such as nickel allergy, are often associated with type IV cutaneous reactions. An orthodontist should be cognizant of the manifestations of these allergies, and interact with a dermatologist or allergy specialist while treating a patient with known allergic tendencies, or upon appearance of allergic symptoms. The confirmation of the allergy can be done with a patch or skin test, and possible precautions can be taken thereafter for prevention of occurrence of such reactions.

Hematological disorders and blood dyscrasias

Hemoglobin synthesis disorders such as thalassemia, sickle cell anemia, nutritional deficiency anemias, red blood cell (RBC) structural defects (e.g. spherocytosis, elliptocytosis), and enzyme deficiencies (e.g. glucose 6-phosphtase deficiency) may lead to repeated episodes of RBC destruction. Patients with thalassemia (Figure 3.5) usually present with poor general growth due to chronic anemia and hyperparathyroidism, apart from iron overload and consequences thereof. Other problems that must be considered in such patients include the propensity for bleeding episodes, frequent infections, spontaneous fractures, and hepatosplenomegaly.

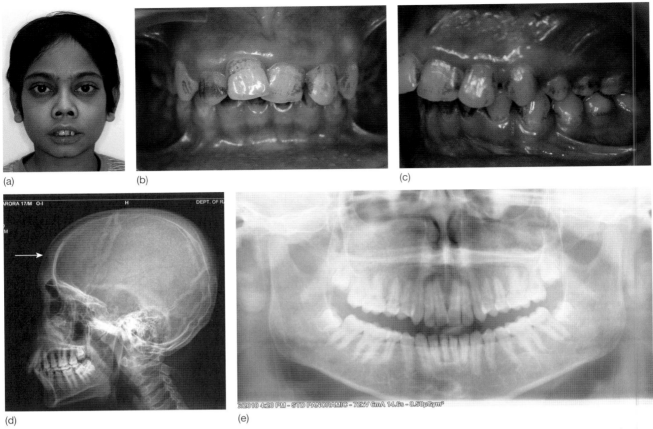

Figure 3.5 (a) Facial photograph of a patient with typical features of thalassemia intermedia: note the prominent midface region, frontal bossing, and convex facial profile due to maxillary excess, which is classically described as 'chipmunk or rodent like'. (b,c) Intraoral pictures show staining of teeth due to repeated bleeding episodes, Class II malocclusion, mild protrusion of anterior teeth, crowding and deep bite. (d,e) Radiographs show typically widened diploic spaces of skull bones (arrow), trabecular rarefaction, loss of bone density, maxillary excess, and obliteration of the maxillary sinus due to erythroid medullary hyperplasia. The classic appearance is often described as 'hair on end' or 'chicken wire appearance'.

Patients with sickle cell anemia (Figure 3.6) usually have impaired growth, delayed maturation, excessive and recurrent hemolytic episodes secondary to sickling crisis, increased propensity to oral infections and jaw osteomyelitis, osteoporosis of bones, and altered splenic and liver function. A sickling crisis can be precipitated by emotional and physical stress, sudden temperature changes, and hypoxia, among other causes, and the associated pain of which in jaw bones may be confused with pulpalgia. As a rule of thumb, extraction of teeth, in such cases, is contraindicated, and, if at all planned, should be done after discussion with the patient's physician and the oral surgeon after evaluation of the coagulation function. Acetylsalicylic acid should be avoided as it interferes with platelet function, and increases chances of gastric ulceration and taxes the already stressed liver. Since such cases might have undergone multiple transfusions, precautions must be taken, keeping in mind the possibility of transmission of bloodborne infective agents.

The compensatory extramedullary erythropoiesis commonly leads to widening of bone marrow spaces and osteoporosis, causing craniofacial deformities such as frontal bossing, maxillary enlargement, and spacing of teeth. Other dental anomalies such as dental hypoplasia and intrinsic staining of teeth are a direct consequence of the hemolytic episodes.

Leukemia

With advances in medical care, children with childhood leukemia/lymphoma have an improved life expectancy, and quite a few such patients in remission may seek orthodontic treatment. While planning their treatment, it must be realized that many of these individuals would have undergone total body irradiation (TBI) and a regimen of cytotoxic drugs. Consequently, secondary to excessive cellular destruction caused by the antineoplastic agents, and due to leukemic infiltration of various organs by the blast cells, generalized growth retardation, bone osteoporosis, prone-

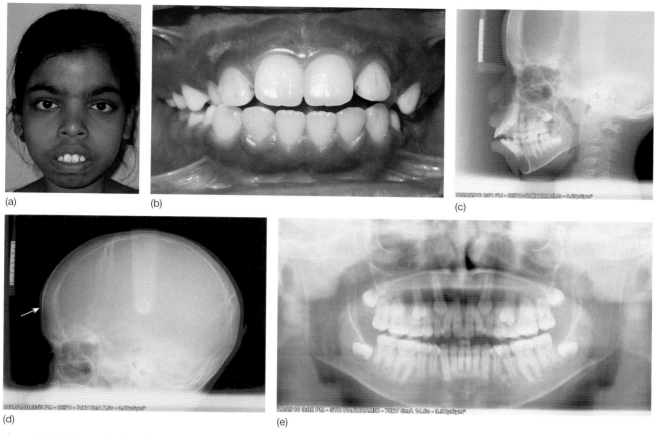

Figure 3.6 A 14-year-old girl with sickle cell anemia. (a) Note the frontal bossing and midface prominence, and icteric sclerae on the facial photograph. (b) Intraoral view shows an anterior open bite. (c) The lateral cephalogram reveals thinned out cortex (arrow) and developing bimaxillary protrusion. Also note the expanded maxillary bone due to medullary hyperplasia. (d) Widened diploic spaces are best recognized on a lateral skull radiograph. (e) The orthopantomogram also shows typical features secondary to marrow hyperplasia.

ness to infections, bleeding episodes, salivary gland dysfunction, dental hypoplasia, reduction in root lengths, and delayed or noneruption can be expected (Nasman et al., 1997). In the light of such findings, growth modulation with functional appliances may have a guarded prognosis (Dahllof and Huggare, 2004).

Conversely, a patient undergoing orthodontic treatment might be diagnosed as having a hematological malignancy (Isaac and Tholouli, 2008). In such cases consultation with the oncologist would be required prior to any further orthodontic procedure because of the deranged physiological conditions.

Bleeding disorders

These can lead to episodes of acute blood loss following minor trauma from orthodontic appliances. The pathophysiology underlying any bleeding disorder is usually related to disorders of the vessel wall, platelets, or the coagulation cascade. Among the inherited bleeding disorders, von Willebrand's disease is the most common type, followed by hemophilia A and B, the three of them account-

ing for 95–97% of all inherited deficiencies of coagulation factors (Tuddenham and Cooper, 1994; Mannucci et al., 2004). Irrespective of the origin of the disorder, a clinical assessment of severity of bleeding is important (Favaloro, 2006; Quiroga et al., 2007) for clinical risk assessment, while advanced tests such as specific factor or component assays may be used for identification of the underlying disorder. Interestingly, many patients with mucocutaneous bleeding may not show evidence of a diagnostically identifiable disease (Flavoro, 2007; Quiroga et al., 2007). Another important consideration in patients with known coagulation disorders is the probable history of blood product infusion, and the consequent risk of viral infections such as hepatitis or HIV. This probability is not only valid for patients with a history of transfusions during the mid-1980s, when virus inactivation procedures for plasma were not in place (Brewer and Correa, 2006), but also for patients undergoing frequent transfusions, as blood transfusion from an infected patient in the window phase is usually difficult to screen for infections, which then often go unnoticed (Jayaraman et al., 2004).

Identifying local dental abnormalities before attempting orthodontic treatment

For the uninformed orthodontist, the intraoral examination would start and end with the classification of malocclusion, and evaluating the patient for either extraction or nonextraction therapy. In such hasty and superficial assessments, the recognition of localized aberrations of the dentition, as contributing factors to the etiology of the malocclusion, may often go unnoticed. A routine examination of the soft and hard tissues is necessary for the identification of lesions, so that a differentiation between infectious diseases, noninfectious diseases, and other mucocutaneous lesions can be made. This knowledge would aid in deciding whether orthodontic treatment can be provided without further delay, or if a referral to a specialist is necessary prior to orthodontic therapy. Hence, an oral examination, in an orderly fashion, is imperative for thorough evaluation of existing conditions and their optimal management.

The intraoral examination should be done in two phases. First, the soft tissues and the hard tissues, both in and around the oral cavity, should be evaluated with an overall view to rule out the presence of any systemic or syndromic conditions, followed by examination of the each tissue individually in detail. The examination should start with a visual screening of the oral soft tissues, such as the vermilion area, lips, buccal mucosa, faucial pillars, tongue and the gingivae, for any physiological or pathological changes, such as discoloration, erythema, petechiae, abnormal keratinization areas, swellings, and sinus tracts. This exploration should be followed by systematic evaluation of the hard tissues, namely the teeth, for number, shape and size, color, and quality of tooth material in each arch. Following the intra-arch examination, an interarch examination should be done to evaluate the occlusion, both dynamic and static, and the relation of the dentitions to each other. The intraoral examination should be supplemented by radiographic examination of the jaw bones, and the clinical and radiographic evaluation of the TMJ. Further advanced investigations should be conducted as and when deemed necessary.

Examination of soft tissues

The presence of patching or crusting on lips or the perioral region may be an indicator of dehydration, a mucosal, dermal, or mucocutaneous disease, or a manifestation of an underlying systemic disorder (Figure 3.7). Nonerythematous pigmentation of the perioral region and the oral mucosa (Kauzman et al., 2004) may be seen in systemic disorders, such as hereditary intestinal polyposis, Gardner syndrome, Addison disease, heavy metal-induced discolorations, smoker's melanosis, and skin diseases. Erythematous pigmentation of the mucosa would usually indicate a hematologic or a bleeding disorder, a hemangioma (see Figure 3.2),

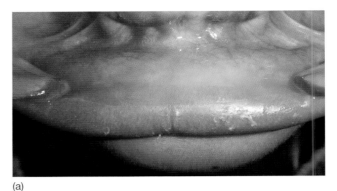

(a)

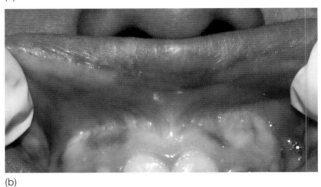

(b)

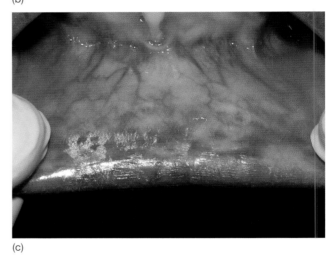

(c)

Figure 3.7 Crusting of the lips. (a) This crusting was the result of chronic lip separation at rest secondary to chronic mouth breathing. (b,c) Lip crusting due to an oral mucosal disease, which makes referral to an oral pathologist necessary.

traumatic injury, or infections, among other possibilities. Erythematous spots on the buccal mucosa or palate may also be seen during the prodromal or initial phase of measles (Koplik spots) or chicken pox, while intraoral petechiae may be seen in viral diseases such as infectious mononucleosis and dengue fever.

Localized white or red mucosal patches in the oral mucosa (Figure 3.8) might occur in a variety of conditions such as erythroplakia, leukoplakia, intraoral hemangiomas,

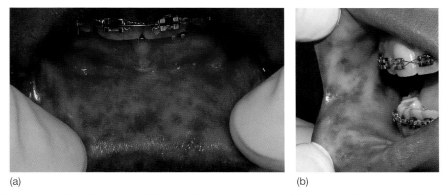

(a)   (b)

Figure 3.8 (a,b) Oral lesions in two patients that developed during orthodontic treatment. Such lesions must be investigated further for the causative factors, including allergy to orthodontic materials, before continuing with the orthodontic treatment.

traumatic injuries, bleeding disorders (Jolly, 1977; Castellanos and Díaz-Guzmán, 2008), various systemic conditions such as vitamin or mineral diseases, endocrinological disorders, and in skin diseases, such as lichen planus, pemphigus, and white sponge nevus (Rajendran, 2009). Since quite a few of these lesions may have carcinogenic potential (Suter et al., 2008), additional history taking and evaluation in the form of a biopsy should be done, along with evaluation by an oral pathologist. Care must be taken to dissociate such lesions from physiological variations such as Fordyce granules and lesions of minor significance, such as those due to chronic cuspal trauma, which manifest as white streaks on the buccal mucosa in the premolar–molar region.

Discoloration of the oral mucosa is seen in several systemic diseases, for example jaundice, heavy metal poisoning, and hypervitaminosis A (Daley and Armstrong, 2007), or as local lesions, such as amalgam tattoos and pigmented nevi. Rarely, the rapid increase in size or pigmentation of a hyperpigmented nevus will be indicative of a developing malignant melanoma (Hicks and Flaitz, 2000). Localized areas of desquamation or ulceration may occur in conditions such as burns (Figure 3.9), allergic reactions (Franz-Montan et al., 2008) and infections such as acute necrotizing ulcerative gingivitis, or secondary to systemic influences such as hormonal imbalances, skin diseases, and drug reactions. Persistent nonhealing ulcers may point towards tuberculosis (Dixit et al., 2008), or even a malignancy (Al-Rawi and Talabani, 2008; Villa et al., 2010), which requires further consideration and referral.

Any intraoral swelling should be first visually inspected followed by palpation to record the color, surface texture, consistency, tenderness, local discharge, and any associated draining sinuses. Lesions with a soft texture or consistency may be either primary soft tissue pathology or the extension of infection/pathology from underlying hard tissues. Inflammation of the mobile mucosa is usually not very painful when compared with lesions of attached mucosa,

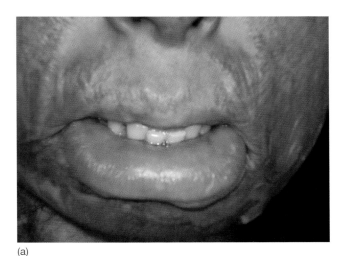

(a)

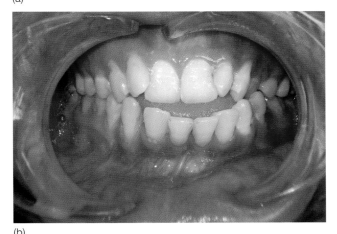

(b)

Figure 3.9 (a,b) A patient with facial scars from burns, showing malocclusion secondary to fibrosis of the facial tissues, loss of tissue elasticity, and loss of lip seal.

which usually exhibit less swelling but are very painful. Long standing soft tissue swellings or lesions may eventually develop fibrosis and/or associated draining sinus tracts. Lesions with a palpably hard surface are usually indicative of a central pathology (bony lesion). Care must be exercised to exclude developmental variations such as benign bony exostoses (tori) from other infective, benign, and malignant lesions. Since tissue enlargement, either bony or soft tissue, may be idiopathic, infectious, allergic, tumorous, or secondary to systemic alterations, or just a physiological variation, it must be carefully evaluated to diagnose the nature and extent of the lesions with the help of appropriate referrals and judicious use of supplemental diagnostic tests.

Tongue examination must include assessment of its size, shape, position, and mobility. Macroglossia may be seen in conditions such as acromegaly, amyloidosis, and lymphangiomas (Figure 3.10), and an altered protrusive tongue position may be particularly noticeable in Down syndrome and other craniosynostosis syndromes. The alterations seen in the tongue in patients with gastrointestinal disorders are described earlier in this chapter.

Evaluation of the periodontal status and oral hygiene

The oral hygiene status reflects many aspects of a patient's personality, physical health, and psychosocial condition. Patients with clinically evident depression or psychiatric disorders, low motivation, low awareness levels, physical deformities, or mental retardation, usually have poor oral hygiene. Certain patients, such as those with obsessive disorders and psychiatric tendencies, malingering or fictitious illness, may complain of nonspecific oro-dental pain or other oral health-related issues, even in its absence. Conversely, there are patients who are extremely conscious of their oral hygiene and might spend a lot of time and money to improve their oral health and dental condition, in the hope that it may lead to changes in their personal or professional life. Extreme care should be exercised when dealing with such unstable personalities. There may also be patients who are poorly informed and are unaware of the benefits of professional care. Even though such patients may present with suboptimal oral health, treating them would usually bring about a rapid and appreciable improvement in their oral health.

Following evaluation of the oral hygiene, a thorough periodontal examination of each tooth, along with charting of all the pockets and lesions should be mandatory. In cases with suspected periodontal bony lesions, the clinical examination should be supplemented with radiographic evaluation of the suspected areas. It must be remembered that, like other craniofacial structures, periodontal health is also governed by local and systemic factors. In a patient with severe generalized periodontitis, apart from local factors, one must look for underlying systemic influences

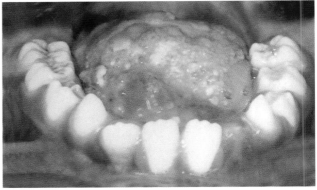

(a)

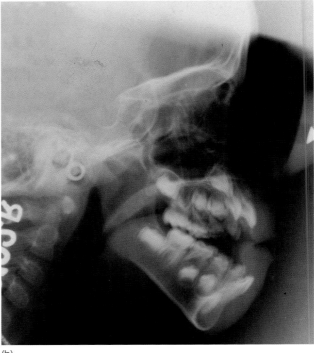

(b)

Figure 3.10 (a,b) Anterior open bite caused by an enlarged and altered position of the tongue. Further investigation in the form of biopsy confirmed the diagnosis of lymphangioma of the tongue, which needed surgical resection. Appropriate referrals were consequently made before orthodontic intervention.

such as diabetes mellitus, neutrophil chemotactic defects, vitamin deficiencies, and hormonal alterations. In contrast, patients with localized aggressive periodontitis usually have alterations in their microbiological flora around specific teeth, mostly the first molars and incisors. Areas of Stillman clefts (Figure 3.11), classically described as being related to traumatic occlusal loading, need consideration regarding the timing of the gingival graft before or after orthodontic treatment. All patients with pathological periodontal involvement require intensive periodontal therapy with the help of or by a competent periodontist, before the onset of the planned orthodontic intervention.

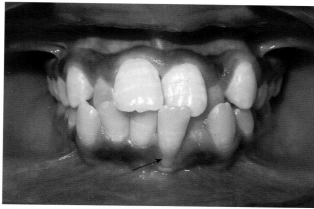

(a)

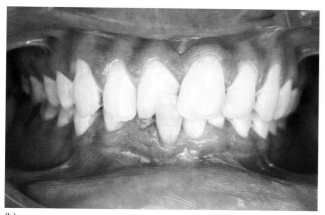

(b)

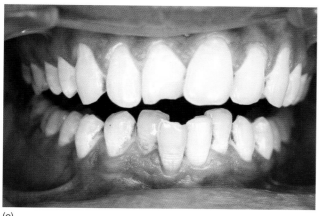

(c)

Figure 3.11 Traumatic occlusion associated with anterior cross bite. (a) Stillman's cleft in left lower central incisor (arrow). (b,c) Loss of tooth substance of anterior teeth and gingival recession of mandibular right central incisor.

Evaluation of the dentition

A planned sequence for examination of the dentition is preferred in the order described below. This examination starts with a note of the number of teeth present (both deciduous and permanent), the maturation status of the dentition, the identification and number of missing teeth, followed by a note on the presence of dental abnormalities such as enamel defects, pathologies of individual teeth, color changes, attrition, irregularities in dental size or shape and pathological migration, and the presence of prosthetic devices.

Maturation of the dentition and its correlation with chronologic age

This is very important to gain insight into the existence of any developmental and growth-related problems (Figure 3.12). It is also essential to assess the status of unerupted teeth, with respect to formation of root/apex and plan appropriate timing management strategies.

Changes in the number of teeth

Both hypodontia and supernumerary teeth are common occurrences in the permanent dentition, and both phenomena may occur as isolated events or as a part of syndromes. The prevalence of hypodontia across the world varies between 1.6% and 9.6% (excluding the third molar) (Fekonja, 2005). As a rule, if a deciduous tooth is missing, its succedaneous counterpart would be missing as well (Hall, 1983). In the permanent dentition, the most frequently missing teeth are the upper lateral incisor (Figure 3.13a,b) and lower second premolar (when the third molar is excluded) (Figure 3.13c,d). As a general rule, if only one or a few teeth are missing, the absent tooth will be the most distal tooth of any given type (Jorgenson, 1980). Interestingly, patients with generalized hypodontia may also manifest a tendency toward Class III malocclusion (Figure 3.14) (Chung et al., 2000). Supernumerary teeth have a reported prevalence of 0.8% in primary dentitions and 2.1% in permanent dentitions (Brook, 1974). They may occur singly or as multiple teeth, unilaterally or bilateral, may be erupted or impacted, and occur in one or both jaws (Figure 3.15a–c). Such teeth usually have a conical, tuberculate, supplemental or odontome morphology (Mitchell, 1996). They may be asymptomatic (Figure 3.1d) or may cause failure of eruption of a permanent tooth, displacement of an adjacent tooth (Figure 3.15a), crowding, cyst formation and, in rare cases, root resorption. The most common location is the anterior maxilla (Altug-Atac and Erdem, 2007), with mesiodens being the most common example (Basdra et al., 2001).

Dental caries and associated morbidity

A complete charting of the carious teeth should be done in an orderly fashion. The extent and the location of the carious lesions can give an insight into the oral health status, the susceptibility of the individual to caries attacks, and his or her dietary habits. Patients with learning disabilities, those with salivary gland dysfunctions, and those with low motivational levels usually experience increased

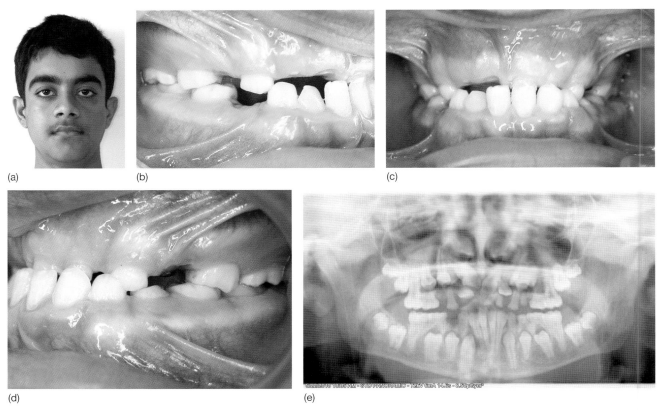

(a)　　　　　(b)　　　　　　　　　(c)

(d)　　　　　　　　　　　　(e)

Figure 3.12 (a–e) A 13-year-old boy with delayed maturation of the dentition. Investigations revealed no apparent systemic problems. Note the excessive attrition of the deciduous teeth and the typical denture-look during smiling due to hypodontia and loss of vertical dimension.

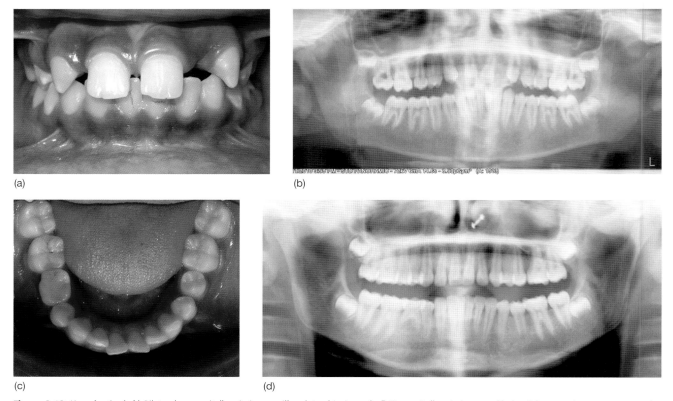

(a)　　　　　　　　　　(b)

(c)　　　　　　　　　　(d)

Figure 3.13 Hypodontia. (a,b) Bilateral congenitally missing maxillary lateral incisors. (c,d) Congenitally missing mandibular right second permanent premolar and an over-retained deciduous second molar.

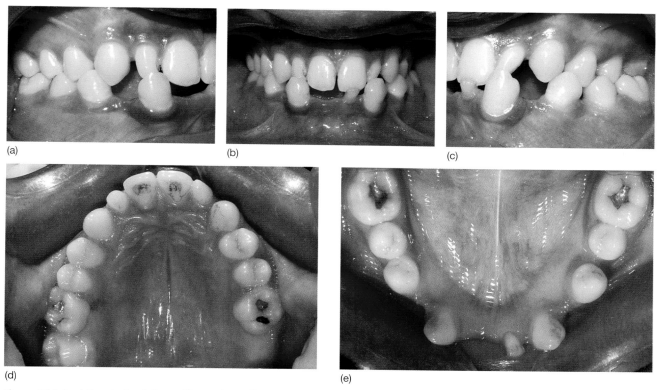

Figure 3.14 (a–e) Hypodontia of the maxillary and mandibular dentition with a typical Class III presentation. Also note the microdontic maxillary lateral incisors.

caries incidence. Loss of tooth structure leads to migration of teeth, which is associated with loss of arch length, and/or supraeruption of opposing tooth (Figure 3.16). Similarly, extension of caries periapically can lead to localized destruction of jaw bone, root resorption, and osteomyelitis in susceptible cases. In certain instances, the status (health) of a tooth's crown or root may influence the decision regarding extraction of teeth for orthodontic treatment (Figure 3.17). Patients with increased caries susceptibility require a complete radiographic evaluation of the jaws and teeth for anticipated interproximal lesions and periapical involvement. Additional help from an endodontist may be sought for proper management of these patients. Moreover, many patients with this tendency may be good candidates for application of caries protective varnishes, which would require interaction with a pediatric/community dentist. Interestingly, application of fluoride varnish and sealants has not been shown to reduce the attachment bond strength (Kimura et al., 2004; Bishara et al., 2005; El Bokle and Munir, 2008; Keçik et al., 2008).

Anomalies of size

Microdontia (Figure 3.18) is a relatively common condition affecting the permanent dentition and has a reported prevalence between 0.8% and 8.4% in various populations

(Neville et al., 2005; Guttal et al., 2010). It most commonly affects the maxillary lateral incisors, apart from the third molars. In contrast, macrodontia is a relatively rare condition of the permanent dentition. True generalized macrodontia is observed only in cases of pituitary gigantism and pineal hyperplasia (Neville et al., 2005), while localized macrodontia is seen in conditions such as unilateral facial hyperplasia, hemifacial hypertrophy, and oculo-facial-cardio-dental syndrome (Turkkahraman and Sarıoglu, 2006). Both microdontic and macrodontic teeth contribute to a Bolton's discrepancy, thus creating treatment finishing and esthetic problems (Figure 3.19).

Anomalies of shape

These include dens invaginatus, talon cusps, dens evaginatus, gemination, fusion, root dilacerations, taurodontism, and concrescence. Size and shape changes may be related to genetic influences or systemic conditions such as malnutrition or endocrinopathies, systemic fluorosis, infectious diseases such as congenital syphilis and rubella, local infections (Turner hypoplasia), trauma, or mechanical obstruction leading to dilacerations. Dens invaginatus has population prevalence between 0.25% and 5.1% (Mupparapu and Singer, 2004) and is usually seen in the maxillary lateral incisor region. Talon cusp (Figure 3.20) has a prevalence of

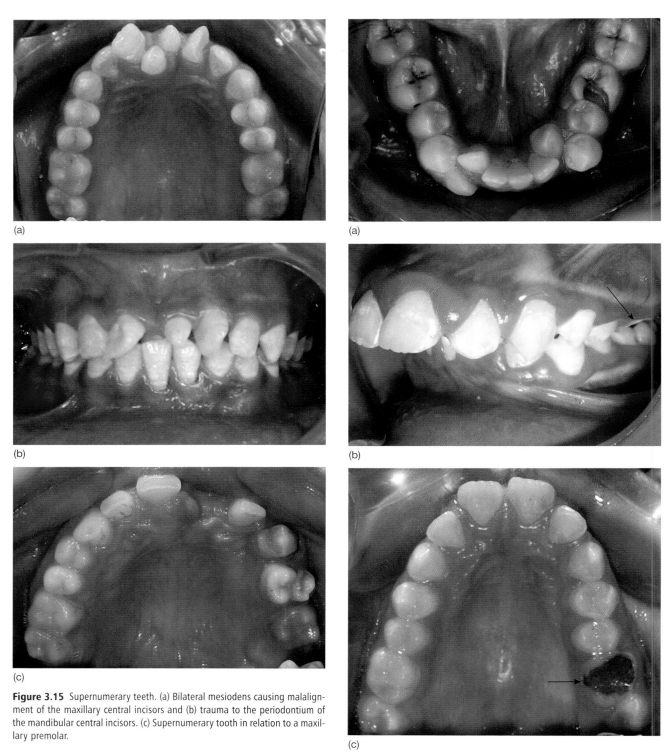

(a)

(b)

(c)

(a)

(b)

(c)

Figure 3.15 Supernumerary teeth. (a) Bilateral mesiodens causing malalignment of the maxillary central incisors and (b) trauma to the periodontium of the mandibular central incisors. (c) Supernumerary tooth in relation to a maxillary premolar.

Figure 3.16 Loss of arch integrity due to caries. (a) A nonrestored mandibular left first molar has led to mesial migration of the molars. (b,c) The poorly restored occlusal surface of the maxillary left first molar (arrow) has allowed the lower molar to supraerupt.

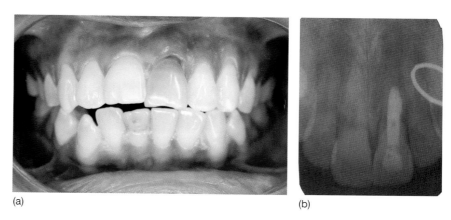

Figure 3.17 A case with bimaxillary protrusion and an endodontically treated upper left central incisor. The radiograph reveals a poorly developed root of the concerned tooth, which makes the long-term prognosis of the tooth uncertain and its response to orthodontic forces unpredictable. The extraction plan in such patients may be modified to extract the tooth with poor prognosis (i.e. the incisor) instead of a healthy premolar. Also note the crown dilaceration of the lower right central incisor.

(a)

(b)

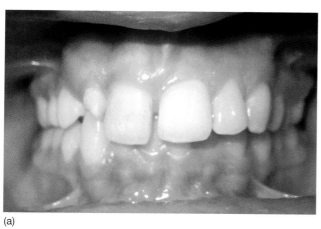

(a)

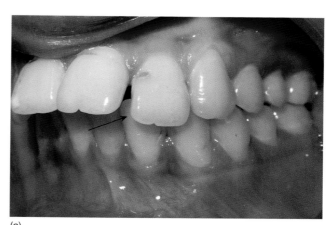

(a)

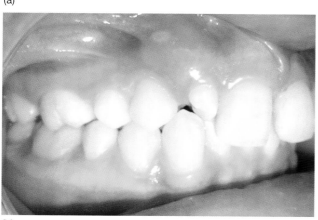

(b)

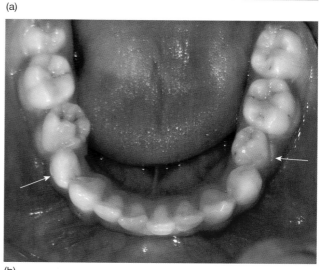

(b)

Figure 3.19 Abnormal size and shape of teeth (arrows). During orthodontic finishing, problems can be anticipated with (a) esthetics and overjet-related issue, and (b) intercuspation.

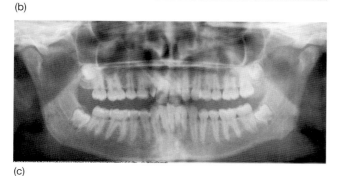

(c)

Figure 3.18 (a–c) A malformed maxillary right lateral incisor with associated canine impaction. Occurrence of malformed laterals is well known in cases of maxillary canine impaction. Also note the supraeruption and the distal inclination of the crown of the maxillary right central incisor due to the pressure on the root from the impacted canine.

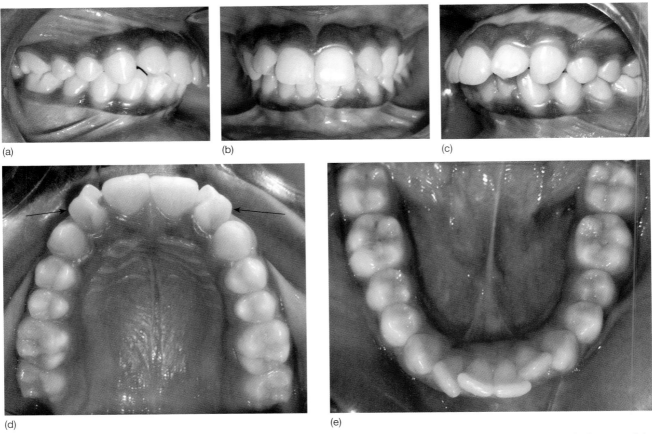

(a) (b) (c)

(d) (e)

Figure 3.20 (a–e) Bilateral talon cusps on the maxillary lateral incisors (arrows) leading to protrusion of the affected teeth and lingual displacement of the lower incisors. An endodontist should be consulted before reduction of talon cusps due to the risk of pulp exposure.

1–8% (Dash et al., 2004) and again the maxillary lateral incisors are most commonly affected, followed by the central incisors and canines. Talon cusps can lead to occlusal interferences, thus acting as an impediment to achieving ideal overjet and overbite and compromised esthetics, caries and periapical pathologies, and periodontal problems (Juan and Jiménez-Rubio, 1999). Similarly, fusion and gemination (Figure 3.21) can affect esthetics, and may lead to dental crowding. The management concerns include esthetics and asymmetric tooth material, re-shaping after intentional endodontic therapy or prosthetic rehabilitation.

Change in color

Systemic disorders such as porphyria, jaundice, heavy metal poisonings, systemic fluorosis (Figure 3.22), vitamin deficiencies, and drugs such as tetracycline (Figure 3.23) can lead to discoloration of teeth (Vogel, 1975; Sulieman, 2005). In addition, local conditions such as traumatic injuries, bacterial pigments, chemicals like chlorhexidine, internal resorption and pulp calcification can also lead to changes in the color of teeth. The orthodontic implications of these findings include the difficulty in bonding to these surfaces

and susceptibility of roots to the resorption process because of underlying defects.

Disorders of eruption

Infraocclusion may occur due to ankylosis, hypercementosis, mechanical obstruction, and habits such as tongue thrusting. Generalized failure of eruption is rare, and is seen as part of hypophosphatasia and primary failure of eruption (PFE) (Figure 3.24). PFE is a unique genetic condition that is characterized by a lack of inherent potential for eruption of teeth. Clinically, the condition presents characteristic features such as generalized lack of contact on posterior teeth, posterior open bite, excessive attrition of anterior teeth, canting and asymmetry of occlusal plane, multiple hypercementosis of teeth and typical changes in the morphology of the mandible. Clinically, an infraerupted tooth would characteristically show a difference in the level of marginal ridges compared with the adjacent teeth, and the opposing tooth would tend to supraerupt, due to loss of occlusal contact. All these factors lead to an imbalance of occlusal forces, anteroposterior space problems, and periodontal problems.

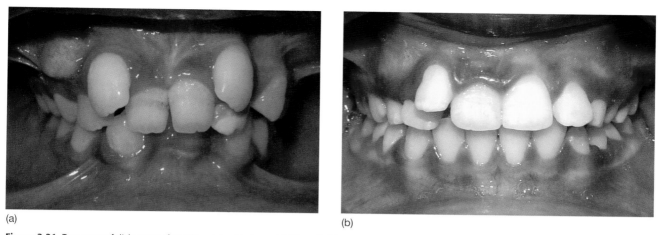

(a)

(b)

Figure 3.21 Two cases of dichotomy of maxillary lateral incisors. (a) Bilateral dichotomous maxillary laterals and (b) dichotomous right maxillary lateral incisor. The decision regarding choice of tooth to be extracted should be based on tooth crown morphology, root morphology, bone support, and location of the tooth. Such cases should undergo a thorough radiographic evaluation for investigating the presence of any other supernumerary teeth, erupted or impacted.

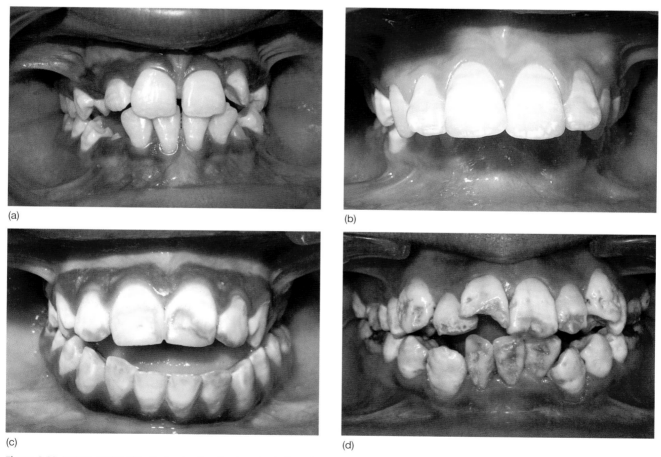

(a)

(b)

(c)

(d)

Figure 3.22 Various grades of tooth discoloration due to systemic fluorosis.

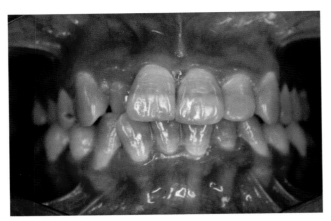

Figure 3.23 Tetracycline discoloration.

Regressive alterations of teeth

Teeth should be inspected for the presence of any attrition, abrasion, or erosions. Although some amount of attrition in the deciduous dentition and in old age is expected, excessive attrition should be particularly investigated (see Figure 3.12). Generalized wear or loss of enamel in the deciduous and permanent dentition may be because of defective dental hard tissue development in conditions such as amelogenesis imperfecta (Figure 3.25) (Crawford et al., 2007), dentinogenesis imperfecta (Barron et al., 2008), and dentine dysplasia (Barron et al., 2008), while generalized attrition in adults may be indicative of bruxism. Localized attrition may occur because of traumatic occlusion, excessive occlusal loading, and improper restorative or prosthetic appliances. Abrasion of teeth, cervical abrasion in particular, may occur with long-term use of abrasive toothpastes, tooth powders, or faulty brushing techniques (Litonjua et al., 2003). Cervical abrasion may also occur due to abfraction (McCoy, 1982), which should alert the orthodontist towards management of occlusal forces. Erosion of teeth may occur in chronic exposure of enamel to acidic substances. Excessive consumption of citrus fruits, gastric reflux disease, and diseases such as anorexia nervosa and bulimia nervosa may be contributory in the etiology of the problem (Daley and Armstrong, 2007).

Evaluation of the occlusion and the temporomandibular joint

A thorough assessment of the TMJ is essential, as many local and systemic processes influence the form and function of this unique ginglymoarthrodial joint. A malocclusion may be an outcome of TMJ pathology resulting from hematogenous spread of infective organisms, or extension of local infections from structures such as the ear (Semlali et al., 2004; Prasad et al., 2007) and the mastoid (Hadlock et al., 2001). Diseases such as rheumatoid arthritis and disorders of bone and joints (for example Ehlers Danlos syn-

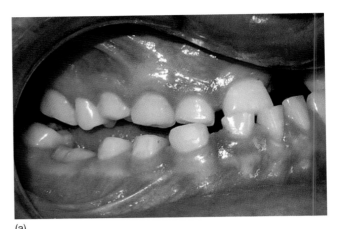

(a)

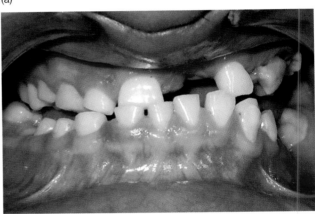

(b)

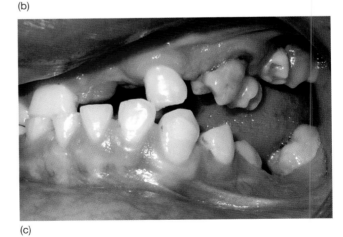

(c)

Figure 3.24 A patient with primary failure of eruption.

drome) can lead to altered function of the TMJ. In many patients, causes of facial pain may reflect as tenderness in the TMJ. Here, it is essential to isolate the pain originating primarily due to internal derangement of the joint, organic or inorganic, from that which occurs due to alterations of the other structures of the craniofacial region. In case an organic disturbance of the joint is suspected, additional

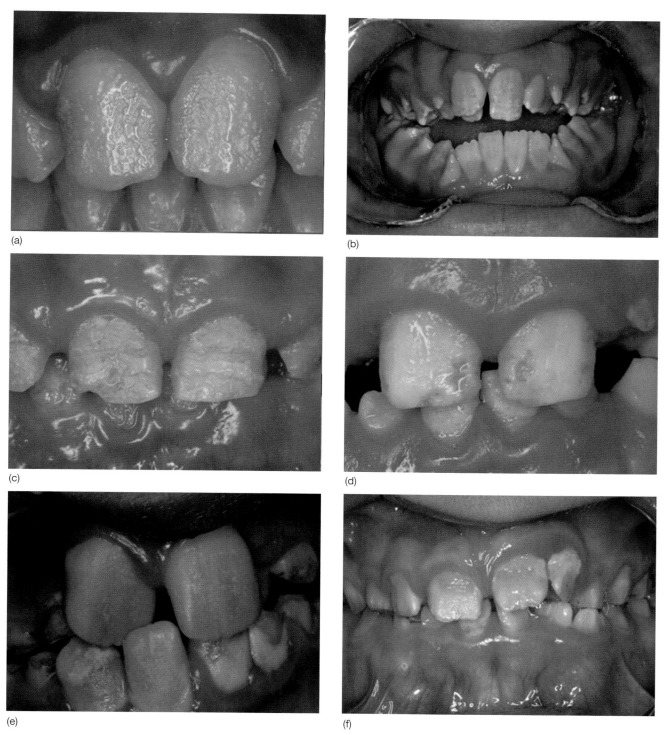

(a)

(b)

(c)

(d)

(e)

(f)

Figure 3.25 Phenotypic variations of amelogenesis imperfecta. Amelogenesis imperfecta may be subdivided at the clinical level into various forms depending on the type of defect and stages of enamel formation affected: hypoplastic (a–d), dysmineralized (e,f), hypomature (g,h). Note the pitted and ridged appearance of the enamel in (a); the association of pitted enamel and open bite in (b–d) are slightly different phenotypic manifestations in a sister (showing a horizontal banding pattern) and brother. In the hypomineralized form (e,f) the enamel is rough, soft, and discolored. Amelogenesis imperfecta may be part of a syndrome as in (f), a case of amelogenesis imperfecta and cone rod dystrophy. Various enamel defects (both hypoplastic and hypomineralized) may coexist in the same patient or even the same tooth (f). The hypomaturation forms (g,h) display enamel of normal thickness and hardness but with a whitish surface. They may be mistaken for fluorosis. (Images reproduced from and text adapted from Crawford et al. (2007) Orphanet, *J Rare Dis* 2: 17.)

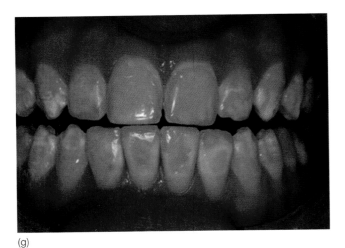

(g)

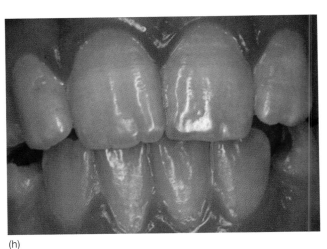

(h)

Figure 3.25 (*Continued*)

radiographic aids may be used to delineate the pathology of the condyle from those of the articular disc and the glenoid fossa, as the problem in each of these structures may be affected by specific systemic and/or local influences.

Similarly, examination of the occlusion, both static and dynamic, forms an important aspect of orthodontic diagnosis. Examination of the centric relation, centric occlusion, the centric shift, and the protrusive and laterotrusive shifts (Figure 3.26) help in assessment of the synchronicity of the movements of the TMJ. This examination is particularly useful in patients with an existing TMJ disorder, those with a mutilated dentition, and those requiring alteration of the occlusal scheme.

Radiographic examination of the jaws

Clinical examination of the jaws should always be supplemented with standard radiographs before crafting a diagnosis and treatment plan for each individual patient, no matter how simple the case seems to be. Many developmental aberrations may become evident only on radiographs, for example cervical spine fusion (Figure 3.27), root dilacerations, hypercementosis, supernumerary and impacted teeth, jaw bone pathologies such as cysts (Figure 3.28), tumors, secondaries of systemic tumors, hyperostotic or resorptive bone lesions, tooth-related pathologies such as a periapical abscess or cyst, idiopathic root resorption, and internal resorption. Skull radiographs may reveal bony lesions secondary to systemic ailments such as thalassemia, leukemias, and multiple myeloma (Shimano 1995; Neyaz et al., 2008), and are also helpful in the evaluation of sinus pathologies, craniosynostoses, and pathologies of the TMJ. Advanced diagnostic techniques such as cone-beam computed tomography (CBCT) are useful in

the assessment of bone pathologies, hard tissue architecture, and assessment of bone density. In patients with suspected hyperactivity or hypoactivity of an organ (e.g. condylar hyperplasia), radionuclide imaging with the isotope ^{99m}Tc is useful (Henderson et al., 2009). MRI is a useful aid in the assessment of the anatomy, function, and pathologies of soft tissues such as the condylar disk, salivary glands, and the sinuses.

Conclusions

Orthodontics is a healthcare specialty concerned with the development of and clinical application of effective means of identifying, diagnosing, and correcting deviations from normal orofacial form and function. The process of orthodontic diagnosis and treatment planning is not merely a detailed description of the dental malocclusion, but also a representation of a broad search for causative factors, both local and systemic.

An orthodontist should be aware that no single patient has orthodontic needs in isolation. Although a few patients can perhaps be managed by the orthodontist alone, most require interactions with the family physician or other medical or dental specialists, for achieving optimum oral health (Figure 3.29). However, ongoing research in clinical and basic sciences continually produces new findings that augment the potential to improve the quality of orthodontic diagnosis and treatment planning. Therefore, it is imperative that practicing orthodontists stay abreast of emerging new knowledge in biological and material sciences and, above all, establish and maintain channels of collaboration and interaction with all other specialists in dentistry and medicine, thereby advancing their capabilities at all times, to the benefit of each of their patients.

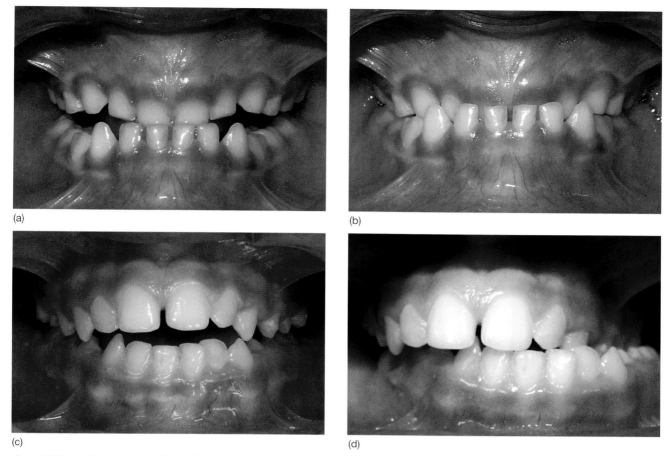

Figure 3.26 Functional occlusion shifts. (a,b) Anterior shift in the deciduous dentition leading to a pseudo-Class III malocclusion, and (c,d) lateral shift in the early permanent dentition. Such pathological shifts may contribute to regressive alterations within the temporomandibular joint.

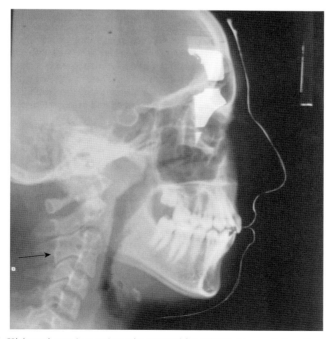

Figure 3.27 Cervical spine fusion (C2–C3) (arrow) seen in a patient who reported for orthodontic consultation. The patient was asymptomatic and the fusion was detected on routine orthodontic investigation. C2–C3 fusion is seen in 0.4–0.7% of the population; there is no sex predilection. The anomaly occurs in the 3rd to 8th week of prenatal development due to reduction in blood supply. Patients are generally asymptomatic, but with age or injury, premature degenerative changes may be seen at adjoining motion segments due to greater biomechanical stress on them. Diskal tears, rupture of the transverse ligament, fractures of the odontoid process, and spondylosis are common consequences. An orthodontist should be cognizant of abnormalities in the cervical spine and should make a referral to a specialist even in the absence of symptoms.

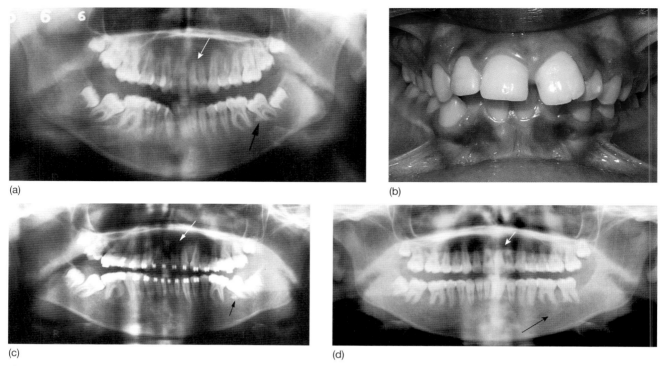

Figure 3.28 A case with a developing cystic lesion in relation to the mesial root of the mandibular left second molar associated with a radiopaque mass (black arrow in (a,c) and root dilaceration of the maxillary left central incisor. Both the conditions, unfortunately, were not noticed during the initial examination. Note the distal tilt in the inclination of the upper left central incisor (b) which should have aroused the suspicion of a potential dilaceration as such conditions are common in the upper central incisors. (c) shows a cyst (white arrow), which was noted on routine radiographic examination 8 months into treatment. The cyst had enlarged significantly in size. The case was discussed with an oral surgeon, and enucleation of the lesion led to successful resolution of the lesion (d). Endodontic therapy was not required for the second molar. (d) also depicts root resorption of the dilacerated central incisor, which occurred as bracket placement did not take into consideration its altered morphology.

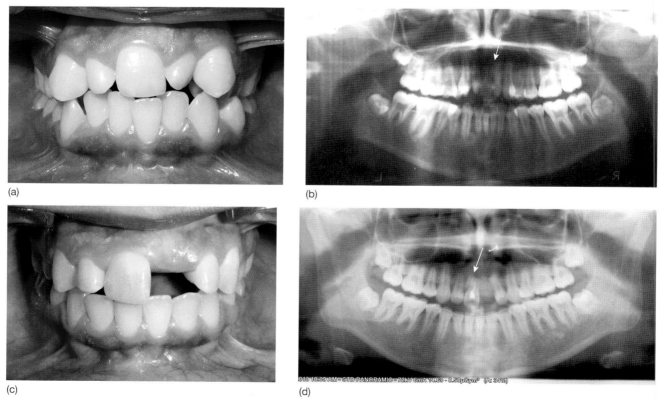

Figure 3.29 (a,b) Traumatic loss of upper left central incisor during childhood. The right central incisor showed calcification of the root canal (arrow). No endodontic intervention was sought for the upper right central incisor prior to orthodontic treatment. (c,d) During the later stages of treatment when the tooth was undergoing torquing, it developed severe sensitivity and root resorption and had to be endodontically treated (arrow). These sequelae could perhaps have been prevented by considering endodontic treatment prior to orthodontic therapy.

References

Abu Alhaija ES, Aldaikki A, Al-Omairi MK, et al. (2010) The relationship between personality traits, pain perception and attitude toward orthodontic treatment. *Angle Orthodontist* 80: 1141–9.

Accurso B, Allem CM (2010) Multiple endocrine neoplasia-2B presenting with orthodontic relapse. *Angle Orthodontist* 80: 585–90.

Adler P, Wegner H, Bohatka L (1973) Influence of age and duration of diabetes on dental development in diabetic children. *Journal of Dental Research* 52: 535–7.

Al Nowaiser A, Roberts GJ, Trompeter RS, et al. (2003) Oral health in children with chronic renal failure. *Pediatric Nephrology* 18: 39–45.

Al-Omiri MK, Alhaija ESA (2006) Factors affecting patient satisfaction after orthodontic treatment. *Angle Orthodontist* 76: 422–31.

Al-Rawi NH, Talabani NG (2008) Squamous cell carcinoma of the oral cavity: a case series analysis of clinical presentation and histological grading of 1,425 cases from Iraq. *Clinical Oral Investigations* 2(1): 15–18.

Altug-Atac AT, Erdem D (2007) Prevalence and distribution of dental anomalies in orthodontic patients. *American Journal of Orthodontics and Dentofacial Orthopedics* 131: 510–14.

Alvear J, Artaza C, Vial M, et al. (1986) Physical growth and bone age of survivors of protein energy malnutrition. *Archives of Disease in Childhood* 61: 257–62.

Annegers JF (1997) The epidemiology of epilepsy. In: E Wyllie (ed.) *The Treatment of Epilepsy: Principles and Practice*, 2nd edn. Baltimore, MD: Lippincott Williams & Wilkins, pp. 165–72.

Ansell D, Feest T, Calvani M (2002) *UK Renal Registry Report 2002*. Bristol: Bristol University.

Babuccu B, Babuccu O, Yurdakan G, et al. (2009) The effect of the Botulinum toxin-A on craniofacial development: an experimental study. *Annals of Plastic Surgery* 63(4): 449–56.

Barron MJ, McDonnell ST, Mackie I, et al. (2008) Hereditary dentine disorders: dentinogenesis imperfecta and dentine dysplasia. *Orphanet Journal of Rare Diseases* 3: 31.

Bartley AJ, Jones DW, Weinberger DR (1997) Genetic variability of human brain size and cortical gyral patterns. *Brain* 120 (Pt 2): 257–69.

Basdra EK, Kiokpasoglou MN, Komposch G (2001) Congenital tooth anomalies and malocclusions: a genetic link? *European Journal of Orthodontics* 23: 145–52.

Bassett JHD, Nordstrom K, Boyde A, et al. (2007) Thyroid status during skeletal development determines adult bone structure and mineralization. *Molecular Endocrinology* 21(8): 1893–904.

Biondi B, Cooper DS (2008) The clinical significance of subclinical thyroid dysfunction. *Endocrine Reviews* 29: 76–131.

Bishara SE, Oonsombat C, Soliman MM, et al. (2005) Effects of using a new protective sealant on the bond strength of orthodontic brackets. *Angle Orthodontist* 75(2): 243–6.

Brambilla F, Cocchi D, Nobile P, et al. (1981) Anterior pituitary responsiveness to hypothalamic hormones in anorexia nervosa. *Neuropsychobiology* 7: 225–37.

Brewer A, Correa ME (2006) *Guidelines for Dental Treatment of Patients with Inherited Bleeding Disorders*. World Federation of Hemophilia Pub., Montreal, Canada, No. 40.

Brook AH (1974) Dental anomalies of number, form and size: their prevalence in British schoolchildren. *Journal of the International Association of Dentistry for Children* 5: 37–53.

Cabell CH, Jollis JG, Peterson GE, et al. (2002) Changing patient characteristics and the effect on mortality in endocarditis. *Archives of Internal Medicine* 162: 90–4.

Canaris GJ, Manowitz NR, Mayor G, et al. (2000) The Colorado thyroid disease prevalence study. *Archives of Internal Medicine* 160: 526–34.

Cantu G, Buschang PH, Gonzalez JL (1997) Differential growth and maturation in idiopathic growth-hormone-deficient children. *European Journal of Orthodontics* 19: 131–9.

Carek PJ, Dickerson LM, Sack JL (2001) Diagnosis and management of osteomyelitis. *American Family Physician* 63(12): 2413–20.

Carmichael DT, Williams CA, Aller MS (1995) Renal dysplasia with secondary hyperparathyroidism and loose teeth in a young dog. *Journal of Veterinary Dentistry* 12: 143–6.

Cascino GD, Luckstein RR, Sharbrough FW, et al. (1993) Facial asymmetry, hippocampal pathology, and remote symptomatic seizures: a temporal lobe epileptic syndrome. *Neurology* 43(4): 725–7.

Cassidy L, Jellinek M (1998) Approaches to recognition and management of childhood psychiatric disorders in pediatric primary care. *Pediatric Clinics of North America* 45: 1037–52.

Castellanos JL, Díaz-Guzmán L (2008) Lesions of the oral mucosa: an epidemiological study of 23785 Mexican patients. *Oral Surgery, Oral Medicine, Oral Pathology, Oral Radiology, and Endodontology* 105(1): 79–85.

Centers for Disease Control and Prevention (1989) Guidelines for prevention and transmission of HIV and HBV to health care and public safety workers. *Morbidity and Mortality Weekly Report (MMWR)* 38: 1–37.

Chung LK, Hobson RS, Nunn JH, et al. (2000) An analysis of the skeletal relationships in a group of young people with hypodontia. *Journal of Orthodontics* 27: 315–18.

Cohen RB, Wilcox CW (1993) A case of acromegaly identified after patient complaint of apertognathia. *Oral Surgery, Oral Medicine, Oral Pathology, Oral Radiology, and Endodontology* 75: 583–6.

Collins MK, Sinclair PM (1988) The local use of vitamin D to increase the rate of orthodontic tooth movement. *American Journal of Orthodontics and Dentofacial Orthopedics* 94(4): 278–84.

Colvard MD, Bishop J, Weissman D, et al. (1986) Cardiazem-induced gingival hyperplasia. *Periodontal Case Reports* 8: 67–8.

Crawford PJ, Aldred M, Bloch-Zupan A (2007) Amelogenesis imperfecta. *Orphanet Journal of Rare Diseases* 2: 17.

Crocetti M, Barone MA (Adapted from Plotnick LP) (2004) Growth disorders. In M Crocetti, MA Barone (eds.) *Oski's Essential Pediatrics*, 2nd edn. USA: Lippincott Williams & Wilkins, pp. 567.

Dahllof G, Huggare J (2004) Orthodontic considerations in the pediatric cancer patients: a review. *Seminars in Orthodontics* 10: 266–76.

Daley TD, Armstrong JE (2007) Oral manifestations of gastrointestinal diseases. *Canadian Journal of Gastroenterology* 21(4): 241–4.

Dash JK, Sahoo PK, Das SN (2004) Talon cusp associated with other dental anomalies: a case report. *International Journal of Paediatric Dentistry* 14: 295–300.

Davidovitch Z, Krishnan V (2009) Role of basic biological sciences in clinical orthodontics: a case series. *American Journal of Orthodontics and Dentofacial Orthopedics* 135(2): 222–31.

Davies TI, Rayner PH (1995) Functional appliance therapy in conjunction with growth hormone treatment: A case report. *British Journal of Orthodontics* 22: 361–5.

Dixit R, Sharma S, Nuwal P (2008) Tuberculosis of oral cavity. *Indian Journal of Tuberculosis* 55(1): 51–3.

Dreizen S, Spirakis CN, Stone RE (1967). A comparison of skeletal growth and maturation in undernourished and well-nourished girls before and after menarche. *Journal of Pediatrics* 70(2): 256–63.

El Bokle D, Munir H (2008) An in vitro study of the effect of Pro Seal varnish on the shear bond strength of orthodontic brackets. *World Journal of Orthodontics* 9(2): 141–6.

Elia J, Ambrosini P, Rapoport J (1999) Treatment of attention deficit hyperactivity disorder. *New England Journal of Medicine* 340: 780–8.

Engström C, Linde A, Thilander B (1982a) Craniofacial morphology and growth in the rat. Cephalometric analysis of the effects of a low calcium and vitamin D-deficient diet. *Journal of Anatomy* 134(Pt 2): 299–314.

Engström C, Magnusson BC, Linde A (1982b) Changes in craniofacial suture metabolism in rats fed a low calcium and vitamin D-deficient diet. *Journal of Anatomy* 134: 443–58.

Eugster EA, Pescovitz OH (1999) Gigantism. *Journal of Clinical Endocrinology and Metabolism* 84: 4379–84.

Fabe SS (1950) Acute hematogenous osteomyelitis of the mandible; report of a case. *Oral Surgery, Oral Medicine, Oral Pathology, Oral Radiology, and Endodontology* 3(1): 22–6.

Favaloro EJ (2006) Laboratory identification of von Willebrand disease: technical and scientific perspectives. *Seminars in Thrombosis and Hemostasis* 32: 456–71.

Fekonja A (2005) Hypodontia in orthodontically treated children. *European Journal of Orthodontics* 27: 457–60.

Field EA, Speechley JA, Rugman FR, et al. (1995) Oral signs and symptoms in patients with undiagnosed B12 deficiency. *Journal of Oral Pathology and Medicine* 24: 68–70.

Finkelstein MW (2001) Overview of general embryology and head and neck development. In: SE Bishara (ed.) *Textbook of Orthodontics*. Philadelphia, PN: WB Saunders, pp. 2–24.

Flavoro EJ (2007) Investigating people with mucocutaneous bleeding suggestive of primary hemostatic defects: a low likelihood of a definitive diagnosis? *Hematologica* 92: 292–6.

Fong GC, Mak YF, Swartz BE, et al. (2003) Body part asymmetry in partial seizure. *Seizure* 12(8): 606–12.

Franz-Montan M, Ranali J, Ramacciato JC, et al. (2008) Ulceration of gingival mucosa after topical application of EMLA: report of four cases. *British Dental Journal* 204(3): 133–4.

Fujieda K, Tanaka T (2007) Diagnosis of children with short stature: Insights from KIGS. In MB Ranke, DA Price, EO Reiter (eds.) *Growth Hormone Therapy in Pediatrics: 20 Years of KIGS*. Basel, Switzerland: Karger AG, pp. 16.

Galili D, Berger E, Kaufman E (1991) Pulp narrowing in renal end stage and transplanted patients. *Journal of Endodontics* 17: 442–3.

Garrow JS, Pike MC (1967) The long-term prognosis of severe infantile malnutrition. *Lancet* i: 1–4.

George A, Johnson M, Blinkhorn A, et al. (2010) Promoting oral health during pregnancy: current evidence and implications for Australian midwives. *Journal of Clinical Nursing* (in press).

Gillchrist JA (1999) Hepatitis viruses A, B, C, D, E and G: Implications for dental personnel. *Journal of the American Dental Association* 130: 509–20.

Gosau M, Vogel C, Moralis A, et al. (2009) Mandibular prognathism caused by acromegaly – a surgical orthodontic case. *Head and Face Medicine* 5: 16.

Gould FK, Elliott TS, Foweraker J, et al. (2006) Guidelines for the prevention of endocarditis: report of the Working Party of the British Society for Antimicrobial Chemotherapy. *Journal of Antimicrobial Chemotherapy* 57(6): 1035–42.

Graham GG, Adrianzen BT (1972). Late catch up growth after severe infantile malnutrition. *Johns Hopkins Medical Journal* 131: 204–11.

Guttal KS, Naikmasurb VG, Bhargava P, et al. (2010) Frequency of Developmental Dental Anomalies in the Indian Population. *European Journal of Dentistry* 4: 263–9.

Hadlock TA, Ferraro NF, Rahbar R (2001) Acute mastoiditis with temporomandibular joint effusion. *Otolaryngology Head and Neck Surgery* 125(1): 111–12.

Hall RK (1983) Congenitally missing teeth – A diagnostic feature in many syndromes of the head and neck. *Journal of the International Association of Dentistry for Children* 14: 69–75.

Harvey CB, O'Shea PJ, Scott AJ, et al. (2002) Molecular mechanisms of thyroid hormone effects on bone growth and function. *Molecular Genetics and Metabolism* 75: 17–30.

Henderson M, Wastie M, Bromige M, et al. (2009) Technetium-99m bone scintigraphy and mandibular condylar hyperplasia. *Clinical Radiology* 41(6): 411–14.

Hicks MJ, Flaitz CM (2000) Oral mucosal melanoma: epidemiology and pathobiology. *Oral Oncology* 36(2): 152–69.

Hollowell JG, Staehling NW, Flanders WD, et al. (2002) Serum TSH, T(4), and thyroid antibodies in the United States population (1988 to 1994): National Health and Nutrition Examination Survey (NHANES III). *Journal of Clinical Endocrinology and Metabolism* 87(2): 489–99.

Hwang CJ, Cha JY (2004) Orthodontic treatment with growth hormone therapy in a girl of short stature. *American Journal of Orthodontics and Dentofacial Orthopedics* 126: 118–26.

Isaac AM, Tholouli E (2008) Orthodontic treatment for a patient who developed acute myeloid leukemia. *American Journal of Orthodontics and Dentofacial Orthopedics* 134(5): 684–8.

Jaffe EC, Roberts J, Chantler C, et al. (1990) Dental maturity in children with chronic renal failure assessed from dental panoramic tomographs. *Journal of the International Association of Dentistry for Children* 20: 54–8.

Jayaraman GC, Bush KR, Lee B, et al. (2004) Magnitude and determinants of first-time and repeat testing among individuals with newly diagnosed HIV infection between 2000 and 2001 in Alberta, Canada: results from population-based laboratory surveillance. *Journal of Acquired Immune Deficiency Syndromes* 37(5): 1651–6.

Johnstone SC, Barnard KM, Harrison VE (1999) Recognizing and caring for the medically compromised child: 4. Children with other chronic medical conditions. *Dental Update* 26(1): 21–6.

Jolly M (1977) White lesions of the mouth. *International Journal of Dermatology* 16(9): 713–25.

Jorgenson RJ (1980) Clinicians' view of hypodontia. *Journal of the American Dental Association* 101: 283–6.

Juan JS, Jiménez-Rubio A (1999) Talon cusp affecting permanent maxillary lateral incisors in 2 family members. *Oral Surgery, Oral Medicine, Oral Pathology, Oral Radiology, and Endodontology* 88: 90–2.

Kauzman A, Pavone M, Blanas N, et al. (2004) Pigmented lesions of the oral cavity: review, differential diagnosis, and case presentations. *Journal of Canadian Dental Association* 70(10): 682–3.

Keçik D, Cehreli SB, Sar C, et al. (2008) Effect of acidulated phosphate fluoride and casein phosphopeptide-amorphous calcium phosphate application on shear bond strength of orthodontic brackets. *Angle Orthodontist* 78(1): 129–33.

Kennedy DS, Linden GJ (2000) Resolution of gingival overgrowth following change from ciclosporin to tacrolimus therapy in a renal transplant patient. *Journal of Irish Dental Association* 46: 3–4.

Kharbanda OP (2009) Steps and treatment stages in contemporary orthodontic treatment. In: OP Kharbanda (ed.) *Orthodontics Diagnosis and Management of Malocclusion and Dentofacial Deformities*. India: Elsevier Publishing, p. 311.

Kho H, Lee S, Chung SC, et al. (1999) Oral manifestations and salivary flow rate, pH, and buffer capacity in patients with end-stage renal disease undergoing haemodialysis. *Oral Surgery, Oral Medicine, Oral Pathology, Oral Radiology, and Endodontology* 88: 316–19.

Kimura T, Dunn WJ, Taloumis LJ (2004) Effect of fluoride varnish on the in vitro bond strength of orthodontic brackets using a self-etching primer system. *American Journal of Orthodontics and Dentofacial Orthopedics* 125(3): 351–6.

Krishnan V, Davidovitch Z (2006) The effect of drugs on orthodontic tooth movement. *Journal of Orthodontics and Craniofacial Research* 9: 163–71.

Krueger RH (1969). Some long-term effects of severe malnutrition in early life. *Lancet* 2: 514–17.

Kumar P (2008) Dysmorphology. In: P Kumar, K Barbara (eds) *Congenital Malformations: Evidence Based Evaluation and Management*. USA: McGraw Publishing, p. 6.

Lamster IB, Lalla E, Borgnakke WS, et al. (2008) The relationship between oral health and diabetes mellitus. *Journal of the American Dental Association* 139(5)(Suppl): 19–24.

Laurikainen K, Kuusisto P (1998) Comparison of the oral health status and salivary flow rate of asthmatic patients with those of nonasthmatic adults – results of a pilot study. *Allergy* 53: 316–19.

Leukefeld CG, Battjes BJ, Amsel Z (1990) AIDS and intravenous drug use: Future directions for community-based prevention research. *NIDA Research Monograph 93*, Washington DC, US Government printing office.

Lip GYH, Beevers DG (2005) Hypertensive emergencies and urgencies. In: DA Warrell, TM Cox, JD Firth, et al. (eds) *Oxford Textbook of Medicine*, 4th edn, vol 2. Oxford: Oxford University Press, pp. 1194.

Litonjua LA, Andreana S, Bush PJ, et al. (2003) Noncarious cervical lesions and abfractions: a re-evaluation. *Journal of the American Dental Association* 134(7): 845–50.

Little JW (2002) Eating disorders: Dental implications. *Oral Surgery, Oral Medicine, Oral Pathology, Oral Radiology, and Endodontology* 93: 138–43.

Litton SF (1974) Orthodontic tooth movement during an ascorbic acid deficiency. *American Journal of Orthodontics* 65(3): 290–302.

Lux CJ, Kugel B, Komposch G, et al. (2005) Orthodontic treatment in a patient with Papillon-Lefèvre syndrome. *Journal of Periodontology* 76: 642–50.

Mannucci PM, Duga S, Peyvandi F (2004) Recessively inherited coagulation disorders. *Blood* 104: 1243–52.

Marik PE, Varon J (2007) Hypertensive crises: management and challenges. *Chest* 131: 1949–62.

Matfin G (2009) Disorders of endocrine control of growth and metabolism. In: RA Hannon, C Pooler, CM Porth (eds) *Porth Pathophysiology: Concepts of Altered Health States*. Canada: Lippincott Williams & Wilkins, p. 986.

McConkey EH (2004) In Lecture 4: Therapy of genetic disorders. In: EH McConkey (ed.) *How the Human Genome Works*. Canada: Jones and Bartlett, p. 66.

McCoy G (1982) The etiology of gingival erosion. *Journal of Oral Implantology* 10: 361–2.

McNab S, Battistutta D, Taverne A, et al. (1999) External apical root resorption of posterior teeth in asthmatics after orthodontic treatment. *American Journal of Orthodontics and Dentofacial Orthopedics* 116: 545–51.

Mitchell L (1996) *An Introduction to Orthodontics*. Oxford: Oxford University Press, pp. 23–5.

Morrison NA, Yeoman R, Kelly PJ, et al. (1992) Contribution of trans-acting factor alleles to normal physiological variability: vitamin D receptor gene polymorphism and circulating osteocalcin. *Proceedings of the National Academy of Sciences of the United States of America* 89: 6665–9.

Mupparapu M, Singer SR (2004) A rare presentation of dens invaginatus in a mandibular lateral incisor occurring concurrently with bilateral maxillary dens invaginatus: Case report and review of literature. *Australian Dental Journal* 49: 90–3.

Murphy E, Williams GR (2004) The thyroid and the skeleton. *Clinical Endocrinology (Oxford)* 61: 285–98.

Nadimi H, Bergamini J, Lilien B (1993) Uremic mixed bone disease. A case report. *International Journal of Maxillofacial Surgery* 22: 268–70.

Nasman M, Forsberg CM, Dahllof G (1997) Disturbances in dental development in long-term survivors after pediatric malignant diseases. *European Journal of Orthodontics* 19: 151–9.

Nasstrom K (1996) Dentin formation after corticosteroid treatment. A clinical study and an experimental study on rats. *Swedish Dental Journal* 115: 1–45.

Nasstrom K, Forsberg B, Petersson A, et al. (1985) Narrowing of the dental pulp chamber in patients with renal diseases. *Oral Surgery, Oral Medicine, Oral Pathology, Oral Radiology, and Endodontology* 59: 242–6.

Neeley WW, Kleumper GT, Hays LR (2006a) Psychiatry in orthodontics. Part I: Typical adolescent psychiatric disorders and their relevance to orthodontic practice. *American Journal of Orthodontics and Dentofacial Orthopedics* 129: 176–84.

Neeley WW, Kleumper GT, Hays LR (2006b) Psychiatry in orthodontics. Part II: substance abuse among adolescents and its relevance to orthodontic practice. *American Journal of Orthodontics and Dentofacial Orthopedics* 129: 185–93.

Neville DW, Damm DD, Allen CM, et al. (2005) Abnormalities of teeth. In: DW Neville, DD Damm, CM Allen, et al. (eds) *Oral and Maxillofacial Pathology*. Philadelphia, PA: Elsevier, pp. 49–89.

Neyaz Z, Gadodia A, Gamanagatti S, et al. (2008) Radiographical approach to jaw lesions. *Singapore Medical Journal* 49(2): 165.

Okada H, Davies JE, Yamamoto H (2000) Brown tumor of the maxilla in a patient with secondary hyperparathyroidism: a case study involving immunohistochemistry and electron microscopy. *Journal of Oral and Maxillofacial Surgery* 58: 233–8.

Orbak R, Simsek S, Orbak Z, et al. (2008) The influence of type-1 diabetes mellitus on dentition and oral health in children and adolescents. *Yonsei Medical Journal* 49: 357–65.

Patel A, Burden DJ, Sandler J (2009) Medical disorders and orthodontics. *Journal of Orthodontics* 36(Suppl): 1–21.

Poley GE Jr, Slater JE (2000) Latex allergy. *Journal of Allergy and Clinical Immunology* 105: 1054–62.

Portelli M, Matarese G, Militi A, et al. (2009) Myotonic dystrophy and craniofacial morphology: clinical and instrumental study. *European Journal of Paediatric Dentistry* 10(1): 19–22.

Prasad KC, Sreedharan S, Prasad SC, et al. (2007) Tuberculosis of the temporomandibular joint and parotid secondary to tuberculous otitis media. *Otolaryngology Head and Neck Surgery* 137(6): 974–5.

Prendergast BD (2006) The changing face of infective endocarditis. *Heart* 92: 879–85.

Proctor R, Kumar N, Stein A, et al. (2005) Oral and dental aspects of chronic renal failure. *Journal of Dental Research* 84: 199–208.

Quiroga T, Goycoolea M, Panes O, et al. (2007) High prevalence of bleeders of unknown cause among patients with inherited mucocutaneous bleeding. Prospective study of 280 patients and 299 controls. *Haematologica* 92: 356–64.

Rajendran R (2009) Diseases of skin. In: R Rajendran, B Sivapathasundharam (eds) *Shafer's Textbook of Oral Pathology*, 6th edn. India: Elsevier, pp. 797–843.

Ren Y, Maltha JC, Kuijpers-Jagtman AM (2003) Optimum force magnitude for orthodontic tooth movement: a systematic literature review. *Angle Orthodontist* 73: 86–92.

Rivkees SA, Bode HH, Crawford JD (1988) Long-term growth in juvenile acquired hypothyroidism: the failure to achieve normal adult stature. *New England Journal of Medicine* 318: 599–602.

Ruiz-Roca JA, Berini-Aytes L, Gay-Escoda C (2005) Pyostomatitis vegetans: Report of two cases and review of the literature. *Oral Surgery, Oral Medicine, Oral Pathology, Oral Radiology, and Endodontology* 99: 447–54.

Sadowsky PL, Bernreuter W, Lakshminarayanan AV, et al. (1988) Orthodontic appliances and magnetic resonance imaging of the brain and temporomandibular joint. *Angle Orthodontist* 58(1): 9–20.

Salerno F, Cocchi D, Lampertico M, et al. (1982) Growth hormone response to thyrotropin-releasing hormone in liver cirrhosis: unique alteration in anterior pituitary responsiveness to hypothalamic hormones. *Hormone Metabolism Research* 14: 482–6.

Semlali S, Nassar I, Fikri M, et al. (2004) Candida arthritis of the TM joint complicating chronic otitis media. *Journal of Radiology* 85(11): 1953–5.

Setian N (2007) Hypothyroidism in children: diagnosis and treatment. *Jornal de Pediatria* 83(5 Suppl): s209–16:

Sheller B (2004) Orthodontic management of patients with seizure disorders. *Seminars in Orthodontics* 10: 247–51.

Shepard CW, Simard EP, Finelli L, et al. (2006) Hepatitis B virus infection: epidemiology and vaccination. *Epidemiologic Reviews* 28: 112–25.

Sheth RD (2004) Metabolic concerns associated with antiepileptic medications. *Neurology* 63(10)(Suppl 4): S24–9.

Shimano T (1995) Radiographic diagnosis of systemic diseases in dentistry. *Oral Radiology* 11(2): 1–19.

Shirazi M, Dehpour AR, Jafari F (1999) The effect of thyroid hormone on orthodontic tooth movement in rats. *Journal of Clinical Pediatric Dentistry* 23: 259–64.

Sidell FR, Kaminskis A (1975) Temporal intrapersonal physiological variability of cholinesterase activity in human plasma and erythrocytes. *Clinical Chemistry* 21:1961–3.

Sonis S (2004) Orthodontic management of selected medically compromised patients: cardiac disease, bleeding disorders, and asthma. *Seminars in Orthodontics* 10: 277–80.

Sonneveld MJ, Janssen HLA (2010) Pros and cons of peginterferon versus nucleos(t)ide analogues for treatment of chronic Hepatitis B. *Current Hepatitis Reports* 9: 91–8.

Sperber GH, Gutterman GD, Sperber SM (eds) (2001) *Craniofacial Development*, vol 1. Ontario: BC Decker.

Sulieman M (2005) An overview of tooth discoloration: extrinsic, intrinsic and internalized stains. *Dental Update* 32(8): 463–4, 466–8, 471.

Suter VG, Morger R, Altermatt HJ, et al. (2008) Oral erythroplakia and erythroleukoplakia: red and red-white dysplastic lesions of the oral mucosa-part 1: epidemiology, etiology, histopathology and differential diagnosis. *Schweiz Monatsschr Zahnmed* 118(5): 390–7.

Teng L, Bui H, Bachrach L, et al. (2004) Catch-up growth in severe juvenile hypothyroidism: treatment with a GnRH analog. *Journal of Pediatric Endocrinology and Metabolism* 17: 345–54.

The Task Force on Infective Endocarditis of the European Society of Cardiology (2004) Guidelines on prevention, diagnosis and treatment of infective endocarditis: executive summary. *European Heart Journal* 25: 267–76.

Tinuper P, Plazzi G, Provini F, et al. (1992) Facial asymmetry in partial epilepsies. *Epilepsia* 33(6): 1097–100.

Trujillo R Jr, Fontão FN, de Sousa SM (2002) Unilateral masseter muscle hypertrophy: a case report. *Quintessence International* 33(10): 776–9.

Tsai CY, Yang LY, Chen KT, et al. (2010) The influence of masticatory hypofunction on developing rat craniofacial structure. *International Journal of Oral Maxillofacial Surgery* 39(6): 593–8.

Tuddenham EGD, Cooper DN (1994) The molecular genetics of haemostasis and its inherited disorders. In: *Oxford Monograph on Medical Genetics No. 25*. Oxford: Oxford Medical Publication.

Turkkahraman H, Sarıoglu M (2006) Oculo-facio-cardio-dental syndrome: report of a rare case. *Angle Orthodontist* 76: 184–6.

Van Erum R, Mulier G, Carels C, et al. (1998) Craniofacial growth and dental maturation in short children born small for gestational age: effect of growth hormone treatment. Own observations and review of the literature. *Hormone Research* 50: 141–6.

van Venrooy JR, Proffit WR (1985) Orthodontic care for medically compromised patients: possibilities and limitations. *Journal of the American Dental Association* 111: 262–6.

Verna C, Dalstra M, Melsen B (2000) The rate and the type of orthodontic tooth movement is influenced by bone turnover in a rat model. *European Journal of Orthodontics* 22: 343–52.

Vernillo AT (2001) Diabetes mellitus: Relevance to dental treatment. *Oral Surgery, Oral Medicine, Oral Pathology, Oral Radiology, and Endodontology* 91(3): 263–70.

Villa A, Mariani U, Villa F (2010) T-cell lymphoma of the oral cavity: a case report. *Australian Orthodontic Journal* 55(2): 203–6.

Vitral RW, Tanaka OM, Fraga MR, et al. (2006) Acromegaly in an orthodontic patient. *American Journal of Orthodontics and Dentofacial Orthopedics* 130: 388–90.

Vogel RI (1975) Intrinsic and extrinsic discoloration of the dentition (a literature review). *Journal of Oral Medicine* 30(4): 99–104.

Walker MR, Lovel SF, Melrose CA (2007) Orthodontic treatment of a patient with a renal transplant and drug-induced gingival overgrowth: a case report. *Journal of Orthodontics* 34(4): 220–8.

Warburton G, Caccamese JF Jr (2006) Valvular heart disease and heart failure: dental management considerations. *Dental Clinics of North America* 50(4): 493–512.

Williams DA (2008) Drug metabolism. In: TL Lemke, DA Williams (eds) *Foye's Principles of Medicinal Chemistry*, 6th edn. Philadelphia: Lippincott William & Wilkins, p. 253.

Wittmann AL (1977) Macroglossia in acromegaly and hypothyroidism. *Virchow's Archives* 373: 353–60.

Yagi T, Kawakami M, Takada K (2004) Surgical orthodontic correction of acromegaly with mandibular prognathism. *Angle Orthodontist* 74: 125–31.

Yasny J (2010) The importance of oral health for cardiothoracic and vascular patients. *Seminars in Cardiothoracic and Vascular Anesthesia* 14: 38–40.

4

Psychosocial Factors in Motivation, Treatment, Compliance, and Satisfaction with Orthodontic Care

Donald B Giddon, Nina K Anderson

Summary

This chapter describes what is known by social scientists and epidemiologists about why and when individuals seek orthodontic care; the cognitive, affective, and behavioral factors involved in becoming an orthodontic patient; and behaviors appropriate during treatment and subsequent compliance. The authors present some of their own work on using a range of acceptability rather than a static image between patient and clinician to communicate about what is in a patient's mind or the perception of changes in facial morphology to achieve a satisfactory treatment outcome. The influence of ethno-cultural differences, effective communication, and health literacy are discussed. Finally, recommendations are offered for managing psychosocial problems when the process and outcome do not progress as planned for patients, parents, and clinicians.

Introduction

Not too long ago, orthodontists, of all the dental specialties, had to deal with the most complex psychosocial issues because most orthodontic patients were children and adolescents who were working out conflicts with authority figures such as parents and teachers as well as the orthodontist, who like other doctors, were perceived to be in charge (Miller and Larson, 1979). Parents, usually the mother, also had to interact with their children and the clinician in making decisions about orthodontic treatment. Orthodontists actually shared the burden with parents for motivating their children to comply with the requirements of orthodontic treatment. Modern orthodontics, however, has progressed beyond 'beware of children' to interacting, complementing, and even competing with other dental and medical specialists involved in the increasing complexities of overall health care.

Motivation for orthodontic care

Relationship of the morphology and function of the orofacial area to quality of life

Although not everyone agrees that orthodontic treatment improves physical and mental health as part of overall quality of life (Kenealy et al., 2007), few doubt that the orofacial-cranial area is the most important part of the body, the rest being a support system. Following from Maslow's (1943, 1970) hierarchy of needs and more recent revisions (Kenrick et al., 2010), the orofacial area is essential for survival as the portal for food and water, as well as security or defense; then for communication using the lips, tongue, teeth, and muscles of facial expressions for verbal and nonverbal communication. After meeting these basic biosocial needs, the orofacial area is available for satisfying higher-order hedonic, esthetic, gustatory, sensual, and intellectual activities (Giddon, 1999; Jones, 2009).

While the eyes may be the window to the soul, the mouth is also a window to the body's physical and mental health (Giddon, 1999). The genetically determined, ontological sequence further supports the intimate relationship of the intraoral structures to the developing brain, face, and cranial soft and hard tissues as does the disproportionate neuroanatomical and physiological representation of the orofacial area in the sensory and motor homunculi, including the muscles of mastication and facial expression

Integrated Clinical Orthodontics, First Edition. Edited by Vinod Krishnan, Ze'ev Davidovitch.
© 2012 Blackwell Publishing Ltd. Published 2012 by Blackwell Publishing Ltd.

(Penfield and Rasmussen, 1978). Thus there is all the more reason for preserving the structure and function of the muscles of facial expression, which 'constitute the most highly differentiated and versatile set of neuromuscular mechanisms in man' (Izard, 1971). Recent functional magnetic resonance imaging (fMRI) studies have also documented activation of specific areas of the brain in response to noxious stimulation of the orofacial area (Kitada et al., 2010). A related earlier observation is the apparent need for some periodic oral activity, such as speaking, eating, drinking, chewing gum, smoking, smiling, kissing, yawning, laughing, frowning, and clenching on average every 96 minutes (Friedman and Fisher, 1967).

Given that the major motivation for orthodontic treatment is to improve physical appearance as a means to enhance social acceptance and quality of life (Baldwin, 1980; Giddon and Anderson, 2006), the orthodontist and referring dentist should discuss any concerns about the teeth and surrounding orofacial area in relation to body image, self-concept, and quality of life before deciding if and when to begin orthodontic treatment. Possible loss of teeth or orofacial mutilation can also be a concern, whether from trauma, multiple extractions, or orthognathic surgery (Giddon, 1999). As Cervantes notes through Don Quixote, 'I had rather they had tore off an arm, provided it were not the sword arm; for, Sancho, you must know, that a mouth without grinders is like a mill without & [sic] stone; and a diamond is not so precious as a tooth' (Cervantes).

For children, a loose tooth is an exciting event. The child continues to pull at it until the primary tooth loosens up and falls into their hands. The child then slips it under the pillow with anticipation that the tooth fairy is on the way to replace the tooth with money while they are sleeping. Thoughts or dreams of losing teeth, having teeth crumble, rot or grow crooked are frequently reported. Fear of losing teeth in dental patients due to biomechanical tooth movement or gingival recession may have a major impact on patients' perceptions of their appearance and quality of life because people cannot change the appearance of missing teeth. According to Freud, Jung, and others (Lorand and Feldman, 1955), thoughts of losing teeth may be symbolic of loss of power or fear that some permanent part of a person's life is about to change or is under threat. The fear of loss of teeth may also represent a retreat to infancy (i.e., when, toothless, the mother was the source of nourishment and comfort), and hence a refusal to face reality. Fears of tooth loss have also been theorized to be important symbols of fear of castration, sexual repression, or masturbatory desires during puberty. Jung (2010) attributed fear of losing teeth in woman to parturition.

Example of patient with underlying 'tooth fairy' issues

Patient LF, being treated by an orthodontist after a fall, displaced her maxillary incisors palatally.

- The teeth were realigned but the patient became very anxious at thought of debonding.
- The orthodontist removed the archwires several months before debonding
- They then sent LF back to the prosthodontist for reassurance that teeth would be healthy enough to continue treatment.

Suggestions

- Acknowledge patient's fears about the fall and the importance of the teeth for survival, social interactions, and physical appearance.
- Provide resources to look up the work of Freud, Jung, and others about the symbolism of teeth.
- Urge patient to 'test' his or her tooth strength by eating foods which require biting or tearing, such as dried meats, apples, chewing gum.
- Proceed slowly as above by removing wires, then debonding.
- Arrange for ways that the patient can receive appropriate attention.

Need versus demand for orthodontic care

Objective measures of malocclusion or need for orthodontic treatment does not translate directly into perceived demand, which may or may not result in actual care. Nevertheless, the demand for orthodontic treatment continues to increase for both children and adults. The American Association of Orthodontists reports a 37% increase from 1994 to 2004 in the number of adult patients in the United States (Bick, 2007). It is estimated that, with cost barriers removed, 60% of the population would be interested in receiving orthodontic care (King, n.d.), and that 77% of Americans agree that straightening 'crooked teeth' is one of the best investments a person can make in improving his or her appearance (Anon, 2005). While the relative shortage of orthodontists explains some of the discrepancy between need and demand, psychosocial and economic variables provide the most likely explanation of the discrepancy. In other words, the difference between demands or the desire to seek orthodontic treatment and actually receiving it is a function of acceptability based on the willingness to comply with temporal and financial requirements of a successful outcome.

Based on oral health-related quality of life measures, differences in emotional and social wellbeing were found between children with malocclusions and acceptable occlusions, even though there were no differences in oral function (Kiyak, 2008). Perceived benefits also differ between referring dentists and orthodontists. In Northern Ireland, both groups agreed on the top five benefits as physical attractiveness, self-esteem and self-confidence, less teasing, and easier-to-clean teeth. As expected, general dentists saw greater benefits for oral function and health than the spe-

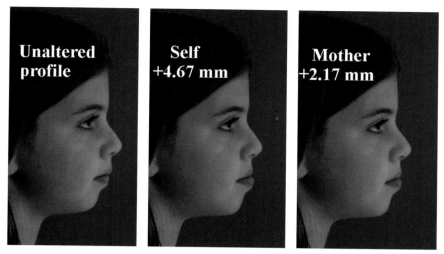

Figure 4.1 Results for most accurate task displaying least accurate patient/mother. (Source: Miner et al., 2007; courtesy of The EH Angle Education and Research Foundation.)

cialists' and patients' perception of the psychosocial benefits of orthodontic treatment (Kiyak, 2008). Thus, what the clinician thinks is best for the patient is not necessarily what the patient and/or parent wants. Note, for example, Miner et al. (2007), who found differences among the perceived preferences of patients, parents, and clinicians, as shown in Figure 4.1. In addition to the assumed skill of the clinician, the actual and perceived behaviors of the orthodontist and staff, including physical appearance, are major factors (Urban et al., 2009), for example, politeness, providing accurate information to enhance health literacy, reassurance, etc. Such demonstration of concern is significantly correlated with compliance and ultimately patient satisfaction (Sinha et al., 1996).

Cognitions, emotions, and behavior influencing motivation for orthodontic treatment

The psychosocial variables intervening between need and demand for treatment can be conceptualized into three domains: *cognition*, which includes memories and perceptions or what we think about verbal or nonverbal communications between patients and clinicians, the accuracy of which is as noted in the next section 'Communication and health literacy'. The *affective* domain includes emotion and associated neurophysiological responses, including facial expression, or *how* we feel about the communication. Emotions also provide cues to intended behaviors regarding whether or not to seek treatment. Attitudes then denote the directionality and magnitude of feeling about the transferred information. Beliefs reflect the influence of age, gender, ethno-cultural and socioeconomic variables determining personal values indicating *why* we feel the way we do about changes in the facial morphology. Emotions certainly enter into a child's decision to accept treatment

because of being teased or bullied related to his or her Class II malocclusion, or reject treatment because braces make him or her look different. Of course, the negative emotional state may be overcome by a promised trip to Disney World.

The *behavioral* domain has three clinically distinct categories: volitional, semi-volitional, and nonvolitional. Volitional behaviors refer to an individual's intended actions mediated by the somatic nervous system, e.g. for speech, preventive oral health, keeping appointments; or conversely, noncompliant actions such as not wearing headgear or elastics, making inappropriate verbal comments, or unreasonable demands such as debonding before an important social event. Also mediated by the somatic nervous system are the semi-volitional behaviors, such as breathing, facial expressions, and most pernicious habits, such as tongue thrusting, nail biting, clenching, smoking, and gum chewing or gagging. Nonvolitional behaviors are primarily under the control of the autonomic nervous and neurohormonal system, of which the patient is not usually aware, such as changes in salivary flow, diaphoretic activity on the upper lip and ventral surface of the hand, pupillary dilation, palpitations, and other responses associated with anxiety, depression, or discomfort related to mechanical tooth movement (Giddon et al., 2007).

Each individual in fact has a unique and consistent pattern of responses across different stressors (Sternbach, 1966; Bakal, 1992; Belsky and Pluess, 2009). The magnitude and duration of these responses may vary on a continuum from simple annoyance to severely disruptive psychopathology. Of relevance to orthodontists is the demonstration of greater psychophysiological responses to simulated distortion of one's own profile than found with distortion of a neutral profile (Amram et al., 1998).

Communication and health literacy

The first step in motivating patients to participate in orthodontic treatment should be to facilitate effective communication among patients, surrogates, and clinicians about the importance of morphology and function of the orofacial area to overall physical and mental health (Colgate, 2006; Jontell and Glick, 2009); the second step is to discuss the advantages and disadvantages of orthodontic treatment. Specifically, does the patient understand the importance of a realistic treatment and is the patient willing to do what is necessary to comply with treatment protocols.

Health literacy is defined as 'the degree to which individuals have the capacity to obtain, process, and understand basic health information and services needed to make appropriate health decisions' (US Department of Health and Human Services, 2000). Deficiencies in health literacy are now a concern of all healthcare professionals (Anderson and Giddon, 2010). Poor health literacy is estimated to affect 90 million Americans (Nielsen-Bohlman and Institute of Medicine (US) Committee on Health Literacy, 2004) and costs the healthcare system US$73 billion annually (in 1998 dollars) (National Academy on an Aging Society, 2009). Poor health literacy is a better predictor of poor health status than age, income, employment, education level, or race (Kutner et al., 2006).

As orthodontic treatment may be uncomfortable, inconvenient, or costly, patients with low health literacy may not fully comprehend the biological reasons for orthodontic treatment. Such patients also may not appreciate the esthetic and oral health benefits or the importance of keeping appointments. As any orthodontist knows, such behaviors occur among affluent and health-literate patients as well, exemplified in the case of a Class II Division 1, 11-year-old patient, the son of two dentists, who was referred for orthodontic treatment. He resisted doing anything other than appearing for the orthodontic consultation. He could not care less about the likely benefits or compliance. In spite of much cajoling by the orthodontist, he discontinued treatment with apparently no psychosocial consequences of a lifelong Class II malocclusion – he became a very successful 'buck-toothed' president of a bank.

As noted by Will (in press), patients do not always understand or remember what they have been told about their malocclusion or the orthodontic treatment plan. After discussing the reasons for the proposed treatment, risks, likely treatment outcome, and responsibilities of patients and clinicians noted in the informed consent form, Mortensen et al. (2003) interviewed children and their parents. Only an average of 1.5 risks out of 4.5 mentioned were recalled by the parents, with less than one by the children. Similarly, of 2.3 reasons for treatment, the parents remembered an average of 1.7 and the children 1.1. Clearly, most of what is important is not remembered by patients or parents.

Perhaps the most critical information to be communicated for a successful treatment outcome is the need for the patient to understand the differences between objective cephalometric data and subjectively determined profile preferences, that is, this distinction is necessary to determine the patient's self-perception of his or her actual facial configuration relative to what changes are being planned and why; and then how the patient feels about these proposed changes. Unfortunately, many misunderstandings about expected changes become examples of deficiencies in health literacy or rather illiteracy. Even the meaning of words used to describe existing and/or desired changes may differ between patient and clinician. To overcome this problem a simple binary classification is suggested, similar to that used with the quantitative, psychophysical facial perception PERCEPTOMETRICS™ method. Thus, negative words such as 'ugly', 'awful', 'grotesque', or 'unattractive' are all classified as 'unacceptable', while positive terms such as 'pretty', 'cute', 'attractive', 'gorgeous', or 'beautiful', or referring to specific features as 'symmetrical', 'protrusive', etc., are classified as 'acceptable' (Giddon, 1995). The same approach can be used to determine the precise anthropometric basis for each one of these negative or positive esthetic descriptors.

What is considered attractive or preferred obviously differs among dental health professionals and lay persons (Prahl-Anderson et al., 1979; Cochrane, et al., 1999). In addition to maximizing cooperation and mutual satisfaction, the use of quantitative methods to establish a range of proposed or preferred changes, rather than a series of single static photo images, will reduce the risk of medicolegal action resulting from unfulfilled expectations which may well have been unrealistic. Thus, it behooves the orthodontist to provide the patient with enough understandable information to agree with an acceptable and realistic expectation of treatment outcome. The treatment process itself can also be the source of disruptive and unnecessary agitation. For example, the problem may simply be due to the failure to explain that biomechanical movement of teeth can cause unpleasantness or pain as the result of unexpected stimulation of tactile or proprioceptive receptors in the periodontal membrane (Giddon et al., 2007). To anticipate problems with patients, it is essential to obtain a detailed medical and social history with a list of medications together with clinical observations and laboratory data as an essential part of effective communication between patient and clinician.

Sensation and perception

Very simply stated, perception begins with sensation, which is objectively defined as the recognition that the sensory receptors have received input from the internal and external environment. Perception may then be defined as a central nervous system process of providing organization and meaning to the incoming sensory information. The quantitative relation of sensation to perception can then be determined mathematically with psychophysical methods (Giddon, 1995; Treutwein, 1995).

Except for expected universal responses to cataclysmic events, there are large individual differences in perception of sensory input which run the gamut from noxious stimulation to the stressor of being different by virtue of being unattractive (McEwen and Gianaros, 2010).

Physical basis of perception of attractiveness

While beauty is traditionally considered to be in the eyes of the beholder, there is increasing evidence of a specific and almost universally agreed-upon configuration of hard and soft tissues being judged as attractive (Jones and Hill, 1993; Anderson and Giddon, 2005; Giddon et al., 2007). As noted by Giddon (1995) and others, the key to understanding the responses to physical appearance is not the actual morphology but the perception by self and significant others as well as the clinician.

An extensive literature exists on improved facial attractiveness as the most important motivation for obtaining orthodontic treatment; for example, some of the benefits attributed to a more attractive face include the perception by others of greater cognitive ability, intelligence, and social skills. Dion et al. (1972) found that attractive individuals were seen as more successful and as achieving higher socioeconomic status and greater marital happiness than those whose faces were judged as unattractive. Subsequent research (Patzer, 1985; Alley, 1988; Wood and Eagly, 2002) provides a consensus across gender, ethnic, and age groups that what is beautiful is good. Compared with unattractive counterparts, attractive individuals receive better grades, higher salaries, shorter prison sentences, and are considered to be more competent, successful, confident, assertive, and likeable, with better mental/physical health. Individuals with attractive dentitions are viewed as more desirable as friends, intelligent, and less likely to behave aggressively than those with unattractive dentitions (Zhang et al., 2006; Jung, 2010).

Perception of facial attractiveness

As noted earlier by Baldwin (1980), approximately 80% of those seeking orthodontic treatment do so for esthetic rather than functional reasons. Potential patients judge their appearance by looking at a reflection of their full face, while the orthodontists base their assessments primarily on the profile, which is not easily viewed by the patient. Hershon and Giddon (1980) pointed out that most people, in fact, have no idea about their own profiles. The fact that perceived personality and other characteristics attributed to the profile differ from those for the full frontal face only adds more complexity and possible shortcomings to the two-dimensional (2D) representations of faces (Bruce et al., 1991; Hancock et al., 2000).

While the orofacial area is more important than the rest of the body in judging overall attractiveness and ultimately self-concept (Currie and Little, 2009), the mouth itself is second only to the eyes in focus of attention (Hassebrauck, 1998). Jornung and Fardal (2007), however, found that patients rated teeth as the most important feature in judging facial attractiveness, with no gender difference (York and Holtzman, 1999). There are many computer methods to derive the ideal face, as shown in Figure 4.2, in which both the male and female faces with shortened lower jaw are considered more attractive than the face with average proportions.

Facial perception *per se* differs from perception in general only in complexity of cognitive, affective, and behavioral responses to objective visual, sensory input; for example, gaze aversion or increasing interpersonal distance from people with craniofacial anomalies (Giddon, 1995). The cognitive, affective, and behavioral responses to perceived anomalies can often have disproportionately greater impact than the actual magnitude of the disfigurement. Individuals with 'mild' dysmorphias as classified by the clinician may be at greater risk for developing psychological problems than those with severe dysmorphias (MacGregor et al., 1953); that is, patients with mild to moderate facial deformities who perceive themselves as near normal may actually experience greater psychological distress than those with more severe anomalies. As shown by Bruun et al. (2008), there is some disagreement even among clinicians about what is classified as mild, moderate, or severe. In general, however, the more severe the deformity, the more consistent and predictable are the negative, often stereotypical, reactions. Such patients may in fact develop a subculture with different methods for coping with social inequities.

The consequences of having more severe craniofacial anomalies such as cleft lip and palate or other relatively severe physical and mental deviations from 'normal' can evoke cognitive, affective, and behavioral responses to being different, whether because of craniofacial anomalies only, or being challenged intellectually or physically, or because of ethnicity/color, size and shape, etc. Encounters such as bullying, isolation, avoidance, and other antisocial behaviors, can result in physical and verbal abuse, adding even more to the decrement in the quality of life compared with unaffected controls (Collett and Speltz, 2007). Day-to-day interactions with peers can be hindered by a poor self-image and resulting low self-esteem. The self-perception of being physically unattractive thus negatively affects a patient's mental health (Giddon and Anderson, 2006).

Patients with visible facial disfigurements tend to be judged as less intelligent, and less athletic, with attributes such as untrustworthiness and dishonesty (MacGregor et al., 1953; Stricker et al., 1979). Even parents may view their unilateral cleft lip and palate children (UCLP) negatively, with a greater likelihood of sexual or physical abuse than non-UCLP children (Sullivan et al., 1991). Children with

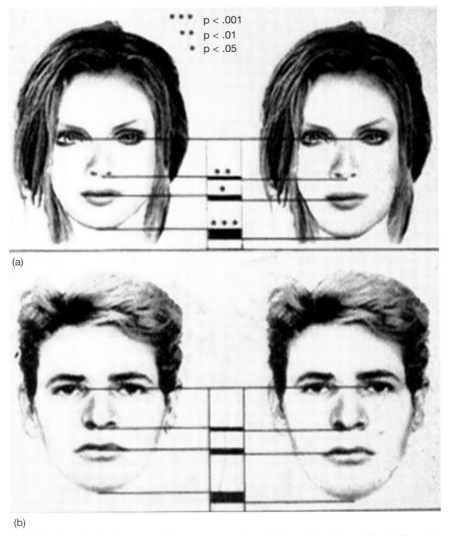

Figure 4.2 Computer-generated female and male faces, one with average proportions (right panels) and one with short lower jaw proportions (left panels). (Source: Johnston and Oliver-Rodriguez, 1997. Available at: www.informaworld.com. Courtesy of Taylor and Francis.)

anomalies often have a lower frustration tolerance, resulting in behavior which increases the household stress and the risk of being maltreated by parents or trusted adults such as teachers (Polnay, 1993). One recognized risk for child abuse is early separation from the parents during hospitalization for primary repair of cleft lip/palate (Sullivan et al., 1991). Also, children with UCLP often have behavioral problems with parents and teachers (Collett and Speltz, 2007), which may become internalized with psycho-physiological manifestations of stress.

Quantitative methods for determining the anthropometric bases for perception of attractiveness

As noted earlier (Albino et al., 1981; Giddon, 1995), the most important psychosocial variable influencing the deci-

sion to seek and comply with orthodontic treatment is the patient's perception of what he or she prefers to accomplish following treatment; in other words, what is in the patient's head or the ideational representation, which the clinician can attempt to elicit by conversation but is more likely to be obtained or inferred from the responses to manipulation of quantitative measures of anthropometric data.

Because most people cannot recall or reproduce their own profiles (Hershon and Giddon, 1980), it is first necessary to determine the accuracy of patients' self-perceptions by comparison with their actual cephalometrically determined data, such as the soft tissue profile, prior to establishing their post-treatment preferred profile. A variety of quantitative methods are now available to assess the physical bases of perceived morphology, many of which use standardized images (e.g. Index of Orthodontic Treatment

Need (IOTN) (Brook and Shaw, 1989). Others use 2D or 3D imaging methods to display anthropometric information for determining the accuracy of the self-perception as well as preferences for post-treatment changes in the soft-tissue profile, e.g. 3DMD, Dolphin Imaging (Sarver, 1993; Berco et al., 2009; Lamichane et al., 2009). Most of these newer techniques, however, still provide a series of static images from which patients can select. In contrast, the psychophysical method of Giddon (1995) and Giddon et al. (1996a,b) used computer morphing of the continuously changing profile image to provide a range rather than a series of discrete images of the preferred outcome of treatment. Specifically, the PERCEPTOMETRICS™ method presents computer-altered photographic images of selected features of the soft tissue profile which are continually morphed in counterbalanced order between retrusive and protrusive extremes of the maxilla and mandible. Patients press the mouse button to indicate the beginning of the acceptable range of changes in profiles and release the button when the changes are no longer acceptable, from which the midpoint of the range in millimeters corrected for actual size can be determined.

The PERCEPTOMETRICS™ method has been used to explore the influence of several psychosocial variables among various patient and clinician groups (Arpino et al., 1998; Kitay et al.. 1999). Hier et al. (1999), for example, compared the preferences for lip fullness between orthodontic patients and untreated subjects, finding that for both genders the untreated subjects preferred fuller lips than orthodontically treated patients. In a comparison of the self-perception of child patients with their mothers and the treating clinicians, Miner et al. (2007) found that both patients and mothers overestimated the protrusiveness of the child's actual mandible, which was consistent with both groups preferring a more protrusive profile for the child than the neutral face. In addition, the mothers had the smallest zone of acceptability or tolerance for change in the soft tissue profile. Similarly, Reluga et al. (2002) confirmed that females had a significantly smaller zone of acceptability than males for tolerance of changes in self-perceived profiles.

These PERCEPTOMETRICS™ studies thus demonstrate the importance of considering racial and cultural influences on the esthetic preferences of orthodontic patients. As noted by Will (in press), such studies point out the inherent inaccuracies of patients' perceptions of themselves relative to the actual cephalometrics (Giddon et al., 1974; Hershon and Giddon, 1980) and serve to remind orthodontists of the need to be sensitive to differences between what the patients themselves prefer to change and the clinician's preferred outcome.

A related concern is the difference in the adjustment of the self-concept between patients undergoing the relatively slower change in the soft tissue profile obtained with the biomechanical movement of teeth and the rapid changes in facial morphology obtained with orthognathic surgery (Arpino et al., 1998), that is, some patients may have considerable difficulty in adjusting their self-image to the sudden improvement in appearance as the result of surgery (MacGregor, 1979). As an example, rhinoplasty patients often continue to hold onto their negative presurgical self-image, until they realize that they can no longer blame continuing social problems on their previously dysmorphic nose. Unfortunately both patients and/or clinicians can be misled by the emotional appeal of the patient about having too large a nose, when in fact, it is their lower facial proportions relative to the nose which may be responsible for the facial disharmony.

Ethno-cultural differences in facial perception

Motivation for orthodontic treatment is also linked to the perception of how much dentofacial appearance deviates from social and cultural norms (Mantzikos, 1998). Americans are more critical than other national groups in judging their own and others' appearance (Cons and Jenny, 1994). In comparing adolescents in the United States with those in Japan and China, it was noted that appearance was the primary characteristic noticed by Americans, with Japanese and Chinese students more focused on specific behaviors. Similarly, Caucasian Americans were the most self-critical of body image and therefore may be at higher risk for becoming 'never satisfied' patients or possibly developing a body dysmorphic disorder (BDD). It is therefore incumbent on orthodontists to determine the reference norms used by patients when discussing the range of acceptable changes in the soft tissue profile.

Given that the differences between Asians and Caucasians in the preferred change in the soft tissue profile are difficult to discern with simple conversation, the use of quantitative psychophysical methods should be considered, particularly for individuals seeking esthetic change outside their country of origin. Regardless of ethnicity, parents in general consistently expect more improvement than their children expect in oral health, function, and quality of life. Non-Hispanic children and their parents expected greater improvement in appearance than other ethnic groups while Latino and African American children expected improved social acceptance from treatment, while all three ethnic groups expected improvement in oral function (Kiyak, 2008). Children of Asian American and mixed ethnicity, followed by Caucasian children, were more likely than any other group to prefer an ideal occlusion (Reichmuth et al., 2005). Although there is no objective evidence that Hispanic children had more severe malocclusions than the other ethnic groups, Hispanic children accepted a larger range of faces as attractive.

Using the PERCEPTOMETRICS™ method for determining ethno-cultural differences, Mexican Americans in general preferred less protrusive lips than Caucasians, which did not hold for the more highly acculturated

Mexican Americans, who may have assimilated more American cultural esthetic values than those who preferred less protrusion (Mejia-Maidel et al., 2005). Compared with Caucasian and Asian American orthodontists, the parents and siblings of Korean American orthodontic patients with previous orthodontic treatment were less likely to expect an ideal occlusion than those without previous treatment; that is, they were more accepting of some malocclusions such as an excessive overbite or overjet (Park et al., 2006). These outcomes again underscore the importance of identifying any ethnically specific factors that may influence an individual patient's motivation and expectations for treatment outcome.

Influence of personality variables in motivation

The relation of facial morphology to personality and other attributes has a long history. 'Personality' as a construct is a constellation of traits and related cognitions, emotions, and behavior. In contrast to more transient psychological states, personality traits are unique to each individual and endure throughout a lifetime.

Personality evolves from the interaction of a genetically determined temperament with the internal and external environments. The influence of temperament throughout life can be seen as early as 4 months (Kagan and Snidman, 2009). Some of the temperament-related responses predictive of subsequent adolescent and adult behavior are activity level, rhythmicity of hunger and sleep, approachability of new stimuli, adaptability to change, threshold for and intensity of reaction, quality of mood, distractibility, and attention (Thomas and Chess, 1977). Historically, there have been many theories about the origin of personality (Adler, 1927; Freud, 1953; Rotter, 1966; Eysenck, 1967; Jung and Campbell, 1971; Hathaway and McKinley, 1983), which in recent years have been factored down to the 'Big Five' (Goldberg, 1993; DeYoung et al., 2010): openness, conscientiousness, extraversion, agreeableness, and neuroticism. The presence of these traits in any given individual is based on their relative positions on a continuum derived from responses to polar opposite scales.

In addition to providing psychobiological information about age, gender, race, fecundity, physical and mental health, the morphology of the orofacial area provides cues to personality and related social behavior. For example, early Greek philosophers attributed related temperaments and dispositions to various geometric facial configurations. In later years, Spurzheim and Gall (1815) suggested that intentions, emotions, and behavior were determined by the distribution of brain tissue, which was reflected in the shape of the skull. They attributed different characteristics (hunger, greed, aggression, and timidity) to specific areas of the brain, which became one of the principal tenets of phrenology or the 'science' of relating personality to head shape. Apparently a version of phrenology continues to be of interest in at least Korea.

Following from phrenology and the relation of morphology to personality, perceptions of brachycephalic persons were compared with dolichocephalic persons (Schack, 2001; Stirrat and Perrett, 2010), finding that brachycephalic faces were perceived as significantly less 'adaptable', 'likeable', and 'honest', and more 'proud' and 'dominant' than the mesofacial and dolichocephalic faces. The attractiveness of dental appearance *per se* has been found to influence perception of intelligence and honesty (Newton et al., 2003; Kershaw et al., 2008).

Child and adolescent development

Stages of development in relation to onset of treatment

When a child is 'ready' to begin treatment depends on where the child is in the physical and mental maturation sequence, that is, the cognitive, emotional, and social developmental stages including behavioral repertoire. According to Piaget et al. (1929), preadolescence is marked by the following stages:

- Preoperational (ages 2–7 years):
  - Learns to use language and to represent objects by images and words
  - Thinking is still egocentric: has difficulty taking the viewpoint of others
  - Classifies objects by a single feature: e.g. groups together all the red blocks regardless of shape
- Concrete operational (ages 7–11 years):
  - Can think logically about objects and events
  - Achieves conservation of number (age 6), mass (age 7), and weight (age 9)
  - Classifies objects according to several features and can order them in series along a single dimension such as size
- Formal operational (ages 11 years +):
  - Can think logically about abstract propositions and test hypotheses systematically
  - Become concerned with the hypothetical relationships among factual information, the future, and ideology.

For most children, orthodontic procedures begin during the concrete operational stage. While children can think logically about events, there is a marked inability to think abstractly, thus limiting the ability to integrate or visualize changes associated with post-treatment outcomes. In the concrete stage, children focus on social and academic skills, compare themselves with their peers in sports and academic skills, friends, and physical appearance. Compared to the pediatrician and general dentist, who focus on functional issues, the orthodontists are sought out because they are the first medical professional in a child's life in the unique position to improve appearance.

Many other recurrent issues exist for children, for example, the attitudes of the media, entertainment, and fashion industries, and dieting continue to contribute to anorexia and bulimia (Giddon, 1985). There is no evidence, however, implicating orthodontic treatment in the propensity of children to develop an eating disorder.

The adolescent orthodontic patient

The teen years are formative in both physical and mental development. Teenagers are discerning their roles in life, struggling with acceptance by peers, and dealing with issues of self-esteem. Adolescence is associated with the stage of 'ego identity vs. role confusion,' (Erikson, 1980) when the child develops his or her unique self-concept. At the same time as great changes are occurring in their bodies and minds, 14–20% of American children and adolescents are being diagnosed with psychiatric disorders, with upwards of 5% of orthodontic patients being diagnosed and/or treated for attention-deficit hyperactivity disorder (ADHD; Neeley et al., 2006a). Orthodontists, more than almost any other health practitioners, should take advantage of their many office visits to be a helpful influence on adolescents during these developmental years.

Given these concerns, the clinician should consider beginning treatment at an earlier stage if self-consciousness about dento-facial appearance is an issue. However, it is also possible that orthodontic appliances might make a child feel different from his peers, in which case the child may not be ready for treatment.

Psychosocial variables influencing compliance

What are some of the most important psychosocial variables facilitating patient cooperation and compliance, which are so essential for a successful treatment outcome? Attitude toward oral health and its relation to adherence to oral health preventive behavior is a major variable. According to social-learning theory, patients with internal loci of control (Rotter, 1966), who believe that their oral health depends on their own efforts, report increased oral health behaviors. Preventive oral health behavior includes the adherence to professional instructions and practicing self-help procedures. Self-efficacy (Bandura, 1977) and later health self-efficacy have been used to explain perceived ability to perform preventive behaviors. Patients considered to have good dental esthetics have greater dentofacial awareness and engage in preventive behaviors more than those with less attractive dentitions. These observations are consistent with recent studies (Johnston et al., 2010) finding that physically attractive people enhance their self-esteem by looking at their own images in the mirror for comparison with others, compared with less attractive individuals who avoid such comparisons. An additional benefit of orthodontic treatment, therefore, may be that monitoring of oral hygiene during orthodontic treatment facilitates maintenance of oral health behaviors.

Using questionnaires (Cucalon and Smith, 1990; Feldmann et al., 2007) and interviews (Albino et al., 1990),

it was found that the more positive the attitude of the parents towards braces, the greater the compliance of the child. Cucalon and Smith (1990) found that being female, with high self-esteem and socioeconomic status, academic performance, involvement in social activities, and relationship with parents was all predictive of patient compliance, with the most compliant patients also being obedient, accommodating, self-confident, polite, and self-conscious (Mehra et al., 1998). Based on two personality measurements, the most cooperative patient was 14 years or younger, enthusiastic, outgoing, hard-working, forthright, and obliging (Allan and Hodgson, 1968), whereas uncooperative patients were those older than 14 years, with superior intelligence, hard-headed, self-sufficient, intolerant, individualistic, impatient, etc. Other variables which correlated with compliance with wearing of headgears and intraoral elastics clustered weakly into four factors:

- Personality type, pain thresholds, inconvenience, and dysfunction
- General health awareness
- Specific dental knowledge
- Personal oral embarrassment.

Girls were generally more cooperative than boys in wearing headgear, which correlated with their need for improved dentofacial esthetics. A good parent–child relationship also appears to facilitate treatment compliance (Kreit et al., 1968). Unfortunately, patients who most needed to wear their headgear were the most troublesome. The authors have also recently attempted to adapt the Frankl Score to predict compliance (Pillar, 2010).

Compliance issues of adolescents at risk for substance abuse

In contrast to its survival role, the oral cavity also serves as a portal of entry for microbial infections, as well as participating in pernicious volitional behaviors such as smoking or recreational drugs. As many as 40% of tenth graders will use an illicit drug at some time in their lives, and 18% within the next 30 days, with an increased risk of suicide and depression (Neeley et al., 2006b). In 2004, the lifetime prevalence for using any illicit drug was estimated at 21.5% in eighth graders and 39.8% in tenth graders (Neeley et al., 2006b).

Again, the frequency of office visits and duration of orthodontic treatment give the orthodontist an opportunity and responsibility to note intraoral and behavioral signs of substance abuse. A few flecks of silver paint around the nose or a propensity for smooth surface caries suggests further enquiry. Behaviorally, patients may begin to miss appointments, have sudden changes in treatment compliance, or become uncharacteristically moody, unruly, or unkempt with poor oral hygiene. Given that orthodontists treat many patients in their formative years, it is appropriate to discuss their observations with the patients' physicians and/or refer them to a mental health professional, particularly when there is a high index of suspicion of abuse.

Identification and management of difficult patients

A difficult patient is one who triggers negative feelings with the potential for unpleasant reaction by the clinician. Having a bad day may be one excuse, but the more likely explanation is that the clinician has some unmet personal needs. Thus, to help to establish the source of the problem, the first requirement for managing difficult patients is to 'know thyself' and become aware of one's own limitations. Until that occurs, the clinician needs to be initially dispassionate and nonjudgmental. Clinicians must recognize that being a difficult patient is a clinical sign of some underlying medical or psychological problem. A wall of indifference does not protect the clinician from overt or covert feelings of his or her own vulnerability. The inability to accept one's own needs and associated anxiety may explain why clinicians who ask psychologists how to manage the apprehensive patient are really asking how to manage the apprehensive clinician.

The prevalence of patients judged as difficult in medical settings is 15–20% (Sharpe et al., 1994; Jackson and Kroenke, 1999), many of whom may display functional symptoms, 'dependent', or 'borderline' personality disorders (Hahn et al., 1994), and are often perceived as untruthful (Woolley and Clements, 1997). Others may simply have had a stigmatizing life, such as prison, substance abuse, or an unattractive physical appearance. Although occasional disruptive episodes can be tolerated, clinicians and staff should be alert to the possibility of frequent atypical behaviors, such as being scheduled more often than needed or missing appointments. Some patients may ultimately be diagnosed with schizophrenia or a social phobia.

Owing to the frequency of visits, orthodontists must assume responsibility for the welfare of children and adolescents during office visits. Continued monitoring is essential for identifying high-risk children by eliciting information about being bullied, disordered eating, depression, substance abuse, and, especially, suicidal ideation. The clinician can minimize the likelihood of stressful doctor–patient interactions from becoming irreversible by setting appropriate limits on the patient's behavior. As noted earlier, one of the best ways to prevent discord is to do whatever is necessary to ensure that the patient has realistic expectations about the treatment and outcome. However, if the intransigence continues, clinicians should not hesitate to refer patients to a mental health professional.

To help the orthodontist understand and communicate with other health professionals about particular patients who may have one of the more frequently encountered mental disorders, a brief description is provided of the American Psychiatric Association system (1994) for classifying mental disorders. These five *Diagnostic and Statistical Manual of Mental Disorders* (DSM) 'axes' are used to place psychiatric diagnoses in a biopsychosocial context: primary/major psychiatric diagnosis on Axis I, pervasive symptomatology (personality disorders and mental retardation) on Axis II, comorbid medical conditions on Axis III, psychosocial environmental factors on Axis IV, and global assessment of functioning on Axis V. While this system is useful for mental health professionals, specialized training is required for accurate nosological distinction among patients.

When the clinician suspects a psychiatric problem, it is essential to review the medical and social history, together with prescription and over-the-counter medications. Because some of the medications affect the structure and function of the orofacial area as well as behavior during orthodontic treatment, it may be useful to divide the drugs into three categories, that is, those used for:

- Comorbid medical conditions
- Psychiatric disorders, which patients often are unwilling to disclose
- Recreational drugs, with similar prohibition on disclosure.

Neeley et al.'s (2006b) publication is an excellent resource for understanding the effects of many of these drugs affecting behavior and/or manifesting in the orofacial area is. In addition to the recognized increase in patients with ADHD and possibly autism spectrum disorders in orthodontic practice noted earlier (Neeley et al., 2006a), the clinician should be aware of the most frequently occurring difficulties with patients, some of whom may have psychiatric disorders. Some examples of problem patients, with suggested recommendations, follow.

The perfectionist patient

Similar to the dissatisfied or malcontent patient, perfectionists have unrealistic expectations of treatment outcomes, but not to the same extent as those with BDD (briefly described later), who are consumed by their obsessions and who may be delusional. Perfectionists are always comparing themselves to an 'ideal' which by definition cannot be achieved. The initial interview should be of sufficient depth to establish the extent to which a patient has consulted other dentists and a multitude of orthodontists. The clinician should ensure that the patient understands the goals of the treatment. Be wary of, 'I am happy, but . . .', not accepting even minor asymmetries or deviations from their expectations.

Example of perfectionist patient

Patient CP, 40-year-old business woman who needed extractions of all four premolar for protrusion, mild crowding.

- CP was concerned with appearance.
- She was 'obsessed' about incomplete space closure, slowness of treatment, with concern about occlusion.

- She insisted on frequent visits to attempt to remedy the problem.
- She was finally dismissed from the practice.

Suggestions

- The anticipated post-treatment extra time and frustration can be minimized by providing a more in-depth initial interview to elicit examples of problems with other healthcare providers and/or self-described examples of obsessive tendencies.
- Use of software (PERCEPTOMETRICS)™ or other morphing methods to provide gradations of photo images helps separate realistic from unrealistic expectations.
- The clinician should modify his or her method for obtaining informed consent from the patient to include a range of expected outcomes rather than an unattainable static image.

Even though orthodontists may not initially recognize such potentially difficult patients, those with borderline personality disorder (BPD) or BDD can be particularly troublesome.

The body dysmorphic disorder patient

A more extreme variant of the perfectionist is the BDD patient. First seen in early childhood and adolescence, the BDD patient is consumed by the obsessive concern with an actual or perceived imperfection in some body part, usually of the orofacial area (Veale, 2004). In addition to obsessive–compulsive disorder and possible hallucinations, a BDD patient may also be depressed with substance abuse problems. Although there is little research on the impact of BDD on orthodontic practice, the clinician should carefully consider whether to treat BDD patients, who unfortunately never appear to be satisfied. Moreover, similar to the perfectionist, actual or attempted correction of one feature often leads to obsessing with another feature (Hepburn and Cunningham, 2006).

The borderline personality disorder patient

BPD is a serious mental disorder which often is unrecognized by the orthodontist, except for some inappropriate behaviors. When suspected, the clinician must be mindful of the patient's seductive, manipulative behaviors (Hannig, n.d.), avoiding disclosure of personal information while clearly establishing that socially inappropriate behaviors will not be tolerated. However, 'don't be surprised or take it personally if the patient shifts from being very positive to a very critical attitude', yet expecting only the best care and very critical of anything less (FE Yeomans, 2010, personal communication). Orthodontists also must be alert to the increase in depression and suicidal ideation in BPD patients (up to 33%) (Neeley et al., 2006a). In patients with suicidal ideation, 55–65% have been found to have a personality disorder (Loochtan and Cole, 1991).

The narcissistic patient

Narcissistic patients possess an enhanced sense of entitlement, particularly in an American culture in which children are increasingly told that they are 'special'. Because of their overinflated sense of importance, narcissistic adult patients feel that they deserve special treatment, even at the expense of others. These patients are often tardy, repeatedly rescheduling or canceling appointments, and despite acknowledging disruptive office behavior, expect special treatment. Narcissistic patients believe that they can only be understood and helped by those with high status; they exhibit discourteous behavior toward those with lesser status, only wanting to see the orthodontist. Patients may engage in provocative behaviors, such as touching the orthodontist in an attempt to gain special treatment. They also cite their influential stature in the community, which can be used to increase the orthodontist's practice. When dissatisfied, narcissists are less likely to forgive delayed treatment, even when due to their own noncompliance with keeping appointments, or not wearing elastics or retainers.

Moreover, meeting their initial demands can result in a pattern of behaviors in which they dominate the office. Patients who are extraordinarily demanding often have a history of unsatisfied need and may have been overly indulged as children. Frustration and anger only add to the discomfort of the office staff, often evoking hostility towards these patients. Consistent with the psychoanalytic theory of countertransference, everyone, including patients, can have attributes and behaviors that clinicians may find detestable (Winnicott, 1949). While feeling angry and hostile toward a patient is acceptable, acting hostile, mean or varying treatment plans to retaliate is not. Tolerating aberrant patient behavior does not mean passive acceptance; rather it should mean just a holding pattern until limits are discussed with the difficult patient. Noncompliant and argumentative patients can and should be confronted, pointing out their provocative or disruptive behaviors. Regardless of excellent treatment outcomes, such patients are never pleased with the efforts of the orthodontist or anyone else.

Example of a narcissistic patient

AA, an adult female patient, had minor malalignment of front teeth with good Class I buccal occlusion. Alignment was not good enough and she frequently complained to other dentists.

- Patient told occlusion was fine.
- Finally agreed to debond; then went through many retainers.

Suggestions

- Validate the patient's anger by remaining nondefensive and agreeing with the demand for a high quality of care.

- Remember that the patient's real problem may be an underlying fear of losing control, etc.
- Help the patient communicate more effectively.
- Establish limits and maintain consistency throughout your practice by ensuring that no staff members are granting special favors, either because of bullying or actually believing that the narcissistic patient is special.
- Patient needs to be instructed when to call and for what reason.
- Do not anticipate gratitude for granting special favors; moreover, once one demand is met, another will follow.
- Personnel changes may cause problems with patients accustomed to getting special favors from previous employees.
- Take extra precautions with the narcissistic patient to ensure that they understand, and obtain a witnessed signature attesting that they understand the informed consent form and billing process, including fee schedule and penalties.

The search engine patient

A search engine patient presents for treatment armed with a packet of photographs of desired outcomes and stacks of articles regarding orthodontic treatment which they obtained via internet searches. They are inherently poor listeners, being fixated and eager to share their own theories about the orthodontic treatment plan. During the pretreatment consult they may frequently interrupt and dominate the interaction, soliciting information already provided. They may give the impression of not having comprehended much of the information being presented by the orthodontist. These interactions can also become extremely frustrating and time-consuming for the orthodontist and office staff, who can look 'forward' to each appointment bringing new search engine questions. After the treatment the orthodontists should be prepared for the patient, who has been unrealistic about the outcome, to accuse them of not fully explaining the initial treatment plan.

Suggestions

- Acknowledge the patient's 'research' efforts.
- Reinforce your credentials as a trained orthodontist without sounding defensive or pretentious.
- Point out why the patient's comprehension and application of his/her acquired information may not be applicable to your own treatment plan.
- Be direct even if bordering on rudeness.
- Provide your own written materials about the proposed treatment, which you should review with the patient.
- Before obtaining the patient's signature on the informed consent form, make sure to note any variation in proposed treatment plans.

Conclusion

In summary, the authors have discussed the role of many of the most important psychosocial factors involved in the diagnosis, implementation, and problems of compliance with orthodontic treatment.

References

Adler A (1927) *The Practice and Theory of Individual Psychology.* New York, NY: Harcourt.

Albino JE, Cunat JJ, Fox RN, et al. (1981) Variables discriminating individuals who seek orthodontic treatment. *Journal of Dental Research* 60: 1661–7.

Albino JE, Alley TR, Tedesco LA, et al. (1990) Esthetic issues in behavioral dentistry. *Annals of Behavioral Medicine* 12: 148–55.

Allan TK, Hodgson EW (1968) The use of personality measurements as a determinant of patient cooperation in an orthodontic practice. *American Journal of Orthodontics* 54: 433–40.

Alley TR (1988) *Social and Applied Aspects of Perceiving Faces.* Hillsdale, NJ: Lawrence Erlbaum Assoc.

American Psychiatric Association (1994) *Quick Reference to the Diagnostic Criteria from DSM-IV.* Washington, DC: American Psychiatric Association.

Amram D, Anderson NK, Giddon DB (1998) Affective and physiological responses to self-confrontation with computer displayed profile images. *Psychophysiology* 35: S16.

Anderson N, Giddon D (2005) What is beauty? The discourse continues. *Global Health Nexus (published by NYU College of Dentistry)* 7: 84–7.

Anderson NK, Giddon DB (2010) Comparing state CHIP dental literature reading levels to literacy rates. *Journal of Dental Research* 89: Spec Iss A.

Anon (2005) *Crooked Teeth Leave Negative First Impression.* Available at: www.dentalplans.com/articles/2285/crooked-teeth-leave-negative-first-impression.html (accessed 6 June 2010).

Arpino V, Giddon DB, BeGole EA, et al. (1998) Presurgical profile preference of patients and clinicians. *American Journal of Orthodontics and Dentofacial Orthopedics* 114: 631–7.

Bakal DA (1992) *Understanding Stress, in Psychology and Health,* 2nd edn. New York, NY: Springer Publishing Co., pp. 67–105.

Baldwin DC (1980) Appearance and aesthetics in oral health. *Community Dentistry and Oral Epidemiology* 9: 244–56.

Bandura A (1977) Self-efficacy: toward a unifying theory of behavioral change. *Psychological Review* 84: 191–215.

Belsky J, Pluess M (2009) Beyond diathesis stress: Differential susceptibility to environmental influences. *Psychological Bulletin* 135: 885–908.

Berco M, Rigali PH Jr, Miner RM, et al. (2009) Accuracy and reliability of linear cephalometric measurements from cone-beam computed tomography scans of a dry human skull. *American Journal of Orthodontics and Dentofacial Orthopedics* 136: 17 e1–9; discussion 17–18.

Bick J (2007) A badge of childhood, now worn by more adults. *The New York Times,* January 14, 6.

Brook PH, Shaw WC (1989) The development of an index of orthodontic treatment priority. *European Journal of Orthodontics* 11: 309–20.

Bruce V, Doyle T, Dench N, et al. (1991) Remembering facial configurations. *Cognition* 38: 109–44.

Bruun R, Chima K, Hocking C, et al. (2008) *Perception of the Severity of Treated Unilateral Cleft Lip and Palate Patients (UCLP) Among Providers, Parents and Educators.* Chapel Hill, NC: American Cleft Palate Association.

Cervantes M. *Don Quixote de la Mancha.* Trans. C Jarvis. (1819) Available at: http://books.google.com (accessed 20 August 2010).

Cochrane S, Cunningham S, Hunt N (1999) A comparison of the perception of facial profiles by the general public and 3 groups of clinicians. *International Journal of Adult Orthodontics and Orthognathic Surgery* 14: 291–5.

Colgate (2006) White papers: new research and commentary on the oral-systemic relationship – periodontal microbiota and carotid intima-media thickness – the oral infections and vascular disease epidemiology study (INVEST), reprinted from *Circulation* 111: 576–82, 2005, vol 1, issue 2. Yardley, PA: Professional Audience Communications, Inc.

Collett BR, Speltz ML (2007) A developmental approach to mental health for children and adolescents with orofacial clefts. *Orthodontics and Craniofacial Research* 10: 138–48.

Cons NC, Jenny J (1994) Comparing perceptions of dental aesthetics in the USA with those in eleven ethnic groups. *International Dental Journal* 44: 489–94.

Cucalon A 3rd, Smith RJ (1990) Relationship between compliance by adolescent orthodontic patients and performance on psychological tests. *Angle Orthodontist* 60: 107–14.

Currie TE, Little A (2009) The relative importance of the face and body in judgments of human physical attractiveness. *Evolution and Human Behavior* 30: 409–16.

DeYoung CG, Hirsh JB, Shane MS, et al. (2010) Testing predictions from personality neuroscience: brain structure and the big five. *Psychological Science* 21: 820–8.

Dion K, Berscheid E, Walster E (1972) What is beautiful is good. *Journal of Personality and Social Psychology* 24(3): 285–90.

Erikson EH (1980) *Identity and the Life Cycle.* New York, NY: Norton.

Eysenck HJ (1967) *The Biological Basis of Personality.* Springfield, IL: Charles C Thomas.

Feldmann I, List T, John MT, et al. (2007) Reliability of a questionnaire assessing experiences of adolescents in orthodontic treatment. *Angle Orthodontist* 77: 311–17.

Freud S (1953) *A General Introduction to Psychoanalysis.* New York, NY: Washington Square Press.

Friedman S, Fisher C (1967) On the presence of a rhythmic, diurnal, oral instinctual drive cycle in man: A preliminary report. *Journal of the American Psychoanalytic Association* 15: 317–43.

Giddon DB (1985) Ethical considerations for the fashion industry. In: MR Solomon (ed.) *The Psychology of Fashion.* Lexington, MA: DC Heath Company, pp. 225–32.

Giddon DB (1995) Orthodontic applications of psychological and perceptual studies of facial esthetics. *Seminars in Orthodontics* 1: 82–93.

Giddon DB (1999) Mental-dental interface: window to the psyche and soma. *Perspectives in Biology and Medicine* 43: 84–97.

Giddon D, Anderson N (2006) The oral and craniofacial area and interpersonal attraction. In: D Mostofsky, A Forgione, D Giddon (eds) *Behavioral Dentistry.* Ames, IA: Blackwell Publishing, pp. 3–17.

Giddon DB, Hershon LE, Lennartsson B (1974) Discrepancy between objective and subjective profile measures. *Scandinavian Journal of Dental Research* 82: 527–35.

Giddon DB, Bernier DL, Kinchen JA, et al. (1996a) Comparison of two computer-animated imaging programs for quantifying facial profile preference. *Perceptual and Motor Skills* 82: 1251–64.

Giddon DB, Sconzo R, Kinchen JA, et al. (1996b) Quantitative comparison of computerized discrete and animated profile preferences. *Angle Orthodontist* 66: 419–26.

Giddon DB, Anderson NK, Will LA (2007) Cognitive, affective, and behavioral responses associated with mechanical tooth movement. *Seminars in Orthodontics* 13: 212–19.

Goldberg LR (1993) The structure of phenotypic personality traits. *American Psychologist* 48: 26–34.

Hahn SR, Thompson KS, Wills TA, et al. (1994) The difficult doctor-patient relationship: somatization, personality and psychopathology. *Journal of Clinical Epidemiology* 47: 647–57.

Hancock PJ, Bruce VV, Burton AM (2000) Recognition of unfamiliar faces. *Trends in Cognitive Science* 4: 330–7.

Hannig PJ (n.d.) Borderline personality disorder: profile and process of therapy. (First published in *Primal Renaissance: The Journal of Primal Psychology* 1995; 1: 54–71.) Available at: www.primals.org/articles/hannig03.html (accessed 7 January 2010).

Hassebrauck M (1998) The visual process method: a new method to study physical attractiveness. *Evolution and Human Behavior* 19: 111–23.

Hathaway SR, McKinley JC (1983) *The Minnesota Multiphasic Personality Inventory.* New York, NY: Psychological Corporation.

Hepburn S, Cunningham S (2006) Body dysmorphic disorder in adult orthodontic patients, *American Journal of Orthodontics and Dentofacial Orthopedics* 130: 569–74.

Hershon LE, Giddon DB (1980) Determinants of facial profile self-perception. *American Journal of Orthodontics* 78: 279–95.

Hier LA, Evans CA, BeGole EA, et al. (1999) Comparison of preferences in lip position using computer animated imaging. *Angle Orthodontist* 69: 231–8.

Izard CE (1971) *The Face of Emotion.* East Norwalk, CT: Appleton-Century-Crofts.

Jackson JL, Kroenke K (1999) Difficult patient encounters in the ambulatory clinic: clinical predictors and outcomes. *Archives of Internal Medicine* 159: 1069–75.

Johnston C, Hunt O, Burden D, et al. (2010) Self-perception of dentofacial attractiveness among patients requiring orthognathic surgery. *Angle Orthodontist* 80: 361–6.

Johnston VS, Oliver-Rodriguez JC (1997) Facial beauty and the late positive component of event related potentials. *Journal of Sex Research* 34: 188–98.

Jones D (2009) *Relating Self-Reported Orofacial Behaviors to Standardized Psychometric Scales.* DMD thesis. Harvard School of Dental Medicine, Boston, MA.

Jones D, Hill K (1993) Criteria of facial attractiveness in five populations. *Human Nature* 4: 271–96.

Jontell M, Glick M (2009) Oral health care professionals' identification of cardiovascular disease risk among patients in private dental offices in Sweden. *Journal of the American Dental Association* 140: 1385–91.

Jornung J, Fardal O (2007) Perceptions of patients' smiles: a comparison of patients' and dentists' opinions. *Journal of the American Dental Association* 138: 1544–53; quiz 1613–14.

Jung CG, Campbell J (eds) (1971) *The Portable Jung.* New York, NY: Viking Press.

Jung MH (2010) Evaluation of the effects of malocclusion and orthodontic treatment on self-esteem in an adolescent population. *American Journal of Orthodontics and Dentofacial Orthopedics* 138: 160–6.

Kagan J, Snidman N (2009) *The Long Shadow of Temperament.* Cambridge, MA: Belknap Press of Harvard University.

Kenealy PM, Kingdon A, Richmond S, et al. (2007) The Cardiff dental study: a 20-year critical evaluation of the psychological health gain from orthodontic treatment. *British Journal of Health Psychology* 12: 17–49.

Kenrick DT, Griskevicius V, Neuberg SL, et al. (2010) Renovating the pyramid of needs: Contemporary extensions built upon ancient foundations. *Perspectives on Psychological Science* 5: 292–314.

Kershaw S, Newton JT, Williams DM (2008) The influence of tooth colour on the perceptions of personal characteristics among female dental patients: comparisons of unmodified, decayed and 'whitened' teeth. *British Dental Journal* 204: E9; discussion 256–7.

King G (n.d.) *Access to Orthodontic Services in the US.* Available at: www.aaomembers.org/mtgs/upload/King-Access-to-Orthodontic-Care-The-Problem-and-Some-Solutions.pdf (accessed 28 June 2010).

Kitada R, Johnsrude IS, Kochiyama T, et al. (2010) Brain networks involved in haptic and visual identification of facial expressions of emotion: An fMRI study. *Neuroimage* 49: 1677–89.

Kitay D, BeGole EA, Evans CA, et al. (1999) Computer animated comparison of self perception with actual profiles of orthodontic and nonorthodontic subjects. *International Journal of Adult Orthodontics and Orthognathic Surgery* 14: 125–34.

Kiyak HA (2008) Does orthodontic treatment affect patients' quality of life? *Journal of Dental Education* 72: 886–94.

Kreit LH, Burstone C, Delman L (1968) Patient cooperation in orthodontic treatment. *Journal of the American College of Dentists* 35: 327–32.

Kutner M, Greenberg E, Jin Y, et al. (2006) *The Health Literacy of America's Adults: Results from the 2003 National Assessment of Adult Literacy.* US Department of Education, National Center for Education Statistics, Washington, DC.

Lamichane M, Anderson NK, Rigali PH, et al. (2009) Accuracy of reconstructed images from cone-beam computed tomography scans. *American Journal of Orthodontics and Dentofacial Orthopedics* 136: 156 e1–6; discussion 156–7.

Loochtan RM, Cole RM (1991) Adolescent suicide in orthodontics: results of a survey. *American Journal of Orthodontics and Dentofacial Orthopedics* 100: 180–7.

Lorand S, Feldman S (1955) The symbolism of teeth in dreams. *International Journal of Psycho-Analysis* 36: 145–60.

MacGregor FC (1979) *After Plastic Surgery: Adaptation and Adjustment.* New York, NY: Praeger.

MacGregor FC, Abel TM, Bryt A, et al. (1953) *Facial Deformities and Plastic Surgery: A Psychosocial Study.* Springfield, IL: Charles C. Thomas.

Mantzikos T (1998) Esthetic soft tissue profile preferences among the Japanese population. *American Journal of Orthodontics and Dentofacial Orthopedics* 114: 1–7.

Maslow A (1943) A theory of human motivation. *Psychological Review* 50: 370–96.

Maslow A (1970) *Motivation and Personality*, 2nd edn. New York, NY: Harper and Row, Inc.

McEwen BS, Gianaros PJ (2010) Central role of the brain in stress and adaptation: links to socioeconomic status, health, and disease. *Annals of the New York Academy of Sciences* 1186: 190–222.

Mehra T, Nanda RS, Sinha PK (1998) Orthodontists' assessment and management of patient compliance. *Angle Orthodontist* 68: 115–22.

Mejia-Maidel M, Evans CA, Viana G, et al. (2005) Preferences for Mexican facial profiles between Mexica Americans and Caucasians. *Angle Orthodontist* 75: 763–8.

Miller ES, Larson LL (1979) A theory of psycho-orthodontics with practical application to office techniques. *Angle Orthodontist* 49: 85–91.

Miner RM, Anderson N, Evans C, et al. (2007) The perception of children's computer-imaged facial profiles by patients, mothers and clinicians. *Angle Orthodontist* 77: 1034–9.

Mortensen MG, Kiyak HA, Omnell L (2003) Patient and parent understanding of informed consent in orthodontics. *American Journal of Orthodontics and Dentofacial Orthopedics* 124: 541–50.

National Academy on an Aging Society (2009). *Fact Sheet: Low Health Literacy Skills Increase Annual Health Care Expenditures by $73 billion.* Available at: www.agingsociety.org/agingsociety/publications/fact/fact_low.html (accessed 23 June 2010).

Neeley WW 2nd, Kluemper GT, Hays LR (2006a) Psychiatry in orthodontics. Part 1: Typical adolescent psychiatric disorders and their relevance to orthodontic practice. *American Journal of Orthodontics and Dentofacial Orthopedics* 129: 176–84.

Neeley WW 2nd, Kluemper GT, Hays LR (2006b) Psychiatry in orthodontics. Part 2: Substance abuse among adolescents and its relevance to orthodontic practice. *American Journal of Orthodontics and Dentofacial Orthopedics* 129: 185–93.

Newton JT, Prabhu N, Robinson, PG (2003) The impact of dental appearance on the appraisal of personal characteristics. *International Journal of Prosthodontics* 16: 429–34.

Nielsen-Bohlman L, Institute of Medicine (US) Committee on Health Literacy (2004) *Health Literacy: a Prescription to End Confusion.* Washington, DC: National Academies Press.

Park YS, Evans CA, Viana G, et al. (2006) Profile preferences of Korean American orthodontic patients and orthodontists. *World Journal of Orthodontics* 7: 286–92.

Patzer GL (1985) *The Physical Attractiveness Phenomena.* New York, NY: Plenum Press.

Penfield W, Rasmussen T (1978) *The Cerebral Cortex of Man: A Clinical Study of Localization of Function.* New York, NY: Macmillan Publishing Co.

Piaget J, Tomlinson J, Tomlinson A (1929). *The Child's Conception of the World.* London: K Paul, Trench, Trubner and Co., Harcourt, Brace and Company.

Pillar A (2010) *An Evaluation of the Efficacy of the Frankl Behavior Rating Scale in an orthodontic Setting.* Postdoctoral thesis, Stony Brook University School of Dental Medicine, New York, NY.

Polnay L (1993) *Manual of Community Paediatrics*, 2nd edn. Edinburgh: WB Saunders.

Prahl-Anderson B, Boersma H, van der Linden FPGM, et al. (1979) Perceptions of dentofacial morphology by laypersons, general dentists, and orthodontists. *Journal of the American Dental Association* 98: 209–12.

Reichmuth M, Greene KA, Orsini MG, et al. (2005) Occlusal perceptions of children seeking orthodontic treatment: impact of ethnicity and socioeconomic status. *American Journal of Orthodontics and Dentofacial Orthopedics* 128: 575–82.

Reluga KC, Anderson NK, Giddon DB (2002) Gender differences in computer-animated profile self-perception. *Journal of Dental Research* 81: 153.

Rotter JB (1966) Generalized expectancies for internal versus external control of reinforcement. *Psychological Monographs* 80: 1–28.

Sarver DM (1993) Videoimaging: The pros and cons. *Angle Orthodontist* 63: 167–70.

Schack K (2001) *Personality and Craniofacial Morphometry.* Postdoctoral thesis, Harvard School of Dental Medicine, Boston, MA.

Sharpe M, Mayou R, Seagroatt V, et al. (1994) Why do doctors find some patients difficult to help? *Quarterly Journal of Medicine* 87: 187–93.

Sinha PK, Nanda RS, McNeil DW (1996) Perceived orthodontist behaviors that predict patient satisfaction, orthodontist-patient relationship, and patient adherence in orthodontic treatment. *American Journal of Orthodontics and Dentofacial Orthopedics* 110: 370–7.

Spurzheim JG (1815) *The Physiognomical System of Drs. Gall and Spurzheim*, 2nd edn. London: Baldwin, Cradock & Joy.

Sternbach RA (1966) Individual response-stereotypy. In: RA Sternbach (ed.) *Principles of Psychophysiology.* New York, NY: Academic Press, pp. 95–109.

Stirrat M, Perrett DI (2010) Valid facial cues to cooperation and trust: Male facial width and trustworthiness. *Psychological Science* 21: 349–54.

Stricker G, Clifford E, Cohen LK, et al. (1979) Psychosocial aspects of craniofacial disfigurement (Proceedings of 1974 Conference). *American Journal of Orthodontics* 76: 410–22.

Sullivan PM, Brookhouser PE, Scanlan JM, et al. (1991) Patterns of physical and sexual abuse of communicatively handicapped children. *Annals of Otology, Rhinology and Laryngology* 100: 188–94.

Thomas A, Chess S (eds) (1977) *Temperament and Development.* New York, NY: Brunner/Mazel.

Treutwein B (1995) Adaptive psychophysical procedures (minireview). *Vision Research* 35(17): 2503–22.

Urban NJ, Anderson NK, Giddon DB (2009) The influence of orthodontists' and dentists' physical attributes on patient selection. *American Association of Orthodontists Annual Meeting*, Boston, MA.

US Department of Health and Human Services (2000) *Healthy People 2010: Understanding and Improving Health*, 2nd edn. Washington, DC: US Government Printing Office.

Veale D (2004) Body dysmorphic disorder. *Postgraduate Medical Journal* 80: 67–71.

Will LA (in press) Psychological aspects of diagnosis and treatment. In: LW Graber, RL Vanardsall and KWL Vig (eds) *Orthodontics: Current Principles and Techniques.* USA: Elsevier/Mosby.

Winnicott D (1949) Hate in the counter transference. *International Journal of Psycho-Analysis* 30: 69–75.

Wood W, Eagly AH (2002) A cross-cultural analysis of the behavior of women and men: implications for the origins of sex differences. *Psychological Bulletin* 128(5): 699–727.

Woolley D, Clements T (1997) Family medicine residents' and community physicians' concerns about patient truthfulness. *Academic Medicine* 72: 155–7.

York J, Holtzman J (1999) Facial attractiveness and the aged. *Special Care in Dentistry* 19: 84–8.

Zhang M, McGrath C, Hagg U (2006) The impact of malocclusion and its treatment on quality of life: a literature review. *International Journal of Paediatric Dentistry* 16: 381–7.

5

Nutrition in Orthodontic Practice

Lauren Schindler, Carole A Palmer

Summary

Maintenance of good general dental health and optimal orthodontic outcomes are greatly dependent on adequate nutrition. The development of the oral cavity and its structures is influenced by the nutritional state of an individual and both deficiencies and toxicities may cause malformations. After tooth eruption, nutritional factors influence the teeth topically and have great impact on both the prevention and development of dental caries. Good nutrition can maximize while poor nutrition can undermine the appropriate biological response of the periodontal ligament and alveolar bone to orthodontic forces.

Orthodontic practitioners, by virtue of patient contact at a nutritionally sensitive period, are in a good position to screen/assess for inadequate nutrition and poor eating behaviors. Simple, quick, and routine diet risk assessment tools (which are different from the more extensive nutritional assessments done by dietitians and nutritionists) can be used during the office visit. Depending on the results of this assessment, the practitioner can either choose to provide simple dietary recommendations and guidance to patients or, if more complex nutritional issues or disease is uncovered, refer them to specialists such as physicians, registered dietitians, and/or therapists. The key to effective diet education in the orthodontic office is a logical, ordered approach, which includes patient education, data collection, data evaluation/diagnosis, providing nutrition guidance, follow-up and re-evaluation, and a few key personalized recommendations.

A basic understanding of nutrition as well as good guidance and communication skills, will help orthodontic practitioners to improve their orthodontic outcomes in addition to helping improve the quality of life of their patients.

Introduction: the role of the orthodontist in nutrition

Nutrition, oral health, and general health are inextricably linked. In his 2000 report on *Oral Health in America*, the Surgeon General of the United States emphasized the need for 'all healthcare providers' to play an 'active role in promoting healthy lifestyles … by incorporating nutrition counseling into their practices' (US Department of Health and Human Services et al., 2000). This is particularly important for dental professionals, as oral health plays an important role in nutrition and vice versa. The health of the oral cavity can facilitate or impede the desire and ability to eat. Conversely, diet and nutrition play important roles in oral health promotion and caries prevention.

The orthodontist is well positioned to help screen for dietary issues, as well as provide meaningful dietary advice. Many orthodontists report regularly engaging in dietary discussions with their patients (Huang et al., 2006). Nutrition and diet are relevant topics between practitioner and patient as good nutrition maximizes orthodontic outcomes. Orthodontists usually see patients in childhood or early adolescence. This allows for early detection of and intervention for dietary problems. When nutrition issues relate directly to dental or orthodontic issues, the orthodontist can assist in promoting behavior change for oral health. When nutrition issues are beyond the orthodontic scope of practice, referral can be made to a physician or registered dietitian.

This chapter will review the relevance of nutrition to orthodontics and how the orthodontist can assist in facilitating good nutrition for good oral health. Additionally, this chapter will provide practical advice about delivering patient education designed to promote positive dietary behavior change. A point to note before considering this in more depth is that in casual conversation the terms *diet* and *nutrition* are often used interchangeably. However, particularly in an oral health context, the difference between the two is important. *Diet* is the pattern of food intake, the ways in which people eat. This includes their individual food choices, the frequency of eating, and the underlying values

---

Integrated Clinical Orthodontics, First Edition. Edited by Vinod Krishnan, Ze'ev Davidovitch.
© 2012 Blackwell Publishing Ltd. Published 2012 by Blackwell Publishing Ltd.

that determine what foods are eaten or avoided. This is particularly important in dental caries etiology and prevention. *Nutrition* is the systemic effect of food on the body. *Malnutrition* can mean undernutrition, overnutrition, or nutrition that contributes to ill health such as in cardiovascular disease.

What is an adequate diet?

An adequate diet is a diet that meets all of the known nutritional requirements for health. As knowledge is ever increasing about human nutritional requirements, dietary standards and guidelines are continuously updated to reflect these changes. Known human nutrient requirements are documented in the dietary reference intakes (DRIs) in the United States, and are available in table form (http://fnic.nal.usda.gov). Most countries have similar standards, however, as the standards are listed in physiologically needed amounts (e.g. grams, milligrams, micrograms/day etc.) and not in commonly consumed foods, they are not useful for educating the public. Thus, dietary guidelines and food grouping systems have been devised, as translations of the DRIs into the foods that provide them. Foods are grouped by similar nutrient content. The most recent and most comprehensive food grouping system for the United States is called MyPlate (http://www.choosemyplate.gov Figure 5.1), which not only provides the general diet guidelines for health but also provides specific recommendations based on age, gender, weight, and exercise level. Table 5.1 shows examples of the recommended daily food intake for two teenagers and two adults. The most useful approaches to diet assessment and education in dental practice compare the patient's usual food intakes with these standards to determine general adequacy/potential concerns. The MyPlate website may be appealing for the tech-savvy adolescent age group. See Table 5.2 for a summary of

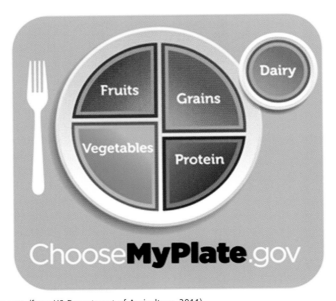

Figure 5.1 http://www.choosemyplate.gov, (from US Department of Agriculture, 2011)

Table 5.1 Recommended daily portions of food groups by age/gender/weight/activity

Person	Grains	Fruits	Vegetables	Dairy	Protein
14-year-old girl, 1.6 m (5′4″), 52 kg (115 lb), mild activity	140 g (5 oz)	1.5 cups	2 cups	3 cups	140 g (5 oz)
14-year-old boy, 1.75 m (5′10″), 68 kg (150 lb), mild activity	198 g (7 oz)	2 cups	3 cups	3 cups	170 g (6 oz)
30-year-old woman, 1.6 m (5′4″), 63 kg (140 lb), minimal activity	170 g (6 oz)	2 cups	2.5 cups	3 cups	156 g (5.5 oz)
45-year-old man, 1.8 m (6′0″), 79.5 kg (175 lb), mild activity	226 g (8 oz)	2 cups	3 cups	3 cups	184 g (6.5 oz)

Source: US Department of Agriculture (2010).

Table 5.2 Guidelines for a healthy diet

Categories	Key recommendations for adults and adolescents	Practical recommendations for patients for improving diet quality
Fruit	2+ cups of fruit per day	Add fresh fruit to cereal, granola, oatmeal, waffles, pancakes, toast, or yogurt
		Eat fruit for snacks
		Eat fruit for dessert with frozen yogurt or whipped topping
		Fresh, canned, frozen, and dried fruits all count, but choose those without added sugar or heavy syrup
Vegetables	2.5+ cups of vegetables per day	Eat fresh vegetables with a dip or hummus for snacking
		Add vegetables to pasta dishes, casseroles, pizza, or stir-fries, sandwiches
		Start meals with a small salad
		Fresh, canned, or frozen vegetables all count, but choose those without add salt or butter or creamy sauces
Dairy	3 cups of low-fat or fat-free dairy per day	Use low-fat or fat-free milk on your cereal
		Snack on low-fat or fat-free yogurt or cheese
		Add low-fat or fat-free cheese to sandwiches or salad
Starches and grains	3–6 28 g (1 oz) servings of whole grains per day with the rest of grains coming from enriched grain products	Choose wholegrain bread products, wholegrain pasta, brown rice, barley, and bulgar for meals
		Choose wholegrain crackers, plain popcorn, or oatmeal cookies for snacks
Fat	Adults: Total fat should comprise 20–35% of the total calories with most coming from monounsaturated fats and polyunsaturated fats Adolescents: Total fat should comprise 25–35% of the total calories with most coming from monounsaturated fats and polyunsaturated fats	Vegetables oils, fatty fish, avocados, nuts, and nut butters are all good sources of mono- and polyunsaturated fats
		Serve salmon for dinner or add it as a protein to a salad
		Add avocado to sandwiches, salads, or eat it as a snack with lemon
		Cook with vegetable oil instead or lard or butter
		Snack on nuts or make a nut butter sandwich
	Saturated fats should be limited to less than 10% of total calories	Limit red meat, lard and full-fat dairy including milk, yogurt, cheese, sour cream, butter, cream, ice cream
	Limit *trans* fat to as low as possible	Limit fried fastfood, commercially prepared bakery goods (pies, donuts, cookies crackers), and shortenings
Protein	114 g (4 oz)/day. Choose lean protein	Lean flesh proteins include: lean cuts of beef (tenderloin, flank steak, roast beef, or London broil); lean cuts of pork (tenderloin or fresh ham); lean cuts of veal and lamb (roast or chop); chicken and turkey meat with skin removed; fish and shellfish, tuna canned in water; sardines; and low-fat luncheon meats
		Lean vegetarian proteins include: tofu, beans, low-fat cheese or cottage cheese, egg whites, and egg substitute
Added sugars	Limit added sugars	Limit general sweets such as cookies, candies and chocolate
		Limit drinking sugar-sweetened beverages including regular soda, sweetened coffee or tea, energy drinks, sports drinks, or imitation fruit drinks
	Practice good dental hygiene and consume sugar- and starch-containing foods less often to reduce the risk of dental caries	Limit sugar-containing foods in between meals
		Limit sucking on hard candies, breath mints or cough drops
		Avoid constantly sipping on sugar sweetened beverages including regular soda, sweetened coffee or tea, energy drink, sports drinks, or imitation fruit drinks
Physical activity	Adults: 30 minutes of moderate- intensity physical activity to reduce the risk of chronic disease and 60 minutes to prevent gradual weight gain into adulthood Adolescents: 60 minutes of physical activity most days of the week	Take the stairs, park further from the store in a parking lot, limit time in front of the television and computer, join a sports team or a gym or walk outside
Minerals	Limit sodium to 2300 mg/day	Limit processed foods such as frozen meals or partially prepared boxed meal starters
		Choose low-sodium or no-salt-added canned foods or rinse regular canned foods
		Avoid adding extra salt during cooking or at the table

Adapted from US Department of Health and Human Services and US Department of Agriculture, 2005. (US Department of Health and Human Services, US Department of Agriculture (2005) *Dietary Guidelines for Americans, 2005.* Washington DC: Government Printing Office.)

the diet recommendations for adolescents and adults along with practical recommendations for meeting these guidelines.

Nutrition and the orthodontic patient

Importance of nutrition during development and for maintenance of oral tissues

Growth and development of all tissues and structures, including that of the oral cavity, directly depend on adequate nutrition. Tooth development begins *in utero* and continues until the third decade of life, when the third molars emerge into the oral cavity, and all teeth complete root formation. Following their emergence into the oral cavity the dental crowns become exposed to the oral environment. At the time of emergence, the dental roots are incomplete, and while the eruptive movement continues, the tissues surrounding the teeth model and remodel, as part of overall growth, and this activity continues in adult life. In both young people and adults, nutrition plays a pivotal role in determining the nature of tissue growth, remodeling, and the individual response to physical and chemical challenges. Thus, all age groups are dependent on consistent good nutrition (Romito, 2003).

Oral development (including tooth mineralization) begins *in utero* and prenatal nutrition of the mother is the first important factor that affects the ultimate oral development of the child (Tinanoff and Palmer, 2000). Maternal deficiencies of folic acid, riboflavin, and zinc during pregnancy can lead to severe craniofacial abnormalities such as cleft lip and palate in the child. General malnutrition and specific nutrient deficiencies (as well as nutrient toxicities) during tooth development can adversely affect tooth size, formation, and eruption pattern. For example, protein deficiency during early childhood can affect the tooth size and eruption sequence. Vitamin C deficiency may alter collagen formation and bone development. In developing countries where malnutrition is rampant, such nutrition-related defects are commonly observed. In developed countries, however, overt malnutrition and specific nutrient deficiencies are less common (Romito, 2003). However, issues related to nutrient toxicity do occur. A few years ago, the accidental over-fortification of milk with vitamin D by a commercial dairy resulted in malformation defects in erupted dentition in a young child (Giunta, 1998). Thus, orthodontists should be aware of the importance of nutrition during oral growth and development, and should counsel pregnant women about the importance of optimal nutrition for the well-being of their unborn child as well as for their own health. They should caution against the random use of nutritional supplements other than multivitamins or calcium/vitamin D supplements, unless they are prescribed by a physician.

Role of diet in dental caries

The orthodontist is in an ideal position to educate patients about diet and dental caries, since orthodontic appliances increase the available surfaces for plaque accumulation, resulting in more areas for caries to occur. Following eruption, teeth are most susceptible to dental caries (2–5 years for deciduous teeth and early adolescence for permanent teeth). Caries is the result of demineralization of tooth enamel and dentin by organic acids formed by bacterial metabolism of dietary sugars. The development of dental caries is influenced primarily by the total amount of time fermentable carbohydrates (simple sugars: mono and disaccharides) are in contact with cariogenic plaque. Thus, the frequency of consumption, form of sugar (indicating retention of sugar in the mouth), and timing of consumption (at or in-between meals) are the important factors in determining caries risk. It is important to remember that the total amount of sugars consumed does not seem to be the most important factor in the cariogenic potential of the diet. Dietary patterns that include frequent snacking/sipping on foods or beverages that contain simple sugars are more conducive to caries development than infrequent snacking (Moynihan and Petersen, 2004). Table 5.3 shows the relative cariogenicity of various foods.

Defining 'sugar'

For the general public, the term *sugar* that is associated with dental caries is often equated with the disaccharide sucrose, or table sugar. However, all monosaccharides (glucose, fructose, galactose) and disaccharides (sucrose, maltose, lactose) have cariogenic potential. In the realm of dental health, the term *fermentable carbohydrate*s is often used for those carbohydrates that can be metabolized by bacteria to produce acid and as a result, increase caries risk (Kandelman, 1997). These are primarily the mono- and disaccharides, but starches can also be cariogenic when held in the mouth long enough for salivary amylase to hydrolyze them to simple sugars.

For simplicity in making recommendations to patients, it is important to communicate that protein, fats, and food

Table 5.3 General cariogenic potential of different types of snack

Cariogenecity		
Low	Moderate	High
Cheese sticks	Chocolate	Dried fruit
Cheese and crackers	Yogurt	Candy, lollipops, hard candy
Nuts	Ice cream	Popsicles
Sugar-free pudding	Fruit	Juice
Vegetables with dip		Soda
Pieces of meat		Cake, cookies, pie
Hard-boiled egg		

fibers are not cariogenic. The only cariogenic foods are those that are composed of one or more of the simple sugars. These include sugars added during manufacturing (formerly sucrose, now primarily high-fructose corn syrup) as well as table sugar added in cooking or at the table and naturally occurring sugar found in fruit, juice, honey, and molasses (Moynihan and Petersen, 2004).

How diet can help protect the teeth against caries
Saliva plays a major role in preventing dental caries by promoting enamel remineralization, cleansing the mouth, and helping neutralize acids. The act of chewing facilitates salivary flow. Many medications, including common over-the-counter ones such as antihistamines, can cause decreased salivary flow or xerostomia. Xerostomia increases the caries risk associated with the diet, due to the loss of the acid-mitigating effects. Thus hydration to maintain salivary flow is vital for caries prevention.

Fluoride is commonly accepted to be the most effective way to protect against dental caries. Fluoride increases the resistance of enamel to demineralization by organic acids following sugar consumption. Frequent exposure to fluoride helps protect enamel against the detrimental effects of acid, but it does not eliminate the risk of developing caries. Overly frequent consumption of cariogenic sugars can overwhelm the benefits of fluoride. The primary source of fluoride is fluoridated community drinking water. Fluoride is also found in tea, but is not present in appreciable amounts in most other foods. Most bottled waters are not good sources of fluoride. The most reliable source is fluoridated drinking water and fluoridated dentifrice (Moynihan and Petersen, 2004).

Some foods may also help protect against enamel demineralization. Studies have shown that cheese, when provided to plaque after a cariogenic challenge such as a cookie, immediately facilitates plaque return to neutral (Kashket and DePaola, 2002). Although the etiological mechanism is not clear, it has been postulated that the salivary stimulating effect of the chewing of these foods, the remineralizing effect of the calcium from the cheese, or the plaque-coating effect of the fat from the cheese or nuts, may be contributing factors. Chewing gum (artificially sweetened) has the same beneficial effect. Gum containing xylitol has a heightened effect as the xylitol itself is cariostatic (Lynch and Milgrom, 2003). Unfortunately, sugar-free chewing gum and nuts may not be appropriate suggestions for orthodontic patients.

Adult dental caries
With increasing age, often gingival recession exposes the less highly mineralized cementum to the oral cavity, leading to increased susceptibility to root caries. Some dietary habits common in adults can increase the risk of root caries. These include use of breath mints or hard candies to sweeten the breath, and constant sipping on sugar-

Box 5.1 Common categories of medications that cause xerostomia, anticholinergics

Antidepressants and antipsychotics
- Selective serotonin-reuptake inhibitors
- Tricyclic antidepressants
- Heterocyclic antidepressants
- Monoamine oxidase inhibitors
- Atypical antidepressants
  Diuretics
  Antihypertensive
  Sedative
  Muscle relaxants
  Antihistamines
  Analgesics

Adapted from Guggenheimer J, Moore PA (2003) Xerostomia: etiology, recognition and treatment. *Journal of the American Dental Association* 134(1): 61–9.

sweetened beverages such as coffee, tea, soda, or juice throughout the day – often to alleviate the effects of xerostomia (Moynihan and Petersen, 2004). Medical conditions associated with xerostomia and an increased caries risk include Sjögren syndrome, therapeutic radiation to the head and neck, and use of pharmacological agents with xerostomic side effects. Common medications that cause xerostomia are shown in Box 5.1. If hydration alone cannot alleviate xerostomia, artificial saliva is available over the counter. Sucking on sugar-free candies or lozenges also helps some patients (Guggenheimer and Moore, 2003).

Importance of nutrition during orthodontic treatment

Not only is adequate nutrition important for proper development and maintenance of the oral cavity, it also plays a role in facilitating the tissue reactions to orthodontic force systems applied to the periodontal ligament and alveolar bone. During orthodontic treatment, applied force systems mechanically induce inflammation to encourage the bone modeling and remodeling process, eventually leading to tooth movement. Appropriate and efficient tooth movement requires a healthy biological response from the alveolar bone and periodontal ligament. This biological response, as well as the bone modeling/remodeling processes, requires adequate nutrition. Theoretically, any nutrient abnormalities (deficiencies or toxicities of carbohydrates, fat, protein, vitamins, minerals and/or water) can influence the proper biological response to applied force systems and undermine orthodontic outcomes.

Studies delineating the specific roles for systemic nutrition and single nutrients during orthodontic treatment are sparse, and many conclusions have been extrapolated from animal studies. Vitamin C deficiency is one classic example of the effects of nutrient deficiency on orthodontic outcomes. A study of lateral forces on guinea pig incisors during vitamin C deficiency resulted in significant alterations to the periodontal ligament and supporting alveolar bone as compared with control animals without deficiency (Litton, 1974). Vitamin C deficiency is theorized to interfere with collagen synthesis, disturbing both the integrity of the periodontal ligament and the formation of osteoid (Hickory and Nanda, 1981).

Additionally, studies outlining the relationship between nutrition and the bone modeling process involved specifically with orthodontic forces are sparse and are also currently limited to animal studies. However, the role of nutrition in general bone modeling/remodeling and bone health is well documented in the literature and can be extrapolated to the bone modeling that occurs during orthodontic tooth movement. Most adult peak bone mass is acquired through bone modeling during childhood and adolescence. Nutritional deficits during this life period may set the stage for poor bone, as well as tooth integrity later in life, leading to osteoporosis or osteopenia. Nutritional deficiencies during more intensive bone modeling – as occurs during orthodontic force application – can greatly influence final outcomes. Many nutrients are important for bone health, including calcium, phosphorus, magnesium, copper, zinc, iron, fluoride, and vitamins D, A, C, and K (Ilich and Kerstetter, 2000).

Most studies conclude that calcium intake is directly correlated with bone mineral density and short-term bone accretion in children and adolescents, although long-term bone accretion is less well understood (Ilich and Kerstetter, 2000; Rizzoli, 2008). Calcium is the bulk cation of which bone is constructed while also indirectly regulating the bone remodeling process. It must be absorbed in sufficient quantities to build bone structure during growth and maintain it in maturity. Although adequate intakes are important for bone health, excessive amounts of calcium (generally >2500 mg/day) may interfere with absorption of other nutrients, such as iron (Roberts et al., 2006).

Animal studies confirm that diets high in phosphorus and low in calcium (much like the common beverage profile of high cola and low dairy intake) are detrimental to bone mass (Calvo, 1994). Magnesium deficiency in animals has resulted in uncoupling of bone resorption and formation (Rude, 1998; Creedon et al., 1999), and poor bone strength and development (Rude et al., 1999). Other studies have found that bone fragility was increased in rats that were iron deficient (Medeiros et al., 1997). Vitamin K deficiency and vitamin A toxicity have been found to increase bone resorption and fragility in humans (Hathcock et al., 1990; Kanai et al., 1997; Feskanich et al., 1999). Energy deficits also adversely affect bone and tooth health. Studies examining patients with anorexia nervosa (characterized by food restriction, dangerously low body weight, amenorrhea, hypoestrogenemia, multiple nutrient deficiencies and general malnutrition) found increased bone resorption and decreased bone formation (Hotta et al., 2000).

> **Box 5.2** Practical dietary recommendations to minimize appliance breakage
>
> - Avoid hard foods such as hard candies or lollipops
> - Avoid crunchy foods such as nuts or popcorn
> - Avoid sticky foods such as taffy or caramels
> - Avoid chewy foods such as gum or chewy fruits snacks
> - Avoid chewing on ice cubes
> - Use caution when eating hard fresh fruits or vegetables. Cut them into small pieces and chew them with your back teeth.
> - Use caution when biting into tough meats, hard cheeses, or crusty breads Cut them into small bites and chew them with your back teeth.

Another principal dietary concern during orthodontic treatment arises from the physical presence of the appliances. Brackets and banding increase surface area and exposure time for debris and demineralization on hard and soft oral tissues. Therefore, eating for general caries prevention becomes an even greater priority. To minimize fixed appliance breakage, a more gentle diet is also recommended. See Box 5.2 for dietary recommendations to minimize appliance breakage.

Age-specific concerns influencing diet and orthodontic treatment

Another important nutritional consideration during orthodontic treatment is the stage of life of patients. Orthodontic patients are often treated during the adolescent growth spurt. This growth period is the time for increased nutritional requirements, making dietary choices even more important (Hickory and Nanda 1981).

The child: the childhood obesity issue

Today, one in three American children is defined as overweight or obese. Childhood obesity has more than tripled in the past 30 years. It is widely understood that obese children are more likely to become obese adults and are more likely to have risk factors for adult onset chronic diseases such as cardiovascular disease and type 2 diabetes (Dietz and Gortmaker, 1985). Obese children are also more likely to have low self-esteem, which may contribute to poor socialization and poor academic performance (Schwartz and Puhl, 2003).

The etiology of obesity is multifactorial and includes genetic and lifestyle components such as diet and physical activity. Other factors contributing to childhood obesity are the home and school environments, the larger community, and societal environments. However, there is current consensus among the scientific community that diet and nutrition play a significant role in childhood obesity. Worsening dietary habits such as eating larger portions, snacking frequently, and consuming sugar-laden beverages are postulated to contribute to childhood obesity (Institute of Medicine, 2005). These dietary patterns are also associated with increased risk of dental caries and therefore can and should be addressed in the orthodontic office. As the US Surgeon General recommended, the entire healthcare team must be willing to address nutrition issues to improve the health of our youth amidst the current childhood obesity epidemic.

The adolescent

Psychosocial influences on food choices

Adolescence encompasses major changes in physical, emotional, psychosocial, and cognitive development. Adolescent girls complete physical growth and begin the process of 'figure development'. As their bodies develop in our modern society that idealizes the 'ultra-thin' (and unrealistic) figure, girls may try out different weight loss techniques (Pinkham, 2005). Many studies show a high prevalence of weight-control behaviors among adolescents, especially girls. One study, Eating Among Teens (Project EAT), found that 45% of adolescent girls were trying to lose weight. Often times, they choose unhealthful weight-loss techniques such as use of diet pills, laxatives, diuretics, or vomiting. Project EAT found that 12% of girls report these extreme weight-loss behaviors. Evidence of these behaviors could indicate more serious psychological conditions such as bulimia or anorexia nervosa. Oftentimes, evidence of eating disorders first appears in the oral cavity. The patient may complain that 'my teeth are flaking off'. When evidence of these behaviors is found, patients should be referred for medical evaluation. Many hospitals now have eating disorders clinics which provide important multidisciplinary care.

Alternatively, adolescent boys' major physical growth continues and calorie requirements increase significantly. Appetite usually increases dramatically, resulting in consumption of large amounts of food. Although more common among girls, dieting and extreme weight-loss behaviors also occur among adolescent boys. Project EAT reports that 21% of boys were currently trying to lose weight while 5% reported using extreme behaviors to achieve weight loss (Neumark-Sztainer et al., 2004).

Typical eating patterns

Among both male and female adolescents, dietary patterns are generally poor. Starting in adolescents, more food is consumed away from the home and teens begin to make their own food choices. Food may be used to establish an independent identity separate from the family unit. As adolescents begin to exert their independence from family life, peer influence becomes more significant and may influence foods choices. Characteristic patterns include (Pinkham, 2005):

- Irregular meals
- Meal skipping
- Frequent snacking
- Vending machine use
- Fast food purchases

- High sugar-sweetened, carbonated, and/or caffeinated beverage intake
- Mindless eating.

These patterns do not align with generally healthful eating recommendations for adolescents and also significantly affect oral health. For example, poor calcium intake is common in girls, precisely during this most important period of bone density accretion. Also, frequent use of sugar-sweetened beverages and frequent snacking can be associated with increased caries risk in teens (Yaghi, 2001). It is important to understand the factors that foster teen eating behaviors in order to be able to be effective in helping teens make diet improvements.

The adult

The demography of orthodontics is changing rapidly. The American Association of Orthodontists now reports that one in five orthodontic patients is an adult. Adult patients can come with their own particular challenges. Typically, adult patients have a more lengthy medical history. Many adults have chronic diseases that may influence treatment. Practitioners should have an understanding of these diseases, their impact on the oral cavity and orthodontic treatment, and refer patients for further care if it appears that these health conditions are not well controlled. For example, type 2 diabetes mellitus is common and often results from adult obesity. If a patient's diabetes is not well controlled, they may have episodes of hypoglycemia or hyperglycemia in the dental office. Quickly absorbed sugar such as fruit juice or cake frosting should be kept on hand for the hypoglycemia that can occur if a patient has not eaten before their appointment. Patients will require medical attention if hyperglycemia is suspected. Those with poorly controlled diabetes may carry hard candies with them to use to overcome hypoglycemia, but if these are used too frequently, dental caries could result. Many adults also take one or more medications with xerostomic side effects and subsequently are at increased risk of root caries and recurrent caries around existing dental restorations.

Effective nutrition management of the orthodontic patient

Practitioner strategies for addressing diet and nutrition

Although adequate nutrition and appropriate dietary choices are essential for effective orthodontic treatment, it is understood that nutrition and dietary discussions are rarely the sole topic during orthodontic visits. They are one of many topics that are covered in a short visit. As expected, dietary discussions in orthodontic offices are less involved than those in dietitians' or nutritionists' offices. However, orthodontists can conduct simple, quick, and routine diet

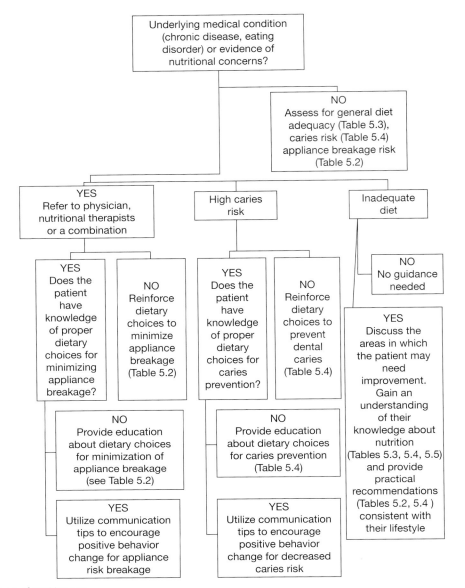

Figure 5.2 Flow diagram of nutrition care.

risk assessments which are very different from full nutritional assessments that are performed by registered dietitians or nutritionists. A diet risk assessment in the orthodontic setting is a quick and simple screening tool used to assess the general diet quality, caries risk, and orthodontic appliance breakage risk. After conducting a diet risk assessment, orthodontic practitioners use information from the assessment to provide simple dietary recommendations and guidance to patients. When there are underlying medical conditions, evidence of nutrient deficiencies or if dietary issues are too complex to address in the orthodontic setting, referrals to appropriate practitioners (registered dietitians, physicians, therapists) can be made (see Figure 5.2).

How to provide meaningful diet and nutrition recommendations and guidance to patients in an orthodontic practice

The key to success in diet education is to have a logical, ordered approach and to personalize recommendations. As with any medical or dental procedure, the following order should be followed.

Patient education

Patients may be surprised to be discussing nutrition and diet during an orthodontic visit. This is a good opportunity for practitioners to explain the importance of dietary choices during orthodontic treatment. An example is provided below. Note that the term *food* is used rather than the term *diet*. Oftentimes for patients, the term diet has a negative connotation and it is usually best to avoid it.

Example

Our number one treatment goal for every patient is to produce a great smile in a reasonable time period. Food choices can have an impact on the outcome of your treatment, so it is important that we don't overlook food as an important factor. I'm going to explain to you how foods can affect your orthodontic care. Then, if you don't mind, we are going to ask you a few questions about the types of foods you eat and how often you eat them. With this information we can provide you with the best possible orthodontic care. Is that all right with you?

This introduction is important as it sets the stage for the care plan which follows and provides the patient with a context for the diet questions.

It is also important to assess the patient's knowledge about diet, and oral and orthodontic health. This can be done with a few simple questions (Box 5.3). This step may appear less critical than others but it is the key to providing efficient and relevant education and recommendations to patients. It is especially important not to waste time teaching patients things they already know.

Box 5.3 Questions to assess patients' knowledge of positive eating behaviors

- What foods do you think can contribute to developing dental caries/cavities? Why?
- What types of foods do you think you should worry about during orthodontic treatment? Why?
- What do you think about your diet?
- What are some healthy things you believe you are doing?
- What are some things you believe you may need to improve about your diet?

Needs assessment/data collection

Generally, two types of data are gathered during the collection stage: subjective data and objective data.

Subjective data

Subjective data are data that the patient reports, such as the history, and does not include anything the practitioner observes directly. An example is a patient disclosing that she drinks at least 1 L of sugar-sweetened soda each day throughout her afternoon at work.

In the orthodontic setting, a diet risk assessment tool using a few simple questions can quickly capture diet quality. There are three major dietary areas to consider in the orthodontic setting: overall diet adequacy, dietary patterns for caries risk, and food choices for risk of appliance breakage. See Figures 5.3–5.5 for diet assessment tools addressing these major topics. These tools can be handed to patients to fill out on their own before the orthodontic visit. However, it is usually better in developing patient rapport for practitioners to ask the questions directly during the orthodontic visit.

Objective data

Objective data are data that are observed by the practitioner through clinical examination. The oral cavity is particularly sensitive to nutrition, as cell turnover is very rapid (3–7 days). Clinical manifestations of deficiencies or toxicities will appear first in the oral cavity before appearing in other body sites. Thus, the oral examination can be an important tool for early detection of nutritional concerns. For example, clinical signs of vitamin B complex deficiencies include:

- Cracking at the corners of the lips (angular cheilosis)
- Inflammation of the corners of the mouth (angular stomatitis)
- Purple or red swollen or smooth tongue (glossitis)
- Inflammation of the oral mucosa causing painful eating or swallowing
- Secondary infection with fungi or bacteria.

Dietary adequacy		
On a daily basis, do you always have AT LEAST:		
4–6 1 oz servings of grain products? (1 oz = 1 slice of bread, 1/2 cup cereal, pasta, rice)	Yes	No
2 pieces or 1/2 cups of fruit or juice	Yes	No
2, 1/2 cup servings of vegetables	Yes	No
3 servings of milk, cheese, yogurt, or ice cream (1 serving of milk/yogurt = 1 cup, ice cream = 1.5 cups, cheese = 1 oz or 1 slice)	Yes	No
4 oz of meat, poultry, fish, eggs, beans	Yes	No

Note: the serving sizes suggested in this table are appropriate for adults and growing adolescents. Children may require smaller servings.

Results: for any 'No' responses, make suggestions from Table 5.2.

Figure 5.3 Diet risk assessment.

Diet habits that increase caries risk		
On a usual or typical day do you:		
Have more than three between meal snacks (including beverages)	Yes	No
Sip slowly on sweetened beverages between meals (e.g. sodas, juice, sweet coffee/tea/cocoa etc.)	Yes	No
Have snacks that include cake, cookies, candy, pastry more than once	Yes	No
Have sweet beverages more than once	Yes	No
Use hard candies, lollipops, or breath mints between meals	Yes	No

Results: for any 'Yes' responses, make suggestions from Table 5.2.

Figure 5.4 Caries risk assessment questionnaire.

Do you eat:		
Hard foods such as hard candies or lollipops	Yes	No
Crunchy foods such as nuts or popcorn	Yes	No
Sticky foods such as taffy or caramels	Yes	No
Chewy foods such as gum or chewy fruits snacks	Yes	No
Ice cubes	Yes	No
Hard fresh fruits or vegetables	Yes	No
Tough meats, hard cheeses or crusty breads	Yes	No

Results: for any 'Yes' responses, make suggestions from Box 5.3.

Figure 5.5 Orthodontic appliance breakage risk assessment.

Additionally, dental enamel demineralization is usually an indicator of frequent use of acidic beverages and may even be an indicator of the eating disorder bulimia.

It is important to note that clinical manifestations may have many causes beyond nutritional deficiencies. Conversely, a lack of clinical oral manifestations does not definitively rule out nutrient deficiencies. Before a definitive diagnosis of a nutrient deficiency is made, biochemical testing is required.

Data evaluation/diagnosis

Data evaluation is the process of assembling an overall picture of patients' dietary status based on subjective data (as collected from the diet assessment tools) and objective data (as collected from the clinical evaluation). Findings that indicate that there is a significant nutrition problem are usually beyond an orthodontist's scope of practice and indicate that a referral should be made. Figure 5.2 provides a decision tree in the form of a flow diagram to assist in the evaluation process in order to determine the proper path to intervention. For example, finding evidence of nutrition deficiencies or an underlying medical condition such as bulimia nervosa or diabetes mellitus cannot be dealt with in the orthodontic setting. On the other hand, simple suggestions to improve food group intake, or reduce the cari-

ogenic potential of the diet are well within the realm of practice of the orthodontist. The diet risk assessment (Figure 5.3) will provide the appropriate direction for needed interventions.

Example

On performing the clinical examination for a new patient, and going through three quick assessment tools (to evaluate diet adequacy, caries risk, and appliance breakage) and scoring the assessments, the practitioner found that the patient's caries risk was high. The practitioner asked the patient if he knew what kinds of foods contributed to caries and the patient was very knowledgeable.

Practitioner: So, I can see that you know a lot about the kinds of foods that cause dental caries. This is good to hear. However, our questionnaire on dental caries risk shows us that your risk is fairly high due to snacking on candy in-between meals. So, I am interested in when, where, and why you are snacking on candies? (Note: avoiding judgment)

Patient: I snack on chocolate because the secretary at the office always has a huge basket of chocolates out on her desk. Every time I walk to the copy machine, I grab a piece. I can't resist them. Chocolate is one of my favorite foods.

Table 5.4 Practical dietary recommendations for preventing and managing dental caries

Limit	Choose instead
Foods and drinks that contain added sugars to fewer than four times per day, especially in between meals	In between meals, snack on foods with minimal added sugars such as low-fat or fat-free dairy, whole grain crackers, nuts, or fresh fruits and vegetables
Sucking on hard candies, breath mints or cough drops	Sugar-free hard candies, breath mints, cough drops
Constantly sipping on sugar sweetened beverages including regular soda, sweetened coffee or tea, energy drink, sports drinks or imitation fruit drinks	To drink to thirst and hydration needs Water, low-fat or fat-free milk, or sugar-free beverages

Practitioner: Can you explain more about why you have them? Are you hungry? Are you stressed? Is it a mindless action? Or do you really, really enjoy every piece you take?

Patient: I don't know. It's probably a mindless habit. I do love chocolate though.

Practitioner: I can imagine how difficult it is to avoid something as good as chocolate if it's right in front of you all day [note: empathy]. But I have some concern about your caries risk. Snacking on sweets for extended periods of time (for example, throughout the afternoon) puts your teeth at much greater risk for developing caries – even more so than just sitting down and have chocolate at one sitting. Would you be interested in discussing ways to try to avoid eating so much chocolate throughout the afternoon?

Patient: Sure.

Practitioner: Can you think of a goal related to decreasing your chocolate intake throughout the afternoon? It should be a small goal that you believe you can achieve.

Patient: I could avoid the chocolate altogether.

Practitioner: Do you think that is a realistic goal?

Patient: Probably not.

Practitioner: What do you think is a more realistic goal?

Patient: How about I stop for chocolate only once. I think that is realistic.

Practitioner: I think that sounds like a good idea.

Providing nutrition guidance

The guidance needed will be dictated by the findings of the diet risk assessment. The orthodontist should work with the patient to determine appropriate improvements in the form of goals.

Goals should be small and should be set by patients and practitioners collaboratively. This ensures that patients are taking an active part in their treatment (Rollnick et al., 1999). Goals are important for moving the patient in the right direction. It is unrealistic to expect patients to immediately make major changes. Long-term goals can be divided into small, short-term goals that are specific, measurable, achievable, and realistic. The goals for improvement should be based on the findings of the diet assessment and thus personalized to the patients' individual situation. Table 5.2 provides suggestions for general diet improvement. Table 5.4 provides suggestions for decreasing cariogenic risk. Box 5.2 provides guidance on avoiding orthodontic appliance breakage.

Follow-up and reassessment

Re-evaluation is necessary to determine if any progress has been made on the dietary patterns discussed in the previous visit. It is usually best to start by asking patients if they believe they have made any progress with the dietary changes discussed during the last visit. Subjective and objective data can be collected again to gain a more concrete understanding of any progress. Depending on the patient's progress, the practitioner can provide reinforcement on dietary choices or they can discuss barriers that prevent dietary changes from occurring (Palmer, 2007).

An important note on enhancing communication between practitioner and patient

The communication process is complicated and messages can be easily misinterpreted. Success or failure in facilitating behavior change depends primarily on the approach of the practitioner. Thus, good communication skills are essential. The following are some tips for enhancing communication (Rollnick et al., 1999; Palmer, 2007):

- Provide a supportive environment. Make sure the environment is friendly and free of distractions
- Be egalitarian. Treat all with equal respect and dignity
- Be nonjudgmental. Bring up sensitive topics descriptively
- Use active and reflective listening. Acknowledge patients while they talk with verbal and nonverbal feedback
- Maintain eye contact
- Be empathetic
- Ask open-ended questions (how, why, what, could, tell me – questions that do not lead to one word answers)
- Encourage patients to do most of the talking
- Brainstorm solutions. Discuss specifically how patients will undertake behavior change – have patients discuss specific actions they plan to take. Also, explore how they will handle challenging situations
- Examine past efforts, both successes and failures. Discuss techniques that worked for patients in the past. Empower them to try those strategies to change dietary, oral, and orthodontic behaviors

---

Box 5.4 Nutrition resources for the orthodontic practitioner

- Palmer C (2007) *Diet and Nutrition in Oral Health*, 2nd edn. Upper Saddle River NJ: Prentice Hall
- American Dietetic Association: www.Eatright.org
- Food and Nutrition Information Center: http://fnic.nal.usda.gov
- MyPyramid: www.Mypyramid.gov
- National Institutes of Health Office of Dietary Supplements: www.nih.od.gov
- Rollnick S, Mason P, Butler C (1999) *Health Behavior Change: A Guide for Practitioners*. Philadelphia, PA: Churchill Livingstone

---

- Ask patients if they have any concerns about their current behavior
- Try to tap into patients' values. Ask questions that subtly relate their current negative behaviors to their values and allow them to discover discrepancies
- Having patients compare the costs and benefits (or pros and cons) of changing behaviors or staying the same
- Have patients make all of the decisions for change for themselves.

Conclusions

Nutrition is an important factor to consider for all dental professionals, including orthodontists. Adequate nutrition allows for proper growth and development and a proper healing response during applied orthodontic forces. Additionally, dietary patterns greatly influence dental caries risk and development of many chronic diseases, for example type 2 diabetes mellitus, both of which affect the health of the oral cavity. Life stage is another important consideration during orthodontic treatment. Children, adolescents, and adults each come with characteristic eating patterns that may present challenges in the orthodontic setting. However, orthodontists must remember that every patient is an individual. Quick and simple dietary assessments can be used to evaluate individual eating patterns that may affect overall diet adequacy, caries risk, or appliance breakage risk (Figures 5.3–5.5) – those areas relevant to orthodontic outcomes. Then individual recommendations can be made to patients, utilizing effective communication strategies. Box 5.4 provides a list of additional resources on nutrition and oral health, dietary recommendations, dietary supplements, and facilitating patient behavior change.

References

Calvo MS (1994) The effects of high phosphorus intake on calcium homeostasis. *Advances in Nutritional Research* 9: 183–207.

Creedon A, Flynn A, Cashman K (1999) The effect of moderately and severely restricted dietary magnesium intakes on bone composition and bone metabolism in the rat. *British Journal of Nutrition* 82: 63–71.

Dietz WH Jr, Gortmaker SL (1985) Do we fatten our children at the television set? Obesity and television viewing in children and adolescents. *Pediatrics* 75: 807–12.

Feskanich D, Weber P, Willett WC, et al. (1999) Vitamin K intake and hip fractures in women: a prospective study. *American Journal of Clinical Nutrition* 69: 74–9.

Giunta JL (1998) Dental changes in hypervitaminosis D. *Oral Surgery, Oral Medicine, Oral Pathology, Oral Radiology and Endodontics* 85: 410–13.

Guggenheimer J, Moore PA (2003) Xerostomia: etiology, recognition and treatment. *Journal of the American Dental Association* 134: 61–9.

Hathcock JN, Hattan DG, Jenkins MY, et al. (1990) Evaluation of vitamin A toxicity. *American Journal of Clinical Nutrition* 52: 183–202.

Hickory W, Nanda R (1981) Nutritional considerations in orthodontics. *Dental Clinics of North America* 25: 195–201.

Hotta M, Fukuda I, Sato K, et al. (2000) The relationship between bone turnover and body weight, serum insulin-like growth factor (IGF) I, and serum IGF-binding protein levels in patients with anorexia nervosa. *Journal of Clinical Endocrinology and Metabolism* 85: 200–6.

Huang JS, Becerra K, Walker E, et al. (2006) Childhood overweight and orthodontists: results of a survey. *Journal of Public Health Dentistry* 66: 292–4.

Ilich JZ, Kerstetter JE (2000) Nutrition in bone health revisited: a story beyond calcium. *Journal of the American College of Nutrition* 19: 715–37.

Institute of Medicine (2005) *Preventing Childhood Obesity-Health in the Balance.* Washington DC: The National Academic Press.

Kanai T, Takagi T, Masuhiro K, et al. (1997) Serum vitamin K level and bone mineral density in post-menopausal women. *International Journal of Gynaecology and Obstetrics* 56: 25–30.

Kandelman D (1997) Sugar, alternative sweeteners and meal frequency in relation to caries prevention: new perspectives. *British Journal of Nutrition* 77: S121–8.

Kashket S, DePaola DP (2002) Cheese consumption and the development and progression of dental caries. *Nutrition Reviews* 60: 97–103.

Litton SF (1974) Orthodontic tooth movement during an ascorbic acid deficiency. *American Journal of Orthodontics* 65: 290–302.

Lynch H, Milgrom P (2003) Xylitol and dental caries: an overview for clinicians. *Journal of the California Dental Association* 31: 205–9.

Medeiros D, Ilich J, Ireton J, et al. (1997) Femurs from rats fed diets deficient in copper or iron have decreased mechanical strength and altered mineral composition. *Journal of Trace Elements in Experimental Medicine* 10: 197–203.

Moynihan P, Petersen PE (2004) Diet, nutrition and the prevention of dental diseases. *Public Health Nutrition* 7: 201–26.

Neumark-Sztainer D, Hannan PJ, Story M, et al. (2004) Weight-control behaviors among adolescent girls and boys: implications for dietary intake. *Journal of the American Dietetic Association* 104: 913–20.

Palmer CA (2007) Effective communication in dental practice. In: *Diet, Nutrition and Oral Health*, 2nd edn. Upper Saddle River, NJ: Pearson, pp. 409–52.

Pinkham JR (2005) Adolescence: dynamics of change. In: JR Pinkham, PS Casamassimo, HW Fields Jr, et al. (eds) *Pediatric Dentistry: Infancy through Adolescence*, 4th edn. Philadelphia, PA: Elsevier/WB Saunders, pp. 650–60.

Rizzoli R (2008) Nutrition: its role in bone health. *Best Practice and Research Clinical Endocrinology and Metabolism* 22: 813–29.

Roberts WE, Epker BN, Burr DB, et al. (2006) Remodeling of mineralized tissues, part II: control and pathophysiology. *Seminars in Orthodontics* 12: 238–53.

Rollnick S, Mason P, Butler C (1999) *Health Behavior Change: a Guide for Practitioners*. Philadelphia, PA: Churchill Livingstone.

Romito LM (2003) Introduction to nutrition and oral health. *Dental Clinics of North America* 47: 187–207.

Rude RK (1998) Magnesium deficiency: a cause of heterogeneous disease in humans. *Journal of Bone and Mineral Research* 13: 749–58.

Rude RK, Kirchen ME, Gruber HE, et al. (1999) Magnesium deficiency-induced osteoporosis in the rat: uncoupling of bone formation and bone resorption. *Magnesium Research* 12: 257–67.

Schwartz MB, Puhl R (2003) Childhood obesity: a societal problem to solve. *Obesity Reviews* 4: 57–71.

Tinanoff N, Palmer CA (2000) Dietary determinants of dental caries and dietary recommendations for preschool children. *Journal of Public Health Dentistry* 60: 197–206.

US Department of Agriculture (2010) (12 May 2010-last update) *MyPyramid Plan*. Available at: www.mypyramid.gov/mypyramid/index.aspx (accessed 24 April 2010).

US Department of Health and Human Services, US Department of Agriculture (2005) *Dietary Guidelines for Americans, 2005*. Washington DC: Government Printing Office.

US Department of Health and Human Services, National Institute of Dental and Craniofacial Research, National Institutes of Health (2000) *Oral Health in America: A Report of the Surgeon General – Executive Summary*. Washington DC: Government Printing Office.

Yaghi MM (2001) Soda pop and caries. *Journal of the American Dental Association* 132: 578.

6

Anomalies in Growth and Development: The Importance of Consultation with a Pediatrician

Adriana Da Silveira

Summary

Growth and development of the craniofacial complex can be altered by a number of factors including the presence of harmful habits, pathological conditions, and medical problems. The goal of orthodontic treatment is to promote the most favorable craniofacial growth and development and to restore it to its optimal status. For this purpose, orthodontists must rely on consultation with pediatricians for identification of existing diseases and for tailoring treatment according to their patients' conditions. We have assumed that the reader has a good knowledge of normal craniofacial growth, and therefore this chapter focuses on the importance of the interaction between healthcare professionals and highlights instances of anomalies of growth and development requiring consultation with a pediatrician.

Introduction

Pediatricians can play an important role in promoting oral healthcare, and their advice regarding dental procedures or therapies may be solicited. However, a large percentage of the lower socioeconomic population does not have access to a regular dentist. Pediatricians have frequent contact with families during routine preventive visits in the childhood years of life and are in a position to advise families about the prevention of oral diseases in their children and to refer them to an adequate professional. It is important to educate pediatricians with knowledge of craniofacial growth, which may enhance the implementation and eventual success of preventive measures.

There are some recognized problems and habits that should be identified early and discouraged, to allow for optimal craniofacial growth and development, and some that require early referral to the orthodontist. These issues will be discussed in detail in this chapter. Conversely, the orthodontist may be in a position of seeing a patient with craniofacial deviations indicative of medical problems. In the latter cases, the orthodontist should understand the implications of the medical problems in order to formulate an optimal, individualized treatment plan. He or she should also work in close relationship with the pediatrician for elimination of possible causes of harmful craniofacial growth and development.

It is usually uncommon for orthodontists to contact their patients' pediatricians to discuss details of the planned orthodontic treatment. Orthodontists in general rely on parents to disclose their children's medical history at the time of the initial evaluation. Most of the communication regarding a specific patient is between the orthodontist and the general or pediatric dentist, on issues of a dental nature. If the child presents with a complicated medical history, the orthodontist should contact the pediatrician to discuss the implications of orthodontic treatment on the health of the patient, and vice versa. Every initial evaluation should contain a detailed medical history, including questions about overall and dental health, past diseases, and the patient's behavior and development. The medical history should be updated every year. When problems of growth and development or diseases (e.g. history of cancer, failure to thrive, cardiac problems, or bleeding disorders) are detected during the medical history, the orthodontist should contact the pediatrician for a discussion of the patient's needs and a better assessment of the child's overall health.

The orthodontic treatment plan should take into consideration the risks involved in mechanotherapy in individual patients, in light of their health status, and modify the treatment plan accordingly to achieve optimal results, despite the existence of some health challenges. For example, in

Integrated Clinical Orthodontics, First Edition. Edited by Vinod Krishnan, Ze'ev Davidovitch.
© 2012 Blackwell Publishing Ltd. Published 2012 by Blackwell Publishing Ltd.

patients with bleeding disorders (hemophilia, von Willebrand disease and other bleeding problems) the risk of bleeding must be minimized and thus it is likely that surgery will not be recommended. Extractions should be discussed in detail with all healthcare providers involved, the orthodontist, the pediatrician, the hematologist, and the oral surgeon. If possible, the use of metallic bands should be avoided because of the inevitable soft tissue injuries that occur during band fitting. A lengthy discussion about risks and benefits of treatment should take place with the parents prior to initiating any treatment. When cardiac problems are identified at the time of medical history, it is important to determine if the patient requires antibiotic prophylaxis prior to placement of bands or any procedure that creates a high risk for bleeding. Again, effective communication with the pediatrician is important.

One should not assume that effective communication always occurs naturally. Acquiring effective interpersonal skills requires observational practice and application of interpersonal communication principles (Fallowfield et al., 1998). Even when providers come from the same geographical area, they often have different educational, socioeconomic, and cultural backgrounds. The orthodontist may opt to contact the pediatrician directly by phone to obtain more information and discuss specifics of treatment. Requests for copies of medical records including chart entries and past examinations are helpful for formulating a proper diagnosis and plan of treatment. Written documentation is essential for continuity of care as well as for future reference. If additional healthcare providers are consulted, written letters and referrals should be supplied to the patient, as well as to the pediatrician, with copies kept on the patient's chart.

The following disorders are easily diagnosed by the pediatrician or parents and represent conditions in which early intervention might be appropriate to prevent possible future orofacial dysfunction: sucking habits and tongue thrusting persisting beyond 3 years of age, speech problems caused by malocclusions, chronic mouth breathing, sleep apnea, significant deviations from tooth eruption norms, early problems with jaw(s) growth and temporomandibular joint disorder (TMD) dysfunction. In general, preventing orofacial dysfunction should be based on promoting normal growth and craniofacial development and the elimination of potential environmental factors that may harm these processes. The following is a discussion of some of these disorders that affect normal growth.

Pervasive sucking habits and tongue thrusting

Sucking behaviors are common in infants and young children. Use of pacifiers, blankets, and toys, as well as nutritive sucking, such as bottle feeding and breastfeeding, should be encouraged for normal development. Early premature babies often need to learn how to suck properly prior to

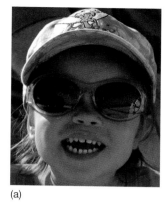 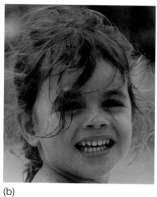

(a)   (b)

Figure 6.1 Two and a half years old girl with a pacifier habit. (a) A dental anterior open bite localized to the right side, where the pacifier usually rested. (b) The pacifier was removed and the habit stopped. Nine months later the open bite closed spontaneously with help from the perioral musculature.

being discharged from the hospital, to enable them to receive adequate nutrition at home. However, prolonged sucking habits should be discouraged after the age of 3 years. If there is an existent open bite at this age, it will usually correct spontaneously if the habit is discontinued, and as long as the perioral musculature is intact and with normal tonicity (Figure 6.1). If the sucking habit persists, there may be negative consequences in the developing orofacial structures, with the severity being dependent on the duration, frequency, and intensity of the habit (Ngan and Fields, 1997).

The literature clearly supports findings of increased severity and frequency of malocclusion, with anterior open bites and posterior crossbites, in children in the late primary dentition period with prolonged sucking habits (Subtelny and Subtelny, 1973; Bishara et al., 2006). It is unlikely that orthodontists will be given an opportunity to evaluate many of these children at this early age. Therefore, it is important to educate pediatricians to recognize these findings for proper referral to a pediatric dentist. Unfortunately, the number of pediatric dentists is inadequate to meet the needs of all children, and many general dentists are not equipped with the skills and training to handle small children. Usually pediatricians see children eight times in the first year of life and 13 times by the age of 3 years and thus have a better chance of recognizing these habits at an earlier age than the dental professionals. Pediatricians can start by discouraging the habit and educating parents on issues such as when to switch from the bottle to the 'sippy cup', and removing the pacifier. A pediatric consultation will be useful for older children with thumb and finger sucking habits, and they can suggest a variety of methods to address such habits, including the use of a number of different commercially available products. Regardless of the existence of a habit, a recommendation to see a pediatric dentist should be made by the pediatrician at early stages of dental development for supervision of oral and dental health.

Thumb sucking or finger sucking is perhaps the most common persistent infant habit beyond the age of 3 years. It has been correlated with an increased prevalence and severity of Class II malocclusions and maxillary protrusion, from the deciduous through the mixed dentition periods (Antonini et al., 2005) (Figure 6.2). Moreover, persistent digit-sucking habits create a mechanical obstacle for the eruption of anterior teeth, which in turn can result in an anterior open bite. Cozza et al. (2005) found that the combination of a persistent sucking habit in a child with a vertical growth pattern can increase the chances of developing an anterior open bite. This finding may explain, at least in part, how external factors can influence or exacerbate the already programmed pattern of facial growth.

Thumb sucking may be an outcome of stress and changes in the child's emotional status, and treatment should be directed at correcting the underlying problem. Therefore, a consultation with the pediatrician is warranted. A risk of reduced social acceptance among school-age children (7 years old) has been implicated in thumb sucking (Friman et al., 1993). In order to stop the habit, a myriad of treatment methods are available, including behavioral conditioning techniques, positive reinforcement, and oral/dental appliances.

Tongue habits, particularly tongue thrusting, have been implicated in the protrusion of lower incisors, and the creation of an anterior open bite (Subtelny and Subtelny, 1973). It seems evident that problems arise from the postural position of the tongue at rest as opposed to during function (Figures 6.3, 6.4). When planning treatment for correction of malocclusions in these patients, a combined approach with a speech pathologist to help train a new tongue position after treatment is recommended. This training may prevent or minimize future relapse tendencies.

Growth-related problems

It is commonly understood that problems with craniofacial growth can result in functional impairments of the masticatory system as well as esthetic concerns. The manifestations of growth-related problems will depend on the craniofacial region or jaw being affected, the direction of growth, and the cause of the problem. Deficiencies such as in cases of Class II malocclusions caused by lack of sufficient growth of the mandible, or too much growth in cases of Class III malocclusions, caused by excessive mandibular growth, are examples of such craniofacial problems. Excessive vertical growth may create an open bite, while deficient vertical growth may create a deep bite. When detected early, growth modification treatment may be a possibility and an option. Because facial growth is the result of the interaction of genetic and environmental factors

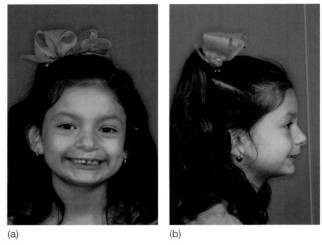

(a)   (b)

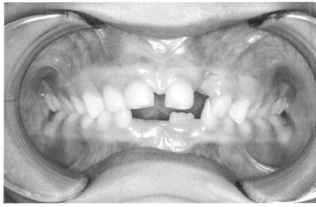

(c)

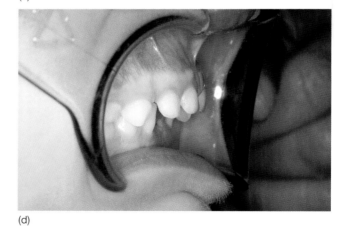

(d)

Figure 6.2 Six-year-old girl with a thumb sucking habit. (a,b) Facial pictures showing protrusion of the upper incisors, and a retrognathic, convex profile. (c,d) Intraoral views showing the dental occlusion with increased overjet and spacing between upper anterior teeth.

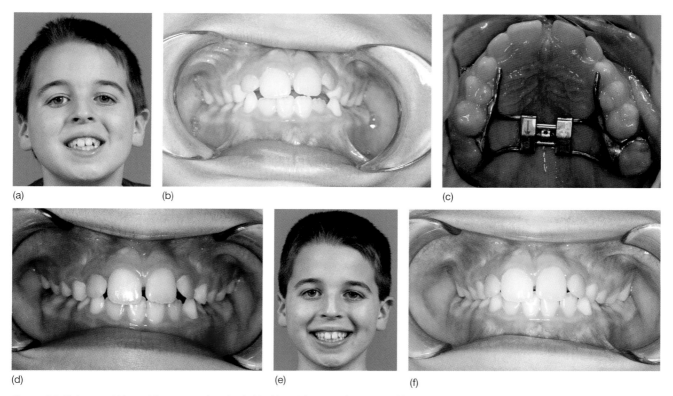

(a)   (b)   (c)

(d)   (e)   (f)

Figure 6.3 Eight-year-old boy with a tongue thrusting habit. (a) Facial picture showing a mild anterior open bite and (b) intraoral view showing the dental occlusion with a mild anterior open bite due to the anterior tongue position, with constricted upper arch and maxilla. (c–e) After expansion treatment, combined with speech therapy to retrain tongue posture, the open bite closed. (f) The patient was followed up for a year, during which no relapse was observed.

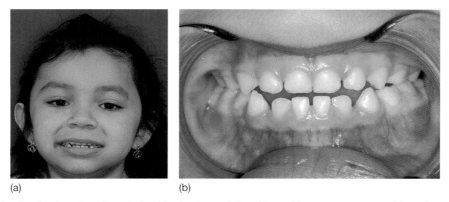

(a)   (b)

Figure 6.4 Four-year-old girl with enlarged tonsils and adenoids, chronic mouth breathing and lower tongue posture. (a) Facial picture showing an enlarged mandible with a deficient maxilla and (b) intraoral view showing the dental occlusion with an anterior crossbite and increased spacing in the lower anterior teeth.

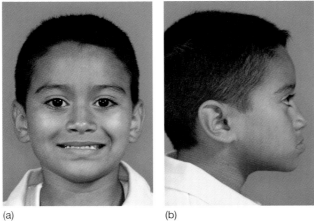

(a)   (b)

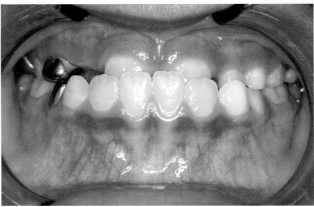

(c)

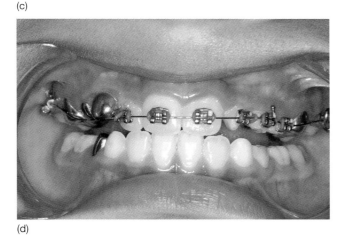

(d)

Figure 6.5 Eight-year-old boy referred by his pediatrician due to problems of jaw growth. The medical history was unremarkable, and on examination, a forward mandibular shift was detected. (a) Frontal facial picture. (b) Profile facial picture. (c) Intraoral view showing the dental occlusion with anterior crossbite. (d) After 6 months of treatment, the mandibular anterior shift was corrected with expansion, and use of a bite block and facemask.

(some of which are functional), if environmental factors are detected early, there is a good chance of improving the facial growth to a more favorable pattern. Therefore, a functional shift resulting from a crossbite should be corrected early, so that unfavorable growth of the mandible can be reduced or even prevented (Figure 6.5). Patients with lateral shifts of the mandible due to bite problems may develop asymmetries in condylar height (Kilic et al., 2008) (Figure 6.6).

Some problems may be treated by a combined approach of surgical and orthodontic means. Continued growth in early adulthood may enhance or negate results from treatment received during childhood or adolescence. If skeletal problems are severe, surgical treatment should be indicated. Although pediatricians are not usually trained to look for alterations in craniofacial growth, they can easily recognize an anterior crossbite or an evident facial asymmetry. Orthodontists should be active in their local communities, providing education to the public and to the local healthcare professionals about recognizing early signs of craniofacial growth problems, for enticing proper referrals. The American Association of Orthodontists recommends that every child should have an evaluation by a trained orthodontist at no later than age 7. This schedule assures that early growth problems are properly recognized and treated, if needed.

Many local and systemic diseases or pathological conditions can alter the growth and development of the craniofacial complex. A child who has had cancer and chemotherapy or radiation therapy at an early age may have alteration of bone quality or dental root formation and development (Avşar et al., 2007). Other systemic diseases can also alter the quality of bone and the development and eruption of teeth (Figures 6.7, 6.8). Local conditions can disturb proper craniofacial growth as well. Hemangiomas and vascular malformations can create enough pressure to modify jaw growth. The severity of the resulting malformation depends on the size of the tumor and the patient's age at the time of its formation (Figures 6.9, 6.10). Restoration to a normal pattern of growth is the main objective of excision of lesions of this nature. Often several surgical procedures will be required for complete removal or correction of functional impairments.

Trauma-related issues

There has been a great improvement in the prevention, diagnosis, and treatment of craniofacial trauma in children. The recommendation to wear safety helmets while practicing sports (skating, bicycling, skiing, baseball) and to use child car seats, have turned out to be excellent measures for prevention of craniofacial trauma. However, accidents involving falls are more frequent than suspected, especially at a young age. The diagnosis of fractures in children is more difficult than in adults and can be easily overlooked (Figure 6.11). The mandibular condyle is fragile at

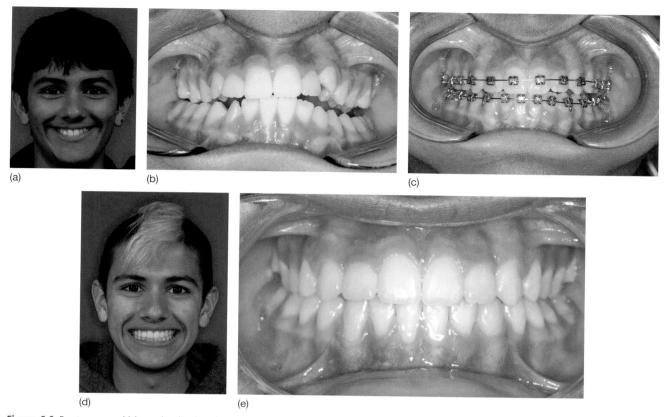

Figure 6.6 Fourteen-year-old boy who developed posterior open bites with mandibular asymmetry over the course of 12 months. The parents could not remember any history of a fall or accident. Maxillary constriction was detected. (a) Facial picture showing lower facial asymmetry with deviation to the left. (b) Intraoral view showing the dental occlusion with posterior open bites, midline discrepancies, and cant of occlusal plane. (c) During treatment, the upper arch was expanded with a fixed expander, and full orthodontic appliances were used to coordinate the arches. (d) Correction of the asymmetry after treatment. (e) Final occlusion after treatment.

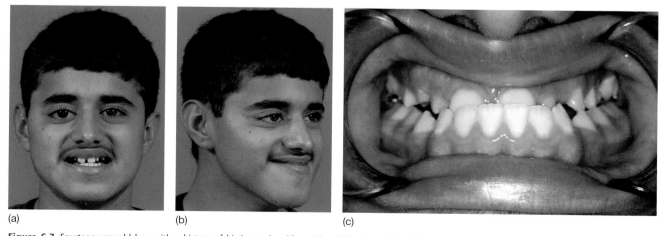

Figure 6.7 Fourteen-year-old boy with a history of histiocytosis with excisional biopsies of the right temporal bone at the ages of 2 and 4 years. (a) Facial picture showing severe maxillary hypoplasia, midface deficiency, and facial asymmetry. Note that the right orbit is lower than the left one. (b) Three-quarter profile view. (c) Dental occlusion showing anterior crossbite and a Class III malocclusion.

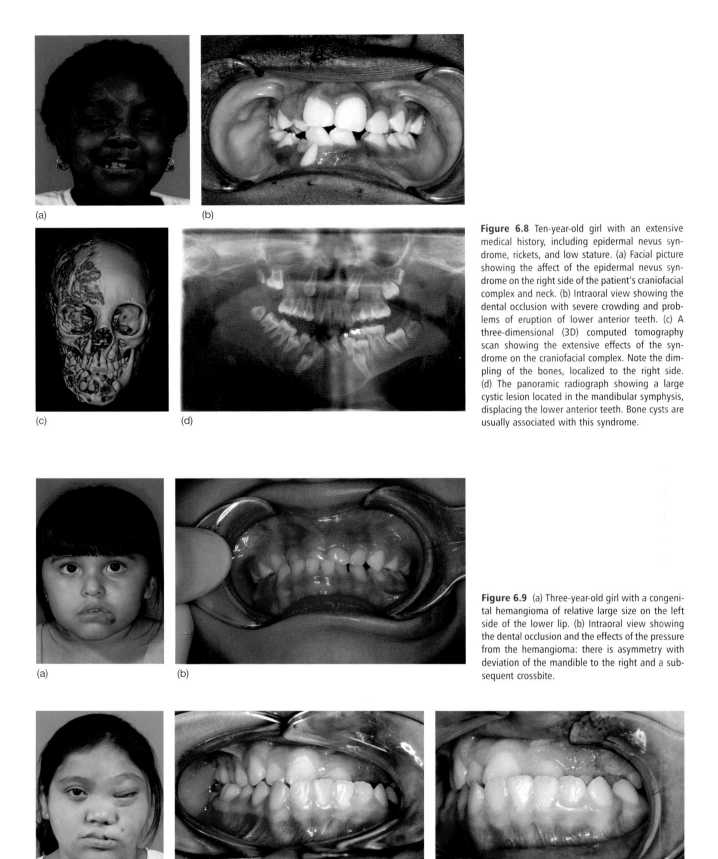

(a)

(b)

Figure 6.8 Ten-year-old girl with an extensive medical history, including epidermal nevus syndrome, rickets, and low stature. (a) Facial picture showing the affect of the epidermal nevus syndrome on the right side of the patient's craniofacial complex and neck. (b) Intraoral view showing the dental occlusion with severe crowding and problems of eruption of lower anterior teeth. (c) A three-dimensional (3D) computed tomography scan showing the extensive effects of the syndrome on the craniofacial complex. Note the dimpling of the bones, localized to the right side. (d) The panoramic radiograph showing a large cystic lesion located in the mandibular symphysis, displacing the lower anterior teeth. Bone cysts are usually associated with this syndrome.

(c)

(d)

(a)

(b)

Figure 6.9 (a) Three-year-old girl with a congenital hemangioma of relative large size on the left side of the lower lip. (b) Intraoral view showing the dental occlusion and the effects of the pressure from the hemangioma: there is asymmetry with deviation of the mandible to the right and a subsequent crossbite.

(a)

(b)

(c)

Figure 6.10 Eleven-year-old girl with history of a complex lymphatic malformation of the left periorbital and malar areas. (a) Due to the malformation, patient's left side is prone to infections, which has caused excessive swelling of the eye and cheek areas. (b) Intraoral view showing the dental occlusion with a crossbite on the left side due to constant pressure from the enlarged tissue. (c) Close-up of the left occlusion, which also shows the involvement of the gingival tissue and lip.

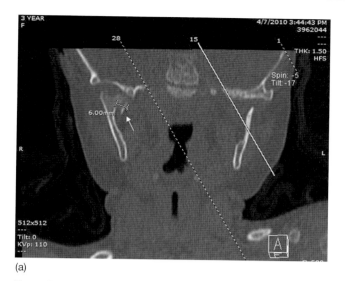
(a)

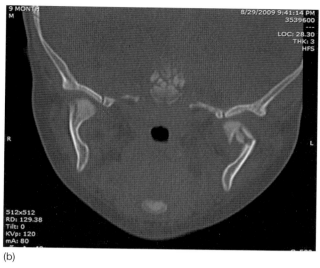
(b)

Figure 6.11 Computed tomography (CT) scans of children with condylar fractures. (a) Right condylar fracture in a 3-year-old girl, who presented to the emergency room many hours after her fall, chiefly for repair of a chin laceration. Condylar fracture with displacement of segment is indicated by the arrow and measures 6 mm. The patient did not report any problems on chewing or moving her jaw and her pain was reported as mild. Observation was the treatment of choice. (b) Nine-month-old baby with multiple condylar head and neck fractures on the left side and multiple fractures of the orbit. The CT scan shows the left condylar head and neck displaced medially compared with the intact right condyle. Treatment included application of a lower splint to allow space for the segments to heal properly, followed by gentle manipulation and observation. The splint was held with a wire for about 4 weeks. Further investigation revealed that the fractures were caused by child abuse by a caregiver.

a young age, and fractures usually happen at this site. Moreover, children require long-term follow-up to monitor potential growth abnormalities. Therefore, it is important to be able to detect traumatic episodes in growing children. Mandibular fracture patterns are affected by the force and direction of impact, as well as the status of osseous development of the child. The younger child has relatively more soft tissue cushioning, and the mandible is in a more protected position. The overall force developed in most childhood falls is low due to children's small stature and weight. Also, in young children the bone is relatively resilient. Therefore, force directed at the chin is transmitted to the condylar heads, which sustain a crush-type injury. As the child becomes older, the fracture sites shift to the mandibular body and ramus, similar to in adults.

The effects of trauma on craniofacial growth and development are thought to be the result of scarring, which restricts further growth. Management of condylar fractures in young children usually does not involve surgery, but rather a careful observation of the healing process, which takes about 8 weeks. It is thought that surgery can do more harm than good, by causing the creation of scars that can prevent joint movements. A balance between restricting movement and preventing temporomandibular joint (TMJ) ankylosis during the healing period is the goal that experienced surgeons and physicians aim to achieve (Aizenbud et al., 2009). The specific treatment of mandibular fractures depends on the location of the fracture, the degree of bony

displacement, alterations in dental occlusion, and the dental age of the child. Methods of fixation differ in accordance with the patient's dental age. An undetected condylar head fracture can result in joint ankylosis, with the possibility of causing abnormal craniofacial growth and development (Figure 6.12) (Proffit et al., 1980). When severe movement restriction occurs, it is usually a 'functional ankylosis', where the condyle can still rotate, but with limited translation. When asymmetrical mandibular growth is encountered, the possibility of a past strike to the facial region should be investigated, especially to the mandible. A detailed medical history taken from the parents, and a possible consultation with the pediatrician for past occurrences may be in order.

In a similar way, patients with a history of severe torticollis and plagiocephaly as infants may have asymmetrical craniofacial growth and development, resulting in facial asymmetry (Kawamoto et al., 2009). Since the underlying causes are different, treatment for these asymmetries may involve a variety of therapies, depending on the degree of severity of the asymmetry. Consultation with the pediatrician for a discussion of symptoms and treatment options is highly recommended in these cases.

Timing of treatment

Pediatricians and other healthcare providers use growth charts to follow a child's growth over time. Growth charts have been constructed by collecting growth data on large

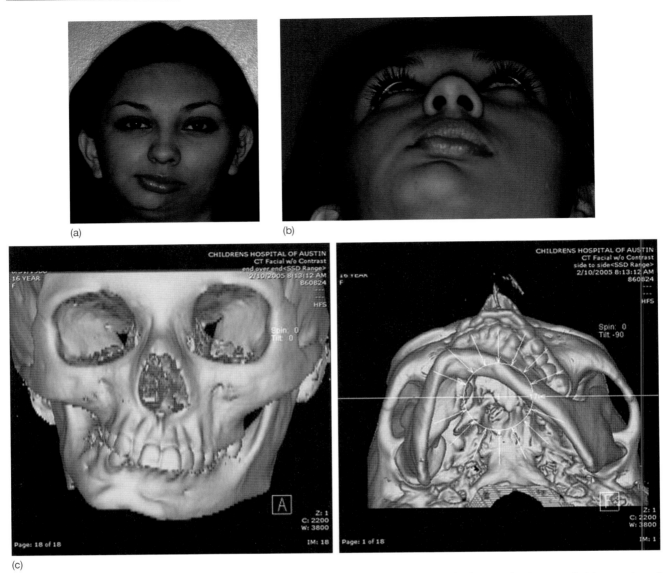

Figure 6.12 Seventeen-year-old girl who was referred to the craniofacial center by a geneticist. (a) Frontal facial picture showing severe facial asymmetry and functional ankylosis of the right condyle and temporomandibular joint (TMJ). The parents could not remember any history of accident. (b) Facial picture showing the severity of her chin deviation. (c) Computed tomography (CT) scan. (d) The patient underwent multiple surgeries including release of the ankylosis and lengthening of the mandible by distraction osteogenesis for partial correction of the asymmetry and deficiency caused by the lack of growth of the affected side. (e) Patient undergoing orthodontic treatment in preparation for a final double jaw surgery for correction of the asymmetries. (f) Intraoral view showing the dental occlusion and severe cant of the occlusal plane. (g) Final facial view after 3 years of treatment. (h) Final dental occlusion.

numbers of normal children over time. The height, weight, and head circumference of a child can be compared with the expected parameters of children of the same age, gender, and ethnic origin, in order to determine whether the child is growing appropriately. Growth charts can also be used to predict the expected adult height and weight of a child, because, in general, children maintain a fairly constant growth curve. When a child deviates from his or her previously established growth curve, investigation into the cause is generally necessary. A decrease in the growth velocity may

indicate the onset of a chronic illness or disease. Growth charts are different for boys and girls, due to differences in the ages at which they reach puberty, and the differences in their final adult height.

The best way to assess the period of peak growth velocity of the craniofacial structures is by evaluating the maturation of cervical vertebrae on serial lateral cephalometric radiographs or by analyzing the hand and wrist growth plates. These are helpful methods for predicting the timing of growth velocity, which in turn allows a decision to be

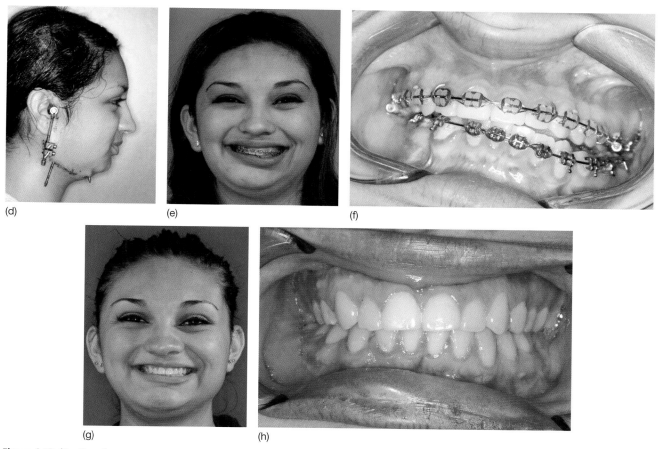

(d)   (e)   (f)

(g)   (h)

Figure 6.12 (*Continued*)

made about whether early functional treatment can be attempted (Wong et al., 2009). Additional questions may be asked of the parents about overall growth events, such as recent, frequent changes in their child's shoe or pants (trousers) size. For more significant data on the onset of puberty, information is sought from the parents about changes in the child's body hair, and voice quality in boys and menarche status in girls. When required, a bone density test can be requested by the pediatrician to allow assessment of skeletal growth and detection of growth impairments. Therefore, communication between the orthodontist and the pediatrician in these cases is extremely important.

Craniofacial growth differs from the growth of long bones. This difference is particularly evident in children born with achondroplasia, a genetic condition of failure of growth of the cartilages of the limbs and cranial base. The resultant presentation is of a small child with very short arms and legs. Growth of the mandible is unaffected, since cartilaginous growth in the condyles is secondary, while the rest of the mandible undergoes membranous bone formation, which involves growth and remodeling independently of the condylar cartilage. The overall facial appearance is that of mid-face deficiency because of lack of growth of the cartilaginous elements of the fetal cranial base (Figure 6.13).

It is not uncommon to encounter patients receiving growth hormone therapy, mostly for an idiopathic short stature. A few studies have examined the effect of growth hormone therapy on growth of the craniofacial complex and found that it can induce catch-up growth of the cranial skeleton, thus improving occlusion and the facial profile (Funatsu et al., 2006; Kjellberg and Wikland, 2007). Growth hormones also may be useful for correcting a convex facial profile, which is frequently because of the presence of a small, retrognathic mandible. In order to effectively address systemic and craniofacial growth-related issues, it is strongly recommended that the orthodontist interact with a pediatrician and an endocrinologist to reach a well-coordinated diagnosis and treatment plan. This interaction should continue throughout the periods of active orthodontic treatment and retention.

Analysis of serial annual lateral cephalometric radiographs can provide valuable information about an individual's pattern of craniofacial growth. Superimposition

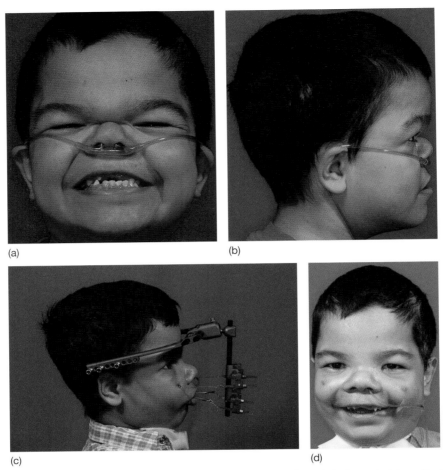

(a) (b)

(c) (d)

Figure 6.13 Fifteen-year-old boy with achondroplasia. (a,b) There is severe midface deficiency due to lack of growth of the cartilaginous sutures of the cranial base and normal mandibular growth. Notice the concave profile and short nose. He also had severe obstructive sleep apnea. (c) The patient underwent midface distraction with a fixed external device. (d) After distraction, the midface was brought forward considerably, improving his facial appearance and airway.

of the tracings of these radiographs can reveal the annual incremental growth of each jaw, as well as the direction of facial growth in the vertical and anteroposterior dimensions. Likewise, frontal cephalometric radiographs are a useful tool for the assessment of facial growth in the transverse plane. When the treatment plan includes surgical intervention, it is advisable, in most cases, to defer treatment until facial growth and development are complete. Such a situation may cause deferral of treatment until late adolescence (Figure 6.14). This delay may create problems with social adjustment at a very sensitive time of life. However, it has been reported that patients who have undergone orthognathic surgery experience psychosocial benefits as a result of the operation, including improved self-confidence, body and facial image, and social adjustment (Hunt et al., 2001). The literature also suggests that patients requiring jaw surgery are not only self-

conscious about their dental appearance, but that existing or presurgical functional problems may lead to social embarrassment in a group setting, such as when eating in public (Williams et al., 2005). Other studies propose that in children with low self-concept or low self-esteem, the child's own perception of the severity of his or her malocclusion, and not the malocclusion itself, is the most important contributing factor to the low self-concept and self-esteem (Rivera et al., 2000). The impact of psychosocial issues in adolescents waiting for jaw surgery needs to be carefully monitored by all involved: parents, orthodontists, and pediatricians.

Conclusions

From the above discussion it is apparent that communication between the orthodontist and the pediatrician is

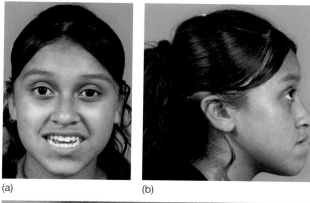

(a)   (b)

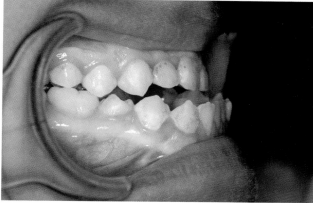

(c)

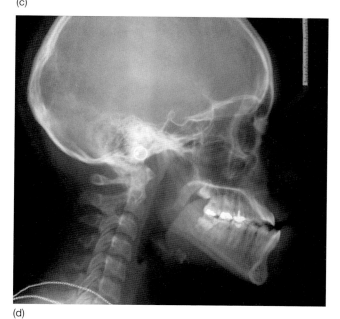

(d)

Figure 6.14 Fourteen-year-old girl with craniofacial growth problems who presented to the craniofacial center. Due to the advanced stage of her growth and severity of the problem, bimaxillary surgery is being planned. (a,b) Facial pictures showing prognathic concave profile with a combination of maxillary deficiency and prognathism, (c) the dental occlusion with Class III malocclusion, anterior crossbite and open bite, and (d) the lateral cephalogram radiograph showing the extent of her skeletal problems.

recommended in most cases, and essential in cases of existing medical conditions and past complex medical history. Facial growth is the result of the interaction between genetic and environmental factors (some of which are functional), and if environmental factors such as harmful habits are detected early, there is a good chance of improving the facial growth to a more favorable pattern. However, our understanding of how anomalies of growth and development can arise in the absence of any environmental factors or known genetic disorders is still scarce. Early orthodontic treatment is recommended to help stimulate the growth of the jaws or decrease excessive growth of the jaws, but this approach has met with limited success, which is usually patient dependent. Understanding patients' needs and how their conditions affect their overall health and craniofacial growth allows for planning and execution of the appropriate treatment. Communicating effectively with the pediatrician, other healthcare providers caring for the patient, and the family is key in these cases.

References

Aizenbud D, Hazan-Molina H, Emodi O, et al. (2009) The management of mandibular body fractures in young children. *Dental Traumatology* 25: 565–70.

Antonini A, Marinelli A, Baroni G, et al. (2005) Class II malocclusion with maxillary protrusion from the deciduous through the mixed dentition: a longitudinal study. *Angle Orthodontist* 75(6): 980–6.

Avşar A, Elli M, Darka O, et al. (2007) Long-term effects of chemotherapy on caries formation, dental development, and salivary factors in childhood cancer survivors. *Oral Surgery, Oral Medicine, Oral Pathology, Oral Radiology and Endodontics* 104(6): 781–9.

Bishara SE, Warren JJ, Broffitt B, et al. (2006) Changes in the prevalence of nonnutritive sucking patterns in the first 8 years of life. *American Journal of Orthodontics and Dentofacial Orthopedics* 130(1): 31–6.

Cozza P, Baccetti T, Franchi L, et al. (2005) Sucking habits and facial hyperdivergency as risk factors for anterior open bite in the mixed dentition. *American Journal of Orthodontics and Dentofacial Orthopedics* 128(4): 517–19.

Fallowfield L, Lipkin M, Hall A (1998) Teaching senior oncologists communication skills: results from phase I of a comprehensive longitudinal program in the United Kingdom. *Journal of Clinical Oncology* 16(5): 1961–8.

Friman PC, McPherson KM, Warzak WJ, et al. (1993) Influence of thumb sucking on peer social acceptance in first-grade children. *Pediatrics* 91(4): 784–6.

Funatsu M, Sato K, Mitani H (2006) Effects of growth hormone on craniofacial growth. *Angle Orthodontist* 76(6): 970–7.

Hunt OT, Johnston CD, Hepper PG, et al. (2001) The psychosocial impact of orthognathic surgery: a systematic review. *American Journal of Orthodontics and Dentofacial Orthopedics* 120(5): 490–7.

Kawamoto HK, Kim SS, Jarrahy R, et al. (2009) Differential diagnosis of the idiopathic laterally deviated mandible. *Plastic and Reconstructive Surgery* 124(5): 1599–609.

Kilic N, Kiki A, Oktay H (2008) Condylar asymmetry in unilateral posterior crossbite patients. *American Journal of Orthodontics and Dentofacial Orthopedics* 133(3): 382–7.

Kjellberg H, Wikland KA (2007) A longitudinal study of craniofacial growth in idiopathic short stature and growth hormone-deficient boys treated with growth hormone. *European Journal of Orthodontics* 29(3): 243–50.

Ngan P, Fields HW (1997) Open bite: a review of etiology and management. *Pediatric Dental Journal* 19(2): 91–8.

Proffit WR, Vig KW, Turvey TA (1980) Early fracture of the mandibular condyles: frequently an unsuspected cause of growth disturbances. *American Journal of Orthodontics* 78(1): 1–24.

Rivera SM, Hatch JP, Rugh JD (2000) Psychological factors associated with orthodontic and orthognathic surgical treatment. *Seminars in Orthodontics* 6: 259–69.

Subtelny JD, Subtelny JD (1973) Oral habits – studies in form, function, and therapy. *Angle Orthodontist* 43(4): 349–83.

Williams AC, Shah H, Sandy JR, et al. (2005) Patients' motivations for treatment and their experiences of orthodontic preparation for orthognathic surgery. *Journal of Orthodontics* 32(3): 191–202.

Wong RW, Alkhal HA, Rabie AB (2009) Use of cervical vertebral maturation to determine skeletal age. *American Journal of Orthodontics and Dentofacial Orthopedics* 136(4): 484.e1–484.e6.

7

The Benefits of Obtaining the Opinion of a Clinical Geneticist Regarding Orthodontic Patients

James K Hartsfield Jr

Summary

This chapter is designed to help educate the dental clinician as to the valuable role that a clinical geneticist can play in the diagnosis and treatment of patients. It describes the evolution of the medical and clinical genetics disciplines and how that evolution impacted certification of dentists in clinical genetics. Discussion addresses the question of when a patient case should be referred to a clinical geneticist, followed by a review of selected syndromes that may affect the craniofacial region and the oral tissues. The chapter closes with lists of selected syndromes that may be associated with traits such as premature tooth exfoliation, delayed tooth eruption, hypodontia/oligodontia, supernumerary teeth, taurodontism, mandibular deficiency, cleft lip and palate, cleft palate alone, median cleft lip, midface deficiency, mandibular prognathism, long anterior facial height, facial asymmetry, ocular hypertelorism, amelogenesis imperfecta and enamel hypoplasia, dentinogenesis imperfecta, and other dentin anomalies.

Introduction

In the field of dentistry, and specifically within the discipline of orthodontics, patients with notable or unique skeletal and/or craniofacial features are occasionally identified. As craniofacial growth and development specialists, orthodontists must be familiar with many of the relatively common medical conditions/syndromes their patients may have, and understand how these may affect a patient's treatment. In addition, the orthodontist should recognize when a patient has an unusual pattern, two or more signs, which may represent an undiagnosed syndrome (Vig, 1990).

In the notable or unique cases, consultation with a clinical geneticist can provide valuable insight into a patient's condition, particularly when the less common cases or cases with multiple complexities are encountered in the clinic. The benefits of such a consultation can include: (1) having a previously unrecognized or developing genetic condition diagnosed with appropriate further referral and counseling, and (2) the clinician orthodontist gaining a better understanding of the patient's condition and how it may affect dental and/or orthodontic treatment (Roberts and Hartsfield, 1997).

Interaction with the clinical geneticist

A referral may be made for evaluation by a clinical geneticist by calling the number given on the American College of Medical Genetics or GeneTests websites after searching for a board certified geneticist or genetics clinic (see the additional resources section at the end of the chapter). Although the orthodontist's staff may schedule the appointment, unless the patient or parent is present at the time of scheduling, availability of the family for appointments may not be known. Alternatively, the phone number of the clinical geneticist or genetics clinic may be given to the family. Family members, however, may not be able to fully convey what the patient is being referred for, and with internet accessibility prevalent, any condition mentioned (even as a clinical possibility to rule out) may be read about in detail without anxiety-relieving clarification.

Perhaps the best approach is for the orthodontist's staff to call the clinical geneticist/genetics clinic to make the referral, giving pertinent information including your name and address, the patient's name and address, and the reason for the referral. This does not necessarily have to be to rule out a named syndrome. A list of your concerns or findings, including reported medical history such as a heart defect, hearing deficit, or diabetes mellitus, etc., will be most helpful for the clinical geneticist's pre-appointment preparation.

It is suggested for convenience and confidentiality that you or your office tell the clinical geneticist/genetics clinic that you will give their number to the patient/family to call for an appointment, and give any additional information such as family history, primary or other physicians and dentists involved in their care, and insurance coverage. Some clinical geneticists/genetics clinics will call the patient/family for an appointment themselves. The clinical geneticist/genetics clinic may send out a family questionnaire form to the patient and/or family to ask about medical history, and to construct a family tree called a 'pedigree'. If not done beforehand, it is expected that this will be done at the time of the visit to the clinical geneticist, which will typically take an hour or more for an initial visit.

The clinical geneticist/genetics clinic may ask for radiographs, and/or may request medical records from other involved health professionals. As most physicians and PhDs do not routinely look at pan-oral, periapical or lateral cephalometric radiographs, providing a brief description of pertinent findings for some of the syndromes, especially pathology or deviations from normal, may be useful.

Following the visit of your patient to the clinical geneticist, expect a letter summarizing the family history, medical history, examination, discussion, diagnosis or differential diagnosis, genetic counseling if given, and recommendations. The latter are more likely to be for any genetic testing or further medical referral than for any specific type of orthodontic treatment.

Evolution of the clinical (medical) geneticist specialist

The American Board of Medical Genetics (ABMG), which was founded in 1980, historically recognized several genetic disciplines pertaining to direct patient care and laboratory services. These disciples included medical, clinical, and laboratory genetics as well as genetic counseling. Initially a 'medical geneticist' was defined by the ABMG as an individual holding a PhD, who had completed the required ABMG-certified medical genetics education, training and experience (including some clinical genetics activity), and had passed the ABMG medical geneticist examination (consisting of the general genetics examination for all ABMG diplomats, and a specialized examination for medical geneticists). Since the ABMG-certified medical

genetics education and training required the genetic assessment of at least 50 clinical cases, it was not unusual for a 'medical geneticist' with a PhD to see and counsel patients regularly after achieving ABMG diplomate status. Over time, relatively few individuals pursued the designation of 'medical geneticist' and, hence, education and training programs for this discipline were subsequently dropped by the ABMG.

In contrast, the ABMG originally defined a 'clinical geneticist' as an individual who held a clinical degree (MD, DO, DDS, or DMD), had also completed the required ABMG-certified clinical genetics education and training, and had passed the ABMG clinical geneticist examination consisting of the general genetics examination for all ABMG diplomates and the specific examination for the designation 'clinical geneticist'. Clinical or medical geneticists, who see patients and examine them for unusual physical features, particularly those that may occur with a congenital abnormality or in a pattern recognized as some syndrome, are often referred to as dysmorphologists.

One of the first members of the ABMG was Dr Robert J Gorlin, DDS, MS (1923–2006), an oral pathologist and well-known author and clinical geneticist/dysmorphologist. Another early diplomate of the ABMG was Dr David Bixler, DDS, PhD (1929–2005), the first president of the Society of Craniofacial Genetics and the founder of the Oral Facial (Craniofacial) Genetics Training Program at Indiana University, Indianapolis, USA. Thus, at the inception of the ABMG, dentists along with physicians played key roles in defining and establishing the functions of a geneticist in patient care. At that time, both dental and medical professionals could be accepted into ABMG-approved clinical genetics fellowship programs and could achieve ABMG diplomate status. These programs were stipulated by the ABMG to be at least 2 years in length with a wide range of clinical experience in genetics, not just of the craniofacies. A handful of dentists also pursued this goal and became diplomates of the ABMG as clinical geneticists.

Early on, one goal of the ABMG was to become recognized as a member of the American Board of Medical Specialties (ABMS), thus helping to recognize and legitimatize the specialty, as well as to foster improved reimbursement for services provided. In 1991, this goal was achieved and the ABMG became a member of the ABMS. The stand was taken that the ABMS is involved in medical specialties and therefore would certify only medical doctors (physicians and osteopaths) and not dentists. Today, to be an active candidate for ABMG certification as a clinical geneticist, the individual must hold a US- or Canadian-earned or the equivalent of an earned MD or DO degree, have had 2 years in an Accreditation Council for Graduate Medical Education (ACGME)-accredited clinical residency program in another medical specialty, had 2 years in an ACGME-accredited residency in clinical genetics (or 4 years in an accredited clinical genetics residency program), have a valid medical license, and have demonstrated competence to provide comprehensive genetic diagnostic, management, therapeutic, and counseling services. Thus even if a dentist with another specialty went into what was now a recognized specialty (medical genetics) in medicine, they could not become a diplomate of that specialty. Unfortunately what was a move forward for the ABMG proved to be exclusionary for dentists who wished to go into this specialty.

Clinical geneticists (including those who had been certified as medical geneticists) are typically located at major medical centers, especially children's hospitals. While they will typically have a wide range of experience in genetic conditions, including craniofacial anomalies, they may not be as familiar with those that are predominantly of the oral cavity. Since ABMG-certified dentists are rare, and none will be certified in the future unless they also have a medical degree, where does the orthodontist send a patient for a referral? The recommendation is to refer to a clinical geneticist if possible.

Clicking on 'Find A Certified Geneticist' on the homepage (www.abmg.org) of the ABMG will take you to a webpage where you may search by name or locale. An additional source of genetics clinics and geneticists may be found by clicking on 'Clinic Directory' at the GeneTests website (www.ncbi.nlm.nih.gov/sites/GeneTests). If the medical geneticist can make or rule out a diagnosis, then the knowledge of the orthodontist, perhaps with a bit of reading in the literature (see the additional resources section at the end of chapter) on the particular condition, can fill in what the clinical geneticist cannot tell you about the effect of the condition on craniofacial growth and other aspects of orthodontic care. Likewise referral to a specific oral pathologist, pediatric dentist, or specialist in oral medicine, or other practitioner who has the interest and experience to be of help, may also supplement the orthodontist's knowledge.

When to refer?

How do you recognize when to seek this referral? We all vary from one another, without it usually being a concern. One of the difficult tasks faced by any practitioner, orthodontist, or medical geneticist, is how to discern normal variation from minor anomaly (Vig, 1990). A minor anomaly is a structural feature seen in less than 4% of the general population, which is of no cosmetic or functional significance to the affected individual. Minor anomalies may or may not have diagnostic significance.

Even major anomalies or signs (those that require medical/surgical intervention) vary among individuals with the same etiological syndrome, meaning clinical diagnosis is generally made on the basis of total pattern of signs or anomalies. Advancements in genetic testing for those conditions that, because of their etiology, are amenable can

make/confirm the diagnosis in some conditions. The clinical geneticist will order or recommend such tests when indicated. However, there is often no single genetic test that can be relied on to make a diagnosis independent of clinical correlation.

In medical genetics, minor anomalies (unusual morphological features that are of no serious medical or cosmetic consequence to the patient) have been useful in three ways. First, some minor anomalies have been external markers of specific 'occult' or hidden major anomalies. In addition, the vast majority of malformation syndromes in clinical genetics are recognizable as patterns of minor anomalies. Finally, although 15% of normal newborns have one or more minor anomalies, finding three or more minor anomalies is unusual, occurring in 0.5% of newborns. The risk of having a major 'hidden' abnormality increases proportionately with the number of minor anomalies present, with three or more signaling a 90% risk of one or more major structural defect, which is an indication for evaluation (Hoyme, 1993; Jones and Smith, 2006).

Minor anomalies may occur in any part of the body. While it would not be expected for the orthodontist to physically examine all body areas, he or she is expected to examine the craniofacies as well as intraorally, and may readily observe the hands as well, where most minor anomalies occur (Jones and Smith, 2006). A familial pattern may be superficially ascertained promptly by asking if anyone else in the family has a similar feature of interest, or by asking who in the family the patient most resembles, and in what way (stature, similar eyes, jaw profile, etc.). In addition, subjective evaluation of the patient's ability to function, as well as a general medical surgery history and questions about the patient being or having been in 'special' classes, may indicate that a medical genetics referral is warranted. This may require some explanation to the patient and/or family members as the orthodontist is typically not in a position to make a diagnosis, or answer all the questions that inevitably follow. One way to approach this is a general discussion of the orthodontist's need to know anything that may affect treatment, noting the potential factors that could be ruled out by consultation with a specialist in medical genetics.

Depending on the patient's insurance, this will often be covered at least partially by medical insurance, but may require the orthodontist to call or send a letter to the primary physician explaining concerns, and that you would like a referral for your patient in common to the medical geneticist because of the listed signs, and to perhaps also rule out a specific syndrome, or of course follow up on whatever referrals the medical geneticist recommends for diagnosis or treatment besides orthodontics. The primary physician may already have some diagnostic information useful to the orthodontist.

As an educator I have often been asked by students: 'What do we need to know?' My response has been, 'Tell me about all the patients you will ever see, and then we can start from there.' No one knows every condition or syndrome that any of our patients may present to us, but we can be aware of when something seems out of the usual range of variation, particularly if more than one unusual feature is present. The following is a *selective and incomplete* survey of conditions/syndromes with brief descriptions regarding each one of them. The list is incomplete and there are many more conditions, which can be referenced with the help of the additional resources provided at the end of this chapter. While typically no single malformation or sign is pathognomonic, it may direct us to consider the referral and differential diagnosis (Cohen, 1980; Babic et al., 1993; Hartsfield, 1994, L Suri et al., 2004; Schulman et al., 2005; Jones and Smith, 2006; Bailleul-Forestier et al., 2008; Fleming et al., 2010). Some of the conditions are rare, and some are only relatively rare, although any of them may be presently recognized or unrecognized in your practice. Box 7.1 and resources noted later may also be useful if a patient comes to you with a particular diagnosis already made. Although not every patient will manifest what is expected of someone with a particular diagnosis, these resources can help the practitioner better understand a patient's condition and how it may affect treatment and how treatment may affect the patient.

Radiographic signs

Odontoma

The presence of an odontoma should alert the practitioner to inquire about the concurrent presence of dysphagia (difficulty in swallowing) or a family history of dysphagia that is perhaps due to hypertrophy of the smooth muscles of the esophagus as a part of the rare autosomal dominant odontoma–dysphagia syndrome (Bader, 1967).

Odontogenic keratocyst

See nevoid basal cell carcinoma (Gorlin) syndrome in maxillary hypoplasia section.

Taurodontism

Found in about 2.5% of Caucasian adults as an isolated (nonsyndromic) trait (Jaspers and Witkop, 1980). Individuals with nonsyndromic hypodontia are more likely to show taurodontism of the permanent first molars, whereas children with nonsyndromic supernumerary teeth are not (Kan et al., 2010). It can also be found in several conditions and syndromes, including the following syndromes.

Trichodentoosseous syndrome (TDO)
The features of TDO include variably kinky curly hair at birth, which straightens about half of the time after infancy; thin, pitted enamel, taurodontism; and, in approximately 80% of affected individuals, thickening of cortical bone (including of the skull). The natural straightening of the hair during infancy complicates the diagnosis of TDO and makes differentiating between TDO and amelogenesis imperfecta with taurodontism difficult in many cases. While TDO is caused by mutations in the *DLX3* gene, it is not clear if at least some cases of amelogenesis imperfecta with taurodontism are also caused by mutations in *DLX3*, or actually represent milder cases of TDO (Bloch-Zupan and Goodman, 2006; Visinoni et al., 2009).

The teeth are typically small, and often have a slight yellow-brown coloration, although there can be considerable variability in the clinical appearance of the teeth in affected individuals even within the same family. The teeth maybe mildly affected with normal color and a slight size reduction, to severe enamel hypoplasia and markedly reduced size. The incidence of dental abscesses is increased, and hypodontia may be present (Wright et al., 1997). The eruption of teeth may also be delayed (Suri et al., 2004). A detailed cephalometric analysis of the craniofacial structures in individuals with TDO did not establish a distinct craniofacial phenotype, although the cranial base length, cranial base angle, and length of the body of the mandible were all increased compared with unaffected relatives (Lichtenstein et al., 1972).

Otodental dysplasia
Features of this syndrome include grossly enlarged molars (globodontia), taurodontism, high-frequency sensorineural hearing deficit, and eye coloboma (part of the eye does not form due to failure of fusion of the intraocular fissure, and may be apparent externally as a 'notch' in the iris). Tooth eruption may also be delayed (Suri et al., 2004). Dental management has been described as interdisciplinary and complex, including regular follow-up, extraction of teeth as indicated and orthodontic treatment (Bloch-Zupan and Goodman, 2006).

Sex chromosome aneuplodies/anomalies
Sex chromosome aneuplodies/anomalies involve deviation from the normal XY chromosomes in males and XX chromosomes in females. The positive predictive value for Klinefelter syndrome (47, XXY, i.e. a male with an extra X chromosome that affects approximately 1.2 in 1000 males), given a male patient with taurodontism and a learning disability, is 84% (Schulman et al., 2005). In addition to tall stature for the family, a tendency toward mandibular prognathism and decreased facial height may also be present.

In contrast to the increase in taurodontism with an extra X chromosome, females lacking an X chromosome (Turner syndrome, 45, X and variations, occurs in 1 in 2500 females) appear not to have an increased incidence of taurodontism, although they may show increased variation in root morphology, including short roots (Varrela et al., 1990; Midtbo and Halse, 1994). Patients with Turner syndrome show

Box 7.1 Selected traits in selected syndromes and conditions[a]

Premature tooth exfoliation

Occurs often
- Early-onset periodontitis
- Hajdu–Cheney syndrome
- Hypophosphatasia
- Papillon–Lefèvre syndrome
- Singleton–Merten syndrome

Occurs occasionally
- Chédiak–Higashi syndrome
- Cherubism
- Coffin–Lowry syndrome
- Down syndrome
- Ehlers–Danlos syndrome
- Hypophosphatemia

Delayed tooth eruption
- Apert syndrome
- Amelo-onychohypohydrotic dysplasia
- Carpenter syndrome
- Cherubism
- Chondroectodermal dysplasia (Ellis–van Creveld syndrome)
- Cleidocranial dysplasia
- Coffin-Lowry syndrome
- Congenital hypertrichosis lanuginosa
- Cross syndrome (has gingival fibromatosis)
- Dentin dysplasia
- De Lange syndrome
- Down syndrome
- Dyskeratosis congenita
- Ectodermal dysplasias (some types)
- Ekman–Westborg–Julin syndrome
- Enamel agenesis and nephrocalcinosis
- Epidermolysis bullosa
- GAPO syndrome (growth retardation, alopecia, pseudoanodontia, and optic atrophy)
- Gardner syndrome
- Gaucher disease
- Gingival fibromatosis with sensorineural hearing loss
- Gingival fibromatosis with growth hormone deficiency
- Nevoid basal cell carcinoma (Gorlin) syndrome
- Hallermann–Streiff syndrome
- Hemifacial microsomia (Goldenhar syndrome, oculoauriculovertebral spectrum)
- Hurler–Scheie syndrome (a type of mucopolysaccharidosis [MPS], MPS I-H/S)
- Hurler syndrome (MPS I-H)
- Hunter syndrome (MPS II)
- Hyperimmunoglobulinemia E (Buckley syndrome)
- I-cell disease (mucolipidosis II)
- Incontinentia pigmenti (Bloch–Sulzberger syndrome)
- Laband syndrome (has gingival fibromatosis)
- Maroteaux–Lamy syndrome (MPS IV)
- Pyknodysostosis
- McCune–Albright syndrome (polyostotic fibrous dysplasia)
- Menke kinky hair syndrome
- Murray–Puretic–Drescher syndrome (has gingival fibromatosis)
- Neurofibromatosis
- Osteoglophonic dysplasia
- Osteopathia striata with cranial stenosis
- Osteopetrosis (marble bone disease)
- Osteogenesis imperfecta (variable)
- Otodental dysplasia
- Parry–Romberg syndrome (progressive hemifacial atrophy)
- Progeria (Hutchinson–Gilford syndrome)
- Rutherford syndrome (has gingival fibromatosis)
- Ramon syndrome (has gingival fibromatosis)

- Rothmund–Thompson syndrome
- Sclerosteosis
- SHORT syndrome
- Singleton–Merten syndrome
- Trichodentoosseous syndrome
- Velocardiofacial syndrome

Supernumerary teeth
- Chondroectodermal dysplasia (Ellis–van Creveld syndrome)
- Cleidocranial dysplasia
- Ehlers–Danlos vascular type (IV)
- Fabry disease
- Familial adenomatous polyposis (Gardner syndrome)
- Incontinentia pigmenti (Bloch–Sulzberger syndrome)
- Nance–Horan syndrome
- Saethre–Chotzen syndrome
- Trichorhinophalangeal syndrome type I (occasionally)

Taurodontism
- Down syndrome (occasionally)
- Ectodermal dysplasias (some occasionally)
- Lowe syndrome (occasionally)
- Oral-facial-digital II syndrome (occasionally)
- Otodental dysplasia
- Sex chromosome aneuplodies/anomalies with one or more extra X chromosome (e.g. Klinefelter syndrome)
- Seckel syndrome (occasionally)
- Trichodentoosseous syndrome
- Trisomy 18 (occasionally)
- Williams syndrome
- X-linked hypophosphatemic rickets (occasionally)

Odontoma
- Gardner syndrome
- Odontoma-dysphagia syndrome

Mandibular deficiency
- Hallermann–Streiff syndrome
- Hemifacial microsomia (Goldenhar syndrome, oculoauriculovertebral spectrum)
- Moebius (Mobius) syndrome
- Nager acrofacial dysostosis
- Robin sequence
- Treacher Collins syndrome
- Velocardiofacial syndrome
- Wildervanck–Smith syndrome

Cleft lip and or cleft palate[b]
- Apert syndrome
- Cleidocranial dysostosis (dysplasia)
- Diastrophic dwarfism
- Nevoid basal cell carcinoma (Gorlin) syndrome
- Ectrodactyly – ectodermal dysplasia – clefting (EEC) syndrome
- Fetal alcohol syndrome
- Fetal hydantoin syndrome
- Hemifacial microsomia (Goldenhar syndrome, oculoauriculovertebral spectrum)
- Larsen syndrome
- Marfan syndrome
- Nager acrofacial dysostosis
- Oral-facial-digital syndrome I
- Oral-facial-digital syndrome II
- Otopalatodigital syndrome
- Popliteal pterygia syndrome
- Single median maxillary central incisor
- Stickler syndrome
- Treacher Collins syndrome

(Continued)

- van der Woude syndrome
- Velocardiofacial syndrome
- Waardenburg syndrome

Median cleft lip[c]
- Frontonasal dysplasia
- Oral-facial-digital syndrome I
- Oral-facial-digital syndrome II
- Premaxillary agenesis syndrome
- 18p-karyotype

Midface (malar) deficiency
- Aarskog syndrome
- Achondroplasia
- Cleidocranial dysplasia (dysostosis)
- Coffin–Lowry syndrome
- Craniosynostoses (including Apert, Crouzon, Peiffer, Muenke and Saethre–Chotzen syndromes)
- Down syndrome
- Hajdu–Cheney syndrome
- Marshall syndrome
- Maxillonasal dysplasia (Binder syndrome)
- Singleton–Merten syndrome
- Stickler syndrome
- Trichorhinophalangeal syndrome I
- Velocardiofacial syndrome

Mandibular prognathism[d]
- Aarskog syndrome
- Chondroectodermal dysplasia (Ellis-van Crevald syndrome, occasionally)
- Cleidocranial dysplasia (dysostosis)
- Coffin–Lowry syndrome
- Down syndrome
- Fabry disease (occasionally)
- Fragile X syndrome
- Klinefelter syndrome and other sex chromosome aneuplodies in males)
- Marfan syndrome
- Maxillonasal dysplasia (Binder syndrome)
- Nevoid basal cell carcinoma (Gorlin) syndrome
- Osteogenesis imperfecta (types III and IV often)
- Papillon-Lefèvre and Haim–Munk syndromes
- Singleton–Merton syndrome (occasionally)

Long anterior facial height[e]
- Amelogenesis imperfecta
- Beckwith–Wiedemann syndrome (associated with macroglossia)
- Fragile X syndrome
- Klinefelter syndrome and other sex chromosome aneuplodies in males)
- Marfan syndrome
- Velocardiofacial syndrome
- Facial asymmetry
- Hemifacial microsomia (Goldenhar syndrome, oculoauriculovertebral spectrum)
- Hemihypertrophy
- Neurofibromatosis (occasionally)
- Parry–Romberg syndrome
- Saethre–Chotzen syndrome (nasal deviation common)
- Velocardiofacial syndrome

Ocular hypertelorism[f]
- Aarskog syndrome
- Apert syndrome
- Nevoid basal cell carcinoma (Gorlin) syndrome
- Crouzon syndrome
- Fetal face syndrome
- Frontonasal dysplasia
- Hypertelorism-hypospadias syndrome
- Leopard syndrome
- Noonan syndrome
- Oral-facial-digital syndrome I

- Pfeiffer syndrome
- Waardenburg syndrome

Syndromes associated with dental dysplasias (amelogenesis imperfecta, dentinogenesis imperfecta and dentin dysplasia)
- Amelogenesis imperfecta with nephrocalcinosis (McGibbon syndrome)
- Autoimmune polyendocrinopathy
- Cone–rod dystrophy and amelogenesis imperfecta
- Ehlers–Danlos syndrome (some types)
- Familial hypophosphatemic vitamin D-resistant rickets
- Goldblatt syndrome
- Hyperphosphatemic familial tumoral calcinosis (HFTC)
- Kohlschütter–Tönz syndrome
- Osteogenesis imperfecta (some in type I, mostly in types III and IV)
- Schimke immunoosseous dysplasia (SIOD)
- Seckel syndrome
- Trichodentoosseous syndrome
- Vitamin D-dependent rickets
- Vitamin D-resistant rickets

Supernumerary teeth (hyperdontia)
- Cleidocranial dysplasia (dysostosis)
- Fabry disease (occasionally)
- Familial adenomatous polyposis (FAP), Gardner syndrome
- Nance–Horan syndrome

Dental agenesis[g]
- Aarskog syndrome
- Axenfeld–Rieger malformation and Rieger syndrome
- Cancer (colorectal, epithelial ovarian, rare?)
- Chondroectodermal dysplasia (Ellis-van Crevald syndrome)
- Coffin–Lowry syndrome
- Down syndrome
- Fabry disease (occasionally)
- Kallmann syndrome
- Ectodermal dysplasias
- Hallermann–Strieff syndrome
- Hypohidrotic ectodermal dysplasia (HED)
- Incontinentia pigmenti
- Hypohidrotic ectodermal dysplasia and immune deficiency (HED-ID)
- p63 mutation-related syndromes
- Lacrimo-auriculo-dento-digital syndrome
- Johansson–Blizzard syndrome
- Single median maxillary central incisor (SMMCI)
- Trichodentoosseous syndrome
- Wilkie oculo-facio-cardio-dental syndrome
- Williams syndrome
- Wolf–Hirschhorn syndrome

[a]A syndrome or condition listed under a trait may not always, or even often, show the trait in every affected individual. Some syndromes/conditions are listed under more than one trait, which may help in forming a differential diagnosis if the patient has more than one trait and two or more are found in the same condition.

[b]There are over 300 'clefting syndromes'.

[c]In the middle of the upper lip, developmentally between the medial nasal prominences, in contrast to the more common cleft lip that is paramedian (lateral) to the midsagittal plane.

[d]May be, at least partially, maxillary hypoplasia.

[e]May be with open bite tendency.

[f]Increased distance between the eyes, real or apparent.

[g]Besides the third molars; avoid the term congenital absence as the teeth are typically absent at birth anyway, at least clinically, and most radiographically as well. Can variably be in families or just one family member. Being associated with some other anomaly, especially in more than one family member, is an indication for clinical genetics referral.

Sources: Hartsfield (1994), L Suri et al. (2004), Fleming et al. (2010), Bailleul-Forestier et al. (2008), Cohen (1980), Jones and Smith (2006), Hennekam et al. (2010), Babic et al. (1993), Schulman et al. (2005).

variable short stature, low hairline, low-set ears, and broad necks. These patients typically experience gonadal dysfunction (nonworking ovaries), which results in amenorrhea (absence of menstrual cycle) (Bader, 1967).

Depending on the sex, lack of an X chromosome or the presence of an extra X chromosome produces opposite effects on cranial base flexion, jaw displacement, and maxillary and mandibular inclination to the anterior cranial base. An extra X chromosome in males affected the jaw relationship in the sagittal plane, typically increasing the length of the mandible, while an extra X chromosome in females resulted in shorter lengths of the anterior and posterior cranial bases, the calvarium, mandibular ramus, and the posterior and upper anterior face.

The lack of an X chromosome in females (Turner syndrome) results predominantly in cranial base changes, so that the mandible is short in the sagittal plane, whereas the maxilla is of normal length. The extra Y chromosome in 47, XYY males results in larger craniofacial dimensions than in normal males, without substantial effects on dimensional ratios and plane angles. In general, there is a skeletal height and craniofacial growth-promoting effect from an extra Y chromosome, and a delaying effect from an extra X chromosome (Babic et al., 1993; Krusinskiene et al., 2005; Alvesalo, 2009).

Williams syndrome

Physical features of this condition include characteristic facial features with full prominent cheeks, wide mouth, long philtrum, small nose with depressed nasal bridge, heavy orbital ridges, medial eyebrow flare, dental abnormalities, hoarse voice, growth retardation, and cardiovascular abnormalities (most commonly supravalvular aortic stenosis and/or peripheral pulmonary artery stenosis). The cognitive profile is distinctive, consisting of strengths in auditory memory, language, and face-processing, but extreme weakness in visual-spatial, numerical, and problem-solving abilities.

Cephalometric analysis shows the anterior and posterior cranial bases are shorter in individuals with Williams syndrome, although the cranial base angle is normal. The frontal and occipital bones are thicker, and the shape of the sella turcica may be unusual. Marked deficiency of the bony chin in combination with a large mandibular plane angle can give the impression of a retrusive mandible. Hypodontia is frequent, and the teeth tend to be small. Maxillary and mandibular incisors in both jaws are often tapered towards the incisal edge (screwdriver-shaped). Most of the molars deemed as being taurodontic have short total tooth lengths and can thus be defined as having taurodontism without meeting the classical definition (Axelsson, 2005).

Other conditions in which taurodontism is seen more commonly than in the general population include trisomy 18, some types of ectodermal dysplasia, Down syndrome,

Mohr (oral-facial-digital, type II) syndrome, Seckel syndrome, Lowe syndrome, and X-linked hypophosphatemic rickets (X-linked hypophosphatemia; see under conditions in which premature tooth exfoliation may occur occasionally) (Cichon and Pack, 1985; Kan et al., 2010).

History of premature tooth exfoliation

A history of primary teeth exfoliation prior to the age of 5 years in the absence of trauma is an indication to investigate further, as a number of conditions that concern orthodontists include the risk of additional tooth loss. The early exfoliation of primary teeth resulting from periodontitis has been observed occasionally in children. Along with hypophosphatasia, early-onset periodontitis appears to be the most common cause of premature exfoliation of the primary teeth, especially in girls (Hartsfield, 1994).

Hypophosphatasia

The disease is characterized by improper mineralization of bone caused by deficient tissue nonspecific alkaline phosphatase activity in serum, liver, bone, and kidney. Increased levels of urinary phosphoethanolamine are also seen. Diagnostic tests should include the determination of serum alkaline phosphatase levels for parents and siblings (Hu et al., 1996).

The typical dental finding diagnostic of hypophosphatasia in children is premature exfoliation of the anterior primary teeth associated with deficient cementum. The loss of teeth in the young child may be spontaneous or may result from a slight trauma. Early exfoliation of the primary teeth is usually associated with the juvenile type of hypophosphatasia, although such a history may also be present in the adult type. Severe gingival inflammation will be absent. The loss of alveolar bone may be limited to the anterior region. Treatment of patients with hypophosphatasia may be problematic because of the risk of permanent tooth loosening during orthodontic procedures (Macfarlane and Swart, 1989).

Early-onset periodontitis

This may occur in the primary dentition (prepubertal periodontitis), develop during puberty (juvenile periodontitis, JP), or may be characterized by exceedingly rapid loss of alveolar bone (rapidly progressive periodontitis). Because several forms of early-onset periodontitis (e.g. localized prepubertal periodontitis, localized JP, and generalized JP) can be found in the same family, the expression of the underlying genetic etiology appears to have the potential to be influenced by other genetic and environmental factors (Schenkein, 1998).

Early-onset periodontitis may occur by itself (nonsyndromic), or as a part of a syndrome. For example, leukocyte adhesion deficiency (LAD) types I and II are autosomal recessive disorders of the leukocyte adhesion cascade. LAD type I has abnormalities in the integrin receptors of leukocytes, leading to impaired adhesion and chemotaxis, which results in an increased susceptibility for severe infections and early-onset (prepubertal) periodontitis (Meyle and Gonzales, 2001). In LAD type II, the severity of the general infectious episodes is much milder than those observed in LAD type I, although there is chronic severe periodontitis. Furthermore, patients with LAD type II, present other abnormal features, such as growth and mental retardation, which are related to the primary defect in fucose metabolism or specific transporter of GDP-fucose into the Golgi apparatus causing no fucolysation and no surface expression (Etzioni and Tonetti, 2000).

Orthodontic movement of teeth into previously affected areas has been reported to be successful after a short healing period following extractions secondary to periodontal disease, crowding, to correct anteroposterior discrepancies, or reduce bimaxillary protrusion (McLain et al., 1983). Teeth that have lost periodontal support may be indicated in particular for extraction. For example, it has been claimed that after orthodontic space closure, bony contours and attachment levels on repositioned second and third molars will be superior to those possible if the affected first molars were retained and treated.

As for any patient, each case is unique, and the treatment plan depends on close collaboration with the periodontist, the stability of the remaining teeth, and possible substitutions that would result in a functional occlusion. Periodontal evaluations should be scheduled as often as orthodontic appointments to monitor the condition during tooth movement (McLain et al., 1983).

Papillon–Lefèvre and Haim–Munk syndromes

Two of the many different types of palmoplantar keratoderma (thickened skin over the palms and soles of the feet that may appear to be darkened or 'dirty') differ from the others by the occurrence of severe early-onset periodontitis with premature loss of the primary and permanent dentition. Lateral cephalometric analysis of eight patients with Papillon-Lefèvre syndrome revealed a tendency toward a Class III skeletal relationship with maxillary retrognathia, decreased lower facial height, retroclined mandibular incisors, and upper lip retrusion (Bindayel et al., 2008).

It has been reported that following a successful combined mechanical and antibiotic therapy of periodontitis associated with the Papillon–Lefèvre syndrome, moderate orthodontic tooth movements may be possible within a complex interdisciplinary treatment regimen (Lux et al., 2005). Haim–Munk syndrome is characterized in addition to features seen in Papillon-Lefèvre syndrome by arachnodactyly (long and thin fingers and toes), acroosteolysis (destruction of the digit tips, including the bone,), and onychogryphosis (hypertrophy and curving of the nails, giving them a claw-like appearance) (Hart et al., 1997).

Singleton–Merten syndrome

A rare condition with dentin dysplasia and poor dental root development, progressive calcification of the thoracic aorta, calcific aortic stenosis, osteoporosis, and expansion of the marrow cavities in hand bones like that observed in anemia. Generalized muscle weakness and atrophy may also be present. Maxillary hypoplasia has also been noted (Singleton and Merten, 1973; Feigenbaum et al., 1988).

Hajdu–Cheney syndrome

A heritable, rare disorder of bone metabolism, associated with acroosteolysis, short stature, distinctive craniofacial and skull changes, periodontitis, and premature tooth loss. Bazopoulou-Kyrkanidou et al. (2007) reported the case of a 22-year-old affected woman, who presented characteristic clinical features including short stature, small face, prominent epicanthal folds, thin lips, small mouth, and short hands. Biochemical, hematological, and hormonal parameters were normal. Tests for bone mineral density were indicative of osteoporosis. Cephalometric analysis revealed hypoplasia of the mid-face and increased cranial base angle; the maxilla and the mandible were set posterior. The sella turcica was enlarged, elongated, and wide open with slender clinoids.

The mandible may be underdeveloped as well as the maxilla and mid-face. Le Fort III maxillary distraction osteogenesis and advancement genioplasty followed by orthodontia were successfully performed for a mid-facial retrusion and to eliminate severe snoring during sleep in a reported case (Satoh et al., 2002).

Conditions in which premature tooth exfoliation may occur occasionally

Ehlers–Danlos syndrome

See 'Connective tissue dysplasia' section later in the chapter.

X-linked hypophosphatemic rickets (X-linked hypophosphatemia)

In addition to short stature and bowing of the lower extremities, there are often dental manifestations, including apical radiolucencies, abscesses (that may result in premature exfoliation of teeth), and fistulas associated with pulp exposures in the primary and permanent teeth. The pulp exposures relate to the pulp horns extending to the dentinoenamel junction or even to the external surface of the tooth. The thin, hypomineralized enamel may abrade easily, exposing the pulp. Dental radiographs show rickety bone trabeculations and absent or abnormal lamina dura (Smith and Steinhauser, 1971; Hartsfield, 1994).

There are other types of hypophosphatemia with overlapping clinical features and different modes of inheritance and genes involved. Generally, the more severe and earlier the onset, the more severe dental manifestations will be. In contrast, vitamin D-deficient rickets does not show the dental abnormalities found in X-linked hypophosphatemic rickets (Hartsfield, 1994). Recently, dental abnormalities in patients with familial hypophosphatemic vitamin D-resistant rickets were prevented or diminished by early treatment with 1-hydroxyvitamin D (Chaussain-Miller et al., 2003). Successful treatment of a relatively mild case with Class II Division 2 malocclusion with severe anterior crowding and lack of mandibular growth with a functional appliance, followed by the extraction of four premolars and the use of edgewise appliances has been reported. No unfavorable root resorption or bone defect occurred (Kawakami and Takano-Yamamoto, 1997).

Coffin–Lowry syndrome

This X-linked condition typically affects boys (although girls may be affected less severely), with developmental delay/usually severe mental deficiency, hypotonia (muscle weakness), laterally downslanting palpebral fissures (eye openings), maxillary hypoplasia, prominent lips and anterior open bite tendency, short stature, and thick soft hands with tapering fingers. Sensorineural hearing deficit, cataracts, and retinal changes are occasional abnormalities. In addition to hypodontia with dental spacing and large maxillary central incisors, late eruption and premature loss of primary teeth are common (Hartsfield et al., 1993).

Down syndrome

This results from trisomy of all or a large part of chromosome 21, occurring in 1 in 660 births. There are many variable features associated with Down syndrome, including laterally up-slanting palpebral fissures, flat facial profile (europrosopic with brachycephaly), hypotonia (which tends to improve with age), joint hyperflexibility, developmental delay/some degree of mental deficiency, and excess neck skin.

Periodontal disease is common in the older patient, especially in the anterior mandibular region. Paradoxically they may have fewer dental caries, although baby bottle caries may be a concern. The tongue is often positioned partially outside the mouth (particularly when young), giving the impression that it is enlarged, although it is likely to be a posture secondary to hypotonia of the tongue and the facial musculature, and the relatively small size of the oral cavity (Hartsfield, 1994; Hennequin et al., 1999).

It has been claimed that almost all individuals with Down syndrome have a significant malocclusion, typically a maxillary hypoplasia, Class III malocclusion with anterior open bite, often with hypodontia, tooth size discrepancy, and occasionally with impacted or transposed teeth. Considerations in the treatment of individuals with Down syndrome include a two-phase or multiphase plan to assist in early correction of maxillary transverse deficiency and Class III malocclusion.

As with any individual with developmental delay/mental deficiency, cooperation and tolerance of the discomforts associated with orthodontic appliances and procedures are necessary for effective treatment (Hennequin et al., 1999; Musich, 2006). Cooperation may occur after some initial difficulty, but sometimes it is just not possible. Some procedures may be done in the operating room, but not orthodontic treatment on a continuing basis.

Treatment considerations include taking impressions using quick-set materials with flavors that may reduce the tendency to gag that is frequently experienced by Down syndrome patients, bonding brackets instead of banding, using a self-etching primer with a glass ionomer cement that can be used in the oral environment when it is difficult to maintain a dry field for several minutes at a time, using nickel-titanium wires when and for as long as possible allowing a longer interval between appointments, and considering the use of implants while treatment planning to replace agenic teeth and temporary anchorage devices to minimize the need for compliance (Musich, 2006).

The stages of eruption and development of teeth are often delayed in children with Down syndrome. It has been recommended that regular radiographic screening, in order to intervene as indicated to guide impacted teeth to their appropriate locations, might prevent or diminish malocclusion and lead to optimal bone height. It is also important to note that growth stature is slower than usual during childhood, the adolescent period is shorter, and that skeletal maturation is delayed, taking place around 15–17 years of age (Reuland-Bosma et al., 2010).

De Moura et al. (2008) found that Down syndrome patients who underwent rapid maxillary expansion showed a reduction in hearing deficit, the yearly rate of ear, nose, and throat infections, and parentally assessed symptoms of upper airway obstruction compared with Down syndrome children who received no treatment. They concluded that these findings were probably related to increased oronasal space secondary to the expansion.

Chédiak–Higashi syndrome

This rare autosomal recessive disorder has frequently been linked with severe periodontitis (Meyle and Gonzales, 2001). It is characterized by oculocutaneous hypopigmentation, severe immunological deficiency with neutropenia and lack of natural killer cells, a bleeding tendency, and neurologic abnormalities (Nagle et al., 1996).

Cherubism

This rare childhood disease may be so variable that a clinically normal-appearing parent may have a history of prominent facial swellings or radiographic evidence of abnormal bone pattern in the mandible. Although the progression of bone destruction typically stabilizes or even regresses after puberty, a few very aggressive cases, sometimes producing morbid results, have been reported (Ayoub and El-Mofty, 1993; Timosca et al., 2000; Silva et al., 2002). Teeth in the involved area are frequently exfoliated prematurely as a result of the loss of support or root resorption or, in permanent teeth, as a result of interference in the development of roots. Spontaneous loss of teeth may occur, or the child may pick teeth out of the soft tissue (McDonald et al., 2011). Delay in tooth eruption may also occur (Suri et al., 2004). Reossification of cystic areas within the jaws therefore usually occurs spontaneously, and dislocated teeth have subsequently been realigned orthodontically. Advancements in virtual three-dimensional (3D) reconstruction of anatomical structures based on computed tomography (CT) or cone-beam CT data have provided for more predictable individual treatment planning (Pierce et al., 1996; Holst et al., 2009).

Supernumerary teeth and hypodontia (oligodontia)

It is rare to find *multiple* supernumeraries in individuals with no other associated disease or syndrome, although some individual cases have been reported (Fleming et al., 2010). Thus the presence of multiple supernumerary teeth is a strong indication for further diagnostic evaluation, especially if any other anomalies are present.

Cleidocranial dysplasia (dysostosis)

Cleidocranial dysplasia or dysostosis is characterized by agenesis or hypoplasia of the clavicles (allowing the shoulders to be rolled to the body midline in the more severe cases), delayed and imperfect ossification of the cranium (with variable persistence of open fontanels and sutures), moderately short stature, and a variety of other skeletal abnormalities; although clinical variation may be seen even among affected members of the same family (Golan et al., 2002; Farronato et al., 2009).

As the frontal, parietal, and occipital bones are prominent, the skull tends to be brachycephalic, with the face appearing small relative to the cranium with hypoplastic maxillary, lachrymal, nasal, and zygomatic bones. The maxillary and/or paranasal sinuses may be underdeveloped. The maxillary hypoplasia results in a relative mandibular protrusion. Occasionally cleft palate has been reported. The dental manifestations are a delayed exfoliation of primary teeth, a lack of or delayed eruption of the permanent dentition which may appear without radiography to be hypodontia, and multiple supernumerary teeth (Farronato et al., 2009).

Patients with cleidocranial dysostosis benefit from a team approach with good cooperation and communication within the team and with the patient and family (Farronato et al., 2009). As with any patient with a hypoplastic/retrusive

maxilla, timing of a dentofacial orthopedic intervention to bring the maxilla ventrally is critical, usually before the age of 10 years, depending on skeletal maturation (Macfarlane and Swart, 1989; Kim et al., 1999; Clocheret et al., 2003).

The most effective therapeutic approach for the early treatment of the dentofacial problems in cleidocranial dysplasia is to start with the protraction of the maxilla, followed by orthodontic and surgical treatments as indicated. Further orthodontic treatment and surgery may be required following the pubertal growth spurt. Although there are abundant teeth, sometimes they cannot be moved or placed in an acceptable position, which may necessitate prosthetics with or without surgery.

Several methods, surgical and/or prosthetic, have been put forth for oral-facial treatment in cleidocranial dysplasia. An early diagnosis is helpful so that early surgical intervention may be undertaken, typically in a more aggressive fashion than previously, in order to facilitate dental eruption. Although application of a protocol depends on individual patient needs, it has been stated that the 'Jerusalem' protocol is recommended as an initial consideration. This protocol involves two surgeries (anterior and posterior) under general anesthesia at the stage when the root development of unerupted teeth is at least two-thirds of the final estimated length. The first surgery is performed at the chronological age of 10–12 years, which with the usual dental development delay in cleidocranial dysplasia corresponds to a dental age of 7–8 years. In addition to the extraction of deciduous incisors and supernumerary unerupted teeth in both arches, unerupted permanent incisors are exposed and have attachments bonded to them, followed by primary closure of the surgical flaps. The immature posterior permanent teeth are not exposed or their dental follicles disturbed at this stage.

In the second operation (chronological age of at least 13 years; dental age of 10–11 years), deciduous canines and molars are extracted, permanent canines and premolars are exposed in both arches, attachments are bonded and the surgical flap is closed. Care should be taken in the extraction of supernumerary unerupted teeth and the exposure of permanent unerupted teeth in order to maintain the integrity of vestibular and lingual/palatal bone plates. Bone is only removed around the crowns of the permanent teeth as needed for the bonding of attachments. In order to encourage healing by first intention, the flap is repositioned so as to completely cover the wound, without compresses/pressure.

Traction is placed by the application of low extrusion forces using rigid upper and lower arches, and anterior box elastic between the two arches to oppose the possible distortions caused by the excess of space in the arch and the resistance to extrusion. Further details of the treatment protocol may be found in the cited papers by

Becker et al. (Becker et al., 1997a,b; D'Alessandro et al., 2010).

Nance–Horan syndrome

This is an X-linked condition typically affecting males, although as with many X-linked recessive conditions, females may be affected to some degree. The typical pattern is the presence of congenital cataracts (with vision impairment, particularly in males), anteverted (folded outward) external ears, shortened metacarpal bones, and dental anomalies including screwdriver-shaped incisors (crown form tapering towards the incisal edge resembling a flat screwdriver head), maxillary midline diastema, mesiodens, and mulberry (multilobed crown) molars. Thirty percent of those affected have some mental impairment. Although some affected males do not have mesiodens, there appears to be a positive correlation in severity between the eye and dental findings (Bixler et al., 1984; Toutain et al., 2002).

Chondroectodermal dysplasia (Ellis–van Creveld syndrome)

This is an autosomal recessive disorder with postaxial polydactyly (extra digit on the little finger side), short limb dwarfism, dysplastic (small and/or misshapen) fingernails, and prominent and additional oral frenula along with serrations of the alveolar ridge. There may be neonatal teeth, hypodontia, small teeth, or delayed eruption of teeth. The upper lip may be short, and more tightly bound to the alveolar ridge because of the frenula (Varela and Ramos, 1996).

Malocclusions are common in Ellis–van Creveld syndrome, albeit inconsistent in type. Many of these patients show normal cephalometric parameters, although hypoplasia of the anterior maxilla with relative prognathism of the mandible has been found in some individuals. A large gonial angle with increased anterior lower face height has also been shown in this syndrome (Prabhu et al., 1978, Varela and Ramos, 1996). Other syndromes that are associated with short stature, polydactyly, and orofacial abnormalities include oral-facial-digital syndromes I and II, and asphyxiating thoracic dystrophy (Varela and Ramos, 1996).

Gardner syndrome (familial adenomatous polyposis)

See section 'Supernumerary teeth or hypodontia (oligodontia)' later in the chapter.

Fabry disease

An X-linked metabolic disorder caused by a deficiency of the lysosomal enzyme α-galactosidase A. The deficit of this catabolic enzyme causes a progressive accumulation of glycosphingolipids containing α-galactosyl residues in multiple organs. Although some patients may be diagnosed in adulthood, the first symptoms of Fabry disease are usually noticed during childhood, when the patient typically experiences febrile episodes, painful acroparesthesia (burning feeling of the hands and feet), and gastrointestinal upset.

The accumulation of glycophospholipids leads to numerous systemic manifestations, including cutaneous angiokeratomas (lesions of capillaries, resulting in small marks of red to blue color and characterized by hyperkeratosis), fever from anhidrosis (lack of sweating) due to sweat gland failure, stroke at a young age, cardiovascular disease, renal dysfunction, and corneal dystrophy (Baccaglini et al., 2001).

Malocclusion has been reported to be common, with variable skeletal bimaxillary protrusion, and molar Class III, I, or rarely II. Both supernumerary teeth and, less commonly, hypodontia have been present in affected individuals. Diastemata may be present. Xerostomia has been reported, which if present may complicate oral hygiene during orthodontic treatment (Baccaglini et al., 2001).

Incontinentia pigmenti (Bloch–Sulzberger syndrome)

This is a genodermatosis that segregates as an X-linked dominant disorder and is usually lethal prenatally in males. In affected females it causes highly variable abnormalities of the skin, hair, nails, teeth, eyes, and central nervous system (Smahi et al., 2000). In the fully developed disease, the skin shows swirling patterns of melanin pigmentation, especially on the trunk, although this may fade with age. Hypodontia and peg-shaped teeth are characteristic, with some cases exhibiting delayed dental eruption as well. The lack of vertical support from hypodontia of the posterior arches may result in forward rotation of the mandible. A combined orthodontic and prosthetic treatment plan is often needed. Treatment may be complicated by the ability of the patient to cooperate, which can vary (Yamashiro et al., 1998).

Trichorhinophalangeal syndrome type I (TRPS type I)

Impacted supernumerary teeth have occasionally been described in TRPS type I (Gorlin et al., 1969; Karacay et al., 2007). Affected individuals have characteristic facies with sparse scalp hair, bulbous tip of the nose, long flat philtrum, thin upper vermilion border, and protruding ears. Axial skeletal abnormalities include cone-shaped epiphyses at the phalanges, hip malformations, and short stature (Momeni et al., 2000). A lateral cephalometric study found them to have a shortened posterior face height associated with a short mandibular ramus, as well as a reduced and superiorly deflected posterior cranial base. These craniofacial findings were associated with a steep inclination of the lower border of the mandible (King and Frias, 1979).

Midface hypoplasia has also been noted (Hennekam et al., 2010).

Syndromic hypodontia

A search on missing permanent teeth, and oligodontia/anodontia, on the 'POSSUM Web' subscription syndrome identification program (Murdoch Childrens Research Institute, Royal Childrens Hospital, Melbourne, Australia, www.possum.net.au) identified 288 syndromes/conditions in which this phenomenon may occur, including trichodentoosseous syndrome, Williams syndrome, Coffin–Lowry syndrome, Down syndrome, Ellis–van Crevald syndrome, Fabry syndrome, incontinentia pigmenti, and many types of ectodermal dysplasia.

Single median maxillary incisor

A unique form of hypodontia that may be of significant medical importance is the presence of a single primary and permanent maxillary central incisor. Although it may at first appear to be a product of fusion, if the single tooth is in the midline, and symmetrical with normal crown, root shape, and size, then it may be an isolated (nonsyndromic) finding, or may be part of the solitary median maxillary central incisor (SMMCI) syndrome. This is a heterogeneous condition which may include midline developmental abnormalities of the brain and other structures due to mutation in the sonic hedgehog (*SHH*) gene, *SIX3*, or other genetic abnormality (Nanni et al., 2001).

SMMCI is estimated to occur in 1:50 000 live births. Congenital nasal malformation (choanal atresia, midnasal or pyriform aperture stenosis) is positively associated with SMMCI. The presence of SMMCI can predict associated anomalies and in particular the serious developmental brain anomaly holoprosencephaly, which is often, but not always, associated with ocular hypotelorism (decreased distance between the eyes). Common developmental anomalies associated with SMMCI are severe to mild intellectual disability, congenital heart disease, and cleft lip and/or palate. Less frequently, microcephaly, hypopituitarism, hypotelorism, convergent strabismus, esophageal and duodenal atresia, cervical hemivertebrae, cervical dermoid, hypothyroidism, scoliosis, absent kidney, micropenis, and ambiguous genitalia are present. Notably, short stature is present in half the children with SMMCI (Hall et al., 1997).

The SMMCI tooth itself is mainly an esthetic problem, which is ideally managed by combined orthodontic, prosthodontic, and oral surgical treatment; alternatively, it can be left untreated. Thus the importance of the orthodontist recognizing and referring the patient and family for evaluation is primarily that SMMCI, even in the absence of any other clinical signs, can be the mildest expression of a strong family tendency to pass on developmental abnor-

malities that may range from just the SMMCI, to other anomalies such as holoprosencephaly. The orthodontist may be responsible for diagnosing cases of SMMCI with no obvious (traumatic) cause, and in these subjects due consideration should be given to referral for the appropriate genetic testing and counseling (Hall et al., 1997; Kjaer et al., 2001; DiBiase and Cobourne, 2008).

Aarskog syndrome

This condition most severely affects males, although carrier females may show milder signs (especially in the facies and hands) with X-linked recessive inheritance. In males, features include slight to moderate short stature, shortened fingers with mild webbing, ocular hypertelorism (increased distance between the eyes), and other findings; the midface and maxilla are often hypoplastic, resulting in a Class III malocclusion, for which orthodontic treatment is often indicated. Delayed dental development and eruption may be found, although it tends to be delayed less than height for chronological age and bone age. In addition to an increase in malocclusion compared with the general population, there is an increased prevalence of hypodontia and caries (Halse et al., 1979).

Supernumerary teeth or hypodontia (oligodontia) and cancer

The association of supernumerary teeth or hypodontia (oligodontia) with cancer may be part of a syndrome, an autosomal dominant trait by itself, or what appears to be a nonsyndromic positive but not absolute correlation.

Gardner syndrome (familial adenomatous polyposis)

Familial adenomatous polyposis (FAP) is an autosomal dominant disorder characterized by predisposition to cancer. Affected individuals usually develop hundreds to thousands of adenomatous polyps of the colon and rectum, a small proportion of which will progress to colorectal carcinoma if not surgically treated. Gardner syndrome is a variant of FAP in which desmoid tumors (fibrous neoplasms originating from musculo-aponeurotic structures), osteomas, and other neoplasms occur together with multiple adenomas of the colon and rectum (Nishisho et al., 1991).

The skull, mandible, facial bones, and paranasal sinuses are the most common sites for the associated osteomas (Ishikawa et al., 1986; Lew et al., 1999). The early detection of osteomas is critical, as they always precede the presentation of intestinal polyps, which may transform into colorectal cancers (Katou et al., 1989; Nandakumar et al., 2004).

The dental abnormalities in Gardner syndrome include multiple ectopic teeth, impacted permanent teeth, supernumerary teeth, retained primary teeth, hypercementosis, and odontomas (Thomas and Smith, 1981; Carl and

Herrera, 1987). Dental eruption may be delayed as well (Suri et al., 2004). Although pan-oral radiographs may be useful for early detection of osteomas, they may be of limited use. Since the size and location of odontomas may act as a complicating factor in the dental management of a case, it has been proposed that cone-beam CT scans would be beneficial (Kamel et al., 2009).

The variation in the location and size of the osteomas requires evaluation and possibly different treatment plans for those affected, even within the same family. Difficulty in moving teeth through bone with increased density may be ascertained by an initial stage of treatment. The hyper-cementosis may complicate tooth extraction. All of these factors necessitate close consultation and cooperation between the oral maxillofacial surgeon and orthodontist, along with the general dentist and/or prosthodontists as needed (Kamel et al., 2009).

Oligodontia-colorectal cancer syndrome

A striking example of autosomal dominant inheritance was reported in a Finnish family in which oligodontia and colorectal cancer were associated with each other. The oligodontia and cancer predisposition were caused by a mutation in the *AXIN2* gene. Colorectal cancer or precancerous lesions in the family were found only in association with oligodontia and the *AXIN2* mutation, and affected all those of the oldest generation who had the mutation (Lammi et al., 2004).

Hypodontia and epithelial ovarian cancer

Further support for the proposition that hypodontia can be developmentally associated with cancer comes from a University of Kentucky report that women with epithelial ovarian cancer (EOC) are 8.1 times more likely to have hypodontia than are women without EOC. In contrast to the oligodontia reported with the specific mutations in *AXIN2*, the severity of hypodontia was similar between the two groups (affected and nonaffected) in the Kentucky study, with one or two teeth being agenic. Maxillary lateral incisors, followed by second premolars, were the most frequently affected teeth (Chalothorn et al., 2008).

This is not to say that everyone who has hypodontia, or even oligodontia, is going to, or is even at increased risk to, develop cancer. To suggest so to young patients and/or their families would only lead to needless worry, unless there is a striking family history of cancer in the individual with hypodontia/oligodontia. In that case, referral to a clinical geneticist, especially one who deals with familial cancer, would be indicated if the family had not previously been evaluated. Future studies into the family history and genetic analysis of individuals with hypodontia will help illustrate what the relative risk may be of individuals or family members developing cancer associated with hypodontia in the general population.

Failure of dental eruption

Primary failure of eruption (nonsyndromic)

In contrast to failure of teeth to erupt associated with mechanical failure of eruption (e.g. cysts, gingival fibromatosis, and impeding adjacent teeth) or with syndromes such as cleidocranial dysplasia, primary failure of eruption (PFE) is a condition in which all teeth distal to the most mesial involved tooth do not erupt *or* respond to orthodontic force. The familial occurrence of this phenomenon in approximately one-quarter of cases facilitated the investigation and discovery of *PTHR1* involvement (Decker et al., 2008; Proffit and Frazier-Bowers, 2009). In addition to diagnosis of individuals who are likely to develop or have PFE, further advancements in this area could potentially result in a treatment for PFE, as well as the molecular manipulation of selective tooth eruption rates to enhance treatment protocols (Wise et al., 2002; Stellzig-Eisenhauer et al., 2010).

The clinical impact of PFE is frequently very severe. Alveolar bone growth is impaired in the affected areas. The affected teeth appear at the base of a large vertical defect and often present dilacerations. The result is a severe lateral open bite. Unfortunately, affected teeth typically become ankylosed as soon as orthodontic force is applied (Proffit and Vig, 1981; Raghoebar et al., 1989). It is not clear why highly variable clinical expressivity is observed in PFE, with some persons affected bilaterally and others affected unilaterally in the same family. Likewise, there is no apparent explanation for why the posterior dentition is preferentially affected. To date, there are only a few anecdotal cases of successful extrusion of teeth affected with PFE. Thus, any attempt at early orthodontic intervention involving affected teeth for these patients has been said to be futile, and may even make the situation worse if the force increases the occurrence of ankylosis (Frazier-Bowers et al., 2010).

Once growth is complete with the expected posterior open bite, single-tooth or multiple-tooth osteotomies or selective extractions followed by implants can often result in a functional occlusion. The advantage of making an early diagnosis of PFE is that the clinician may observe the unfavorable growth changes that inevitably take place, and can then explain to the patient and family that this is preferred over useless and potentially damaging early orthodontic intervention involving those teeth. The best treatment for an accurately established early diagnosis of PFE is initially no treatment of the affected teeth, reserving the multidisciplinary options for affected patients for a later time after the completion of growth (Frazier-Bowers et al., 2010).

Gingival fibromatosis (hyperplasia)

Generalized gingival enlargement can be caused by a variety of factors. It can be inherited as a nonsyndromic trait (hereditary gingival fibromatosis, HGF), associated with other diseases characterizing a syndrome or, most commonly, induced as a side effect of medications such as phenytoin, ciclosporin, or nifedipine. Regardless of the etiology, the increased thickness and firmness of the overlying gingiva may impede and/or alter the course of dental eruption. Interestingly its occurrence is coincident usually, but not always, with the eruption of teeth, particularly of the permanent dentition (Hartsfield et al., 1985; Suri et al., 2004; Coletta and Graner, 2006).

Excision of the hyperplastic tissue is indicated for esthetic or functional reasons, including facilitation of tooth eruption and good oral hygiene. Unfortunately, reports about recurrence rates are conflicting, and so the long-term benefit (chance of recurrence) of gingival resection and other periodontal surgical outcomes cannot be predicted, which the patient must be made aware of prior to gingivectomy. It has been recommended that gingivectomy should only be carried out wherever orthodontic treatment is about to be, or has been, initiated in order to reduce the recurrence of gingival hypertrophy. Although personal experience would indicate otherwise, it has been said that it is not clear if the additional oral hygiene burden from fixed orthodontic appliances increases the severity of the hyperplasia, or its postsurgical recurrence. Regardless, monthly periodontal check-ups with scaling and polishing as indicated are recommended to counteract gingival inflammation (Kelekis-Cholakis et al., 2002; Clocheret et al., 2003).

Searching POSSUM Web for 'thickened gingivae' yields 84 syndromes/conditions with which it may be associated, including gingival fibromatosis with sensorineural hearing loss. In this condition with autosomal dominant inheritance, all individuals with hearing loss/deafness had gingival fibromatosis, although not all who have gingival fibromatosis will have hearing loss (Hartsfield et al., 1985).

Soft and hard tissue asymmetry

Hemifacial microsomia

(See also see 'Craniofacial/hemifacial microsomia' in Chapter 8.)

Hemifacial microsomia is a congenital asymmetry of the lower face that may be associated with other cranial and extracranial anomalies. Assessment of facial symmetry involves a conscious or subconscious threshold above which the patient is recognized as having a functional and/or esthetic asymmetry. Recognizing the variable expression of hemifacial microsomia versus garden variety nonsyndromic facial asymmetry can be facilitated by noting involvement of not only the face, but the symmetrical formation of the external ears, cant of the occlusal plane, vertical position of the orbits, and eye abnormalities, as well as a medical history of skeletal, heart, kidney, or other developmental anomaly (Hartsfield, 2007). On occasion,

eruption of teeth may also be delayed (Suri et al., 2004). For a detailed description of the clinical manifestations, see Chapter 8.

The etiology is often stated to be a perturbation of embryonic blood flow in the developing region, although other factors may also play a role in some cases. It can clearly be heterogeneous. In some animal models and human families there is an apparent influence of genetic factors on phenotype, perhaps through alteration of mesodermal development, or indirectly through increased susceptibility to vascular disruption. Depending on what is considered to be minimum criteria for affected classification, what is often to be presumed to be a sporadic event in a family may be the more severe manifestation of a familial condition, in which family members who are minimally affected may, for example, have a slightly smaller ear on one side, a small preauricular tag, or slight facial asymmetry (Hartsfield, 2007).

Parry–Romberg (Romberg) syndrome

In contrast to the congenital nature of hemifacial microsomia, Parry–Romberg syndrome, also known as hemifacial progressive atrophy, is characterized by a slowly progressive atrophy of the soft tissues of essentially half the face, accompanied usually by contralateral Jacksonian epilepsy, trigeminal neuralgia, and changes in the eyes and hair. The process typically begins in the first or second decade of life, and may occur in association with localized scleroderma or a 'coup de sabre' anomaly with thinning of the skin and subcutaneous fat. The condition may extend to the jaws resulting in a unilateral hypoplasia of the maxilla and mandible, producing a malocclusion with an occlusal cant (Anderson et al., 2005).

Without any orthodontic and orthopedic therapy during craniofacial growth in the patient with Parry–Romberg syndrome, the mandible will become asymmetrical, with a longer ramus and condyle on the healthy side of the face with respect to the other side, as the maxilla is affected. Although it is not possible to arrest the progression of the atrophy in the affected area, it is possible to limit the effect secondarily caused by this process on the mandible. Thus, as vertical facial growth slows, an open bite, caused by hypoplasia of the maxilla, is evident on the affected side.

A removable acrylic appliance with a maxillary labial bow stretches the soft tissue on the affected side by keeping the maxillary and mandibular teeth apart on the affected side more than on the normal side. It is used to counteract the asymmetrical growth pattern, similar to what might be used in hemifacial microsomia. In order to be effective, the young patient must keep the appliance in place using muscular force for at least 12–14 hours per day. The treatment must be constantly maintained during the growth period until the end of puberty.

Monitoring the patient monthly, the appliance may require frequent revision by changing the thickness of the inner layer of acrylic interposed between dental arches when a lateral deviation in opening the mouth is detected because of progressive atrophy of the affected area. Grooves and guiding surfaces may be placed in the acrylic appliance to allow and guide dental eruption as needed (Grippaudo et al., 2004).

Saethre–Chotzen syndrome

Although cranial and associated facial asymmetry may occur with any asymmetrical craniosynostosis (see 'Craniosynostosis' later in this chapter for the definition and further information, and also Chapter 8), one type in particular, Saethre–Chotzen syndrome (caused by a mutation in *TWIST1*) may result in cranial asymmetry (plagiocephaly), as well as facial asymmetry (particularly in individuals with unilateral coronal synostosis). Ironically, for a condition associated with asymmetrical premature closure of some sutures, the anterior fontanel (soft spot) closure may be delayed. As part of a differential diagnosis, another condition that often presents with a persistently open anterior fontanel is cleidocranial dysostosis. Saethre–Chotzen syndrome has autosomal dominant inheritance, and variable expressivity and associated findings include ptosis ('drooping' upper eyelids), low frontal hairline, deviated nasal septum, and partial soft tissue syndactyly (Jones and Smith, 2006; Cunningham et al., 2007). Midface hypoplasia, narrow palate, and supernumerary teeth may also be present (Hennekam et al., 2010).

Maxillary hypoplasia

Maxillonasal dysplasia (Binder syndrome)

Some do not consider this a true syndrome, but rather a nonspecific abnormality of the nasomaxillary complex that may possibly be related in some cases to prenatal deficiency of vitamin K or actually a manifestation of chondrodysplasia punctata. Clinically, the nose is notably flattened, the anterior nasal spine is absent or hypoplastic, and the labial bone overlying the maxillary incisors may be thin on radiographs. Because of premaxillary hypoplasia and maxillary sagittal shortening, patients typically have relative mandibular prognathism (Hennekam et al., 2010).

Fragile X (Martin–Bell) syndrome

The frequency of occurrence of X-linked mental retardation, Down syndrome, and fetal alcohol syndrome is similar, with fragile X syndrome being the most common inherited form of mental retardation. As noted before for X-linked conditions, although males are affected more often and more severely than females, the latter can be affected as well. The face tends to be long and narrow in approximately 70%

of postpubertal males with fragile X syndrome. The maxilla can be hypoplastic with mandibular prognathism, and crossbite and anterior open bite are relatively common. Increased occlusal wear has also been described. Although the cognitive abilities of affected males are often severely affected, the IQs of affected females can range from 50 to normal, with an average of 81. Joint laxity, recurrent middle ear infections, and prominent ears are also common (Shellhart et al., 1986; Hennekam et al., 2010).

Nevoid basal cell carcinoma (Gorlin) syndrome

This condition combines variable manifestations including numerous basal cell cancers, epidermal cysts of the skin, odontogenic keratocysts of the jaws, other tumors and cancers, rib and vertebral anomalies, cleft lip and/or palate, with autosomal dominant inheritance, although approximately one-third to one-half of cases are the result of new mutations. Mandibular prognathism may be mild (Hennekam et al., 2010).

Craniosynostosis

This is the premature closure of some or all cranial sutures, occurring in 1 in 2500 children. The discovery of mutations in *MSX2*, *FGFR1*, *FGFR2*, *FGFR3*, and *TWIST1* (as mentioned above in the section on Saethre–Chotzen syndrome), and *EFNB1* in both syndromic and nonsyndromic cases has led to considerable insights into the etiology, classification and developmental pathology of these disorders (Morriss-Kay and Wilkie, 2005). Depending on the sutures involved, the resulting cranial shape may be long and narrow anterior to posterior (dolichocephaly) or scaphocephaly), or relatively short anterior to posterior and broad transverse (brachycephaly). The latter may also be associated with a pronounced increase in the vertical face height from nasion to bregma, resulting in turricephaly. Most instances of craniosynostosis are nonsyndromic, although there are over 100 craniosynostosis syndromes, the most common of which have a known genetic etiology (Boyadjiev, 2007). Craniosynostosis, particularly involving the coronal sutures, often results in maxillary hypoplasia and a Class III malocclusion secondary to the effect on craniofacial growth and development. The clinical features of this syndrome are given in detail in Chapter 8.

A generally extreme phenotype associated with an autosomal dominant mutation can be markedly variable, even within those who are to some degree affected in a family. Simply discovering the gene mutation might be indicative of a future effect on craniofacial growth and development but will not necessarily predict the precise effect, and the severity present in any one patient may be relatively mild and overlooked (Hartsfield, 2005). The overlap of clinical presentations for different, and even the same, mutations in one of the *FGFR* genes has led some to refer to this group of conditions, along with the conditions involving short stature that may also affect facial growth (such as achondroplasia, the most common type of short-limbed 'dwarfism'), also resulting from mutations in the *FGFR* genes, as the fibroblast growth factor receptor (FGFR) syndromes. (See also fibroblast growth factor related short limbed syndrome [achondroplasia/hypochondroplasia in Chapter 8.)

Functional (neuromuscular) asymmetry

Muscle function can influence facial morphology, from overcontraction (e.g. torticollis, sometimes called a 'wry' neck), or cerebral palsy, or a lack of muscle tone/strength (hypotonia). Many syndromes, such as Down syndrome, may often include hypotonia. If the syndrome is of neurological or muscular etiology, or the hypotonia is central or systematic, the effect is likely to be generally symmetrical, e.g. in myotonic dystrophy; the muscular dystrophies that affect to some degree the muscles of mastication or facial expression often directly or indirectly lead to an anterior open bite. If the muscular and/or neurological abnormality is generally unilateral, as in hemifacial microsomia, then the effect will typically be asymmetry.

A symmetrical or asymmetrical lack of facial expression may be due to hypoplasia of cranial nerve ganglia affecting to a variable degree the facial, external eye, and tongue musculature called Moebius (Mobius) sequence (also referred to as syndrome). The cause is heterogeneous, although one mechanism may be a tendency for vascular bleeding to occur, and may be associated with limb reduction and other developmental anomalies beyond the face (Hennekam et al., 2010).

Mandibular retrognathism

Robin sequence

The congenital retrognathic appearance in this condition may be due to mandibular micrognathia or retrognathia relative to the maxilla. If this position of the mandible was present when the palatal shelves were closing, a cleft palate (particularly of the posterior) may result. After birth, the position of the tongue secondary to the small mandible may obstruct the airway (glossoptosis). Thus the sequence of events, mandibular size/position, and resulting cleft palate and glossoptosis are the classic triad of the (Pierre) Robin sequence. The prevalence of Robin sequence has been estimated to be 1/3000 to 1/5000 (Jones and Smith, 2006). During childhood some 'catch-up growth' has been reported, but appears to be variable (Figueroa et al., 1991). Cephalometric analysis at an adolescent age may show a decreased SNB angle, high mandibular plane angle, and short ramus height. The gonial angle may be increased, and the mandibular body may or may not be short in length. There may be an increase in hypodontia, particularly of the

mandibular second premolars or incisors (Matsuda et al., 2006).

The Robin sequence may be nonsyndromic or a part of over 40 conditions, including Stickler syndrome, velocardiofacial syndrome, and the Mobius sequence (Hennekam et al., 2010). The medical geneticist can investigate whether the Robin sequence is part of a syndrome, and may clarify mandibular growth expectations in the presence or lack of hypodontia. For example, children with nonsyndromic Robin sequence with mandibular hypodontia have been shown to have smaller mandibles than children with non-syndromic Robin sequence and no mandibular hypodontia. A comparison of the average growth pattern in nonsyndromic Robin sequence patients with and without mandibular hypodontia revealed that the average growth pattern of the nonsyndromic Robin sequence subjects with mandibular hypodontia did not improve during adolescence, and the magnitude of differences between the two groups increased (Suri et al., 2006). Ultimately, orthodontic treatment with or without orthognathic surgery will depend on the individual case (Suri et al., 2006).

The mean mandibular length is shorter than normal in nonsyndromic and syndromic (Stickler, velocardiofacial, Treacher Collins, and bilateral facial microsomia) Robin sequence patients, although more significantly in the latter group, and varies considerably in the different syndromes. The sagittal position of the mandible is relatively normal on average in the nonsyndromic and Stickler and velocardiofacial syndromic patients, in contrast to the Treacher Collins and bilateral facial microsomia patients, who tend to have more of an abnormal mandibular shape. Thus, it has been recommended that mandibular distraction should be considered in selective Robin sequence patients, such as those with Treacher Collins syndrome or bilateral facial microsomia, because they are unlikely to achieve relatively normal mandibular growth and position (Rogers et al., 2009). Rogers et al. did not provide an analysis or discuss the possible effects of hypodontia in these groups.

Velocardiofacial (Shprintzen or del22q11) syndrome

(See also 'DiGeorge syndrome/velocardiofacial syndrome/Takao syndrome' in Chapter 8.)

This extremely variable spectrum of conditions with autosomal dominant inheritance is usually due to a relatively small deletion on part of the long arm of the number 22 chromosome. It is not rare, as it accounts for 8% of cleft palate patients, and is second only to Stickler syndrome for syndrome-associated Robin sequence. However, cases do not have to have cleft palate or marked developmental delay, and may only show mild problems at school due to submucous cleft and/or nasal speech. Facial asymmetry is not unusual, along with upslanting palpebral fissures, increased anterior vertical face height, malar hypoplasia, and mandibular retrognathia. A history of congenital heart disease may also be a part of the condition (Hennekam et al., 2010).

Hallermann–Strieff syndrome

Almost all cases of this condition have been sporadic, i.e. only one member in each family has been affected. It is characterized by dyscephaly, hypotrichosis, microphthalmia, congenital cataracts, beaked nose, marked retrognathia (especially of the mandible, which may exacerbate respiratory problems), and proportionate short stature (Hennekam et al., 2010).

Abadi et al. (2009) reported the case of a19-year-old man with severe mandibular retrognathia, maxillary transverse hypoplasia, oligodontia, and ankylosed primary teeth. He was treated by surgically assisted rapid palatal expansion, fixed orthodontic therapy, orthognathic surgery, and prosthodontic rehabilitation with implant retained fixed partial dentures.

Connective tissue dysplasia

Ehlers–Danlos syndromes

The Ehlers–Danlos syndromes (EDS) are a heterogeneous group of heritable connective tissue disorders characterized by articular hypermobility, skin extensibility, and tissue fragility. Other manifestations, including periodontal disease, can vary according to EDS type, and thus it is important to distinguish the EDS type. The classification has been revised from at least 10 types, most of which were designated by Roman numerals, to six main types (plus 'other forms') which are based primarily on the etiology:

- Classical type (formally gravis [EDS type I] and mitis [EDS type II])
- Hypermobility type (formally hypermobile [EDS type III])
- Vascular type (formally arterial-ecchymotic [EDS type IV])
- Kyphoscoliosis type (ocular-scoliotic [EDS type VI])
- Arthrochalasia type (arthrochalasis multiplex congenita [EDS types VIIA and VIIB])
- Dermatosparaxis type (human dermatosparaxis [EDS type VIIC]).

Other forms include X-linked EDS (now called EDS type V), periodontitis type (EDS type VIII), fibronectin-deficient EDS (EDS type X), familial hypermobility syndrome (EDS type XI), progeroid EDS, and other unspecified forms (Beighton et al., 1998).

Dental concerns in EDS have included hypermobility of the temporomandibular joint (TMJ), with an increased incidence of subluxation, fragile oral mucosa, early-onset periodontitis, high cusps and deep fissures on the crowns of teeth, high incidence of enamel and dental fractures, stunted roots or dilacerations, coronal pulp stones, aberrant

dentinal tubules, pulpal vascular lesions and denticles, increased rate of tooth movement in response to orthodontic forces, and increased need for and duration of orthodontic retention (Norton and Assael, 1997).

In a subjective survey, patients with EDS were compared with a control sample of patients without EDS, with respect to their orthodontic and temporomandibular disorder experiences. The results indicated that the majority of those with EDS types I, III, and VI experienced difficulty in their orthodontic treatment. Those with EDS type II found it tolerable, with a 25% split between easy and difficult. This compared with a control group that unanimously reported orthodontic treatment as being either easy or tolerable. Frequent subluxation of the TMJ was found in all patients with EDS. This is a particular problem in EDS types II, IV, V, and VI patients (Norton and Assael, 1997).

Although not exclusively, major periodontal concerns in EDS are primarily related to the periodontal and the vascular types. In addition to early-onset periodontitis, the periodontal-type patients have variable hyperextensibility of the skin, ecchymotic pretibial (purple discoloration of the shin) lesions of the skin, variable bruising besides the pretibial ecchymosis, minimal to moderate joint hypermobility of the digits, and 'cigarette-paper' scars (in which the skin looks thin and crinkled) (Stewart et al., 1977; Linch and Acton, 1979; Hartsfield and Kousseff, 1990).

The outcome of orthodontic treatment in at least two cases of periodontal-type EDS is the basis for the recommendation that these patients be considered high risk for orthodontia, in respect not only to alveolar bone loss, but also to enhanced external apical root resorption. For example, prior to starting orthodontic treatment, one patient had, since the age of 5 years, atrophic, hyperpigmented scars on his shins, as well as bruising from mild trauma. He reportedly had gingival bleeding for many years. Four first premolars had been extracted at the beginning of orthodontic treatment. Unfortunately, periodontal status deteriorated after orthodontic treatment with fixed appliances began (Karrer et al., 2000; Buckel and Zaenglein, 2007).

Early periodontal disease may also be found in patients with vascular-type EDS. This type has some overlap clinically with the periodontal type, as evidenced by the finding of skin hyperextensibility, ecchymotic pretibial lesions, easy bruisibility, cigarette-paper scars, joint hypermobility of the digits, pes planus (flat feet), and of special importance arterial and intestinal ruptures, the last two features being major characteristics for diagnosis and prognosis (Hartsfield and Kousseff, 1990).

Osteogenesis imperfecta

Osteogenesis imperfecta is a heterogeneous group of conditions affecting bone mass and fragility. It is a highly variable disease that is usually secondary to an abnormality in type I collagen synthesis or extracellular secretion. However, some osteogenesis imperfecta patients with normal type I collagen apparently have mutations affecting other bone proteins. The hallmark sign of osteogenesis imperfecta ('brittle bone disease') is an increased incidence or history of bone fracture, usually resulting from minimal if any trauma. In addition to a variable decrease in bone mass, there is abnormal tissue organization and aberrant morphology (size and shape) of bones. There are associated craniofacial and dental manifestations that may include dentinogenesis imperfecta, a hypoplastic maxilla, and hypodontia, among others.

Variable expression of dentin developmental defects has been documented, with approximately one-fourth to three-fourths of the cases showing some manifestation of dentinogenesis imperfecta, depending to a degree on the type of osteogenesis imperfecta. To control the elevated rate of bone remodeling, some osteogenesis imperfecta patients are treated with bisphosphonates, drugs that inhibit osteoclastic resorption. Bisphosphonate treatment may introduce additional problems, which have been observed in other patients, such as decreased rates of tooth movement, problems maintaining dental implant integration, or osteonecrosis following dental extractions (Hartsfield et al., 2006).

An information sheet for healthcare professionals and the public on 'Dental care for people with osteogenesis imperfecta' is available online from the Osteogenesis Imperfecta Foundation (www.oif.org/site/DocServer/Dental_Care.pdf?docID=8101; Hartsfield and Schwartz, 2007). However, because of the marked clinical variability both among and within families with osteogenesis imperfecta, comprehensive statements about treatment and prognosis should be understood to be merely guidelines.

There are several types of osteogenesis imperfecta, based on phenotype and to some degree genotype. Taking all the different types and manifestations of osteogenesis imperfecta as a group, the incidence is probably between 1/5000 and 1/10 000 individuals (Byers and Steiner, 1992). Documentation of histological dentin abnormalities, in clinically and radiographically normal teeth, indicates that the effect on dentin development is a continuum. In addition to dentinogenesis imperfecta, the presence of additional dental and craniofacial manifestations has been documented: attrition of teeth and tooth fracture (associated with dentinogenesis imperfecta), thistle-shaped pulp chambers, apically extended pulp chambers (resembling taurodontism), denticles, maxillary lateral incisor invagination, gemination, odontoma, Class II malocclusion, periapical radiolucencies in noncarious teeth, Class III malocclusion (more common than Class II malocclusion), maxillary hypoplasia, anterior and posterior crossbite, anterior and posterior open bite that tends to worsen with age, hypodontia, supernumerary teeth (rare), advanced or delayed dental development, mandibular cysts (rare), and lack of eruption (or ectopic eruption) of the first and/or second permanent molars (Schwartz and Tsipouras, 1984; Lukinmaa et al., 1987a,b; Lund et al., 1998; Petersen and Wetzel, 1998; O'Connell and Marini, 1999; Malmgren and Norgren, 2002).

Bone continues to form during the growth period in patients with osteogenesis imperfecta (Jones et al., 1999). Although all affected patients are said to be osteoporotic, it has not been determined if bone mineralization patterns in the lumbar spine or other locations correlate well with those of the craniofacies. So bone mineral density determinations in other parts of the body may not be informative for orthognathic surgery and other treatment. Healing of fractures occurs within the time frame experienced by patients without osteogenesis imperfecta (O'Connell and Marini, 1999). With regard to tooth movement, rapid palatal expansion, and orthognathic surgery, in general, rapid palatal expansion and tooth movement are not a problem, although the teeth may seem relatively mobile after debanding, and so immediate, long-term, retention is advised.

When present in cases with osteogenesis imperfecta, dentinogenesis imperfecta tends to affect the maxillary anterior teeth the least, and the mandibular arch the most. Care should be taken when debonding brackets from teeth with dentinogenesis imperfecta to minimize the chance of fracture and chipping. Although banding of teeth may be contemplated if some teeth are already chipped or fractured prior to initiating orthodontic treatment, prudence may indicate no orthodontic attachments on those teeth, and possibly some restorative coverage.

The variability of the facial bone quality is so great that prediction of orthognathic surgery outcome can be uncertain until the surgeon actually makes the osteotomies and places the surgical fasteners. Moreover, patients with osteogenesis imperfecta have general anesthesia-related and possible bleeding concerns, of which the anesthesiologist and surgeon should be aware.

Recommendations must be tempered by the particular characteristics and condition of the affected individual. It is imperative that informed consent be given with the clear understanding by the patient and/or family (depending on patient age) that each individual with osteogenesis imperfecta is unique with regard to a particular combination of genes and environmental factors. Presumed collagen or other bone protein mutation(s) may influence the expression of osteogenesis imperfecta and also the response to treatment (Hartsfield et al., 2006; Hartsfield and Schwartz, 2007).

Marfan syndrome

This is estimated to occur in 1 in 5000–10 000 individuals, has autosomal dominant inheritance, and is typically associated with mutations in *FBN1*, thereby affecting fibrillin, an important component of many connective tissues. There is a tendency for those affected to be taller than family members, a tendency to have scoliosis, pectus excavatum or carinatum (indented or ridged sternum), and to variably have long and thin limbs, hands and feet; an overall body build sometimes referred to as a 'Marfanoid' habitus.

Not only is there often an oral facial component from affected growth, but there is significant morbidity from increased likelihood of ectopia lentis (ocular lens displacement), myopia, retinal detachment, and/or aortic dissecting aneurysm, including in those previously undiagnosed and thought to be in good health. Thus, this is a condition in which a diagnosis may not only assist in treatment of malocclusion but also lead to medical care that may save the patient from a sudden premature death.

Malocclusion in this condition often presents as a high and narrow palatal vault (transverse maxillary deficiency), mandibular retrognathia, dental crowding, increased overjet and open bite. In one report on occlusion and cephalometrics in Marfan syndrome patients, 36% (of a total of 76) had undergone orthodontic treatment before a diagnosis or suspicion of the condition (Westling et al., 1998). In addition to these structural concerns, including dolichocephaly, there is also an increased risk for caries, local hypoplastic enamel spots (thought to possibly be related to caries in the deciduous dentition), root deformity, abnormal pulp shape, pulpal inclusions, calculus, elevated gingival indices, and periodontal disease (De Coster et al., 2002; Utreja and Evans, 2009). Severe root resorption and TMJ derangement with some resorption of the condyles have been reported in Marfan syndrome, but it is not clear if these were a pleiotropic effect of, or coincident occurrence with, the condition (Bilodeau, 2010).

Stickler syndrome

This is another connective tissue dysplasia in which the body proportions may be 'Marfanoid'-like with hyperextensible 'loose' joints, which is usually secondary to a mutation in type 2 or 11 collagen. Three types of Stickler syndrome have been described: type 1 – *COL2A1* mutation in 75% of cases overall; type 2 – *COL11A1* mutation; and type 3 – *COL11A2* mutation, generally found to be without ocular involvement. There is often a sensorineural hearing loss, and conductive hearing loss associated with cleft palate, if present, and recurrent otitis (ear infections).

About 20% of type 1 patients have a cleft palate or bifid uvula. As already mentioned, it is also a condition with which the Robin sequence may be associated (Hennekam et al., 2010). Cephalometric findings in Stickler syndrome patients include malar hypoplasia (flat midface), small SNA and SNB angles, steep mandibular planes, enlarged gonial angles, and retroclined incisors in both arches (Kucukyavuz et al., 2006; Suda et al., 2006). As in Marfan syndrome, the vision may be affected, with high myopia (thus the patient may be wearing relatively thick eyeglasses) that may even lead to retinal detachment, but there is no typically increased risk of mortality from aortic aneurysm.

Treacher Collins syndrome

(See also 'Treacher Collins syndrome' in Chapter 8.)

This craniofacial syndrome can vary from very severe to clinically nonpenetrant (skipping a generation), with typical bilateral mandibular deficiency, downslanting palpebral fissures, malformed ears; and one-third with cleft palate. Eye abnormalities may also be present (Hennekam et al., 2010).

Cleft lip and cleft palate

In children with a cleft lip and palate the question of etiology always arises. This is the case, in particular, when the neonatologist discovers or suspects additional malformations. Since neonates with cleft lip and palate are now usually brought for initial treatment to an orthodontist, it is her or his responsibility to inform the parents about the possibility and necessity of genetic counseling and, possibly, to initiate contact with the appropriate institute. This is always the case when the wish for further children is expressed. If the orthodontist recognizes microsymptoms in the parents or finds indications of their occurrence in the family, he or she will strongly recommend such a consultation. With cleft lip and palate patients, the orthodontist should discuss genetic consultation as part of a confidential relationship with the patient so that young patients understand the possible risk for the next generation. This consultation can bring enormous psychological relief for the patient if there is only a slight risk of recurrence (Schwanitz and Zschiesche, 1989). See Chapter 9 for a detailed discussion on interaction of orthodontists with other specialists in the craniofacial team with regard to management of cleft lip and palate patients.

Cleft uvula is a relatively common finding, occurring in every 1 in 75 Caucasians in one group (Meskin et al., 1964, 1965, 1966). Although it has been reported to have familial pattern by itself and also to be a mild expression of the more severe cleft of the entire palate, care must be taken to presume a connection with cleft palate that occurs with an incidence of 1 in 2500. The presence of cleft uvula by itself is unlikely to be of any significance. Its occurrence with a family history of cleft palate may suggest familial cleft palate, or other minor anomalies may suggest it is part of a syndrome (Meskin et al., 1964, 1965, 1966).

Van der Woude syndrome

This is said to be the most common of the over 300 syndromes with oral clefting, occurring in 1:40 000–100 000 stillbirths or live births. In addition, this condition with autosomal dominant inheritance is extremely variable. It is one of a few clefting syndromes in which a cleft lip with or without a cleft palate, or a cleft palate (that may be as mild as a submucous cleft, or cleft uvula) may occur in different members of the same family. It may also skip a generation (nonpenetrance) or only manifest with small paramedian (just to the side of the midsagittal plane) lower lip pits or mounds of tissue (these should not be confused with commissural lip pits that occur at the lateral oral commissures). Thus, a family history of any of these findings should raise suspicion. It has been stated that this syndrome is not associated with a consistent skeletal pattern. This is not surprising given the wide range of clinical expression from normal to cleft lip and palate, so that the skeletal pattern of each patient will be influenced by the particular malformation(s), if any is present (Rizos and Spyropoulos, 2004; Suda et al., 2006; Lam et al., 2010).

Conclusion

Today, understanding the medical/genetic condition of a patient may help the orthodontist to understand how to help and what to expect from the patient. A more common application of genetics to orthodontic practice in the near future may be in how nonsyndromic complex traits – such as external apical root resorption (EARR) associated with orthodontic treatment, Angle's Class III malocclusion and Angle's Class II division 2 malocclusion, and palatally displaced canines – occur and respond to different orthodontic treatment protocols. Other areas that also require more investigation include the application of genetics for better prediction of individual growth during puberty, and when the orthodontist should send a patient with hypodontia to the medical geneticist for cancer risk evaluation (Bader, 1967; Jaspers and Witkop, 1980; McLain et al., 1983; Hartsfield, 2005, 2008, 2009).

Knowledge of the diagnosis, and characteristics, of a genetic condition, or evaluation of genetic factors to better anticipate an individual's risk as opposed to the general population of disease or developmental abnormality, or their growth pattern and/or likely response to a treatment, is termed personalized medicine. Application of this principle to orthodontic practice is 'personalized orthodontics' (Hartsfield, 2005, 2008, 2009; Hartsfield et al., 2010). To use this approach, this chapter can help recognize when to refer a patient to a medical geneticist, and to understand some of the conditions that orthodontists may encounter in their patients.

References

Abadi BJ, Van Sickels JE, McConnell TA, et al. (2009) Implant rehabilitation for a patient with Hallerman-Streiff syndrome: a case report. *Journal of Oral Implantology* 35: 143–7.

Alvesalo L (2009) Human sex chromosomes in oral and craniofacial growth. *Archives of Oral Biology* 54(Suppl 1): S18–24.

Anderson PJ, Molony D, Haan E, et al. (2005) Familial Parry-Romberg disease. *International Journal of Pediatric Otorhinolaryngology* 69: 705–8.

Axelsson S (2005) Variability of the cranial and dental phenotype in Williams syndrome. *Swedish Dental Journal Supplement* 170: 3–67.

Ayoub AF, El-Mofty SS (1993) Cherubism: report of an aggressive case and review of the literature. *Journal of Oral and Maxillofacial Surgery* 51: 702–5.

Babic M, Scepan I, Micic M (1993) Comparative cephalometric analysis in patients with X-chromosome aneuploidy. *Archives of Oral Biology* 38: 179–83.

Baccaglini L, Schiffmann R, Brennan MT, et al. (2001) Oral and craniofacial findings in Fabry's disease: a report of 13 patients. *Oral Surgery, Oral Medicine, Oral Pathology, Oral Radiology, and Endodontics* 92: 415–19.

Bader G (1967) Odontomatosis (multiple odontomas). *Oral Surgery, Oral Medicine, and Oral Pathology* 23: 770–3.

Bailleul-Forestier I, Berdal A, Vinckier F, et al. (2008) The genetic basis of inherited anomalies of the teeth. Part 2: syndromes with significant dental involvement. *European Journal of Medical Genetics* 51: 383–408.

Bazopoulou-Kyrkanidou E, Vrahopoulos TP, Eliades G, et al. (2007) Periodontitis associated with Hajdu-Cheney syndrome. *Journal of Periodontology* 78: 1831–8.

Becker A, Lustmann J, Shteyer A (1997a) Cleidocranial dysplasia: Part 1 – General principles of the orthodontic and surgical treatment modality. *American Journal of Orthodontics and Dentofacial Orthopedics* 111: 28–33.

Becker A, Shteyer A, Bimstein E, et al. (1997b) Cleidocranial dysplasia: Part 2 – Treatment protocol for the orthodontic and surgical modality. *American Journal of Orthodontics and Dentofacial Orthopedics* 111: 173–83.

Beighton P, De Paepe A, Steinmann B, et al. (1998) Ehlers-Danlos syndromes: revised nosology, Villefranche, 1997. Ehlers-Danlos National Foundation (USA) and Ehlers-Danlos Support Group (UK). *American Journal of Medical Genetics* 77: 31–7.

Bilodeau JE (2010) Retreatment of a patient with Marfan syndrome and severe root resorption. *American Journal of Orthodontics and Dentofacial Orthopedics* 137: 123–34.

Bindayel NA, Ullbro C, Suri L, et al. (2008) Cephalometric findings in patients with Papillon-Lefevre syndrome. *American Journal of Orthodontics and Dentofacial Orthopedics* 134: 138–44.

Bixler D, Higgins M, Hartsfield J Jr (1984) The Nance-Horan syndrome: a rare X-linked ocular-dental trait with expression in heterozygous females. *Clinical Genetics* 26: 30–5.

Bloch-Zupan A, Goodman JR (2006) Otodental syndrome. *Orphanet Journal of Rare Diseases* 1: 5.

Boyadjiev SA (2007) Genetic analysis of non-syndromic craniosynostosis. *Orthodontics and Craniofacial Research* 10: 129–37.

Buckel T, Zaenglein AL (2007) What syndrome is this? Ehlers-Danlos syndrome type VIII. *Pediatric Dermatology* 24: 189–91.

Byers PH, Steiner RD (1992) Osteogenesis imperfecta. *Annual Review of Medicine* 43: 269–82.

Carl W, Herrera L (1987) Dental and bone abnormalities in patients with familial polyposis coli. *Seminars in Surgical Oncology* 3: 77–83.

Chalothorn LA, Beeman CS, Ebersole JL, et al. (2008) Hypodontia as a risk marker for epithelial ovarian cancer: a case-controlled study. *Journal of the American Dental Association* 139: 163–9.

Chaussain-Miller C, Sinding C, Wolikow M, et al. (2003) Dental abnormalities in patients with familial hypophosphatemic vitamin D-resistant rickets: prevention by early treatment with 1-hydroxyvitamin D. *Journal of Pediatrics* 142: 324–31.

Cichon JC, Pack RS (1985) Taurodontism: review of literature and report of case. *Journal of the American Dental Association* 111: 453–5.

Clocheret K, Dekeyser C, Carels C, et al. (2003) Idiopathic gingival hyperplasia and orthodontic treatment: a case report. *Journal of Orthodontics* 30: 13–19.

Cohen MM Jr (1980) Craniofacial syndromes. In: WH Bell, WR Proffit, RP WHITE (eds) *Surgical Correction of Dentofacial Deformities*. Philadelphia, PA: WB Saunders.

Coletta RD, Graner E (2006) Hereditary gingival fibromatosis: a systematic review. *Journal of Periodontology* 77: 753–64.

Cunningham ML, Seto ML, Ratisoontorn C, et al. (2007) Syndromic craniosynostosis: from history to hydrogen bonds. *Orthodontics and Craniofacial Research* 10: 67–81.

D'Alessandro G, Tagariello T, Piana G (2010) Craniofacial changes and treatment of the stomatognathic system in subjects with Cleidocranial dysplasia. *European Journal of Paediatric Dentistry* 11: 39–43.

De Coster PJ, Martens LC, De Paepe A (2002) Oral manifestations of patients with Marfan syndrome: a case-control study. *Oral Surgery,*

Oral Medicine, Oral Pathology, Oral Radiology, and Endodontics 93: 564–72.

De Moura CP, Andrade D, Cunha LM, et al. (2008) Down syndrome: otolaryngological effects of rapid maxillary expansion. *Journal of Laryngology and Otology* 122: 1318–24.

Decker E, Stellzig-Eisenhauer A, Fiebig BS, et al. (2008) PTHR1 loss-of-function mutations in familial, nonsyndromic primary failure of tooth eruption. *American Journal of Human Genetics* 83: 781–6.

DiBiase AT, Cobourne MT (2008) Beware the solitary maxillary median central incisor. *Journal of Orthodontics* 35: 16–19.

Etzioni A, Tonetti M (2000) Leukocyte adhesion deficiency II–from A to almost Z. *Immunological Reviews* 178: 138–47.

Farronato G, Maspero C, Farronato D, et al. (2009) Orthodontic treatment in a patient with cleidocranial dysostosis. *Angle Orthodontist* 79: 178–85.

Feigenbaum A, Kumar A, Weksberg R (1988) Singleton-Merten (S-M) syndrome: autosomal dominant transmission with variable expression. *American Journal of Human Genetics* 43: A48.

Figueroa AA, Glupker TJ, Fitz MG, et al. (1991) Mandible, tongue, and airway in Pierre Robin sequence: a longitudinal cephalometric study. *Cleft Palate-Craniofacial Journal* 28: 425–34.

Fleming PS, Xavier GM, DiBiase AT, et al. (2010) Revisiting the supernumerary: the epidemiological and molecular basis of extra teeth. *British Dental Journal* 208: 25–30.

Frazier-Bowers SA, Simmons D, Wright JT, et al. (2010) Primary failure of eruption and PTH1R: the importance of a genetic diagnosis for orthodontic treatment planning. *American Journal of Orthodontics and Dentofacial Orthopedics* 137: 160 e1–7; discussion 160–1.

Golan I, Baumert U, Wagener H, et al. (2002) Evidence of intrafamilial variability of CBFA1/RUNX2 expression in cleidocranial dysplasia – a family study. *Journal of Orofacial Orthopedics* 63: 190–8.

Gorlin RJ, Cohen MM Jr, Wolfson J (1969). Tricho-rhino-phalangeal syndrome. *American Journal of Diseases of Children* 118: 595–9.

Grippaudo C, Deli R, Grippaudo FR, et al. (2004) Management of craniofacial development in the Parry-Romberg syndrome: report of two patients. *Cleft Palate-Craniofacial Journal* 41: 95–104.

Hall RK, Bankier A, Aldred MJ, et al. (1997) Solitary median maxillary central incisor, short stature, choanal atresia/midnasal stenosis (SMMCI) syndrome. *Oral Surgery, Oral Medicine, Oral Pathology, Oral Radiology, and Endodontics* 84: 651–62.

Halse A, Bjorvatn K, Aarskog D (1979) Dental findings in patients with Aarskog syndrome. *Scandinavian Journal of Dental Research* 87: 253–9.

Hart TC, Stabholz A, Meyle J, et al. (1997) Genetic studies of syndromes with severe periodontitis and palmoplantar hyperkeratosis. *Journal of Periodontal Reserach* 32: 81–9.

Hartsfield JK (2007) Review of the etiologic heterogeneity of the oculo-auriculo-vertebral spectrum (Hemifacial Microsomia). *Orthodontics and Craniofacial Research* 10: 121–8.

Hartsfield JK Jr (1994) Premature exfoliation of teeth in childhood and adolescence. *Advances in Pediatrics* 41: 453–70.

Hartsfield JK Jr (2005) Genetics and orthodontics. In: TM Graber, RL Vanarsdall, KWL Vig (eds) *Orthodontics Current Principles and Techniques*, 4th edn. St. Louis, MO: Mosby, Inc.

Hartsfield JK Jr (2008) Personalized orthodontics, the future of genetics in practice. *Seminars in Orthodontics* 14: 166–71.

Hartsfield JK Jr (2009) Pathways in external apical root resorption associated with orthodontia. *Orthodontics and Craniofacial Research* 12: 236–42.

Hartsfield JK Jr, Kousseff BG (1990) Phenotypic overlap of Ehlers-Danlos syndrome types IV and VIII. *American Journal of Medical Genetics* 37: 465–70.

Hartsfield JK Jr, Schwartz S (2007) *Dental Care for People with Osteogenesis Imperfecta*. Gaithersburg, MD: Osteogenesis Imperfecta Foundation. Available at: www.oif.org/site/DocServer/Dental_Care.pdf?docID=8101 (accessed September 2010).

Hartsfield JK Jr, Bixler D, Hazen RH (1985) Gingival fibromatosis with sensorineural hearing loss: an autosomal dominant trait. *American Journal of Medical Genetics* 22: 623–7.

Hartsfield JK Jr, Hall BD, Grix AW, et al. (1993) Pleiotropy in Coffin-Lowry syndrome: sensorineural hearing deficit and premature tooth loss as early manifestations. *American Journal of Medical Genetics* 45: 552–7.

Hartsfield JK Jr, Hohlt WF, Roberts WE (2006) Orthodontic treatment and orthognathic surgery for patients with osteogenesis imperfecta. *Seminars in Orthodontics* 12: 254–71.

Hartsfield JK Jr, Zhou J, Chen S (2010) The importance of analyzing specific genetic factors in facial growth for diagnosis and treatment planning. In: JA Mcnamara, SD Kapila (eds) *Surgical Enhancement of Orthodontic Treatment, Craniofacial Growth Series, Department of Orthodontics and Pediatric Dentistry and Center for Human Growth and Development*. Ann Arbor, MI: The University of Michigan.

Hennekam RCM, Allanson JE, Krantz ID, et al. (2010) *Gorlin's Syndromes of the Head and Neck*. Oxford: Oxford University Press.

Hennequin M, Faulks D, Veyrune JL, et al. (1999) Significance of oral health in persons with Down syndrome: a literature review. *Developmental Medicine and Child Neurology* 41: 275–83.

Holst AI, Hirschfelder U, Holst S (2009) Diagnostic potential of 3D-data-based reconstruction software: an analysis of the rare disease pattern of cherubism. *Cleft Palate-Craniofacial Journal* 46: 215–19.

Hoyme HE (1993) Minor anomalies: diagnostic clues to aberrant human morphogenesis. *Genetica* 89: 307–15.

Hu CC, King DL, Thomas HF, et al. (1996) A clinical and research protocol for characterizing patients with hypophosphatasia. *Pediatric Dentistry* 18: 17–23.

Ishikawa T, Yashima S, Hasan H, et al. (1986) Osteoma of the lateral pterygoid plate of the sphenoid bone. *International Journal of Oral and Maxillofacial Surgery* 15: 786–9.

Jaspers MT, Witkop CJ Jr (1980) Taurodontism, an isolated trait associated with syndromes and X-chromosomal aneuploidy. *American Journal of Human Genetics* 32: 396–413.

Jones KL, Smith DW (2006) *Smith's Recognizable Patterns of Human Malformation*, Philadelphia, PA: Elsevier/WB Saunders.

Jones SJ, Glorieux FH, Travers R, et al. (1999) The microscopic structure of bone in normal children and patients with osteogenesis imperfecta: a survey using backscattered electron imaging. *Calcified Tissue International* 64: 8–17.

Kamel SG, Kau CH, Wong ME, et al. (2009) The role of cone beam CT in the evaluation and management of a family with Gardner's syndrome. *Journal of Cranio-Maxillofacial Surgery* 37: 461–8.

Kan WY, Seow WK, Holcombe T (2010) Taurodontism in children with hypodontia and supernumerary teeth: a case control study. *Pediatric Dentistry* 32: 134–40.

Karacay S, Saygun I, Tunca Y, et al. (2007) Clinical and intraoral findings of a patient with tricho-rhino-phalangeal syndrome type I. *Journal of the Indian Society of Pedodontics and Preventive Dentistry* 25: 43–5.

Karrer S, Landthaler M, Schmalz G (2000) Ehlers-Danlos syndrome type VIII with severe periodontitis and apical root resorption after orthodontic treatment. *Acta Dermato-Venereologica* 80: 56–7.

Katou F, Motegi K, Baba S (1989) Mandibular lesions in patients with adenomatosis coli. *Journal of Cranio-Maxillofacial Surgery* 17: 354–8.

Kawakami M, Takano-Yamamoto T (1997) Orthodontic treatment of a patient with hypophosphatemic vitamin D-resistant rickets. *ASDC Journal of Dentistry for Children* 64: 395–9.

Kelekis-Cholakis A, Wiltshire WA, Birek C (2002) Treatment and long-term follow-up of a patient with hereditary gingival fibromatosis: a case report. *Journal of the Canadian Dental Association* 68: 290–4.

Kim JH, Viana MA, Graber TM, et al. (1999) The effectiveness of protraction face mask therapy: a meta-analysis. *American Journal of Orthodontics and Dentofacial Orthopedics* 115: 675–85.

King GJ, Frias JL (1979) A cephalometric study of the craniofacial skeleton in trichorhinophalangeal syndrome. *American Journal of Orthodontics* 75: 70–7.

Kjaer I, Becktor KB, Lisson J, et al. (2001) Face, palate, and craniofacial morphology in patients with a solitary median maxillary central incisor. *European Journal of Orthodontics* 23: 63–73.

Krusinskiene V, Alvesalo L, Sidlauskas A (2005) The craniofacial complex in 47, XXX females. *European Journal of Orthodontics* 27: 396–401.

Kucukyavuz Z, Ozkaynak O, Tuzuner AM, et al. (2006) Difficulties in anesthetic management of patients with micrognathia: report of a patient with Stickler syndrome. *Oral Surgery, Oral Medicine, Oral Pathology, Oral Radiology, and Endodontics* 102: e33–6.

Lam AK, David DJ, Townsend GC, et al. (2010) Van der Woude syndrome: dentofacial features and implications for clinical practice. *Australian Dental Journal* 55: 51–8.

Lammi L, Arte S, Somer M, et al. (2004) Mutations in AXIN2 cause familial tooth agenesis and predispose to colorectal cancer. *American Journal of Human Genetics* 74: 1043–50.

Lew D, Dewitt A, Hicks RJ, et al. (1999) Osteomas of the condyle associated with Gardner's syndrome causing limited mandibular movement. *Journal of Oral and Maxillofacial Surgery* 57: 1004–9.

Lichtenstein J, Warson R, Jorgenson R, et al. (1972) The tricho-dento-osseous (TDO) syndrome. *American Journal of Human Genetics* 24: 569–82.

Linch DC, Acton CH (1979) Ehlers-Danlos syndrome presenting with juvenile destructive periodontitis. *British Dental Journal* 147: 95–6.

Lukinmaa PL, Ranta H, Ranta K, et al. (1987a) Dental findings in osteogenesis imperfecta: I. Occurrence and expression of type I dentinogenesis imperfecta. *Journal of Craniofacial Genetics and Developmental Biology* 7: 115–25.

Lukinmaa PL, Ranta H, Ranta K, et al. (1987b) Dental findings in osteogenesis imperfecta: II. Dysplastic and other developmental defects. *Journal of Craniofacial Genetics and Developmental Biology* 7: 127–35.

Lund AM, Jensen BM, Nielsen LA, et al. (1998) Dental manifestations of osteogenesis imperfecta and abnormalities of collagen I metabolism. *Journal of Craniofacial Genetics and Developmental Biology* 18: 30–7.

Lux CJ, Kugel B, Komposch G, et al. (2005) Orthodontic treatment in a patient with Papillon-Lefevre syndrome. *Journal of Periodontology* 76: 642–50.

Macfarlane JD, Swart JG (1989) Dental aspects of hypophosphatasia: a case report, family study, and literature review. *Oral Surgery, Oral Medicine, and Oral Pathology* 67: 521–6.

Malmgren B, Norgren S (2002) Dental aberrations in children and adolescents with osteogenesis imperfecta. *Acta Odontologica Scandinavica* 60: 65–71.

Matsuda A, Suda N, Motohashi N, et al. (2006) Skeletal characteristics and treatment outcome of five patients with Robin sequence. *Angle Orthodontist* 76: 898–908.

McDonald RE, Avery DR, Hartsfield JK Jr (2011) Acquired and developmental disturbances of the teeth and associated oral structures. In: JA Dean, DR Avery, RE Mcdonald (eds) *McDonald's and Avery's Dentistry for the Child and Adolescent*, 9th edn. St. Louis, MO: Mosby/Elsevier.

McLain JB, Proffit WR, Davenport RH (1983) Adjunctive orthodontic therapy in the treatment of juvenile periodontitis: report of a case and review of the literature. *American Journal of Orthodontics* 83: 290–8.

Meskin LH, Gorlin RJ, Isaacson RJ (1964) Abnormal morphology of the soft palate. I. The prevalence of cleft uvula. *Cleft Palate Journal* 35: 342–6.

Meskin LH, Gorlin RJ, Isaacson RJ (1965) Abnormal morphology of the soft palate. II. The genetics of cleft uvula. *Cleft Palate Journal* 45: 40–5.

Meskin LH, Gorlin RJ, Isaacson RJ (1966) Cleft uvula – a microform of cleft palate. *Acta Chirurgiae Plasticae* 8: 91–6.

Meyle J, Gonzales JR (2001) Influences of systemic diseases on periodontitis in children and adolescents. *Periodontology* 2000 26: 92–112.

Midtbo M, Halse A (1994) Root length, crown height, and root morphology in Turner syndrome. *Acta Odontologica Scandinavica* 52: 303–14.

Momeni P, Glockner G, Schmidt O, et al. (2000) Mutations in a new gene, encoding a zinc-finger protein, cause tricho-rhino-phalangeal syndrome type I. *Nature Genetics* 24: 71–4.

Morriss-Kay GM, Wilkie AO (2005) Growth of the normal skull vault and its alteration in craniosynostosis: insights from human genetics and experimental studies. *Journal of Anatomy* 207: 637–53.

Musich DR (2006) Orthodontic intervention and patients with Down syndrome. *Angle Orthodontist* 76: 734–5.

Nagle DL, Karim MA, Woolf EA, et al. (1996) Identification and mutation analysis of the complete gene for Chediak-Higashi syndrome. *Nature Genetics* 14: 307–11.

Nandakumar G, Morgan JA, Silverberg D, et al. (2004) Familial polyposis coli: clinical manifestations, evaluation, management and treatment. *Mount Sinai Journal of Medicine, New York* 71: 384–91.

Nanni L, Ming JE, Du Y, et al. (2001) SHH mutation is associated with solitary median maxillary central incisor: a study of 13 patients and review of the literature. *American Journal of Medical Genetics* 102: 1–10.

Nishisho I, Nakamura Y, Miyoshi Y, et al. (1991) Mutations of chromosome 5q21 genes in FAP and colorectal cancer patients. *Science* 253: 665–9.

Norton LA, Assael LA (1997) Orthodontic and temporomandibular joint considerations in treatment of patients with Ehlers-Danlos syndrome. *American Journal of Orthodontics and Dentofacial Orthopedics* 111: 75–84.

O'Connell AC, Marini JC (1999) Evaluation of oral problems in an osteogenesis imperfecta population. *Oral Surgery, Oral Medicine, Oral Pathology, Oral Radiology, and Endodontics* 87: 189–96.

Petersen K, Wetzel WE (1998) Recent findings in classification of osteogenesis imperfecta by means of existing dental symptoms. *ASDC Journal of Dentistry for Children* 65: 305–9, 354.

Pierce AM, Sampson WJ, Wilson DF, et al. (1996) Fifteen-year follow-up of a family with inherited craniofacial fibrous dysplasia. *Journal of Oral and Maxillofacial Surgery* 54: 780–8.

Prabhu SR, Daftary DK, Dholakia HM (1978) Chondroectodermal dysplasia (Ellis-van Creveld syndrome): report of two cases. *Journal of Oral Surgery* 36: 631–7.

Proffit WR, Vig KW (1981) Primary failure of eruption: a possible cause of posterior open-bite. *American Journal of Orthodontics* 80: 173–90.

Proffit WR, Frazier-Bowers SA (2009) Mechanism and control of tooth eruption: overview and clinical implications. *Orthodontics and Craniofacial Research* 12: 59–66.

Raghoebar GM, Boering G, Jansen HW, et al. (1989) Secondary retention of permanent molars: a histologic study. *Journal of Oral Pathology and Medicine* 18: 427–31.

Reuland-Bosma W, Reuland MC, Bronkhorst E, et al. (2010) Patterns of tooth agenesis in patients with Down syndrome in relation to hypothyroidism and congenital heart disease: an aid for treatment planning. *American Journal of Orthodontics and Dentofacial Orthopedics* 137, 584 e1–9; discussion 584–5.

Rizos M, Spyropoulos MN (2004) Van der Woude syndrome: a review. Cardinal signs, epidemiology, associated features, differential diagnosis, expressivity, genetic counselling and treatment. *European Journal of Orthodontics* 26: 17–24.

Roberts WE, Hartsfield JK Jr (1997) Multidisciplinary management of congenital and acquired compensated malocclusions: diagnosis, etiology and treatment planning. *Journal of the Indiana Dental Association* 76: 42–3, 45–8, 50–1.

Rogers GF, Lim AA, Mulliken JB, et al. (2009) Effect of a syndromic diagnosis on mandibular size and sagittal position in Robin sequence. *Journal of Oral and Maxillofacial Surgery* 67: 2323–31.

Satoh K, Tsutsumi K, Tosa Y, et al. (2002) Le Fort III distraction osteogenesis of midface-retrusion in a case of Hajdu Cheny syndrome. *Journal of Craniofacial Surgery* 13: 298–302.

Schenkein HA (1998) Inheritance as a determinant of susceptibility for periodontitis. *Journal of Dental Education* 62: 840–51.

Schulman GS, Redford-Badwal D, Poole A, et al. (2005) Taurodontism and learning disabilities in patients with Klinefelter syndrome. *Pediatric Dentistry* 27: 389–94.

Schwanitz G, Zschiesche S (1989) Consultation for patients with cheilognathopalatoschisis and their family members. Cooperation between orthodontists and human geneticists. *Fortschritte der Kieferorthopädie* 50: 118–26.

Schwartz S, Tsipouras P (1984) Oral findings in osteogenesis imperfecta. *Oral Surgery, Oral Medicine, and Oral Pathology* 57: 161–7.

Shellhart WC, Casamassimo PS, Hagerman RJ, et al. (1986) Oral findings in fragile X syndrome. *American Journal of Medical Genetics* 23: 179–87.

Silva EC, De Souza PE, Barreto DC, et al. (2002) An extreme case of cherubism. *British Journal of Oral and Maxillofacial Surgery* 40: 45–8.

Singleton EB, Merten DF (1973) An unusual syndrome of widened medullary cavities of the metacarpals and phalanges, aortic calcification and abnormal dentition. *Pediatric Radiology* 1: 2–7.

Smahi A, Courtois G, Vabres P, et al. (2000) Genomic rearrangement in NEMO impairs NF-kappaB activation and is a cause of incontinentia pigmenti. The International Incontinentia Pigmenti (IP) Consortium. *Nature* 405: 466–72.

Smith WK, Steinhauser RA (1971) Vitamin D-resistant rickets with dental abnormalities. *Birth Defects Original Article Series* 7: 274–5.

Stellzig-Eisenhauer A, Decker E, Meyer-Marcotty P, et al. (2010) Primary failure of eruption (PFE) – clinical and molecular genetics analysis. *Journal of Orofacial Orthopedics* 71: 6–16.

Stewart RE, Hollister DW, Rimoin DL (1977) A new variant of Ehlers-Danlos syndrome: an autosomal dominant disorder of fragile skin, abnormal scarring, and generalized periodontitis. *Birth Defects Original Article Series* 13: 85–93.

Suda N, Takada J, Ohyama K (2006) Orthodontic treatment in a patient with Van der Woude's syndrome. *American Journal of Orthodontics and Dentofacial Orthopedics* 129: 696–705.

Suri L, Gagari E, Vastardis H (2004) Delayed tooth eruption: pathogenesis, diagnosis, and treatment. A literature review. *American Journal of Orthodontics and Dentofacial Orthopedics* 126: 432–45.

Suri S, Ross RB, Tompson BD (2006) Mandibular morphology and growth with and without hypodontia in subjects with Pierre Robin sequence. *American Journal of Orthodontics and Dentofacial Orthopedics* 130: 37–46.

Thomas JG, Smith HW (1981) Gardner's syndrome. Report of a case. *Oral Surgery, Oral Medicine, and Oral Pathology* 51: 213–14.

Timosca GC, Galesanu RM, Cotutiu C, et al. (2000) Aggressive form of cherubism: report of a case. *Journal of Oral and Maxillofacial Surgery* 58: 336–44.

Toutain A, Dessay B, Ronce N, et al. (2002) Refinement of the NHS locus on chromosome Xp22.13 and analysis of five candidate genes. *European Journal of Human Genetics* 10: 516–20.

Utreja A, Evans CA (2009) Marfan syndrome – an orthodontic perspective. *Angle Orthodontist* 79: 394–400.

Varela M, Ramos C (1996) Chondroectodermal dysplasia (Ellis-van Creveld syndrome): a case report. *European Journal of Orthodontics* 18: 313–18.

Varrela J, Alvesalo L, Mayhall J (1990) Taurodontism in 45, X females. *Journal of Dental Research* 69: 494–5.

Vig KW (1990) Orthodontic considerations applied to craniofacial dysmorphology. *Cleft Palate Journal* 27: 141–5.

Visinoni AF, Lisboa-Costa T, Pagnan NA, et al. (2009) Ectodermal dysplasias: clinical and molecular review. *American Journal of Medical Genetics Part A* 149: 1980–2002.

Westling L, Mohlin B, Bresin A (1998) Craniofacial manifestations in the Marfan syndrome: palatal dimensions and a comparative cephalometric analysis. *Journal of Craniofacial Genetics and Developmental Biology* 18: 211–18.

Wise GE, Frazier-Bowers S, D'Souza RN (2002) Cellular, molecular, and genetic determinants of tooth eruption. *Critical Reviews in Oral Biology and Medicine* 13: 323–34.

Wright JT, Kula K, Hall K, et al. (1997) Analysis of the tricho-dento-osseous syndrome genotype and phenotype. *American Journal of Medical Genetics* 72: 197–204.

Yamashiro T, Nakagawa K, Takada K (1998) Case report: orthodontic treatment of dental problems in incontinentia pigmenti. *Angle Orthodontist* 68: 281–4.

Additional resources

Online

American Board of Medical Genetics (ABMG): www.abmg.org, or specifically for listing of board certified geneticists, see www.abmg.org/pages/searchmem.shtml.

Online Mendelian Inheritance in Man (OMIM): www.ncbi.nlm.nih.gov/omim

OMIM is a United States of America publicly funded comprehensive, authoritative, and timely compendium of human genes and genetic phenotypes. The full-text, referenced overviews in OMIM contain information on all known Mendelian disorders and over 12 000 genes. OMIM focuses on the relationship between phenotype and genotype. It is updated daily, and the entries contain copious links to other genetics resources.

GeneTests: www.ncbi.nlm.nih.gov/sites/GeneTests/?db=GeneTests

This is a United States of America publicly funded medical genetics information resource (including pictures of some individuals for some of the conditions) developed for physicians, other healthcare providers, and researchers, available at no cost to all interested persons. A genetics clinic directory is also searchable at this site.

MedlinePlus: www.nlm.nih.gov/medlineplus/

This is the publicly funded United States of America National Institutes of Health's website for patients and their families and friends that is produced by the National Library of Medicine.

Books

Both these texts have numerous pictures. *Gorlin's Syndromes* (2010) also has sections on most of the conditions specifically concerning the facies and oral manifestations.

Hennekam RCM, Allanson JE, Krantz ID, et al. (2010) *Gorlin's Syndromes of the Head and Neck*. Oxford: Oxford University Press.

Jones KL, Smith DW (2006) *Smith's Recognizable Patterns of Human Malformation*. Philadelphia, PA: Elsevier/WB Saunders.

8

Multidisciplinary Team Management of Congenital Orofacial Deformities

Sherry Peter, Maria J Kuriakose

Summary

The term 'craniofacial anomalies' describes a diverse group of dysmorphic congenital disorders involving abnormalities of craniofacial development that vary from minor changes in the facial features to major abnormalities of craniofacial skeleton and its appendages: that is, ranging from simple craniosynostosis involving single fusions and simple clefts of the lip and palate to complex syndromes marked by multiple sutural fusions, complex facial clefts, branchial arch syndromes, gene depletions, gene mutations, and many more.

The management of children with complex craniofacial anomalies requires the skills of a variety of medical and dental professionals, and includes observation and assessment of their development, and formulation of a comprehensive treatment plan. These children need to be under constant care of this team from birth to adolescence or even beyond. With the emergence of craniofacial orthodontics, orthodontists have become an integral part of the team, providing skills to modify the growth and development of these inherently anomalous conditions. The value brought by the orthodontist to the craniofacial surgery team is clearly enunciated by McCarthy (2009) in his statement that 'no other field of endeavor has brought the medical and dental professions closer together.'

This chapter aims to provide a concise description of the commonly encountered craniofacial anomalies and their multidisciplinary management.

Introduction

Craniofacial orthodontics, an emerging and challenging field, demands creative and innovative thinking to deal with often unique and very difficult clinical problems. According to the American Dental Association, craniofacial orthodontics is the area of orthodontics concerned with the management of patients with congenital and acquired deformities of the integument and its underlying musculoskeletal system within the maxillofacial area and associated structures (Santiago and Grayson, 2009). The world of craniofacial anomalies is complex and children with craniofacial anomalies show wide variations in their cranial and facial features. Management of these anomalies requires expertise as it involves trying to establish a normalcy which was never there. Comprehensive and coordinated care from infancy through adolescence is essential in order to achieve an ideal outcome, and thus people with formal training and experience in all phases of care must be actively involved in the planning, treatment, and long-term follow-up of these patients (Kapp, 1979; Kapp-Simon, 1995).

The presence of a craniofacial anomaly has a devastating effect on the child and the parents. The complex etiology and involvement of multiple anatomical regions complicate the management and necessitate establishment of centralized units to deliver a team-oriented or interdisciplinary approach as the standard of care. With the advances in intrauterine imaging, early identification of congenital deformities is now possible. However, this finding is usually a source of significant concern to the parents psychologically, and numerous centers have established counseling and family support groups. These support groups educate and reassure the parents that their baby will be well cared for in a structured team environment over a number of years, from birth to adulthood. This gaining of trust of the parents forms an essential component of the integrated team approach, because parents need to be active participants in the treatment protocol, and prepare themselves and their child to confront the challenges that might arise in the ensuing years. Parents appreciate discussing issues

Integrated Clinical Orthodontics, First Edition. Edited by Vinod Krishnan, Ze'ev Davidovitch.
© 2012 Blackwell Publishing Ltd. Published 2012 by Blackwell Publishing Ltd.

with others who have had similar experiences, and reviewing pre- and post-treatment records (M Goonewardene, personal communication, 2010). This approach adds to the complex interdisciplinary interaction, which aims to achieve a more complete integration of all parties concerned with care and attention of the needs of the extended family.

A significant number of medical and dental specialties play important roles throughout the course of treatment of the patient with a congenital craniofacial deformity. The initial acute needs are addressed by the neurosurgeon, neonatologist, pediatric surgeon, and a special nursing unit, but the orthodontist and craniofacial surgeon are often also involved early in the course of care. Additional specialist clinicians may play roles at specific times appropriate for the patient's specific needs. These needs are determined and constantly reviewed at regular team meetings of the interdisciplinary group, and this excellent level of coordinated communication is the keystone to interdisciplinary-based, interactive care.

As almost all of the craniofacial anomalies involve jaw deformities, which are amenable to timely functional orthopedic and orthodontic treatments, orthodontists play an intrinsic role in their management (McCarthy, 2007). For example, they are actively involved in infant presurgical orthopedics, early mixed dentition treatment, dentofacial orthopedics and orthodontics, adolescent/adult orthodontics, preprosthetic orthodontics, and pre- and postsurgical orthodontics. The present chapter provides an overview of interdisciplinary team management of the most common craniofacial malformations (except cleft lip and palate, which is covered in Chapter 9). For the purpose of this chapter, the major congenital orofacial malformations are considered under the headings of otofacial malformations, craniosynostosis, achondroplasia/*FGFR3* mutations, and holoprosencephalic disorders.

Otofacial malformations

Craniofacial/hemifacial microsomia

This term describes a sporadic, complex spectrum of congenital anomalies that primarily involve the jaws, other skeletal components, muscles of mastication, ears, the nervous system, and soft tissues derived from the first and second branchial arches, unilaterally or bilaterally (Ross, 1975; Converse et al., 1979; Kaban et al., 1981; Posnick, 2000). It is the second most common congenital syndrome of the head and neck region after cleft lip and palate, with an incidence as high as 1 in 3500 live births (Munro and Lauritzen, 1985). The hypoplasia can manifest itself in any of the structures derived from the first and second branchial arches, accounting for the wide spectrum of deformities observed in this syndrome. This variable expression has resulted in numerous alternative names, such as Goldenhar

syndrome, dysostosis otomandibularis, and oculo-auriculovertebral dysplasia. Gorlin et al. (1990) have suggested that they should all be considered part of the oculo-auriculovertebral group. Over the years, several methods of classification have been developed, describing the anatomical regions and grade of involvement (Posnick, 2000). The most accepted classifications are the orbit, mandible, ear, nerve, and soft tissue (OMENS) classification (Vento et al., 1991) (Box 8.1), and the SAT method, where S stands for skeleton, A for auricle, and T for soft tissue (David et al., 1987).

The etiology of this anomaly has been related to defects in neural crest cells (Johnston and Bronsky, 1995), and the most accepted etiopathogenetic mechanism is that of a vascular insult, with hemorrhage and hematoma formation in the developing stapedial artery in the first and second branchial arches, with subsequent maldevelopment (Poswillo, 1975; Soltan and Holmes, 1986). The mandible has long been considered the 'cornerstone' of hemifacial microsomia (JC Kaban et al., 1981; Vento et al., 1991), as it is always involved and contributes to the natural course of

---

Box 8.1 OMENS classification of craniofacial anomalies

Orbit
- O0: normal orbital size, position
- O1: abnormal orbital size
- O2: abnormal orbital position
- O3: abnormal orbital size and position

Mandible
- M0: normal mandible
- M1: small mandible and glenoid fossa with short ramus
- M2: ramus short and abnormally shaped
  - 2A: glenoid fossa in anatomical acceptable position
  - 2B: temporomandibular joint (TMJ) inferiorly, medially, anteriorly displaced, with severely hypoplastic condyle
- M3: complete absence of ramus, glenoid fossa, and TMJ

Ear
- E0: normal ear
- E1: minor hypoplasia and cupping with all structures present
- E2: absence of external auditory cannel with variable hypoplasia of *the concha*
- E3: malposition of the lobule with absent auricle, lobular remnant usually inferior anteriorly displaced

Facial nerve
- N0: no facial nerve involvement
- N1: upper facial nerve involvement (temporal or zygomatic branches)
- N2: lower facial nerve involvement (buccal, mandibular, or cervical)
- N3: all branches affected

Soft tissue
- S0: no soft tissue or muscle deficiency
- S1: minimal tissue or muscle deficiency
- S2: moderate tissue or muscle deficiency
- S3: severe tissue or muscle deficiency

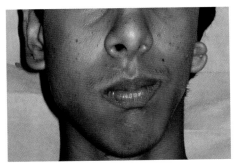

Figure 8.1 Characteristic facial asymmetry in hemifacial microsomia.

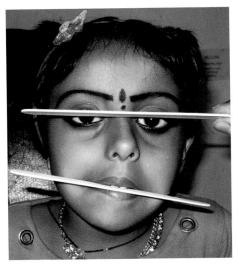

Figure 8.2 Canting of the occlusal plane in a hemifacial microsomia patient.

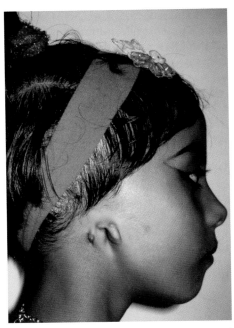

Figure 8.3 Malformation of external ear (microtia), as part of hemifacial microsomia.

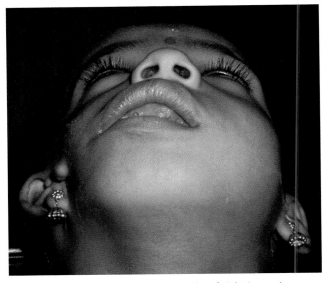

Figure 8.4 Characteristic malar flattening in hemifacial microsomia.

skeletal asymmetry (Kaban et al., 1981; Kaban et al., 1988; Polley et al., 1997; Kearns et al., 2000). The restricted growth potential of the affected hemimandible inhibits ipsilateral vertical maxillary development, resulting in a progressive facial asymmetry (Figure 8.1). The mandibular hypoplasia may range from mild flattening of the condylar head to complete agenesis of the condyle, ascending ramus, and glenoid fossa. Because of the hypoplastic ramus, the mandibular plane angle is increased, the chin deviates toward the affected side, and there is a corresponding cant of the mandibular occlusal plane, which impacts the maxillary occlusal plane as well as the levels of the pyriform apertures (Figure 8.2).

Variable hypoplasia of the ipsilateral zygomatico-orbital region is a common finding, occasionally resulting in orbital dystopia (Gougoutas et al., 2007). Because of their proximity, secondary involvement of skeletal structures not directly derived from first and second branchial arch derivatives, such as the temporal bone, frontal bone, the styloid, mastoid and pterygoid processes, and cervical vertebrae is

inevitable (Converse et al., 1973). The auricle is involved in most patients (Meurman, 1957) (Figure 8.3). A combination of cutaneous and subcutaneous connective and neuromuscular tissue deficiency is most evident in the region of the external ear and eye, and the temporal, malar, and masseteric regions of the face, giving rise to a characteristic temporal hollowing and malar flattening (Figure 8.4). This

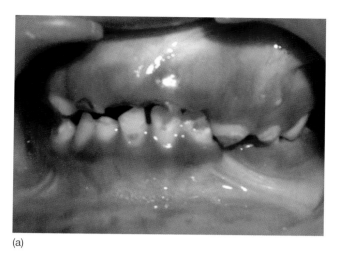

(a)

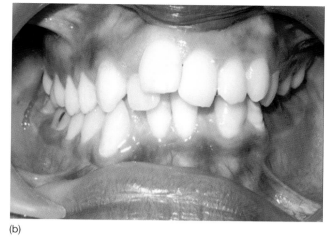

(b)

Figure 8.5 (a,b) Occlusion in two craniofacial microsomia patients.

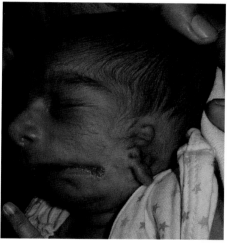

Figure 8.6 Macrostomia and ear anomaly in a baby with craniofacial microsomia.

classic appearance may be accentuated by muscular hypoplasia involving the muscles of mastication. Masticatory muscle function on the affected side may likewise be impaired. The maxillary and mandibular dentoalveolar complexes are reduced in the vertical dimension on the affected side, and exhibit crowding, delayed eruption of the deciduous and permanent teeth, and, occasionally, missing molars (Figure 8.5). Macrostomia or clefting through the oral commissure, and hypoplasia of the parotid gland may also be present (Whitaker and Bartlett, 1990) (Figure 8.6). Facial palsies have been estimated to occur in 22–45% of patients (Figure 8.7) (Bergstrom and Baker, 1981; McCarthy, 1997).

Management

Management of hemifacial microsomia requires a comprehensive evaluation of the extent of the skeletal contribution to the deformity. It is possible that functional appliance treatment and dental compensation may suffice for minor skeletal discrepancies, but moderate to severe skeletal problems will require surgical intervention. The timing of and techniques used for correction will differ from center to center, and from patient to patient. The parents are often in a state of shock, and should be met and counseled by the members of the team during the first visit itself (Barden et al., 1989). Treatment will depend on the severity of the dysmorphism and age of the child (Silvestri et al., 1996).

No surgery is indicated in very young children, unless there is an airway disruption due to mandibular micrognathia, which is usually dealt with by tracheostomy or mandibular distraction (McCarthy et al., 1992, Boston and Rutter, 2003). But often, excision of the preauricular skin tags and cartilage remnants and correction of macrostomia are carried out as this is quite reassuring for the parents because it removes some of the stigmata of the syndrome (McCarthy, 2007) (Figure 8.8). Assessment of hearing and provision of hearing aids also need attention during the early childhood.

The most widely followed treatment protocol is that of Silvestri et al. (1996), based on the SAT classification system (David et al., 1987). It emphasizes functional appliance treatment during growth, followed by surgery to reposition the skeleton, and grafting. The objectives of early intervention include providing a growth stimulus for the affected side of the maxilla, and the associated dentoalveolar and soft tissues. Effective mandibular lengthening and correction of facial asymmetry has been reported with distraction osteogenesis, and this has become the treatment of choice, especially in growing children (McCarthy et al., 1992;

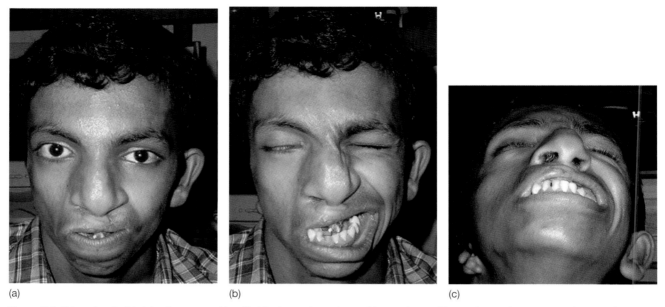

(a)   (b)   (c)

Figure 8.7 This patient had facial palsy as part of hemifacial microsomia syndrome. (a) Frontal view. (b) Frontal view showing incomplete eye closure and deviation of the angle of the mouth towards the normal left side. (c) Worm's eye view showing malar flattening and deviation of the angle of the mouth.

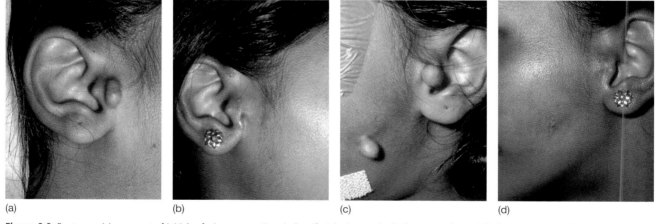

(a)   (b)   (c)   (d)

Figure 8.8 Ear tag excision as part of initial soft tissue corrections in hemifacial microsomia: (a,c) preoperative and (b,d) postoperative photographs.

Cascone et al., 2005). The distraction is beneficial, especially in patients with psychological or functional impairments, as it improves function and appearance during growth, creating an almost normal interim status. Generally, distraction osteogenesis of the mandible is too complicated to perform in children under 2 years of age, because of inaccuracies in the assessment of the location of the tooth germs.

In preadolescent patients, distraction may be performed to open up space vertically and anteroposteriorly for development of the soft tissues, and subsequent secondary maxillary growth. The soft regenerate requires protection from the constricting effects of the healing tissues, so the ortho-dontist will be required to construct a unilateral bite block to maintain the open bite that is created. This bite block may be modified to encourage dental eruption following consolidation of the regenerate. In postadolescent patients, distraction procedures are reserved for the more severe skeletal anomalies, and it is not uncommon for the patient to undergo mandibular distraction as the major defect usually lies in the mandible, followed by maxillary surgery and revision surgery on the mandible, to achieve the final position of the mandible. The maxilla and mandible may be simultaneously distracted to effect three-dimensional changes, if required (Ortiz-Monasterio et al., 1997). There are conflicting reports regarding the growth potential of the

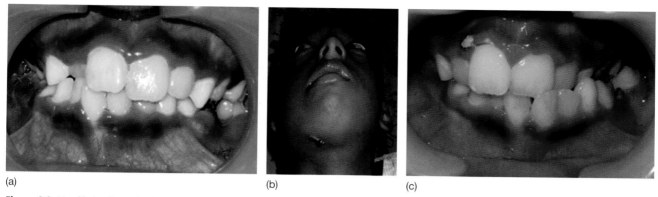

(a) (b) (c)

Figure 8.9 Mandibular distraction in a craniofacial microsomia patient. (a) Pre-distraction occlusion; (b) distractor in place; and (c) post-distraction occlusion.

mandible after initial distraction (Figure 8.9). Though Sheyte et al. (2006) have reported mandibular growth after distraction, usually further surgical management is needed after growth is complete, as the inherent growth potential of the affected side is deficient (Iseri et al., 2008; Nagy et al., 2009). The patient will also require a series of soft tissue procedures to compensate for the hypoplasia and ear malformations (Brent, 1992; Longaker and Siebert, 1995; Wang and Andres, 1999) (Figure 8.10).

Orthodontic treatment in craniofacial microsomia

Orthodontic treatment is carried out in a staged manner. The best possible results are achieved when the orthodontist and the surgeon agree on a carefully designed and customized treatment plan. Both should be aware of the treatment objectives, limitations, and risks. This approach should also be explained to the patient and the family.

The orthodontic treatment phases can be broadly divided into pre-distraction orthodontic treatment, orthodontic treatment during distraction and consolidation, and post-consolidation orthodontics.

Pre-distraction treatment planning and orthodontics

This phase of treatment is carried out in the growing child, where the aim of distraction is to decrease the facial asymmetry. Vector planning is crucial in this stage, depending on the lengthening of the mandible required in the vertical, sagittal, and oblique planes. The decision about the type of movement that would be required, and the associated position of the distractor, is made in a combined clinic between the operating surgeon and orthodontist (Hanson and Melugin, 1999). It is always advantageous to use stabilization appliances as part of pre-distraction, which help in elastic traction (Hanson and Melugin, 1999). This treatment also facilitates control of the force vectors and maintenance of the transverse relationship between the maxilla and mandible, preventing lateral displacement of the dental segment.

Orthodontics during distraction

The aim of orthodontic treatment during the distraction is to control the force vector to direct the growth of the mandible into an advantageous position. As the distraction progresses, the rami lengthen vertically, resulting in a posterior open bite. In this stage, the mandibular occlusal cant is corrected, and vertical symmetry is established. But as the posterior open bite increases, the patient might find it difficult to occlude and so shifts the mandible to the unaffected side. This situation can be observed clinically as shifting of the dental midline away from the distracted side, and as a buccal crossbite on the distracted side. A crossbite develops on the unaffected side, and is termed laterognathism.

Orthopedic forces are required to correct the laterognathism. The direction of force from the elastics may be opposite to that of the distraction forces, and so the distraction force has to be greater than the elastic traction. Elastic traction can also be used to coordinate the dental arches, and correct the dental midline shifts (Figure 8.11). Orthodontists should maintain all records for future re-evaluations and planning treatment progression.

Post-distraction orthodontics

In the growing child, post-distraction orthodontic treatment is extremely important. Guided eruption of the teeth, correction of laterognathism with elastics, and controlled vertical closure of the unilateral posterior open bite are the main objectives of this stage of treatment, along with stabilization of the corrected mandibular occlusal plane. Failure to stabilize the occlusal plane will lead to overeruption of both maxillary and mandibular teeth, and re-establishment of the previous maxillary and mandibular occlusal cant. The corrected mandibular occlusal plane is maintained by the selective eruption of the maxillary teeth, and can be performed with:

- An occlusal acrylic wafer that is reduced one tooth at a time, to allow controlled eruption of the maxillary teeth. Santiago and Grayson (2009) recommend inserting a

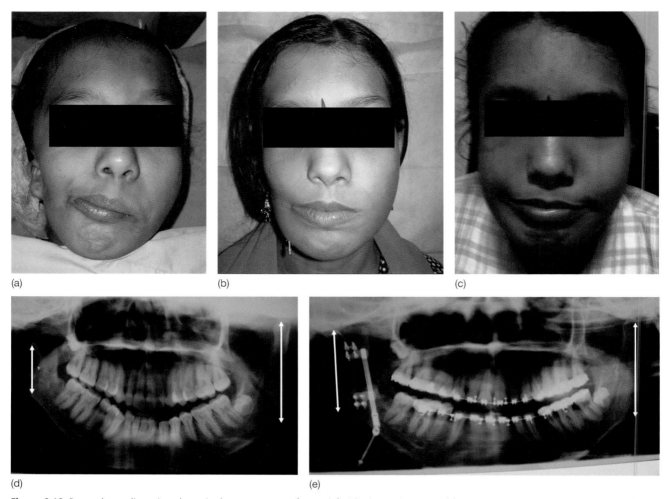

Figure 8.10 Pre- and post-distraction phases in the management of a craniofacial microsomia patient. (a) Pre-treatment extraoral view. (b) Post-distraction extraoral view. (c) Soft tissue corrections performed using a temporoparietal flap. (d) Pretreatment orthopantomogram – note the discrepancy between the right and left mandibular rami in the vertical plane (arrows). (e) Post-distraction orthopantomogram showing nearly symmetrical rami after distraction (arrows).

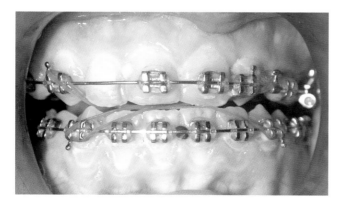

Figure 8.11 Midline oblique elastics to coordinate dental arches during distraction osteogenesis.

bite block that fills the open bite on the distracted side soon after active distraction, providing a bilateral balanced occlusion (Figure 8.12).

- A functional appliance with lingual shields, to provide lateral control of mandibular position. A bite plane is also included, which is adjusted to allow serial eruption of maxillary teeth. Elastic traction is often added to the appliance, which has been shown to decrease treatment time (Hanson and Melugin, 1999).

The role of functional appliances

The aim of functional therapy is to stimulate impaired function of the stomatognathic system, to substitute for absent structures, and stimulate differential growth on the two sides of the face (Silvestri et al., 1996). Functional appliances alone are more effective in patients with the milder form of the malformation than in those with severe malformation, where the functional appliances have to be combined with further orthodontics and surgery. But even in these cases,

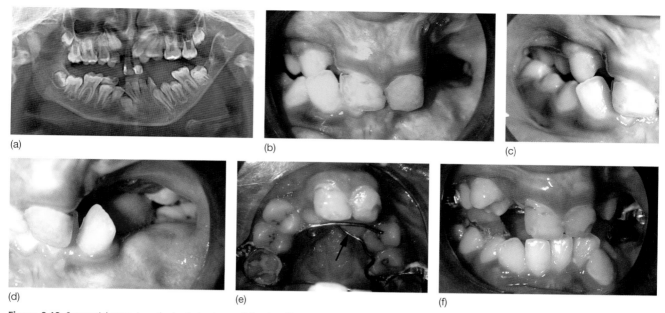

Figure 8.12 Sequential steps in orthodontic treatment following distraction osteogenesis in a growing child with hemifacial microsomia and bilateral cleft palate. (a) Pre-treatment orthopantomogram. (b–d) Occlusion after distraction. Note the bilateral posterior crossbite. (e) Fabrication and placement of a soldered custom-made expansion appliance to procline the central incisors. The right maxillary canine can be seen erupting behind the central incisor (arrow). (f) Bite block in the mandibular arch for promoting controlled eruption of maxillary teeth.

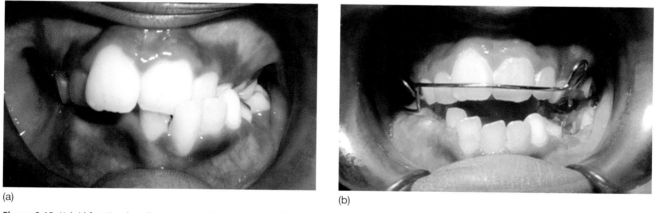

Figure 8.13 Hybrid functional appliance treatment in a growing child with craniofacial microsomia, after distraction. (a) Occlusion after distraction at the start of functional therapy. Note the upper and lower midlines are not coincident. (b) Hybrid functional appliance in place. Note the upper and lower midlines coinciding with the functional appliance in situ.

several authors believe that functional therapy is useful, as it corrects the dentoalveolar disorders, and prepares the neuromuscular system for the new position adopted by the skeletal structures after surgical intervention. The postsurgical open bite, when functional appliance treatment is followed by surgical intervention, can be dealt with with the help of comprehensive orthodontic treatment.

Silvestri et al. (1996) successfully used an asymmetric functional activator (AFA) to induce harmonious maxillomandibular growth. A wax bite is taken with the mandible protruded and deviated contralaterally to the side of the

microsomia, with an occlusal rise greater than the rotation of the occlusal plane. An activator/monobloc is then constructed, which consists of a body with an occlusal rise contralateral to the malformation, which acts as a guide for the mandible when the mouth is closed. To prevent muscular forces from acting on the normal side, the appliance has a shield in the vestibule on the side of the microsomia and also two small inferior shields. In this fashion, all the growth stimuli are directed towards the side of the microsomia, while inhibiting the growth of the maxilla and mandible on the healthy side (Figure 8.13).

Orthodontics in the skeletally mature patient

Distraction is the treatment of choice in skeletally mature patients, when the deformity is severe. Orthodontic treatment in these patients is performed in three stages.

Pre-distraction orthodontics

The aim of the pre-distraction orthodontics is to achieve a functional and esthetic occlusion. It involves moving teeth into ideal positions relative to the basal bone, so that the maxillomandibular skeletal relationship is not compromised by the dental compensations. It is critical to ascertain that the maxillary and mandibular arches are coordinated. For instance, in severe mandibular retrognathia, as the mandible is moved forward, a maxillary transverse deficiency might get unmasked, necessitating a preoperative expansion approach for its correction. Rigid, full-sized rectangular stainless steel archwires that fill the bracket slots should be in place. If possible, lingual cleats needs to be welded to the molar bands, as they may be helpful in using elastics during the distraction phase.

Orthodontics during distraction

This phase involves close monitoring during the distraction process. Any interference with the free movement of the distracted segment might need to be addressed. Bite planes can be used to prevent occlusal interferences and elastic traction can be applied for correcting transverse discrepancy and occlusal cant. Elastics can be used in a cross-arch or midline-oblique fashion. Sometimes, expansion appliances might be needed to correct transverse discrepancies (Figure 8.14).

Post-distraction

Some patients might require further orthognathic surgery to fully correct the deformity. In these instances, the pre-surgical preparation should be commenced. Otherwise, this phase involves correction of transverse discrepancies, midline shifts, and the cant of the occlusal plane. If unilateral mandibular distraction is the treatment choice, controlled vertical closure of the bite, using elastic traction or other means, are performed at this stage (Figure 8.15).

Orthognathic surgery

Many patients treated with early distraction often require an orthognathic surgical procedure at a later stage, as the mandibular asymmetry reappears (Nagy et al., 2009). The role of the orthodontist in this stage involves performing presurgical as well as postsurgical orthodontics.

Treacher Collins syndrome (mandibulofacial dysostosis)

Mandibulofacial dysostosis (MFD), or Treacher Collins syndrome (TCS), is an autosomal dominant disorder that is caused by aberrations in the development of the first and second branchial arches, with an incidence of 1 in 50 000 live births (Gorlin et al., 1990). TCS occurs as a result of destruction of neural crest cells before they migrate to form facial structures (Van Vierzen et al., 1995). TCS is named after Edward Treacher Collins (1862–1932), the English surgeon and ophthalmologist who described two patients with lower eyelid and malar deformities. Tessier (1971a) described TCS as the expression of bilateral 6, 7, and 8 craniofacial clefts, which accounts for the absent or malformed zygomas, eyelid coloboma, and ear and oral malformations (Figure 8.16).

Mandibulofacial dysostosis can be recognized at birth, given the characteristic facial appearance (Trainor et al., 2009). Most frequent clinical characteristics include hypoplasia of facial bones, mandible and zygoma, anti-mongoloid slant of the palpebral fissures, eyelid coloboma, total or partial absence of lower eyelashes, external ear malformations and conductive hearing loss, cleft palate with shortened soft palate, tongue-shaped extension of hair onto the face, macrostomia, and obstructive apnea (25% of cases). The convex profile and the prominent/retrusive chin give the characteristic bird-facies or fish-facies to TCS patients (Franceschetti and Klein, 1949) (Figure 8.17). Dental malalignment with an anterior open bite is also a common feature.

Management

Early diagnosis of TCS allows appropriate treatment for esthetic and functional deficiencies in these patients. It is possible to take advantage of anticipated growth during normal skeletal maturation at this stage in order to obtain better therapeutic results. Ameliorating the outward signs of TCS gives these patients an opportunity for improved social life.

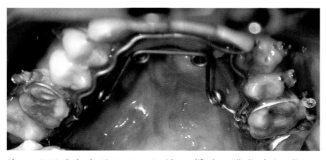

Figure 8.14 Orthodontic treatment with modified quadhelix during distraction to correct transverse discrepancy. A posterior bite plane may be used along with expansion devices to avoid occlusal interferences during the distraction procedures.

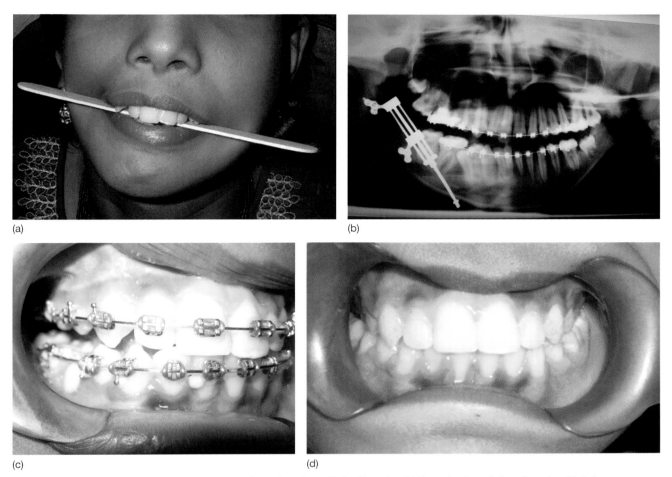

Figure 8.15 Orthodontics in a skeletally mature patient after unilateral mandibular distraction. (a) The occlusal cant before distraction. (b) Orthopantomogram showing the distractor in place. (c,d) Open bite following unilateral distraction, closed with conventional orthodontic treatment and occlusion at debonding.

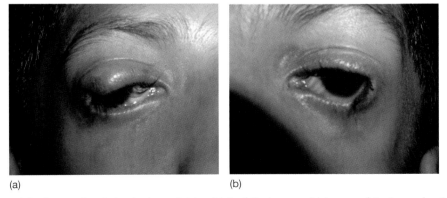

Figure 8.16 (a,b) Characteristic absence of eyelashes in the medial two-thirds of the lower eyelid because of Tessier number 6 cleft in Treacher Collins syndrome.

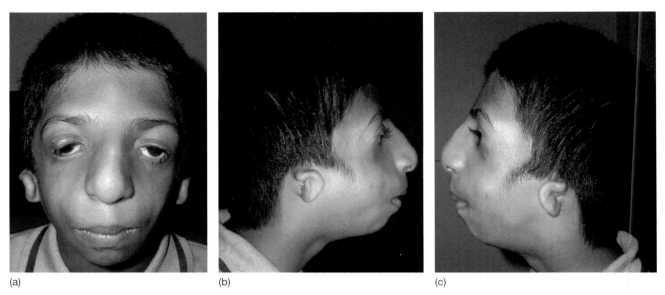

(a) (b) (c)

Figure 8.17 Characteristic facies of Treacher Collins syndrome. (a) Frontal facial photograph showing bilateral malar flattening because of Tessier number 7 cleft and anti-mongoloid slant of the palpebral fissures due to lack of lateral orbital support because of Tessier number 8 cleft. (b,c) Lateral views showing microtia and anterior displacement of side burns because of Tessier number 7 cleft.

All members of the craniofacial team need to evaluate the infant with TCS. The hypoplastic mandible, and sometimes the maxilla, along with pharyngeal incompetence and choanal atresia are reasons for concerns about the pharyngeal airway and oral alimentation (Dufresne, 1992). An experienced pediatric otolaryngologist needs to perform an audiology test to allow early fitting of hearing aids. The speech/swallow team is invaluable for assistance with learning better communication skills. A pediatric neuro-ophthalmologic evaluation of the eyelid deformities, ocular muscles, and visual acuity is important.

Distraction osteogenesis of the mandible in infancy allows issues with breathing and nutrition to be addressed. In the growing child, distraction allows the mandible to move down and forward, theoretically allowing the maxilla to descend vertically. Definitive distraction at skeletal maturity helps resolve the problems with occlusion. Often a maxillary osteotomy is needed for esthetic improvement. Specialized maxillary procedures have been reported to reduce the relative prominence of central midface (Tulane and Tessier, 1986; Fuento del Campo et al., 1994)

Staged repair of ear deformities is usually clubbed with distraction procedures. Split rib and calvarial bone onlay grafts or vascularized bone flaps are needed, depending on the severity of mandibular and zygomatic hypoplasia. Rhinoplasty and genioplasty are usually carried out along with or after the final bone correction procedure

Orthodontic management
An experienced multidisciplinary team comprising orthodontists and maxillofacial surgeons is necessary for good results, since the method of choice in the treatment of TCS is distraction osteogenesis along with preoperative and postoperative orthodontic treatment (Opitz et al., 2004).

The treatment schedule advocated by Opitz et al. (2004) includes therapeutic measures in the following sequence:

1. Preoperative alignment of the maxillary and mandibular dental arches, with extractions if needed to relieve crowding
2. Extraction of all third molars
3. Mandibular advancement by sagittal osteotomy of the ramus
4. Bilateral zygomatic augmentation
5. Genioplasty and rhinoplasty
6. Postoperative adjustment of the occlusion.

Functional appliances for mandibular advancement and protrusion have proved to be only moderately effective. The use of functional appliances during the primary and mixed dentition is often aimed at stimulating mandibular growth and preventing further asymmetrical development in cases of unilateral dysplasia.

Regarding distraction osteogenesis, orthodontists works in close collaboration with the oral and maxillofacial surgeon for precise treatment planning, preoperative alignment of the dental arches, prevention or at least reduction of deviations of the occlusal plane through targeted encouragement of vertical growth, and elimination of dental compensation and crowding in the dental arches (Opitz et al., 2004). Orthodontic treatment is usually performed with acrylic splints or functional appliances with customized bite planes that allow individual occlusal adjustment with selective extrusion of the molars and premolars on the affected side. This also regulates the transverse position of the mandible, especially in cases of unilateral dysplasia. Distraction osteogenesis demands intensive, often long-term orthodontic aftercare to achieve correct alignment of the teeth and controlled closure of lateral open bite. Simultaneous or subsequent treatment with intermaxillary elastics is often used to allow the regenerate bone to be shaped before consolidation according to the needs of the patient.

Presurgical orthodontics commences at around skeletal maturity, and is followed by postsurgical orthodontics after osteotomy, to align the teeth in the best possible relation to the basal bone and to achieve occlusal settling.

DiGeorge syndrome/velocardiofacial syndrome/ Takao syndrome

DiGeorge syndrome (DGS), otherwise known as 22q11.2 deletion syndrome, is the commonest chromosome deletion syndrome, with an incidence of about 1:3000 live births (Goodship et al., 1998). DGS presents with variable clinical features, such as thymus dysfunction, cardiac diseases, immunodeficiency, cleft palate, velopharyngeal insufficiency, and learning disabilities (Kobrynski and Sullivan, 2007). Infections are common in children, due to changes in the immune system's T-cell mediated response, resulting from an absent or hypoplastic thymus. Parathyroid dysfunction may cause hypocalcemia and seizures in the neonatal period. These findings are considered a warning sign, suggestive of DGS. Behavioral, neurological, and psychiatric disorders are frequent in this syndrome (Gothelf et al., 2007). Facial dimorphism, oral defects inclusive of dental malformations, microstomia, micrognathia, ear anomalies, hypertelorism, and strabismus has been reported (Fomin et al., 2010).

There is no genetic cure for 22q11.2 deletion syndrome. Certain individual features are treatable, using standard treatments. The key is to identify all the associated features and manage each using the best available treatments.

Craniosynostoses

Craniosynostoses is characterized by the premature closure of the calvarial sutures. There are over 100 recognized syndromes that include craniosynostoses of various types in their clinical features (Gorlin et al., 1990). Syndromic craniosynostosis is most often genetic in nature. Most craniosynostoses are autosomal dominant, although Carpenter syndrome is a notable exception, being transmitted in an autosomal recessive pattern. The synostosis of the cranial sutures, and probably a mesenchymal defect in the cranial base, contribute to the abnormal craniofacial features in these syndromic children. Out of more than 100 reported, Apert (1 in 25 000 live births), and Crouzon (1 in 25 000 live births) syndromes represent the more commonly identified ones (Cohen, 1986). The craniosynostosis is sometimes present even at birth. All these craniosynostoses may have varying degrees of fusion of the calvarial sutures, which may result in progressive increase in intracranial pressure, and development of characteristic hypertelorism, exophthalmos, midface deficiency, and a Class III malocclusion (Bartlett, 2007) (Figures 8.18 and 8.19).

These familial syndromes share many common craniofacial features, and only the digital anomalies of the hands may be the differentiating feature. Premature fusion of both coronal sutures results in a brachycephalic head, with a flat, elongated forehead with bitemporal widening and occipital flattening (Bartlett, 2007).

As the cranial base sutures are frequently involved, forward translation of the midfacial region/maxilla is restricted, resulting in its hypoplasia. The patients will often present with a concave profile, shallow orbits with

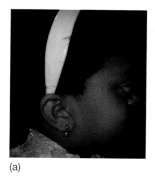 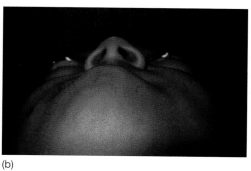 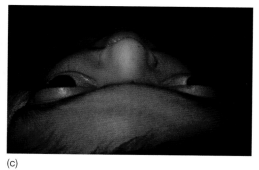

(a) (b) (c)

Figure 8.18 Craniosynostosis – Crouzon syndrome. (a) Lateral view showing midface hypoplasia and exorbitism. (b) Bird's view of the same patient showing retruded position of the forehead and exorbitism. (c) Worm's eye view showing midface hypoplasia and exorbitism.

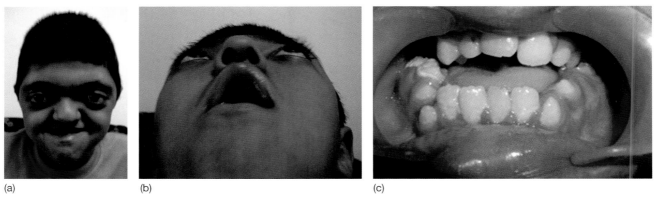

(a)   (b)   (c)

Figure 8.19 Craniosynostosis – Apert's syndrome. (a) Frontal view showing midface hypoplasia and exorbitism. (b) Worm's eye view showing midface hypoplasia and exorbitism. (c) Class III occlusal relationship in the same patient.

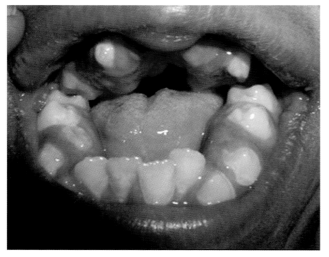

Figure 8.20 Characteristic Class III skeletal relationship with anterior crossbite and open bite in a patient with Apert syndrome.

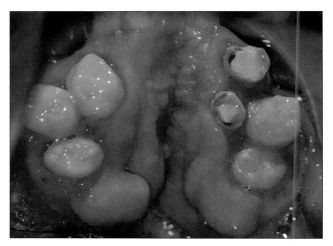

Figure 8.21 Palatal swellings in the same patient as in Figure 8.20.

exorbitism, and obstructive sleep apnea (Nout et al., 2008). A skeletal Class III relationship with anterior crossbite is a common finding (Figure 8.20). The palate is often high arched and constricted, exhibiting lateral palatal swellings containing excess mucopolysaccharides (Solomon et al., 1973; Pruzansky, 1974; MM Cohen 1986; Kreiborg et al., 1992) that increase in size with age, especially in Apert syndrome (Figure 8.21). The hard palate is shorter than normal, and the soft palate is longer and thicker (Peterson-Falzone et al., 1981). Cleft soft palate, or bifid uvula occur in 75% of patients (Kreiborg et al., 1992). As the maxillary arch width is reduced, there is severe crowding and ectopic eruption of teeth (Nurko and Ouinonese, 2004). Associated with the narrow maxilla is a tongue thrust swallow and anterior open bite. In both Apert and Crouzon syndromes,

the saliva is thick and mucinous. Apert syndrome patients exhibit short clinical crowns, along with thick and fibrous gingival tissue.

Apert syndrome in addition also manifests as symmetrical syndactyly of both hands and feet, most often involving fusion of the second, third, and fourth fingers as well as toes. These hand anomalies are so severe and functionally debilitating that referral to a hand surgeon with special expertise in this area is essential (Bartlett, 2007) (Figure 8.22).

Management

Surgical procedures for the correction of craniofacial deformities in patients with syndromic craniosynostosis

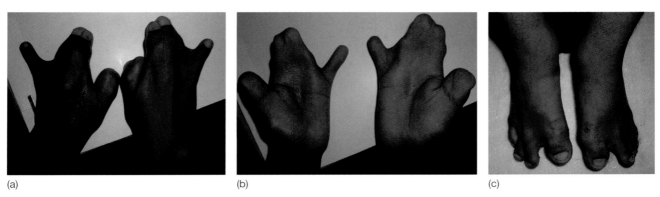

(a)   (b)   (c)

Figure 8.22 a–c Syndactyly in the upper and lower limbs seen in a patient with Apert syndrome.

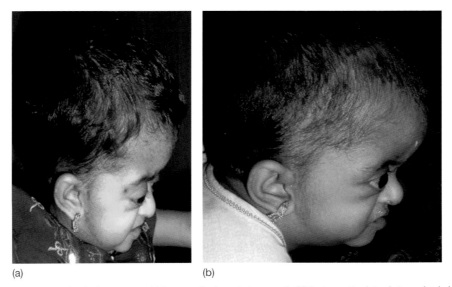

(a)   (b)

Figure 8.23 Craniosynostosis- Fronto-orbital advancement. (a) Preoperative lateral photograph. (b) Postoperative lateral view – healed incision line can be seen and advancement of the fronto-orbital region can be appreciated.

can be divided into procedures that are performed early in life (4–12 months: suture release, cranial vault decompression, and upper orbital reshaping/advancement), and those performed at a later age (4–12 years: for midface deformities at Le Fort III level) and jaw surgery (14–18 years) (Bartlett, 2007). These patients often require multiple surgeries, which may include suture release and fronto-orbital advancement (Tessier, 1971b; Cohen, 1986; Whitaker and Bartlett, 1990) (Figure 8.23), or distraction of the fused sutures to accommodate the enlarging brain (Sugawara et al., 1998; Kobayashi et al., 1999), and advancement of the midface by osteotomy or distraction (Converse and Telsey, 1971; Ortiz-Monasterio et al., 1978; McCarthy et al., 1990; Polley et al., 1995,1997; Cohen et al., 1997) (Figure 8.24).

Definitive surgery is usually carried out in the post-adolescent stage, when a combination of distraction of the maxilla and possibly setback of the mandible, may be considered to establish well or relatively well-balanced skeletal relationships. Definitive surgery to address any residual skeletal issues is dictated by individual morphological needs. The exact timing and sequence of each of the aforementioned surgical procedures depend on both the functional and the psychological needs of the patient (Bartlett, 2007).

Skull deformities may require early intervention by a neurosurgeon, so that the elevated intracranial pressure and papilledema can be effectively managed. Such craniofacial dysostosis patients are at high risk of upper airway

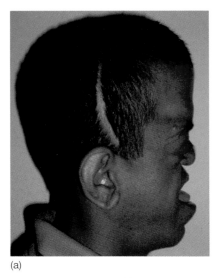 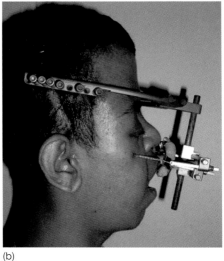

(a)   (b)

Figure 8.24 Midface distraction in Apert syndrome. (a) Pre-distraction photograph. Note the scar of a previous fronto-orbital advancement. (b) Lateral view with distractor for midface advancement.

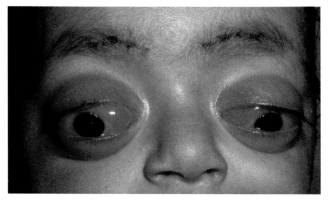

Figure 8.25 Exposure keratitis in a patient with Crouzon syndrome.

obstruction, necessitating tracheostomy or timely advancement of the midface in order to enlarge the nasopharynx and the palatopharyngeal space (Boston and Rutter, 2003; Hoeve et al., 2003; Pijpers et al., 2004). Ocular proptosis in these patients results in exposure keratitis (Figure 8.25), and infection leading to corneal ulceration and cataracts (Khan et al., 2003). Ocular (sub-)luxation requires reduction of the globe and tarsorrhaphy to contain the globe in the most severe cases to prevent development of complications (Figure 8.26) (Tay et al., 2006).

Orthodontic treatment in craniosynostosis
The orthodontist, as part of the team, should be involved right from the beginning of the management, to monitor

the growth and development of the craniofacial complex. It is essential that the child is seen by a pedodontist, and an oral hygiene regimen established. Orthodontic treatment in these patients can be divided into two stages, treatment carried out during childhood and during adolescence. It is to be kept in mind that orthodontic treatment alone will not be enough to correct the skeletal and dental deformities.

Orthodontic treatment during childhood
It is necessary at this stage to keep a close eye on the erupting pattern of teeth. Due to the severe crowding, often it is necessary to extract primary teeth to allow the permanent teeth to erupt. The primary canines are most commonly extracted to make space for the erupting laterals or the permanent canines. Care should be taken that the extraction of the primary teeth does not result in a shift in the midline. When the primary canines are extracted in the mandibular arch, a lingual arch may be needed to prevent loss of space. In the maxilla, expansion is often necessary, and a palatal arch or a trihelix could be used, because jackscrew expansion in these patients is impossible.

During childhood, in some cases, correction of midface deficiency with either Le Fort III osteotomy or distraction is performed, as the change in appearance might have a psychological effect on the child (Tessier, 1971b; McCarthy et al., 1990; Polley and Figueroa, 1997). The aim is to correct the fronto-orbital relationship in these patients. It would be ideal at this stage to wait for the permanent first molars to erupt and for the canines to drop a little so that the teeth are not damaged during osteotomy.

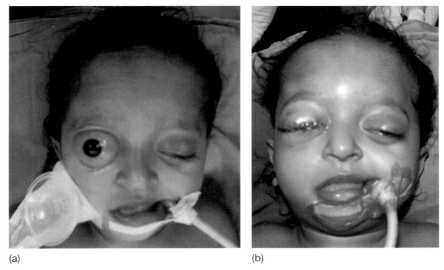

Figure 8.26 Orbital complications as part of Crouzon syndrome. (a) Globe dislocation due to the hypoplastic bony orbits. (b) Post-reduction photograph after tarsorrhaphy to contain the globe.

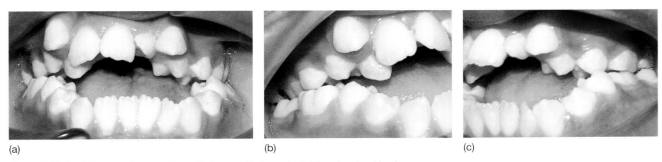

Figure 8.27 (a–c) Apert syndrome patient with the mandibular arch at different occlusal levels.

All orthodontic procedures during this stage are performed with minimal fixed appliances, such as 2 × 4 appliances. Once in rectangular rigid wires, hooks can be attached or a stabilization appliance (Hanson and Melugin, 1999) can be used. These procedures help in the construction of the surgical splint, which is necessary at the time of an osteotomy or distraction, as the case may be. The occlusion is not finalized at this stage.

Orthodontic treatment during adolescence
Once growth is over, a Le Fort I osteotomy to correct the skeletal Class III relationship will be necessary (Bachmayer et al., 1986). Orthodontic decompensation is performed keeping in mind that movement of teeth will be considerably slower than in normal patients. This should be explained to the patient and family before initiating the treatment itself. Sometimes, it is necessary to perform gingivectomy before bonding, as the clinical crowns are small and the gingiva is thick and fibrous. At other times, unerupted teeth might need to be exposed with this procedure. During the course of treatment, the gingivectomy may need to be repeated due to gingival hyperplasia as a result of poor oral hygiene.

Due to pressure from the tongue, the buccal and incisor segments will be at different occlusal levels (Figure 8.27). The alignment procedure in these situations is often initiated with sectional arch orthodontics and gradually progressed to full archwires (Figure 8.28). Occasionally, in extreme cases, orthodontic treatment might have to be finished with sectional mechanics itself. In the maxillary arch, exposure of unerupted teeth with their gradual alignment into the dental arch is a major step. With multiple missing

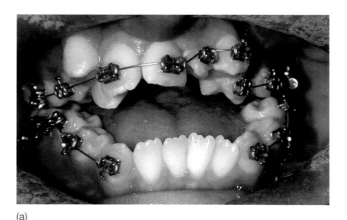

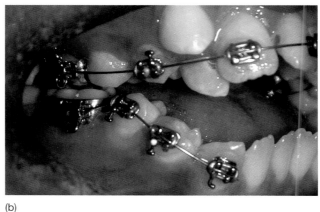

(a)   (b)

Figure 8.28 (a,b) Sectional arch mechanics in an Apert syndrome patient for aligning the different occlusal levels.

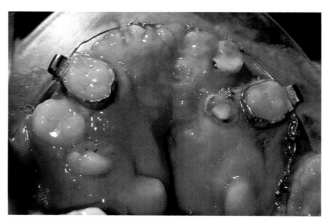

Figure 8.29 Implants in the retromolar area being used as source of anchorage to distalize the left maxillary molar in a patient with Apert syndrome. Note the elastomeric chain placed from the distal of the first molar to the implant.

teeth, more favorable anchorage may be obtained by using implants (Figure 8.29). As in normal decompensation, if there is severe crowding, extractions will be necessary. Correction of midline shifts should be kept in mind while extracting teeth in these patients, making asymmetrical extraction patterns a good option (Figure 8.30). In the mature adolescent child with severe crowding, surgically assisted palatal expansion is a better alternative (Figure 8.31). Once the teeth are aligned, an osteotomy is performed to correct the Class III appearance as well as the decompensated occlusion.

Postsurgical orthodontics

Postsurgical orthodontics is aimed mainly at preventing relapse and coordinating the arches. The archwires might need to be changed from rectangular stabilizing wires to working archwires to achieve good arch coordination and occlusion. Elastics are used in different directions for occlusal settling and to prevent relapse. In Apert and Crouzon patients use of a reverse-pull headgear may help prevent relapse of the Class III skeletal pattern. Box elastics are also used to close open bites and in patients with a tendency towards anterior open bite. For patients with persistent tongue thrusting, habit correction should be considered important (Santiago and Grayson, 2009). Depending on the severity of the initial deformity, the time of postsurgical orthodontics may vary, and the treatment is stopped once the occlusion is stable. Just as in conventional treatment, retention is an important part of treatment of hemifacial microsomia and craniofacial dysostosis and because of the potential for relapse, lifelong retention is recommended.

Achondroplasia/FGFR3 mutations

Achondroplasia, the most common cause of short-limbed dwarfism in humans, has an estimated birth prevalence of 1 in 26000–28000 live births (Orioli et al., 1995). Fibroblast growth factor receptor-3 (FGFR3) genes, which regulate endochondral bone growth, undergo mutations, affecting the cartilaginous development of both the long and flat bones. These individuals have disproportionately short limbs, with an average adult height of 131 cm (4 feet 3.5 inches) for males and 123 cm (4 feet 0.5 inch) for females. In addition, they have macrocephaly, depressed nasal bridge, frontal bossing, and trident-shaped hands. There are significant deficiencies in cranial base and midface development. Since mandibular growth is unaffected, most present with a significant skeletal Class III malocclusion.

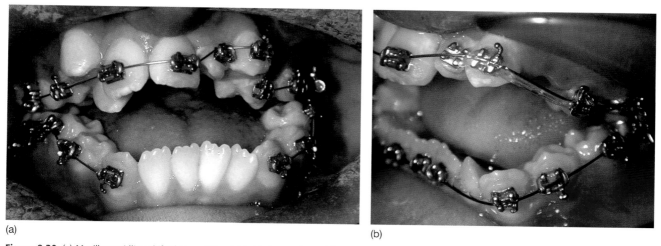

Figure 8.30 (a) Maxillary midline shifted toward the right side in a patient with Apert syndrome. The patient is in the alignment and leveling stage. Note the sectional mechanics being used in the lower arch to level the different occlusal planes anteriorly and posteriorly. (b) Asymmetrical extraction pattern (maxillary first premolar only on left side) to correct the midline.

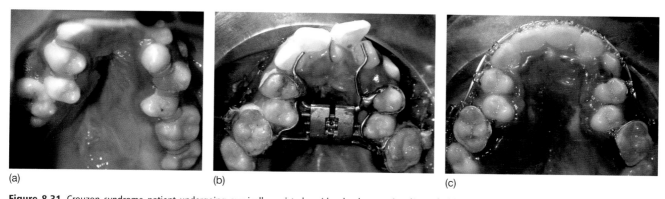

Figure 8.31 Crouzon syndrome patient undergoing surgically assisted rapid palatal expansion (SARPE). (a) Note the severely constricted and high-vaulted palate and the placement of the elastic separators to help in the placement of the bands soldered to a rapid maxillary expansion screw (Hyrax). (b) Hyrax appliance in place. (c) Expansion obtained after SARPE with the Hyrax appliance. An overexpanded rectangular archwire is in place to help maintain the expansion achieved. Note that the maxillary second premolars need to be aligned and there is lack of space to accommodate the right maxillary canine, even after SARPE.

Hertel et al. (2005) showed that 4 years of treatment with growth hormone in children with achondroplasia resulted in an improvement in height without any adverse effect on trunk–leg disproportion. Individuals with these conditions may be considered for routine orthognathic surgery or distraction osteogenesis depending on the extent of their skeletal discrepancy.

Holoprosencephalic disorders

Holoprosencephaly (HPE) is the most common congenital malformation of the human forebrain, with a prevalence of 1 in 250 conceptions and 1 in 10 000–20 000 live births (Roessler and Muenke, 2010). HPE results from incomplete division of the forebrain early in gestation, and is exquisitely sensitive to both genetic and environmental insults during the initial critical period. HPE is traditionally categorized by the degree of anatomical malformations from most severe to least severe. Facial features in patients with HPE range from the most severe form with cyclopia, proboscis, and cleft lip and palate, to less severe microforms, including a single maxillary central incisor, microcephaly, and hypotelorism, but with structurally normal brains on conventional neuroimaging (Muenke and Beachy, 2000).

Severe neurological impairment is found in virtually all patients with brain malformations (Muenke and Beachy, 2000).

A child with a single central incisor should be investigated fully as there is a significant chance that their children will have this genetic defect, and which may have a more severe phenotypic expression. For a detailed description of the single primary and permanent maxillary central incisor condition, see Chapter 7.

Fetal alcohol syndrome

Fetal alcohol syndrome (FAS) is the most common cause of holoprosencephaly and affects 1 in every 500 live births. It is a pattern of mental and physical defects that can develop in a fetus when the mother consumes alcohol during pregnancy. Alcohol crosses the placental barrier and can cause stunting of fetal growth or weight and distinctive facial stigmata, damage the neurons and brain structures and can result in psychological or behavioral problems along with other physical problems. Ethanol is known to impair the development of the frontonasal process in animal models, with significant variations in morphology (Sulik et al., 1981). Several craniofacial abnormalities are often seen in individuals with FAS. The three characteristic FAS facial features are smooth philtrum, thin vermilion, and small palpebral fissures. Major problems such as structural abnormalities of the brain, associated neurological impairments, cardiac, skeletal, renal and ocular problems, and cleft lip with or without a cleft palate occur occasionally.

There is no treatment for FAS, because the central nervous system (CNS) damage creates a permanent disability. Medical and behavioral interventions have been attempted with little success. The esthetic problems associated with facial developmental deviations have been addressed with distraction osteogenesis and routine orthognathic surgery with orthodontic intervention.

Conclusion

Patients with craniofacial anomalies present with multiple skeletal and soft-tissue deformities and medical conditions, and an interdisciplinary team approach is the standard of care in most developed nations. Craniofacial units have been established to centralize care and create a critical mass of resources necessary for efficient coordinated therapy. This interactive effort requires timely and careful consideration towards intervention, supported by specific evidence-based protocols, to ensure that the affected individual receives the best of care possible. The orthodontist plays a unique role in this team, with their expertise in assessing, monitoring, and influencing growth and development of the craniofacial structures. They are active participants in data collection, clinical examination, diagnosis and treatment planning, and have the opportunity to make a significant contribution, at specific times, to the management of the child with a craniofacial anomaly.

References

Bachmayer DI, Ross RB, Munro IR (1986) Maxillary growth following Le Fort III advancement surgery in Crouzon, Apert, and Pfeiffer syndromes. *American Journal of Orthodontics and Dentofacial Orthopedics* 90: 420–30.

Barden RC, Ford ME, Jensen AG, et al. (1989) Effects of craniofacial deformity in infancy on the quality of mother-infant interactions. *Child Development* 60: 819–24.

Bartlett SP (2007) Craniosynostosis syndromes. In: CH Thorne (ed.) *Grabb and Smith's Plastic Surgery*, 6th edn. Philadelphia, PA: Lippincott Williams & Wilkins, pp. 237–47.

Bergstrom L, Baker BB (1981) Syndromes associated with congenital facial paralysis. *Otolaryngology Head and Neck Surgery* 89: 336–42.

Boston M, Rutter MJ (2003) Current airway management in craniofacial anomalies. *Current Opinion in Otolaryngology and Head and Neck Surgery* 11: 428–32.

Brent B (1992) Auricular repair with autogenous rib cartilage grafts: two decades of experience with 600 cases. *Plastic and Reconstructive Surgery* 90: 355–74.

Cascone P, Gennaro P, Spuntarelli G, et al. (2005) Mandibular distraction: evolution of treatment protocols in hemifacial microsomy. *Journal of Craniofacial Surgery* 16: 563–71.

Cohen MM Jr (ed.) (1986) *Craniosynostosis: Diagnosis, Evaluation, and Management*. New York, NY: Raven Press.

Cohen SR, Burstein FD, Stewart MB, et al. (1997) Maxillary-midface distraction in children with cleft lip and palate: a preliminary report. *Plastic and Reconstructive Surgery* 99: 1421–8.

Converse JM, Telsey D (1971) The tripartite osteotomy of the mid-face for orbital expansion and correction of the deformity in craniostenosis. *British Journal of Plastic Surgery* 24: 365–74.

Converse JM, Coccaro PJ, Becker M (1973) On hemifacial microsomia – the first and second branchial arch syndrome. *Plastic and Reconstructive Surgery* 51: 268–79.

Converse JM, McCarthy JG, Coccaro PJ, et al. (1979) Clinical aspects of craniofacial microsomia. In: JM Converse, JG McCarthy, D Wood-Smith (eds) *Symposium on Diagnosis and Treatment of Craniofacial Anomalies*. St Louis, MO: Mosby, pp. 461–2.

David JD, Mahatumarat C, Cooter RD (1987) Hemifacial microsomia: A multi system classification. *Plastic and Reconstructive Surgery* 80: 525–33.

Dufresne C (1992) Treacher Collins syndrome. In: C Dufresne (ed.) *Complex Craniofacial Problems: A Guide to Analysis and Treatment*. New York, NY: Churchill Livingstone.

Fomin ABF, Pastorino AC, Kim CA, et al. (2010) Di George syndrome: a not so rare disease. *Clinics* 65: 865–9.

Franceschetti A, Klein D (1949) The mandibulofacial dysostosis. A new hereditary syndrome. *Acta Ophthalmologica* 27: 143–224.

Fuento del Campo A, Elizondo MM, Arnaud E (1994) Treacher Collins syndrome (mandibulofacial dysostosis). *Clinics of Plastic Surgery* 21: 613–23.

Goodship J, Cross L, LiIing J, et al. (1998) A population study of chromosome 21q11 deletions in infancy. *Archives of Diseases in Childhood* 79: 348–51.

Gorlin RJ, Cohen MM, Levin LS (1990) *Syndromes of the Head and Neck*, 3rd edn. Oxford: Oxford University Press.

Gothelf D, Michaelovsky E, Frish A, et al. (2007) Association of the low activity COMT 158Met allele with ADHD and OCD in subjects with velocardiofacial syndrome. *International Journal of Neuropsychopharmacology* 10: 301–8.

Gougoutas AJ, Singh DJ, Low DW, et al. (2007) Hemifacial microsomia: clinical features and pictographic representations of the OMENS classification system. *Plastic and Reconstructive Surgery* 120: 112e–13e.

Hanson P, Melugin MB (1999) Orthodontic management of the patient undergoing mandibular distraction osteogenesis. *Seminars in Orthodontics* 5: 25–34.

Hertel NT, Eklof O, Ivarsson S, et al. (2005) Growth hormone treatment in 35 prepubertal children with achondroplasia: A five-year dose-response trial. *Acta Paediatrica* 94: 1402–10.

Hoeve LJ, Pijpers M, Joosten KF (2003) OSAS in craniofacial syndromes: an unsolved problem. *International Journal of Pediatric Otorhinolaryngology* 67: S111–13.

Iseri H, Kisnisci R, Altug-Atac AT (2008) Ten-year follow-up of a patient with hemifacial microsomia treated with distraction osteogenesis and orthodontics: An implant analysis. *American Journal of Orthodontics and Dentofacial Orthopedics* 134: 296–304.

Johnston MC, Bronsky PT (1995) Prenatal craniofacial development: new insights on normal and abnormal mechanisms. *Critical Reviews in Oral Biology and Medicine* 6: 368–422.

Kaban JC, Mulliken JB, Murray JE (1981) Three-dimensional approach to analysis and treatment of hemifacial microsomia. *Cleft Palate Journal* 18: 90–9.

Kaban LB, Moses MH, Mulliken JB (1988) Surgical correction of hemifacial microsomia in the growing child. *Plastic and Reconstructive Surgery* 82: 9–19.

Kapp K (1979) Self concept of the cleft lip and or palate child. *Cleft Palate Journal* 16: 171–6.

Kapp-Simon KA (1995) Psychological interventions for the adolescent with cleft lip and palate. *Cleft Palate Craniofacial Journal* 32: 104–8.

Kearns GJ, Padwa BL, Mulliken JB, et al. (2000) Progression of facial asymmetry in hemifacial microsomia. *Plastic and Reconstructive Surgery* 105: 492–8.

Khan SH, Nischal KK, Dean F, et al. (2003) Visual outcomes and amblyogenic risk factors in craniosynostotic syndromes: a review of 141 cases. *British Journal of Ophthalmology* 87: 999–1003.

Kobayashi S, Honda T, Saitoh A, et al. (1999) Unilateral coronal synostosis treated by internal forehead distraction. *Journal of Craniofacial Surgery* 10: 467–72.

Kobrynski LJ, Sullivan KE (2007) Velocardiofacial syndrome, DiGeorge syndrome: the chromosome 22q11.2.2 deletion syndrome. *Lancet* 370: 1443–52.

Kreiborg S, Cohen MM Jr (1992) The oral manifestations of Apert syndrome. *Journal of Craniofacial Genetics and Developmental Biology* 12: 41–8.

Longaker MT, Siebert JW (1995) Microvascular free flap correction of hemifacial atrophy. *Plastic and Reconstructive Surgery* 96: 800–9.

McCarthy JG (1997) Craniofacial microsomia: A primary and secondary surgical treatment plan. *Clinics in Plastic Surgery* 24: 459–74.

McCarthy JG (2007) Craniofacial microsomia. In: CH Thorne (ed.) *Grabb and Smith's Plastic Surgery*, 6th edn. Philadelphia, PA: Lippincott Williams & Wilkins, pp. 248–55.

McCarthy JG (2009) Development of craniofacial orthodontics as a subspecialty at New York University Medical Center. *Seminars in Orthodontics* 15: 221–4.

McCarthy JG, LaTrenta GS, Breitbart AS, et al. (1990) The Le Fort III advancement osteotomy in the child under 7 years of age. *Plastic and Reconstructive Surgery* 86: 633–46.

McCarthy JG, Schreiber JS, Karp NS, et al. (1992) Lengthening of the human mandible by gradual distraction. *Plastic and Reconstructive Surgery* 89: 1–10.

Meurman Y (1957) Congenital microtia and meatal atresia. *AMA Archives of Otolaryngology* 66: 443–63.

Muenke M, Beachy PA (2000) Genetics of ventral forebrain development and holoprosencephaly. *Current Opinion in Genetics and Development* 10: 262–9.

Munro IR, Lauritzen CG (1985) Classification and treatment of hemifacial microsomia. In: EP Caronni (ed.) *Craniofacial Surgery*. Boston, MA: Little, Brown, pp. 391–400.

Nagy K, Kuijpers-Jagtman AM, Mommaerts MY (2009) No evidence for long-term effectiveness of early osteodistraction in hemifacial microsomia. *Plastic and Reconstructive Surgery* 124: 2061–71.

Nout E, Cesteleyn LLM, van der Wal KGH, et al. (2008) Advancement of the midface, from conventional Le Fort III osteotomy to Le Fort III distraction: review of the literature. *International Journal of Oral and Maxillofacial Surgery* 37: 781–9.

Nurko C, Ouinonese R (2004) Dental and orthodontic management of patients with Apert and Crouzon syndromes. *Oral Maxillofacial Surgical Clinics of North America* 16: 541–53.

Opitz C, Ring P, Stoll C (2004) Orthodontic and surgical treatment of patients with congenital unilateral and bilateral mandibulofacial dysostosis. *Journal of Orofacial Orthopedics* 65: 150–63.

Orioli IM, Castilla EE, Scarano G, et al. (1995) Effect of paternal age in achondroplasia, thanatophoric dysplasia, and osteogenesis imperfecta. *American Journal of Medical Genetics* 59: 209–17.

Ortiz-Monasterio F, Molina K, Andrade L, et al. (1997) Simultaneous mandibular and maxillary distraction in hemifacial microsomia in adults: avoiding occlusal disasters. *Plastic and Reconstructive Surgery* 100: 852–61.

Ortiz-Monasterio F, del Campo AF, Carillo A (1978) Advancements of the orbits and the mid-face in one piece, combined with frontal repositioning for the correction of Crouzon's deformities. *Plastic and Reconstructive Surgery* 61: 507–16.

Peterson-Falzone SJ, Pruzansky S, Parris PJ, et al. (1981) Nasopharyngeal dysmorphology in the syndromes of Apert and Crouzon. *Cleft Palate Journal* 18: 237–50.

Pijpers M, Poels PJ, Vaandrager JM, et al. (2004) Undiagnosed obstructive sleep apnea syndrome in children with syndromal craniofacial synostosis. *Journal of Craniofacial Surgery* 15: 670–4.

Polley JW, Figueroa AA (1997) Management of severe maxillary deficiency in childhood and adolescence through distraction osteogenesis with an external adjustable, rigid distraction device. *Journal of Craniofacial Surgery* 8: 181–5.

Polley JW, Figueroa AA, Charbel FT, et al. (1995) Monobloc craniomaxillofacial distraction osteogenesis in a newborn with severe craniofacial synostosis: a preliminary report. *Journal of Craniofacial Surgery* 6: 421–3.

Polley JW, Figueroa AA, Liou EJ, et al. (1997) Longitudinal analysis of mandibular asymmetry in hemifacial microsomia. *Plastic and Reconstructive Surgery* 99: 328–39.

Posnick JC (2000) *Craniofacial and Maxillofacial Surgery in Children and Young Adults*, 1st edn. Philadelphia, PA: WB Saunders, pp. 419–45.

Poswillo D (1975) Hemorrhage in development of the face. *Birth Defects Original Article Series* 11: 61–81.

Pruzansky S (1974) Palatal anomalies in the syndromes of Apert and Crouzon. *Cleft Palate Journal* 11: 394–403.

Roessler E, Muenke M (2010) The molecular genetics of holoprosencephaly. *American Journal of Medical Genetics Part C Seminars in Medical Genetics* 154: 52–61.

Ross RB (1975) Lateral facial dysplasia (first and second brachial arch syndrome, hemifacial microsomia). *Birth Defects* 11: 51–9.

Santiago PE, Grayson BH (2009) Role of the craniofacial orthodontist on the craniofacial and cleft lip and palate team. *Seminars in Orthodontics* 15: 225–43.

Sheyte PR, Grayson BH, Mackool RJ, et al. (2006) Long-term stability and growth following unilateral mandibular distraction in growing children with craniofacial microsomia. *Plastic and Reconstructive Surgery* 118: 985–95.

Silvestri A, Natali G, Iannetti G (1996) Functional therapy in hemifacial microsomia: therapeutic protocol for growing children. *Journal of Oral and Maxillofacial Surgery* 54: 271–8.

Solomon LM, Medenica M, Pruzansky S, et al. (1973) Apert syndrome and palatal mucopolysaccharides. *Teratology* 8: 287–91.

Soltan HC, Holmes LB (1986) Familial occurrence of malformations possibly attributable to vascular abnormalities. *Journal of Pediatrics* 108: 112–14.

Sugawara Y, Hirabayashi S, Sakurai A, et al. (1998) Gradual cranial vault expansion for the treatment of craniofacial synostosis. A preliminary report. *Annals of Plastic Surgery* 40: 554–65.

Sulik KK, Johnston MC, Webb MA (1981) Fetal alcohol syndrome: embryogenesis in a mouse model. *Science* 214: 936–8.

Tay T, Martin F, Rowe N, et al. (2006) Prevalence and causes of visual impairment in craniosynostotic syndromes. *Clinical and Experimental Ophthalmology* 34: 434–40.

Tessier P (1971a) Vertical and oblique facial clefts (orbitofacial fissures). In: IC Mustarde (ed.) *Plastic Surgery in Infancy and Childhood*. Philadelphia, PA: WB Saunders.

Tessier P (1971b) The definitive surgical treatment of the severe facial deformities of craniofacial dysostosis. Crouzon's and Apert's diseases. *Plastic and Reconstructive Surgery* 48: 419–42.

Trainor PA, Dixon J, Dixon MJ (2009) Treacher Collins syndrome: etiology, pathogenesis and prevention. *European Journal of Human Genetics* 17: 275–83.

Tulane IF, Tessier PL (1986) Results of the Tessier integral procedure for correction of Treacher Collins syndrome. *Cleft Palate Journal* 23: 40–9.

Van Vierzen PB, Joosten FBM, Marres HAM, et al. (1995) Mandibulofacial dysostosis: CT findings of the temporal bones. *European Journal of Radiology* 21: 53–7.

Vento AR, LaBrie RA, Mulliken JB (1991). The OMENS classification of hemifacial microsomia. *Cleft Palate Craniofacial Journal* 28: 68–76.

Wang RR, Andres CJ (1999) Hemifacial microsomia and treatment options for auricular replacement: A review of the literature. *Journal of Prosthetic Dentistry* 82: 197–204.

Whitaker LA, Bartlett SP (1990) Craniofacial anomalies. In: MJ Jurkiewicz, TJ Krizek, SJ Mathes, et al. (eds) *Plastic Surgery Principles and Practice*, vol 1, 1st edn. St Louis, MO: Mosby, pp. 99–136.

9

Cleft Lip and Palate: Role of the Orthodontist in the Interdisciplinary Management Team

Anne Marie Kuijpers-Jagtman

Summary

The treatment of patients with cleft lip and palate (CLP) is a challenge. The principal role of the interdisciplinary CLP team is to provide integrated care for children with clefts, and to assure quality and continuity of patient care and longitudinal follow-up. The orthodontist has proven to be an essential partner in the cleft palate team, not only responsible for the orthodontic and facial orthopedic treatment, but more importantly, he or she is also the guardian of the child's maxillofacial growth. By nature, orthodontists have a long-term treatment perspective in mind, which will assist the team in its consideration of treatment techniques, sequence, and timing, in relation to the effect on maxillofacial growth. Moreover, standardized records collected by the orthodontist provide a valuable basis for retrospective studies on treatment outcome and inter-center comparisons. Finally, in recent times orthodontists seem to be quite often the motor behind large-scale inter-center randomized clinical trials in the field of CLP.

Introduction

Cleft lip with or without cleft palate (CL ± P), and isolated cleft palate (CP) are serious birth defects that affect approximately 1 in every 600 newborn babies worldwide. Assuming that 15 000 children are born per hour worldwide, it means that approximately every 2.5 minutes a child is born with a cleft somewhere in the world (World Health Organization, 2002).

It has been recognized for a long time that prevalence varies for the type of cleft, gender, population, and geographical location. Recently, the International Perinatal Database of Typical Orofacial Clefts (IPDTOC), which was established in 2003, published the first results of a global study on the prevalence of cleft lip with and without cleft palate. The data covered at least one complete year during the period 2000–2005 from 54 registries in 30 countries all over the world. Data on a total of 7704 cases of CL ± P, including live births, stillbirths, terminations of pregnancy, and unknown pregnancy outcome, were available, resulting from a total of more than 7.5 million births. The overall estimate of the prevalence of CL ± P turned out to be 9.92 per 10 000 (95% confidence interval [CI] 9.70 to 10.14); that of cleft lip was 3.28 per 10 000 (95% CI 3.15 to 3.41), and that of cleft lip and palate [CLP] 6.64 per 10,000 (95% CI 6.46 to 6.82). Just over three quarters of the cases were isolated, 16% multi-malformed and 7% occurred as part of recognized syndromes (IPDTOC Working Group, 2011).

The healthcare burden of children with clefts and their families is high. Presently, the treatment history often starts with prenatal counseling of the expecting parents as soon as a CLP deformity of the fetus has been detected by ultrasound. Treatment continues from birth until maturity involving, among other actions, feeding counseling and clinical nursing, several surgeries to close the defect, genetic screening, speech and hearing assessments and management of middle ear infections, orthodontic and facial orthopedic management, speech interventions, psychological counseling, and dental and prosthodontic care.

There has been consensus since the early 1950s that children with clefts need comprehensive, coordinated care by an interdisciplinary team. The team should function as an organization with a general policy for the treatment, and each member of the team should have an understanding of the different aspects of treatment. The team provides multidisciplinary treatment and usually includes specialists from the following disciplines: pediatrics and obstetrics, plastic and reconstructive surgery, orthodontics, genetics, social work and/or nursing, ear nose and throat (ENT), speech/language pathology, maxillofacial surgery, (prosthetic) dentistry, and psychology. Consultation with other medical and dental professionals should also be available, if needed.

The aim of the interdisciplinary treatment approach is to create the conditions that allow the affected child to grow up with an esthetically pleasing face, good hearing and speech, properly functioning and esthetically acceptable dentition and, last but not least, harmonious social-psychological development (Kuijpers-Jagtman, 2006).

Interdisciplinary team care

The principal role of the interdisciplinary CLP team is to provide integrated care for children with clefts, and to assure quality and continuity of patient care and longitudinal follow-up. Why do we need interdisciplinary teams instead of multidisciplinary teams? The distinction does seem to be quite arbitrary, but it is not so.

In multidisciplinary teams, specialists work together in a more or less loose connection, treating the various problems of the patient, but not within the framework of a mutually agreed treatment plan. Comparing interdisciplinary and multidisciplinary teams, Day (1981) states: 'A multidisciplinary approach can occur as a series of isolated evaluations by several disciplines and does not imply the merger of evaluative insights or the shared development of a treatment plan, which are the hallmarks of an interdisciplinary team'. An interdisciplinary team, on the other hand, is one in which professionals from different disciplines are involved in conducting a joint evaluation and developing a treatment plan in which expertise is pooled and decision making is collective (Day, 1981; Strauss, 1999). It seems quite obvious that we should aim for the latter team format when treating children with clefts. Joint team consultations, where the patients are examined and discussed by all team members at the same time, are the backbone of well-functioning teams. The patient and the family are the leading figures in the team deliberations. These sessions might be confusing or even overwhelming for the patient and the family. This situation can be prevented by structuring the consultations according to a strict protocol that the patient and the family after a while recognize as a routine, and by having the clinical nurse or social worker, around all the time, to reassure the family. The team coordinator or one of the other designated team specialists then serves at the end to summarize the session for the patient and the family, and to meet any other needs they might have.

The team coordinator and the team leader do not have to be the same person. The role of the team coordinator is to facilitate and coordinate the treatment plan, and to com-

municate it with the patient and the family (Strauss, 1999). The team leader is in charge of the coordination of the activities of the team and the clinic; he or she monitors the functioning and decision-making process of the interdisciplinary team, and represents the team in contacts with the hospital management, health authorities, insurance companies, and patient support organizations. The medical or dental discipline of the team leader is less important than the ability to show leadership in getting the group to function as a team, and resolving slumbering conflicts between disciplines about boundaries and responsibilities.

Members of the cleft lip and palate team and their task

Each patient seen by the team requires comprehensive, interactive treatment planning to achieve maximum habilitation, with efficient use of parent and patient time and resources. The American Cleft Palate Craniofacial Association has described the roles of the team members in a position paper on 'Parameters for Evaluation and Treatment of Patients with Cleft Lip/Palate or Other Craniofacial Anomalies' in 1993, which was revised in 2000 (ACPA 1993, 2000). Below, the role of the team members is described according to the chronology in which they get involved in the treatment of a child with a cleft (Figure 9.1). Not all CLP teams have the same composition. National agreements on which discipline performs which operation, local spearheads, and scientific interests may influence the composition of the team.

Obstetrics

The first report on prenatal detection of a CLP deformity in two fetuses by transabdominal ultrasound was published

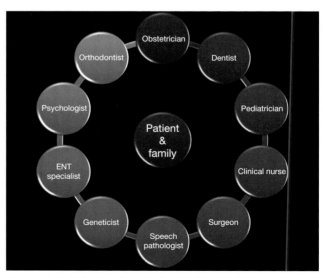

Figure 9.1 Patient-centered care by the cleft lip and palate team.

by Christ and Meininger (1981). Currently, almost all pregnant women receive routine ultrasound screening during their pregnancy. This examination usually involves two-dimensional (2D) ultrasound, and is performed in a primary care setting. The problem is that transabdominal 2D ultrasound screening for orofacial clefts in a low-risk population has relatively low detection rates, ranging from 9% to 100% for cleft lip with or without cleft palate, 0% to 22% for cleft palate only, and 0% to 73% for all types of clefts (Maarse et al., 2010). The favorable result of this finding is that it is associated with few false-positive diagnoses. If there is suspicion of a fetal anomaly, the woman should be referred for more advanced three-dimensional (3D) ultrasound imaging, which has, in high-risk women, much higher detection rates of 100% for cleft lip, and 86% to 90% for CLP. However, cleft palate only is hardly detected on 2D ultrasound, and 3D ultrasound is also unable to arrive at a reliable diagnosis for cleft palate only, as detection rates vary widely from 0% to 89% (Maarse et al., 2010).

Today, in our center, more than 60% of the expecting parents have received a prenatal diagnosis of their child, and have been counseled accordingly. Detection of the facial cleft *in utero* by ultrasound has resulted in an established routine between the referring obstetrician and the CLP team for informing the parents of the deformity and the sequential steps necessary for its correction. Because of the relatively low detection rates at present, parents need to be aware that a negative ultrasound result does not necessarily mean that their unborn child is without an orofacial cleft (Maarse et al., 2010).

Pediatrics

The pediatrician is an essential part of the CLP team, providing initial diagnosis and referral, close monitoring of the day-to-day medical issues including immunizations, management of growth (particularly for infants who have difficulty with feeding and weight gain), treatment of acute ear infections, assessment of development, and family support (Kasten et al., 2008). More importantly, CL ± P may occur in association with other congenital malformations. In a Swedish study, 21% of the infants with clefts had associated malformations that required follow-up treatment. The prevalence of congenital heart disease was 16 times that of the general population (Milerad et al., 1997). A more extensive cleft seems to be associated with a higher risk for associated malformations but, surprisingly, the prevalence of associated anomalies was the highest for female patients with a cleft palate only, increasing to 50%.

Clinical nursing and/or social work

The clinical nurse or social worker is the vital link between the CLP team and the parents and child. He or she guides them through the treatment process from birth until maturity, or sometimes even earlier if she has a role in the prenatal counseling. Because many children have difficulties

nursing from a breast or bottle, the clinical nurse is there to assist the parents directly after birth regarding feeding issues. They provide psychological support for the parents to deal with acceptance of their child with a deformity. He or she assumes the role of 'case manager', organizing and coordinating services throughout the clinical pathway followed by the patient, serving as a walking encyclopedia for questions of the family and the patient. In our experience, the availability of advice and counseling by phone is very helpful, but sometimes home visits are necessary.

The clinical nurse or social worker will organize, if needed, the contacts with social and vocational rehabilitation services, insurance companies, school teachers, and governmental support systems, and provide assistance with family finances. He or she arranges for enrollment in special education programs, in case of learning or behavioral disorders, when necessary (Wellens and Vander Poorten, 2006).

Surgery

Children with a complete unilateral or bilateral cleft, undergo at least three surgical interventions: cleft lip repair, hard and soft palate repair, and alveolar bone grafting. Additional secondary surgery may be needed for velopharyngeal incompetence, skeletal discrepancies, lip revision, and nose correction. It depends on the country and from which discipline the surgeon, who is performing these operations originates. Experience and skills of the surgeon seem to be a major issue in achieving a good treatment outcome. Results from the EUROCLEFT study suggest that decentralized care and low-volume surgeons are associated with low-quality treatment results (Shaw et al., 1992a,b). A study in England and Wales showed that low-volume operators (fewer than 10 cases a year) were less likely to attend joint disciplinary clinics than high-volume operators. None of the low-volume operators collected standardized records for their patients (Williams et al., 1996). This finding emphasizes the great importance of centralized care for children with clefts.

Orthodontics

The orthodontist has an active role in the interdisciplinary care of children with clefts, from birth until they become adults. Longitudinal evaluation, including standardized follow-up documentation, and record taking to provide a general overview of treatment outcomes, is in the hands of the orthodontist. Five distinct stages of orthodontic mechanotherapy can be distinguished. A detailed description of these stages follows below.

Genetics

Genetics is becoming increasingly important in the search for the etiology of orofacial clefts and, therefore, the role of the clinical geneticist in the CLP team increases, as well. All parents expecting a child who has been diagnosed prenatally as having a cleft with associated anomalies should be counseled antenatally by the clinical geneticist. About 3–6 months after birth, all children with clefts are examined by the clinical geneticist. This timing is important, as not all associated congenital malformations may manifest at birth. Parents are also counseled about the risk of having another child with a cleft. Over the years we have learned that adults with CLP who were treated by the team return with questions about their own risk of having a child with a cleft.

ENT

The ENT specialist is responsible for the audiological and otologic management of the children with clefts. The association of the presence of a cleft palate with middle ear effusion is widely recognized (Hubbard et al., 1985; Sheahan et al., 2003). Cleft palate may lead to disruption of the tensor veli palatini muscle, which plays a role in the function of the eustachian tube. Dysfunction of the eustachian tube increases the risk of serous otitis media and more than 90% of patients with cleft palate have middle ear effusions. Placement of ventilating tubes is frequently utilized. Some children require multiple sets of tubes, and there is increased risk of persistent hearing loss. The ENT specialist is responsible for prescribing hearing aids when necessary. He may also address issues of tonsillar and adenoidal hypertrophy, sinusitis, nasal abnormalities, and nasal obstruction (Kasten et al., 2008).

Speech pathology

A speech pathologist, specialized in cleft palate speech, is indispensable in a CLP team. Children with CLP are at a higher risk for speech disorders, and to a lesser degree for language disorders. The speech disorders in children with clefts concern articulation, phonation, and resonance disorders, primarily hypernasality. The speech pathologist treats communication disorders and contributes the necessary information to the team when surgical interventions are considered to improve speech. Careful planning of orthodontic treatment in relation to speech therapy is also needed, as certain developmental stages of the dentition and some orthodontic appliances interfere with speech therapy. The speech pathologist is heavily involved in the care of children with clefts during the first 9 years of life. After that age, most speech problems have already been solved. In some teams, the speech therapist also serves as a lactation consultant or feeding expert, in others this is the role of the clinical nurse.

Dental care

Routine dental care should be provided by the family dentist, in close contact with the CLP team. As many children with clefts have a suboptimal oral hygiene, an oral/dental hygienist could assist the orthodontist in maintaining good oral hygiene through the years of orthodontic treatment. The prosthodontist is responsible for replacement of missing teeth, and embellishment of abnormally shaped teeth, as an adjunct to the orthodontic and surgical treatment plan. Therefore, the prosthodontist always works in close collaboration with the orthodontist and, eventually, the surgeon.

Psychology

Last, but not least, the psychologist is mentioned as an important team member. For some children, psychosocial support is never needed, while others have numerous psychological and social problems. Living with a facial disfigurement is not easy, as the deformity is always visible. This fact may have a severe impact on the wellbeing of the child. Besides, teasing and social rejection at school and by peers can grow into a severe problem that needs to be addressed professionally. Fostering to psychosocial adjustment, positive self-esteem and healthy interpersonal skills are objectives that should be met by the team treatment (Broder et al., 1994).

Orthodontic management

The orthodontist is actively involved in the life of a child born with a cleft, from birth until maturity. Shortly after birth, the child with a cleft is seen by the CLP team, more in particular by the pediatrician, clinical geneticist, plastic surgeon, and orthodontist and, if available, also by the social worker or clinical nurse of the team. From then on, each patient is treated according to the overall comprehensive treatment plan that has been established by the team. The orthodontic procedures focus on monitoring craniofacial growth and development, and on correcting jaw relationships and dental occlusion, in order to achieve optimal function and appearance (ACPA, 1993; Kuijpers-Jagtman, 2006; Santiago and Grayson, 2009). The orthodontic and dentofacial orthopedic treatment of a child with a complete unilateral or bilateral cleft takes many years, and the challenge for the orthodontist is to avoid continuous active orthodontic intervention from birth to the age of permanent dentition. Children become bored of endless treatment, and may develop serious compliance problems. Therefore, it is wise to distinguish five well-defined treatment courses, and try to keep some 'orthodontics-free' time in between. The five-stage treatment includes:

1. Infant orthopedics
2. Early mixed dentition treatment and facial orthopedics
3. Orthodontic treatment in relation to alveolar bone grafting
4. Adolescent orthodontic treatment
5. Combined orthodontic-surgical treatment in early adulthood.

From birth to 7 years of age

At the first visit to the team, a clinical examination is performed, and an initial treatment plan made, aiming at reconstructive surgery of the lip and/or the palate, while infant orthopedics can precede the surgical closure of the lip. Other medical conditions of the child and psychological or social problems of the parents are also integrated in the initial treatment plan.

Baseline documentation is then created, consisting of frontal, right, and left lateral facial views, a close-up of the lips and a worm's eye view (a view of the patient's face from below). It is quite difficult to make standardized pictures of young toddlers. It is easier to photograph them lying down, at least until the age of 6 months, when they begin to sit up by themselves. A palatal intraoral view could be obtained in the operating room. The Institute of Medical Illustrators of the UK has developed an excellent illustrated guideline for photography of patients with clefts, which can be downloaded from its website (lMI, 2004). 3D stereophotogrammetry images are difficult to obtain before the age of 3 months, as head balance has not developed yet before that time, and the parents need to hold the child's head, which may disturb the facial soft tissues. A baseline maxillary dental cast of the unoperated cleft condition has been proven to be very helpful for later ascertainment of the exact diagnosis for research purposes. Due to the risk of respiratory obstructions resulting in cyanotic events or worse, maxillary impressions should only be taken by an orthodontist who is experienced in impression taking in cleft-affected babies. The maxillary impression could be made just prior to the lip repair in the operating room (Figure 9.2a,b). Digitization of the plaster casts will facilitate storage.

In most centers, the first surgical intervention for a child with CL ± P is surgical repair of the lip, followed a couple of months later by palatal repair. To date this is a highly controversial issue and no consensus exists among centers. After the infantile period, the CLP team follows the child on an annual basis. Speech and hearing are the main issues during this period.

Infant orthopedics

Whether infant orthopedics will be part of the treatment plan prior to surgical repair of the lip depends on the treatment protocol of the team. Ever since its introduction by McNeil (1950), it has been a controversial issue. In Europe, about 54% of the operational centers use infant orthopedics (Shaw et al., 2000), while in the USA this approach has always been less popular.

Basically, infant orthopedics aims at molding the alveolar segments into the correct anatomical position, to facilitate lip repair by an intraoral acrylic appliance. Later on, the orthodontic discipline tried to justify early intervention for other reasons. Prahl et al. (2001) summarized the arguments of the proponents of the use of infant orthopedics, who state that this approach allows a more normalized pattern of deglutition while preventing twisting and dorsal position of the tongue in the cleft, improves arch form and position of the alar base, facilitates surgery, and improves outcome in general. Other alleged benefits that became *en vogue* are: reduction of posterior cleft width, prevention of initial collapse after surgery, prevention of crossbites, straightening of the nasal septum, facilitation of feeding, reducing the danger of aspiration, improving speech development, nose breathing, reducing the severity and frequency of middle ear conditions, the extent of orthodontic treatment at later ages, and creating a positive psychological effect in the parents (Kuijpers-Jagtman and Prahl-Andersen, 2006). Most of these benefits could not be substantiated by scientific evidence.

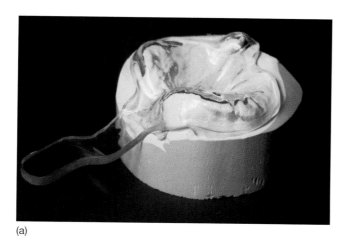

(a)

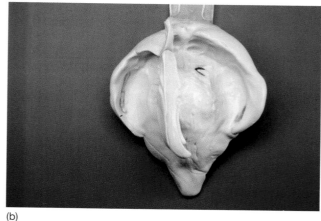

(b)

Figure 9.2 (a) Baby impression tray. (b) Baby impression.

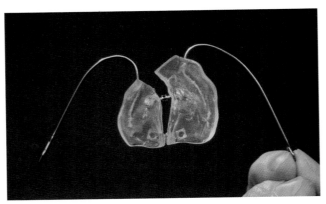

Figure 9.3 Active neonatal appliance with buccal extensions.

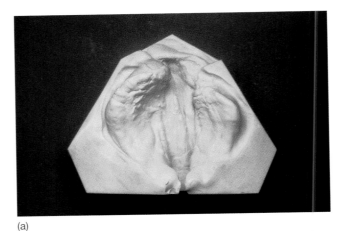

(a)

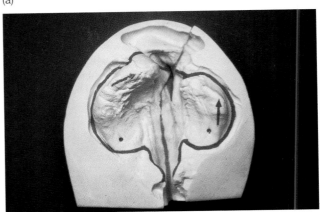

(b)

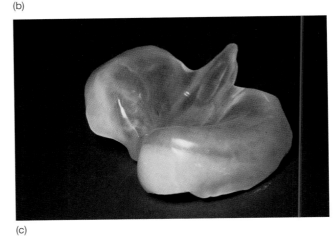

(c)

Figure 9.4 (a) Dental cast – baby. (b) Dental cast – sectioned. (c) Semi-active plate.

A wide range of appliances has been designed for these purposes with pin-retained active appliances at one side of the spectrum (Georgiade et al., 1968; Latham, 1980) and passive appliances at the other side (Hotz and Gnoinski, 1976). Arbitrarily, they fall into three main categories: active, semi-active, and passive appliances (Kuijpers-Jagtman, 2006). *Active* appliances are constructed to apply a force to the maxillary segments, to move them into the desired direction by using an active force delivery system, like springs and screws (Figure 9.3). Additional anchorage can be obtained by pins that are driven into the maxillary bone holding the plate in position. *Semi-active* appliances are constructed by sectioning the dental cast, and reorienting the maxillary segments in a more favorable position. The plate is fabricated on the reconstructed cast, and forces the palatal segments into the predetermined direction when placed in the oral cavity (Figure 9.4). External strapping across the cleft can be part of the treatment protocol. These are the McNeil (1950)-type of appliances. *Passive* appliances that are combined with extraoral strapping also fit into this category. They are supposed to induce arch alignment during growth by grinding away acrylic material in definitive areas of the plate, to ensure a proper spontaneous development of the segments (Figure 9.5). The plate is held in position by suction and adhesion only, and no extraoral strapping is applied. The so-called Zurich approach is the most well-known representative of this kind of neonatal maxillary orthopedic device (Hotz and Gnoinski, 1976).

Many different techniques for infant orthopedics have been described, and therefore it is difficult to compare treatment results. More importantly, treatment for a cleft patient consists of more than infant orthopedics alone. All treatment steps may have an influence on the final treatment outcome, and it is impossible to separate these steps when comparing results in retrospective research (e.g. Ross, 1987; Mølsted et al., 1992). So far only one randomized controlled trial has been performed in this field. From the 6-year results of this three-center trial, named

'DUTCHCLEFT', it can be concluded that infant orthopedics in children with a complete unilateral CLP with a passive appliance as performed in this trial, is not necessary for feeding and nutritional status of the child, parents' satisfaction (Prahl et al., 2005), facial appearance (Bongaarts et al., 2008), facial growth (Bongaarts et al., 2009), or orthodontic reasons (Bongaarts et al., 2004, 2006). Regarding speech, a

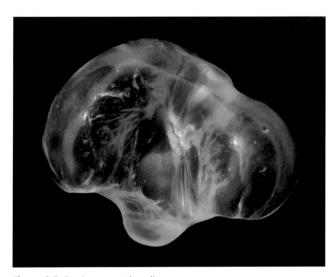

Figure 9.5 Passive neonatal appliance.

positive but very limited effect was found until the age of 2.5 years, but the speech of children with clefts remained far behind that of their non-cleft peers, anyway (Konst et al., 2000, 2003). Relative to the total costs of the treatment of a unilateral CLP patient, the financial investment to reach this effect was rather limited (Konst et al., 2004). However, it is questionable whether this limited effect is important enough to justify infant orthopedics. It should also be taken into consideration that the 6-year results for speech have not been analyzed yet.

For children with bilateral clefts, no evidence-based data from randomized clinical trials are available about the effect of infant orthopedics. Based on experience, it can be stated that with the therapy, good alignment of the maxillary segments can be obtained, which facilitates closure of the lip in one operation. An easier approach is preoperative lip taping only, without an intraoral appliance, which could also assist in reducing a prominent or deviated premaxilla, and is also occasionally applied in wide unilateral clefts. Steri-Strips™ or specially designed commercially available strips can be used for this purpose.

A special type of infant orthopedics that has emerged during the past two decades is nasoalveolar molding. There is a distinct difference between the types of infant orthopedics, as described previously, and the one that has been developed by Grayson and Cutting (Grayson et al., 1993; Cutting et al., 1998; Grayson and Cutting, 2001; Barillas et al., 2009). In the latter method, nasal stents are added to the molding plate. This appliance aims to address correction of the nasal deformity, i.e. to improve nasal tip projection, and septal and lower lateral cartilage position, before cleft repair. In bilateral CLP, the nasal stents can be used to gradually lengthen the deficient columella. The molding plate itself is mainly used to approximate the alveolar

segments, to reduce the nasal deformity to a degree that enables the start of more precise nasal molding with stents (Grayson and Maull, 2006; Santiago and Grayson, 2009). The scientific evidence for nasoalveolar molding needs to be investigated further. The authors rightly state in their 2009 paper that: 'Although these benefits have been demonstrated in multiple clinical publications there is no doubt that a need for long-term and perhaps federally supported clinical trials exists'.

Treatment during the early mixed dentition period

The development of the deciduous dentition, the presence of anterior and/or posterior crossbites, oronasal fistulae in the palate, and midfacial growth are the major concerns of the orthodontist during the annual team visits of the patients.

The early mixed dentition period starts with the emergence of the first permanent molars. In patients with an operated cleft palate, special attention should be given to the first molars, as it happens quite often that their eruption pattern is directed mesially. The permanent molars are disturbed in their eruption pattern, and become entrapped underneath the bulging distal surface of the second deciduous molars, leading to premature distal resorption of the maxillary second deciduous molars. The reason for this undesirable development is probably the scar tissue in the region of the tuberosities, due to the surgical palatal repair. Distal movement with a simple orthodontic device (two brackets and an opening coil) or extraction of the deciduous molars may be required in these cases.

The permanent incisor next to the cleft nearly always erupts into a rotated position. This rotation may cause a functional lateral shift of the mandible. In patients with a unilateral CLP the smaller segment often has a tendency to a crossbite at the deciduous canine and the first deciduous molar, which may lead to a mandibular shift. Another reason for a mandibular shift is a developing midfacial retrusion, with an end-to-end incisor relationship, resulting in an anterior posturing of the mandible. It is not always possible to correct a rotated incisor at this stage, as the root of the tooth is located very close to the alveolar cleft. Early orthodontic correction could move the incisor in the cleft space. Then it would be better to wait and align the incisors after bone grafting of the alveolar cleft at the age of 8–10 years. A posterior crossbite with mandibular shift can be easily corrected with a removable appliance with a fan-shaped expander screw. This appliance rotates around a posterior hinge, resulting in a differential expansion, more in the front than in the back (Figure 9.6).

Large oronasal fistulae in the palate can cause hypernasal speech as air can escape through the nose and create nasal regurgitations. During the team consultation, the speech pathologist provides the team members with the necessary information, to support the decision making regarding

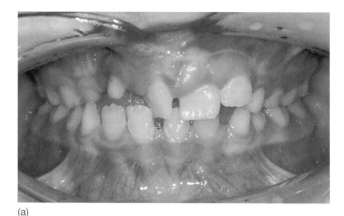

(a)

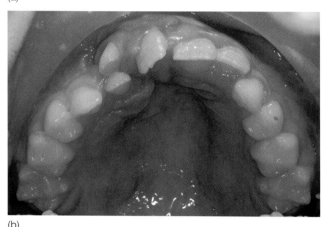

(b)

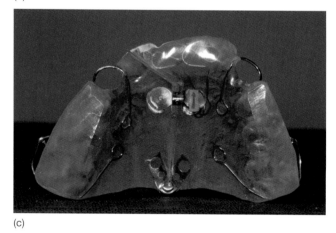

(c)

Figure 9.6 (a) Anterior and lateral crossbite. (b) Palatal view. (c) Expansion appliance.

surgical or orthodontic management at this stage. If it is decided to cover the fistula temporarily, the orthodontist will make a 'speech plate' covering the palate.

Facial orthopedics

Despite careful monitoring of maxillary growth, midfacial retrusion remains a common finding in operated CLP-

patients (Figure 9.7). Delaire and co-workers (1978) have laid down the theoretical basis for the clinical application of maxillary protraction in patients with severe maxillary deficiency. Since then, numerous case reports and case series studies have been published, a majority being concerned with noncleft individuals with Class III malocclusions (Tindlund, 2006). However, studies on CLP patients within homogeneous groups, an adequate sample size, and a long-term follow-up, remain rare (Kuijpers-Jagtman, 2006).

There seems to be general agreement that orthopedic forces to the maxillary complex are more effective at an early age, i.e. in the deciduous and early mixed dentition periods (Tindlund, 2006), taking into consideration the patency of the circum-maxillary sutures. However, no comparative, well-controlled studies on timing of maxillary protraction in patients with CLP could be found. In a noncleft sample, comparing the result of maxillary protraction started between 5 and 8 years of age and between 8 and 12 years, no difference in maxillary skeletal response was found, but the vertical response was greater in the older age group (Merwin et al., 1997).

Most of the more recent studies in patients with CLP have been conducted in Bergen, Norway, but the results published so far cover only a 3-year period after maxillary protraction (Tindlund, 2006). Since 1977, the Bergen rationale has involved transverse expansion, anterior protraction, and fixed retention at the age of 6–7 years. The treatment procedure is assumed to normalize orofacial function and dimensional anatomy, in order to reduce detrimental functional disturbances during further growth. A significant increase of the SNA angle of 0.9° was found, together with a clockwise rotation of the mandible, and an increase in lower facial height. As a result, a mean change of 2.3° in the ANB angle was found. However, the treatment response was highly variable. The short-term effect of maxillary protraction was found to be a maxillary skeletal/dentoalveolar effect, according to a ratio 45%/55% in unilateral CLP and 10%/90% in bilateral CLP (Tindlund and Rygh, 1993). The changes were reflected in the soft-tissue profile as a mild increase in nose prominence and upper lip protrusion, as well as a reduction in lower lip and chin protrusion. During a 3-year follow-up period the initial growth pattern reappeared, but the upper jaw position remained stable. The maxillo-mandibular relationship was impaired because of the normal downward and forward growth of the mandible while the maxillary position relative to anterior cranial base remained constant. Although the effect on the soft tissue profile had diminished, some positive effect still remained (Tindlund, 2006). The results of the Bergen studies have been generally confirmed by studies from a limited number of centers around the world, but mainly short-term results have been published. It is unclear whether the long-term effect is stable and sufficient to avoid surgical advancement of the maxilla after puberty.

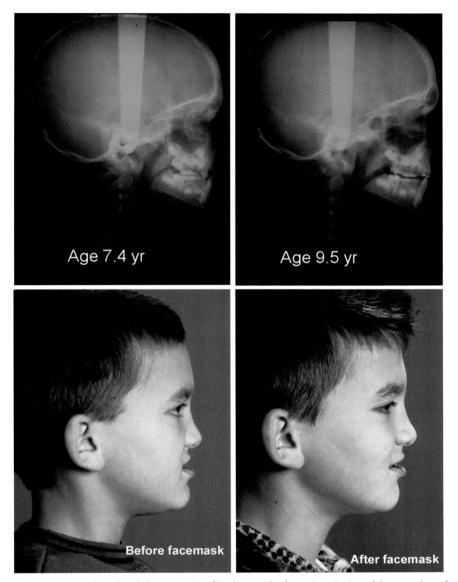

Figure 9.7 Pretreatment and post-treatment lateral cephalogram and profile photograph of a patient. During adolescence the unfavourable growth pattern re-appeared and the patient had a Le Fort I osteotomy after growth had ceased.

In this respect, cost-effectiveness analyses should be carried out, as well.

Recently, DeClerck et al. (2009) presented a new approach to midfacial deficiency, using skeletal anchorage with miniplates in the upper and lower jaws, and class III elastics. These miniplates offer the possibility to apply pure bone-borne orthopedic forces between the maxilla and the mandible, using class III elastics for 24 hours per day, avoiding any dentoalveolar compensations such as lower incisor retroclination or backward rotation of the mandible, as seen when using a facemask. Three preliminary case series studies have shown that intermaxillary class III elastics attached to miniplates can enhance midfacial growth in young maxillary-deficient, noncleft patients

(DeClerck et al., 2009; Cevidanes et al., 2010; Heymann et al., 2010). The reader is referred to these freely available publications (through PubMed) to appreciate the remarkable treatment changes for the maxilla as assessed on 3D overlays of superimposed cone-beam computed tomography (CT) models and visualized with color-coded displacement maps.

However, no reports have been published yet about application of this bone-anchored maxillary protraction system in CLP patients. Miniplate placement surgery in young patients is complicated by the reduced height of the maxillary alveolar bone, and mandibular miniplates cannot be placed before canine emergence, therefore orthopedic traction on miniplates usually cannot start before the age of 10 years. As miniplate surgery in young children has to be performed under general anesthesia, it should be preferably combined with the bone grafting procedure. It seems to be an interesting concept, but many questions are still unanswered, such as the ideal age and force for this type of orthopedic traction, the effect of the direction of force on the rotation of the palatal plane, the possibilities of retention to prevent catch-up growth after treatment, and the possibility of decreased need for orthognathic surgery (DeClerck et al., 2009)

From 8 to 15 years of age

The CLP team continues to follow the patient on an annual basis and closure of the alveolar cleft with an autologous bone graft is the next surgical intervention at this stage. Again, this is a joint decision of the team members and the parents. It is recommended to obtain standardized records at the age of 9 years, before the bone graft operation, consisting of extra- and intraoral pictures, dental casts, a cone-beam CT scan, and a 3D stereophotogrammetry facial image. The recent advances in 3D technology have greatly enhanced our insight into the 3D deformity of the cleft. From a cone-beam CT, a 2D head film can be reconstructed, as well as an orthopantomogram, if there is a need for comparison with earlier conventional cephalometric records that are part of the patient's documentation. It has been shown that there is no clinically relevant difference between angular and linear measurements performed in conventional cephalometric radiographs, compared with measurements in cephalometric radiographs constructed from cone-beam CT scans (Kumar et al., 2008; van Vlijmen et al., 2009). This means that cone-beam CT-reconstructed head films can be used in longitudinal follow-up series in patients who have both 2D and 3D records.

Orthodontic treatment in relation to alveolar bone grafting

When a complete cleft of the alveolus is present, unilateral or bilateral, an early secondary bone graft is recommended between the age of 8 and 11 years, and prior to emergence of the canine at the cleft-affected side. The timing of the procedure is based on the developmental stage of the unerupted canine adjacent to the cleft, whereby its root length should be half to three-quarters of its full length (Da Silva Filho et al., 2000; Matsui et al., 2005). The bone is usually harvested from the iliac crest, and also from other bones such as the tibia, the cranial bones, or the mandibular symphysis (Figure 9.8).

The benefits of reconstruction of the alveolus are appreciated with respect to supporting cleft-adjacent teeth, facilitating eruption of the cleft-side canine, stabilizing the cleft maxillary segments, supporting the alar base, and closing the oronasal communication (Long, 1995). Da Silva Filho et al. (2000) reviewed the literature on eruption of the cleft-side canine after bone grafting. They reported that about 2–56% of the canines that were unerupted before bone grafting needed surgical exposure during the course of orthodontic treatment after the bone grafting procedure. In a recently published study on a large sample (N = 308) it was found that a third of the patients need surgical assistance for eruption of the canine (De Ruiter et al., 2010). These findings mean that the orthodontist should always be aware of eruption disturbances of the cleft-side canine. On the other hand, it is reassuring to know that the treatment of the impacted canine is not much different from that in a noncleft patient.

In their landmark paper, Boyne and Sands (1976) readdressed the bone grafting issue in the mixed dentition with a technique that has become a standard and is still in use today in many centers. As orthodontists are always con-

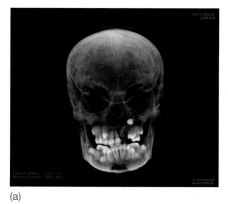
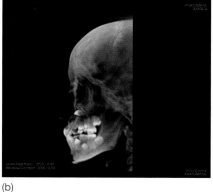
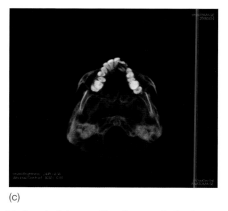

(a)   (b)   (c)

Figure 9.8 (a) Frontal view: bone graft from chin. (b) Lateral view depicting the canine position. (c) Axial view depicting maxillary bone graft. (3D image constructed out of cone-beam computed tomography with the help of InVivoDental software.)

cerned about possible scar-induced growth inhibition of any type of surgery, it remains to be determined whether early secondary bone grafting affects the subsequent growth of the maxilla. A large multicenter cephalometric study found only a minor vertical deficiency of the anterior part of the maxilla (Ross, 1987). Other studies were unable to detect any differences in maxillary size or position in a secondary grafted group when compared with a group of ungrafted matched controls (Semb, 1988; Levitt et al., 1999). In general, despite the absence of any prospective, controlled trials, existing data from retrospective studies on secondary bone grafting would seem to indicate a minimal, if any, effect on maxillofacial growth.

Orthodontic preparation for the bone graft procedure is almost always needed, involving expansion of the maxillary arch to align the maxillary segments in the correct position and relation to each other. This alignment can be performed easily with a removable expander or a quadhelix, in about 6–12 months. Caution should be exercised, however, not to over-expand the arch, as it will be very difficult for the surgeon to close the soft tissues over the bone-grafted area. A successful outcome of this procedure requires a sufficient amount of healthy attached gingiva (Iino et al., 2001). Therefore, a consultation with the surgeon is indicated during the expansion phase, and the degree of expansion should be determined by the surgeon. After the proper maxillary arch form has been achieved, retention is needed. The easiest way to establish retention is to fabricate a surgical acrylic splint that does not touch the soft tissues, and is placed directly after surgery. If a quadhelix is used for the expansion, the device has to be removed before surgery. Due to its flexibility it can be easily replaced 1–2 weeks after surgery.

As was mentioned earlier, the precondition for a successful bone graft is complete soft tissue closure over the bone-grafted area. This result may be difficult to achieve in patients with a wide alveolar cleft. In addition to the conventional segment osteotomy to mesialize the lateral segment, two newer approaches using distraction osteogenesis have been advocated to solve this problem. Liou et al. (2000) proposed interdental distraction osteogenesis within the alveolar process of the lateral segment, to create a new site of alveolar bone and attached gingiva. The osteotomized dental arch is transported forward, minimizing the size of the alveolar cleft. One week after distraction, the teeth adjacent to the distraction site can be moved into the newly generated bone in the dental arch. The remaining cleft is closed in a second procedure using gingivoperiosteoplasty to induce alveolar bone development in that area. The other approach is distraction osteogenesis with a bone-anchored maxillary distractor, to mesialize the lateral segment as a whole. It may be difficult to keep the transverse dimension with such a unilaterally applied distractor, with the potential risk of palatal tilting of the lateral segment during the distraction procedure. However, this movement

can be easily corrected by means of a quadhelix, once the lateral segment has reached its new position with the distractor still in situ (Binger et al., 2003). The success rate of these distraction osteogenesis procedures is still unclear, as long-term results have not been published yet.

Adolescent orthodontic treatment
After bone grafting, the orthodontic treatment continues, with the timing being dependent on the developmental stage of the dentition, especially the emergence of the canine adjacent to the cleft. Fixed appliances are always necessary, and treatment takes several years to be completed. If maxillofacial growth develops favorably, this will be the final orthodontic intervention. After active treatment, lifelong retention is usually necessary, particularly for preserving the maxillary transverse dimension.

The main problems we encounter during adolescent orthodontic treatment concern dental abnormalities, bad oral hygiene, the presence of scar tissue, and borderline skeletal relationships. Dental abnormalities are a common finding in CLP patients. When compared with the general population, subjects with CLP have been found to have a higher prevalence of dental abnormalities, such as variations in tooth number and position, and reduced tooth size, most of which are localized in the area of the cleft defect (Akcam et al., 2010). Lucas et al. (2000) reported a higher prevalence of enamel discoloration in children with a CLP when compared with a control group. A high prevalence of hypodontia of the permanent cleft-side lateral incisor (49.8%) as well as delayed root development in comparison with the contralateral tooth is common (Ribeiro et al., 2002). Akcam et al. (2010) found very high rates of anterior agenesis on the cleft side, varying between 70.8% and 97.1%, depending on the cleft type. Dental anomalies are also more common outside the cleft area. In individuals with CL ± P, the highest incidence of dental anomalies is in the maxillary second premolars, followed by the maxillary lateral incisors and the mandibular second premolars (Menezes and Vieira, 2008). In a case of missing teeth, the orthodontic treatment plan should be developed together with the prosthodontist, who is able to determine the optimal location for future implants, veneers, and other restorations.

Poor oral hygiene, which is quite common in CLP patients, could complicate the orthodontic treatment. For children without clefts and craniofacial anomalies we require good oral hygiene, otherwise orthodontic treatment is contraindicated. However, in children with clefts we tend to stretch thin our criteria for good oral hygiene, because these children have to be treated anyway. Unfortunately, the tolerance of poor oral hygiene can complicate the orthodontic treatment, and frustrate the clinician.

Scar tissue, especially on the palate, is associated with collapse of the transverse maxillary dimensions, and can result in an omega-shaped arch form. However, although the teeth can be aligned to a normal arch form, the tendency for relapse should be anticipated. Nearly all patients with a cleft palate as part of the cleft anomaly show a tendency of transversal relapse, even many years after treatment. Scar tissue in the palate should be considered while planning the retention protocol in cleft patients. In patients with scarred palate, the transverse dimensions need to be retained lifelong. In these patients a canine-to-canine bar, touching the anterior teeth, is indicated together with a Hawley retainer, which has to be worn lifelong at night, or even a retention frame. A preliminary study in our center showed, however, that out of a group of 39 patients with a complete cleft, only six were still wearing the retainer 10 years after the end of orthodontic treatment. In those six patients, the transverse dimensions were unchanged, but in all other patients the transverse dimensions were decreased.

Borderline skeletal relationship is one of the main problems appearing during orthodontic treatment of an adolescent with a cleft. A midfacial deficiency develops gradually during the course of the orthodontic treatment, and at a certain moment the decision has to be made as to whether the objectives still can be achieved by dental compensation only, without compromising facial esthetics. Unfortunately, in a considerable number of patients with clefts, a combined surgical-orthodontic correction of the skeleton is necessary after growth has ceased.

From 16 to 20 years

As stated earlier, the aim of the interdisciplinary treatment approach is to create conditions that allow the affected child to grow up with an esthetically pleasing face, good hearing and speech, properly functioning and esthetically acceptable dentition and, a harmonious social-psychological development. Around the age of 16 years, these goals are reached for most of the children with mild cleft types. They are in the final stage of their treatment, perhaps requiring some minor surgical secondary corrections of the nose and/or lip. Despite careful growth monitoring, however, many patients with complete clefts end up with a midfacial deficiency after puberty. An estimated 10–30% of the children with more severe complete CLP will need a combined surgical-orthodontic treatment to reach these goals. As the patient has now reached the age that he or she can make their own decision, it is important that they participate in the decision-making process, rather than just the parents.

The orthodontist, surgeon, and prosthodontist need extensive documentation to be able to develop a comprehensive treatment plan. This collaborative effort includes, but is not limited to, a thorough clinical examination with all three specialists together, particularly for an assessment of the dynamic aspects of the face, by collecting and evaluating extra- and intraoral pictures, articulated dental casts, cone-beam CT, and 3D stereophotogrammetry images of the face at rest and smiling. Postsurgical records should also

be taken, to evaluate the orthodontic and surgical outcomes (Santiago and Grayson, 2009).

Combined orthodontic-surgical treatment in adulthood

Correction of the jaw deformity is planned for when the permanent dentition has been fully erupted, the dental arches have been aligned orthodontically, and maxillofacial growth has ceased. Unfortunately, it is not so easy to determine the end point of facial growth. Chronological age and hand-wrist radiographs do not provide reliable information. Cervical vertebral maturation could be a good indicator for skeletal maturity, and can be easily assessed, as the vertebrae are visible on almost all lateral cephalograms (Franchi et al., 2000; Baccetti et al., 2005). Although this method seems to be a valid indicator of skeletal growth during the circumpubertal period (Wong et al., 2009), providing information for timing of growth modification, it has been shown to be only modestly effective in determining the amount of postpeak circumpubertal craniofacial growth (Fudalej and Bollen, 2010).

As there is no reliable method to determine the end of facial growth, the decision should be based on individual longitudinal cephalometric data of craniofacial growth. Radiographs should be taken at intervals of at least 6 months, but as the error of the method is large, longer time intervals are to be preferred. Currently, there is a tendency to operate earlier, and not to wait until late adolescence for complete definitive surgery (Posnick and Tiwana, 2006). Clearly, this treatment has psychosocial advantages, as the child will not have to live through puberty with a disfigured face. Furthermore, it means that the orthodontic treatment can be performed in one stage, extending from the period after bone grafting until the surgical correction of the jaw deformity. On the other hand, long-term data on the final outcome of orthognathic surgery or maxillary distraction to correct skeletal malformations in CLP patients before maxillofacial growth has ceased completely, are still lacking.

A wide range of orthopedic and orthodontic appliances may be used in the pre- and postsurgical orthodontic treatment stages. These appliances include fixed appliances, palatal expansion devices, temporary anchorage devices such as mini-screws and mini-plates, inter- and intra-arch elastics, removable appliances to unlock the occlusion or to support occlusal plane changes, and more. When performing midfacial distraction with intraoral distractors, a face-mask is helpful in supporting and controlling movement in the three planes of space, by altering the force vectors.

After the planned presurgical dental relationships have been achieved, new orthodontic records are taken, and a 3D digital surgical plan is worked out by surgeon and orthodontist that takes into consideration the viewpoints of the collaborating team specialists, and discussed with the patient and the patient's family. The final postsurgical orthodontic correction should be carefully planned between all team specialists involved. At this stage, the prosthodontist may want to replace missing teeth or restore hypoplastic incisors, and the plastic surgeon will perform final nose- and lip corrections. A good framework of well-aligned dental arches and an optimal jaw relationship will support these late corrections.

It takes time to reach stability of the facial skeleton after this operation. Usually the skeletal structures become progressively more stable in the 12-month period after surgery. In the postsurgical orthodontic period, emphasis is placed on retaining the surgically repositioned components of the craniofacial skeleton, and refining the dental occlusion. This is especially true for patients who have had large skeletal movements, or when the midface of a patient with a heavily scarred cleft palate was advanced. Therefore, inter-arch elastics and facemask therapy are used to balance relapse as needed. After the orthodontic and postsurgical treatment objectives have been met, fixed appliances are removed and orthodontic retainers placed. The same considerations as explained for the previous stage of adolescent orthodontics are valid. Therefore, increased attention is given to retention appliance design and long-term stability. In view of the potential for relapse in the transverse and sagittal dimensions, lifetime retention is highly recommended (Santiago and Grayson, 2009).

Conclusions

There are few greater challenges in the professional life of an orthodontist than the care for children with orofacial clefts and other craniofacial anomalies. Over the years, the orthodontist has proven to be an essential partner in the cleft palate team, not only responsible for the orthodontic and facial orthopedic treatment, but more importantly, he or she is also the guardian of the child's maxillofacial growth. By nature, orthodontists have a long-term treatment perspective in mind, which will assist the team in its consideration of treatment techniques, sequence, and timing, in relation to the effect on maxillofacial growth. Moreover, standardized records collected by the orthodontist provide a valuable basis for retrospective studies on treatment outcome and inter-center comparisons (Kuijpers-Jagtman, 2006). Finally, in recent times orthodontists seem to be quite often the motor behind large-scale inter-center randomized clinical trials in the field of CLP (Shaw and Semb, 2006).

CLP research and/or the aggregation of existing data into meta-analyses are extremely difficult, because of problems inherent to the CLP material itself, and because of a series of inherent weaknesses in the many studies published so far. As a result of these deficiencies, it would appear as if relatively little has been accomplished over the past 50 years. However, with the negative effects of scar tissue now well accepted, the next challenge is to keep that in balance with the desire to reach outcomes as 'normal'

as possible, as soon as possible. To optimize treatment outcome for patients with clefts, two research approaches need to be pursued: prospective randomized controlled trials, and controlled inter-center outcome studies. This target asks for standardized record taking, so that growth and treatment data between centers is consistent, to facilitate comprehensive data analysis (Kuijpers-Jagtman and Long, 2000).

Over the years, craniofacial orthodontics has developed to a subspecialty of regular orthodontics. Orthodontic residents may be introduced to the field, but are not able to treat these patients independently, without additional training. This has been recognized by the American Association of Orthodontists and the American Dental Association. A Fellowship in Craniofacial and Special Needs Orthodontics has been developed as a post-residency program that contains advanced education and training in a focused area of the specialty of orthodontics, including cleft lip/palate patient care, syndromic patient care, orthognathic surgery, craniofacial surgery and special care orthodontics (ADA, 2009). The contents of this fellowship could serve as an example for other countries desiring to improve the care for patients with clefts and craniofacial anomalies.

References

Akcam MO, Evirgen S, Uslu O, et al. (2010) Dental anomalies in individuals with cleft lip and/or palate. *European Journal of Orthodontics* 32: 207–13.

American Cleft Palate-Craniofacial Association (ACPCA) (1993, 2000) Parameters for the evaluation and treatment of patients with cleft lip/palate or other craniofacial anomalies. *Cleft Palate Craniofacial Journal* 30(Suppl 1): S1–S16. Revised April 2000.

American Dental Association Commission on Dental Accreditation (ADA) (2009) *Accreditation Standards for Clinical Fellowship Training Programs in Craniofacial and Special Care Orthodontics*. Website ADA. Available at: www.ada.org/sections/educationAndCareers/pdfs/ortho_fellowship.pdf (accessed 13 August 2010).

Baccetti T, Franchi L, McNamara JA Jr (2005) The cervical vertebral maturation (CVM) method for the assessment of optimal treatment timing in dentofacial orthopaedics. *Seminars in Orthodontics* 11: 119–29.

Barillas I, Dec W, Warren SM, et al. (2009) Nasoalveolar molding improves long-term nasal symmetry in complete unilateral cleft lip-cleft palate patients. *Plastic and Reconstructive Surgery* 123: 1002–6.

Binger T, Katsaros C, Rücker M, et al. (2003) Segment distraction to reduce a wide alveolar cleft before alveolar bone grafting. *Cleft Palate Craniofacial Journal* 40: 561–5.

Bongaarts CAM, Kuijpers-Jagtman AM, van 't Hof MA, et al. (2004) The effect of infant orthopedics on the occlusion of the deciduous dentition in children with complete unilateral cleft lip and palate (Dutchcleft). *Cleft Palate Craniofacial Journal* 41: 633–41.

Bongaarts CAM, van 't Hof MA, Prahl-Andersen B, et al. (2006) Infant orthopedics (IO) has no effect on maxillary arch dimensions in the deciduous dentition of children with complete unilateral cleft lip and palate (Dutchcleft). *Cleft Palate Craniofacial Journal* 43: 665–72.

Bongaarts CAM, Prahl-Andersen B, Bronkhorst EM, et al. (2008) Effect of infant orthopedics on facial appearance of toddlers with complete unilateral cleft lip and palate (Dutchcleft). *Cleft Palate Craniofacial Journal* 45: 407–13.

Bongaarts CAM, Prahl-Andersen B, Kuijpers-Jagtman AM (2009) Infant orthopedics and facial growth in complete unilateral cleft lip and palate until six years of age (Dutchcleft). *Cleft Palate Craniofacial Journal* 46: 654–63.

Boyne PJ, Sands NR (1976) Combined orthodontic-surgical management of residual palato-alveolar cleft defect. *American Journal of Orthodontics* 70: 20–37.

Broder HL, Smith FB, Strauss RP (1994) Effects of visible and invisible orofacial defects on self-perception and adjustment across developmental eras and gender. *Cleft Palate Craniofacial Journal* 31: 429–36.

Cevidanes L, Baccetti T, Franchi L, et al. (2010) Comparison of two protocols for maxillary protraction: bone anchors versus face mask with rapid maxillary expansion. *Angle Orthodontist* 80: 799–806.

Christ JE, Meininger MG (1981) Ultrasound diagnosis of cleft lip and cleft palate before birth. *Plastic and Reconstructive Surgery* 68: 854–59.

Cutting CB, Grayson BH, Brecht L, et al. (1998) Presurgical columellar elongation and retrograde nasal reconstruction in one-stage bilateral cleft lip and nose repair. *Plastic and Reconstructive Surgery* 101: 630–9.

Da Silva Filho OG, Teles SG, Ozawa TO, et al. (2000) Secondary bone graft and eruption of the permanent canine in patients with alveolar clefts: literature review and case report. *Angle Orthodontist* 70: 174–8.

Day DW (1981) Perspectives on care: the interdisciplinary team approach. *Otolaryngology Clinics of North America* 14: 769–75.

DeClerck HJ, Cornelis MA, Cevidanes LH, et al. (2009) Orthopedic traction of the maxilla with miniplates: a new perspective for treatment of midface deficiency. *Journal of Oral and Maxillofac Surgery* 67: 2123–9.

Delaire J, Verdon P, Flour J (1978) Möglichkeiten und Grenzen extraoraler Züge in postero-anteriorer Richtung unter Verwendung der orthopädischen Maske bei der Behandlung von Fällen der Klasse III. *Fortschritte der Kieferorthopädie* 39: 27–45.

De Ruiter A, van der Bilt A, Meijer G, et al. (2010) Orthodontic treatment results following grafting autologous mandibular bone to the alveolar cleft in patients with a complete unilateral cleft. *Cleft Palate Craniofacial Journal* 47: 35–42.

Franchi L, Baccetti T, McNamara JA Jr (2000) Mandibular growth as related to cervical vertebral maturation and body height. *American Journal of orthodontics and Dentofacial Orthopedics* 118: 335–40.

Fudalej P, Bollen AM (2010) Effectiveness of the cervical vertebral maturation method to predict postpeak circumpubertal growth of craniofacial structures. *American Journal of Orthodontics and Dentofacial Orthopedics* 137: 59–65.

Georgiade NG, Miadick RA, Thorne FL (1968) Positioning of the premaxilla in bilateral cleft lips by oral pinning and traction. *Plastic and Reconstructive Surgery* 41: 240–3.

Grayson BH, Cutting CB (2001) Presurgical nasoalveolar orthopedic molding in primary correction of the nose, lip, and alveolus of infants born with unilateral and bilateral clefts. *Cleft Palate Craniofacial Journal* 38: 193–8.

Grayson BH, Maull D (2006) Nasoalveolar molding for infants born with clefts of the lip, alveolus and palate. In: S Berkowitz (ed.) *Cleft Lip and Palate. Diagnosis and Management.* Berlin: Springer Verlag, pp. 451–8.

Grayson BH, Cutting CB, Wood R (1993) Preoperative columella lengthening in bilateral cleft lip and palate. *Plastic and Reconstructive Surgery* 92: 1422–3.

Heymann GC, Cevidanes L, Cornelis M, et al. (2010) Three-dimensional analysis of maxillary protraction with intermaxillary elastics to miniplates. *American Journal of Orthodontics and Dentofacial Orthopedics* 137: 274–84.

Hotz M, Gnoinski W (1976) Comprehensive care of cleft lip and palate children at Zürich University: a preliminary report. *American Journal of Orthodontics* 70: 481–504.

Hubbard TW, Paradise JL, McWilliams BJ, et al. (1985) Consequences of unremitting middle-ear disease in early life. Otologic, audiologic, and developmental findings in children with cleft palate. *New England Journal of Medicine* 312: 1529–34.

Iino M, Fukuda M, Murakami K, et al. (2001) Vestibuloplasty after secondary alveolar bone grafting. *Cleft Palate Craniofacial Journal* 38: 551–9.

IPDTOC Working Group (International Perinatal Database of Typical Orofacial Clefts Working Group) (2011) Prevalence at birth of cleft lip with or without cleft palate. Data from the International Perinatal Database of Typical Oral Clefts (IPDTOC). *Cleft Palate Craniofacial Journal* 2011;48: 66–84.

Institute of Medical Illustrators (2004) *IMI National Guidelines Photography of Cleft Audit Patients.* Website IMI. Available at: www.imi.org.uk/natguidelines/guidelines01.asp (accessed 13 August 2010).

Kasten EF, Schmidt SP, Zickler CF, et al. (2008) Team care of the patient with cleft lip and palate. *Current Problems in Pediatric and Adolescent Health Care* 38: 138–58.

Konst EM, Weersink-Braks H, Rietveld T, et al. (2000) An intelligibility assessment of toddlers with cleft lip and palate who received and did not receive presurgical infant orthopedic treatment. *Journal of Communication Disorders* 33: 483–501.

Konst EM, Rietveld T, Peters H, et al. (2003) Use of perceptual evaluation instrument to assess the effects of infant orthopedics on the speech of toddlers with cleft lip and palate. *Cleft Palate Craniofacial Journal* 40: 597–605.

Konst EM, Prahl C, Weersink-Braks H, et al. (2004) Cost-effectiveness of infant orthopedic treatment regarding speech in patients with complete unilateral cleft lip and palate: a randomized three-center trial in the Netherlands (Dutchcleft). *Cleft Palate Craniofacial Journal* 41: 71–7.

Kuijpers-Jagtman AM (2006) The orthodontist, an essential partner in CLP treatment. *B-ENT* 2(Suppl 4): 57–62.

Kuijpers-Jagtman AM, Long RE Jr (2000) The influence of surgery and orthopedic treatment on maxillofacial growth and maxillary arch development in patients treated for orofacial clefts. *Cleft Palate Craniofacial Journal* 37: 527/1–527/12.

Kuijpers-Jagtman AM, Prahl-Andersen B (2006) History of neonatal orthopedics: past to present. In: S Berkowitz S (ed.) *Cleft Lip and Palate, Diagnosis and Management.* Berlin: Springer, pp. 395–408.

Kumar V, Ludlow J, Soares Cevidanes LH, et al. (2008) In vivo comparison of conventional and cone beam CT synthesized cephalograms. *Angle Orthodontist* 78: 873–9.

Latham RA (1980) Orthopedic advancement of the cleft maxillary segment: a preliminary report. *Cleft Palate Journal* 17: 227–33.

Levitt T, Long RE Jr, Trotman CA (1999) Maxillary growth in patients with clefts following secondary alveolar bone grafting. *Cleft Palate Craniofacial Journal* 36: 398–406.

Liou EJ, Chen PK, Huang CS, et al. (2000) Interdental distraction osteogenesis and rapid orthodontic tooth movement: a novel approach to approximate a wide alveolar cleft or bony defect. *Plastic and Reconstructive Surgery* 105: 1262–72.

Long RE Jr (1995) Factors affecting the success of secondary alveolar bone grafting in patients with complete clefts of the lip and palate. In: CA Trotman, JA McNamara Jr (eds) *Orthodontic Treatment: Outcome and Effectiveness*, Monograph 30. Craniofacial Growth Series. Ann Arbor, MI: Center for Human Growth and Development, The University of Michigan, pp. 271–95.

Lucas VS, Gupta R, Ololade O, et al. (2000) Dental health indices and caries associated microflora in children with unilateral cleft lip and palate. *Cleft Palate Craniofacial Journal* 37: 447–52.

Maarse W, Bergé SJ, Pistorius L, et al. (2010) Diagnostic accuracy of transabdominal ultrasound in detecting prenatal cleft lip and palate: a systematic review. *Ultrasound in Obstetrics and Gynecology* 35: 495–502.

Matsui K, Echigo S, Kimizuka S, et al. (2005) Clinical study on eruption of permanent canines after secondary alveolar bone grafting. *Cleft Palate Craniofacial Journal* 42: 309–13.

McNeil CK (1950) Orthodontic procedures in the treatment of congenital cleft palate. *Dental Record* 70: 126–32.

Menezes R, Vieira AR (2008) Dental anomalies as part of the cleft spectrum. *Cleft Palate Craniofacial Journal* 45: 414–19.

Merwin D, Ngan P, Hägg U, et al. (1997) Timing for effective application of anteriorly directed orthopedic force to the maxilla. *American Journal of Orthodontics and Dentofacial Orthopedics* 112: 292–9.

Milerad J, Larson O, PhD D, et al. (1997) Associated malformations in infants with cleft lip and palate: a prospective, population-based study. *Pediatrics* 100: 180–6.

Mølsted K, Asher-McDade C, Brattström V, et al. (1992) A six-center international study of treatment outcome in patients with clefts of the lip and palate: Part 2. Craniofacial form and soft tissue profile. *Cleft Palate Craniofacial Journal* 29: 398–404.

Posnick J, Tiwana PS (2006) Cleft-orthognathic surgery. In: S Berkowitz (ed.) *Cleft Lip and Palate, Diagnosis and Management.* Berlin: Springer, pp. 573–85.

Prahl C, Kuijpers-Jagtman AM, Van 't Hof MA, et al. (2001) A randomized prospective clinical trial into the effect of infant orthopedics on maxillary arch dimensions in unilateral cleft lip and palate (Dutchcleft). *European Journal of Oral Sciences* 109: 297–305.

Prahl C, Kuijpers-Jagtman AM, van 't Hof MA, et al. (2005) Infant orthopedics in UCLP: Effect on feeding, weight and length: a randomized clinical trial (Dutchcleft). *Cleft Palate Craniofacial Journal* 42: 171–7.

Ribeiro LL, das Neves LT, Costa B, et al. (2002) Dental development of permanent lateral incisor in complete unilateral cleft lip and palate. *Cleft Palate Craniofacial Journal* 39: 193–6.

Ross RB (1987) Treatment variables affecting facial growth in complete unilateral cleft lip and palate. *Cleft Palate Journal* 24: 5–77.

Santiago PE, Grayson BH (2009) Role of the craniofacial orthodontist on the craniofacial and cleft lip and palate team. *Seminars in Orthodontics* 15: 225–43.

Semb G (1988) Effect of alveolar bone grafting on maxillary growth in unilateral cleft lip and palate patients. *Cleft Palate Journal* 25: 288–95.

Shaw WC, Semb G (2006) Eurocleft – An experiment in intercenter collaboration. In: S Berkowitz (ed.) *Cleft Lip and Palate, Diagnosis and Management*. Berlin: Springer, 765–76.

Shaw WC, Asher-McDade C, Brattström V, et al. (1992a) A six-center international study of treatment outcome in patients with clefts of the lip and palate: Part 1. Principles and study design. *Cleft Palate Craniofacial Journal* 29: 393–7.

Shaw WC, Dahl E, Asher-McDade C, et al. (1992b) A six-center international study of treatment outcome in patients with clefts of the lip and palate: Part 5. General discussion and conclusions. *Cleft Palate Craniofacial Journal* 29: 413–18.

Shaw WC, Semb G, Nelson P, et al. (2000) *The EUROCLEFT Project 1996– 2000. Standards of Care for Cleft Lip and Palate in Europe*. Amsterdam: IOS Press.

Sheahan P, Miller I, Sheahan JN, et al. (2003) Incidence and outcome of middle ear disease in cleft lip and/or cleft palate. *International Journal of Pediatric Otorhinolaryngology* 67: 785–93.

Strauss RP (1999) The organization and delivery of craniofacial health services: The state of the art. *Cleft Palate Craniofacial Journal* 36: 189–95.

Tindlund RS (2006) Protraction facial mask for the correction of midfacial retrusion: the Bergen Rationale. In: S Berkowitz (ed.) *Cleft Lip and Palate, Diagnosis and Management*. Berlin: Springer, 486–502.

Tindlund RS, Rygh P (1993) Maxillary protraction: different effects on facial morphology in unilateral and bilateral cleft lip and palate patients. *Cleft Palate Craniofacial Journal* 30: 208–21.

van Vlijmen OJ, Bergé SJ, Swennen GR, et al. (2009) Comparison of cephalometric radiographs obtained from cone-beam computed tomography scans and conventional radiographs. *Journal of Oral and Maxillofacial Surgery* 67: 92–7.

Wellens W, Vander Poorten V (2006) Keys to a successful cleft lip and palate team. *B-ENT* 2(Suppl 4): 3–10.

Williams AC, Shaw WC, Sandy JR, et al. (1996) The surgical care of cleft lip and palate patients in England and Wales. *British Journal of Plastic Surgery* 49: 150–5.

Wong RW, Alkhal HA, Rabie AB (2009) Use of cervical vertebral maturation to determine skeletal age. *American Journal of Orthodontics and Dentofacial Orthopedics* 136: 484.e1–6.

World Health Organization (2002) *Global Strategies to reduce the Health-Care Burden of Craniofacial Anomalies: Report of WHO Meetings on International Collaborative Research on Craniofacial Anomalies, Geneva, Switzerland, 5–8 November 2000; Park City, Utah, USA, 24–26 May 2001*. World Health Organization, Geneva. Website WHO. Available at: http://whqlibdoc.who.int/publications/9241590386.pdf (accessed 10 August 2010).

10

What can Orthodontists Learn from Orthopaedists Engaged in Basic Research?

Carlalberta Verna, Birte Melsen

Summary

The first part of this chapter focuses on the need for an integration of the terminology used within bone biology into the orthodontic world. According to the appropriate biological terminology, bone modelling is defined as uncoupled resorption and formation activities that occur at different sites, while bone remodelling consists of coupled resorption and formation activities occurring on the same site in a specific sequence, i.e. resorption always preceding formation. While bone modelling occurs mainly during growth, bone remodelling occurs throughout life, and plays a role both in the maintenance of the phosphate–calcium homeostasis and in the repair of bone microdamages. The movement of the teeth 'with' the alveolar bone obtained with orthodontic appliances is a result of bone modelling rather than bone remodelling, although orthodontists generally refer to this phenomenon as remodelling. Bone modelling can be used by the orthodontist for implant site development, by moving a tooth away from the area where new bone has to be created. The bone remodelling rate in fact influences tooth movement rate. The orthodontists may face situations where the bone metabolic rate has changed (due to disease or pharmacological treatment), or may want to accelerate tooth movement rate by producing local bone damage. The latter case will stimulate bone healing, therefore increasing tooth movement rate. Clinical situations with metabolic impairment are exemplified, and related clinical suggestions are given. In the light of the latest morphological and finite element analysis, the pressure–tension theory is no longer valid in the explanations about bone modelling reactions to orthodontic force. This chapter suggests a new paradigm, founded on the assumption that bone cells are able to react to deformation. Finally, the alveolar bone reaction to skeletal temporary anchorage devices is described, and a potential role for them in bone width maintenance is suggested.

A common language

As correctly indicated by the editors of this book, the face is part of a whole body. Therefore, there is no reason to believe that the stomatognathic system would not follow general physiopathological rules applying to the entire body. Basic research carried out by orthopaedists can, therefore, be utilized by orthodontists. However, a precondition for a learning process is a common language.

Modeling

Regarding the biological reaction occurring as a result of orthodontic force systems, there is no lexical consistency between orthodontists and orthopaedists, the former describing it as remodelling, the latter as modelling. In bone-biological terms, bone remodelling and modelling are two distinctly separate processes, with different physiological roles.

Modelling is the term applied to the changes in shape and size of bones (macro-modelling) resulting from resorption and formation activities, and is the dominant biological activity during growth. Modelling also occurs at the trabecular level, the so-called mini-modelling (Frost, 1990). Resorption and formation drifts do not necessarily follow a given sequence, i.e. they are biologically uncoupled. In adult life the physiological mesial drift of the alveolar socket is a result of modelling. Bone modelling reflects the structural adaptation of bone mass and shape to varying demands. It is thus largely controlled by functional and applied loads, and less by systemic metabolic requests. Formation drifts may occur in both lamellar and woven bone. Woven bone is a result of larger strain values than lamellar bone, and usually appears after fracture healing, in response to neoplasms, infections, and in reaction to large mechanical loads produced by orthodontic appliances (Frost, 1994) (Figure 10.1).

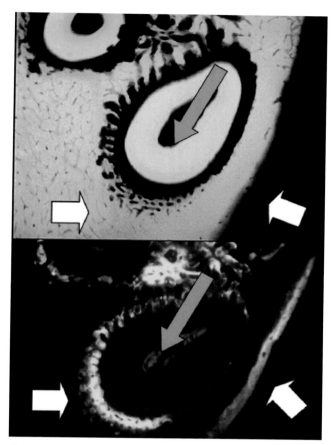

Figure 10.1 Alveolar bone modelling following the application of 25 g of force. After 14 days of treatment, the microradiographic analysis (top) shows new bone formation ahead of the tooth in the direction of the force (red arrow). On the buccal side, new periosteal bone formation is observed, as shown by the wide strips of bone markers (white arrow). (From Verna et al. (1999b) with permission from Elsevier.)

Clinical implications of modelling

When teeth are moved 'with bone', modelling of the alveolar bone occurs, and thus the teeth can be moved beyond the immediate alveolar envelope while maintaining the marginal bone level. This principle underpins the treatment of partially dentate adult patients with atrophied alveolar bone areas (Mantzikos and Shamus, 1999; Chandler and Rongey, 2005). An example of the so-called tooth movement with bone is illustrated in Figure 10.2, where the tooth has been moved into an atrophic edentulous area, with 'rebuilding' of the alveolar process, giving the impression that the tooth has carried the alveolus along to the new position.

When determining the force system necessary for a planned tooth movement, the quantity and the quality of the bone surrounding the tooth should be taken into consideration. High-resolution micro-computed tomography (CT) scans of alveolar bone samples show that the bone surrounding the roots is highly variable in density and that the so-called lamina dura is a non-uniform structure (Dalstra et al., 2006) (Figure 10.3). Therefore, even very light forces may result in overcompression over small surfaces of the alveolar bone. This is in line with the finding that hyalinization is rarely avoidable (von Bohl et al., 2004), although the amount may vary.

Particular attention should be paid to the origin of the cells that will activate the modelling process. In the case of indirect resorption in areas dominated by dense cortical bone, for example in labial movement of lower incisors, tooth movement requires modelling of the cortical bone, and the osteoclasts should originate from the cortical bone, or from the periosteum. Labial tipping of incisors in the presence of thin cortical bone increases the probability

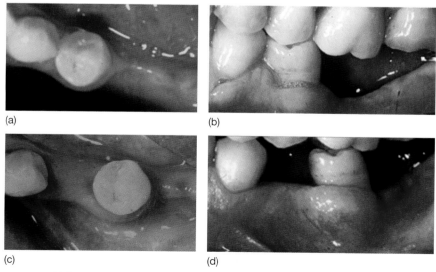

Figure 10.2 (a,b) Tooth movement with bone in an edentulous alveolar crest, where no bone is present. The alveolar drift allows for the movement of the whole alveolus (c,d), and the osteogenic potential of the periodontal ligament is fully expressed in the formation of bone. (From Melsen B, Garbo D [2004] with permission from Quintessence.)

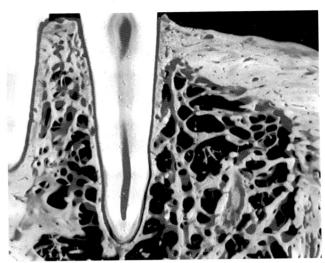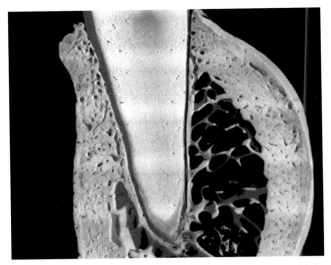

Figure 10.3 Mesiodistal (left) and buccolingual (right) views of the alveolus of the canine. Note the uneven thickness of the alveolar bone proper and the sparse trabecular support. (From Dalstra et al. [2006] with permission from Blackwell Munskgaard.)

of bone fenestration (Baron, 1975). To reduce the risk of iatrogenic dehiscence, the initial force system should be directed at the displacement of the apex of the root, which is usually surrounded by trabecular bone. Thereafter, the bending of the alveolar process will generate formation on the buccal side of the alveolar process. The use of controlled, uniformly distributed, low-magnitude forces is recommended, and, since the modelling rate of cortical bone is slower than that of trabecular bone, adequate time should be allowed for initiation of cellular activation and subsequent bone formation at the periosteal side. An example is shown in Figure 10.4, where the system was checked monthly to adjust the line of action of the force without activation.

In sum, the drift of the alveolar bone occurring following the application of an orthodontic force can be described as modelling, in response to a modified functional demand. Since the anatomy of the teeth differs both within an individual dental arch and between patients, modelling of the alveolar bone without bone loss can only be achieved by use of customized biomechanical systems. However, based on this premise, it is difficult, if not impossible, to agree on absolute standardization of treatments.

Remodeling

As mentioned above, orthodontists do not distinguish between modelling and remodelling. Remodelling is a phenomenon that occurs throughout life in discrete locations in the whole skeleton. It involves cycles of resorption and subsequent formation, spatially and temporally coupled. Remodelling allows bone adaptation to mechanical stresses by minimizing fatigue damages, and is influenced by the action of hormones and cytokines (Burr, 1993; Mori and Burr, 1993; Frost, 1998).

The bone remodelling cycle is carried out by a team of cells called the bone multicellular unit (BMU) (Frost, 1986). The cycle in humans lasts 120–160 days, and is composed of four phases: activation, resorption, reversal, and formation (Eriksen et al., 1984). Although the stimulus necessary for the initiation of a new BMU is still not fully identified, it has been shown that microcracks can initiate remodelling via the sensory input to the osteocytes. In the activation phase, the lining cells, the preosteoblasts, change to a cuboidal shape, and secrete a receptor ligand, RANKL (receptor activator of nuclear factor kappa B ligand), on the cell surface. The preosteoclasts within the bone marrow present receptors for RANKL on their cell membrane, called RANK. The interaction between RANK and RANKL determines the activation of the preosteoclasts, which then fuse and differentiate into mature multinucleated osteoclasts and resorb bone. The resorption of bone also occurs as a result of inhibitory activities directed towards osteoblasts, as in the case of the release of sclerostin (SOST), which inhibits bone formation and enhances osteoblast apoptosis (Winkler et al., 2003). The RANKL present on the cell surface of the preosteoblast is neutralized by a free-floating decoy receptor belonging to the tumour necrosis factor (TNF) family, osteoprotegerin (OPG), thus controlling further activation of the pre-osteoclasts via RANK. Bone resorption lasts for about 2 weeks, after which the osteoclasts undergo programmed cell death or apoptosis.

Following resorption by the osteoclasts, the lacuna is deepened by mononuclear phagocyte cells (Eriksen et al., 1984). At the end of this process the reversal phase is initiated, and further preosteoblasts migrate into the resorbed cavity and differentiate into osteoblasts. The interface between the resorbed old bone and the new-formed bone is called the cement line, or reversal line, and these osteob-

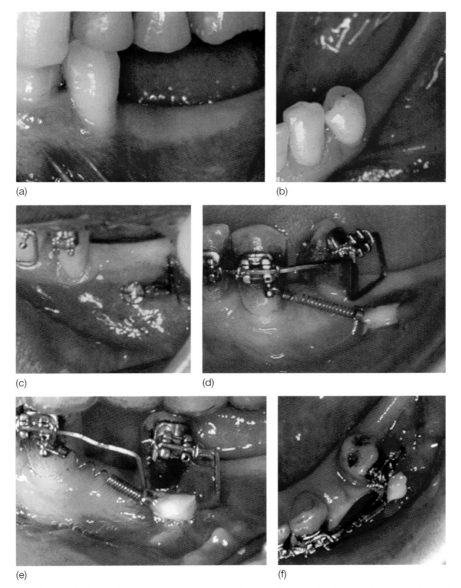

Figure 10.4 (a,b) Modelling of the alveolar bone achieved by bodily movement of a premolar in an atrophic area. (c,d) Following the insertion of a mini-implant (Aarhus System) the biomechanical system consisted of a box loop in a titanium molybdenum in a .017 × .025 inch archwire activated to apply a distal force and uprighting moment. This enabled a bodily tooth movement, with uniform distribution of the force in the periodontal ligament. Anchorage was ensured by the use of a 50 g superelastic coil spring attached to the skeletal anchorage device. (e,f) The same biomechanical system was used to achieve the final displacement, and at each appointment the appliance was adjusted to maintain the force-to-moment ratio for continuation of the translation movement. (From Melsen B, Garbo D [2004] with permission from Quintessence.)

lasts now start to form bone. The precursor preosteoblasts are probably attracted by bone-derived growth factors (such as transforming growth factor-β, TGF-β) and are derived from marrow stromal cells. Through a positive feedback mechanism the preosteoblasts also secrete growth factors, osteopontin, osteocalcin, and other proteins, such as insulin growth factor-1 (IGF-1), interleukin-6 (IL-6), bone morphogenetic proteins (BMPs), and fibroblast growth factors (FGF), all of which enhance the osteoblast's activities. Fibroblasts also migrate towards the cement line and secrete the thin collagen fibrils around which the osteoblasts start synthesizing osteoid. The osteoid is non-mineralized bone matrix that cannot be resorbed by osteoclasts. The mineralization process starts when the osteoid thickness reaches about 6 μm. After about 4 months the resorption cavity is filled with new bone, although not completely, with closely packed mineral crystals and subsequent increase in bone density.

It is essential for the orthodontist to understand the role of remodelling following the application of an orthodontic

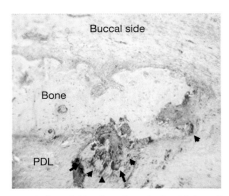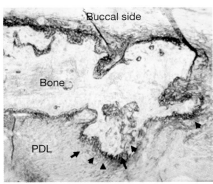

Figure 10.5 Alveolar bone on the buccal side of a rat's tooth after 14 days of orthodontic treatment. On the side facing the periodontal ligament (PDL; arrows), there is staining for alkaline phosphatase (dark blue, right panel) and for acid phosphatase (red, left panel), confirming bone remodelling activities. (From Verna and Melsen [2002] with permission from Libra Ortodonzia.)

load. Bone formation has been observed not only in the periodontal ligament (PDL) tension side, but also in the direction of the force (Mohri et al., 1991; King et al., 1992); bone resorption has also been observed at this site (Mohri et al., 1991; Zaffe and Verna, 1995; Melsen, 1999) (Figure 10.5). The presence of markers of both resorption and formation adjacent to the alveolar wall reflects the coupled activity of osteoclasts and osteoblasts that characterizes what orthopaedists describe as bone remodelling. Synchronized initiation of numerous BMUs results in bone turnover on both the pressure and tension sides in the PDL (Tanne et al., 1990). The RANKL-RANK mechanism has been shown to be active in the PDL and is strengthened by mechanical load (Ogasawara et al., 2004). Tooth movement can be accelerated by local delivery of RANKL (Kanzaki et al., 2006), whereas the delivery of OPG decreases the rate of tooth movement (Oshiro et al., 2002; Kanzaki et al., 2004). A lack of OPG has been found to be associated with a significantly higher level of bone resorption in the compression area, whereas the upregulation of RANKL induced by orthodontic forces depends on the presence of prostaglandin (PG) E_2, which is released by osteoblasts and osteocytes (Kanzaki et al., 2002; Yamaguchi, 2009).

It is clear, therefore, that the application of a mechanical load initiates remodelling as well as bone modelling. The variation in the quality of remodelling between patients may explain the individual variations in tissue response to orthodontic treatment.

Clinical implications of bone remodelling

Cortical anchorage was defined by Ricketts as movement of the roots towards the cortex of the alveolar bone to resist the active force of the appliance (Ricketts, 1998). The biological principle behind cortical anchorage is the utilization of the differential turnover rates of cortical and trabecular bone, the former being 5–10 times slower than the latter (Steineche and Hauge, 2003). Teeth closer to the cortical bone need more time to be moved, but at a later

stage anchorage loss will occur. Absolute anchorage can, however, only be achieved with ankylosed teeth or skeletal anchorage devices (Melsen and Costa, 2000; Melsen and Verna, 2000).

The biological reaction to an orthodontic force system interacts with the already occurring physiological bone turnover. Our knowledge of turnover rate of the bone in the alveolar process is, however, scarce. The sole human histomorphometric study comparing static cortical remodelling in the mandible with that of the iliac crest, which is the most frequent site for bone biopsies, showed that the levels of remodelling parameters were lower in the basal part of the mandible than in bone samples harvested from load-bearing areas, confirming that remodelling is maintained by function (Verna et al., 1999a). Recently, the site-specificity of bone remodelling has been confirmed by Deguchi et al. (2008), who demonstrated faster bone remodelling and faster tooth movement in a dog's maxilla than in the mandible. This is due to not only a different ratio between cortical and trabecular bone in the two anatomical sites, but also differences in remodelling rates. At the clinical level, it is advisable to start the orthodontic treatment in the lower jaw to avoid unnecessary prolongation of treatment time.

The rate of tooth movement is influenced by the rate of bone remodelling. Any substance able to interfere with bone remodelling may, in principle, influence the rate of tooth movement rate. Different substances have been tried experimentally and clinically to increase/decrease the rate of tooth movement, but their use is not recommended in the routine clinical setting. On the other hand, as clinicians, we need to know whether substances that may interfere with orthodontic treatment are being taken by our patients. Non-steroidal anti-inflammatory drugs, vitamin D, estrogen, and doxycycline are known to interfere with bone remodelling and to decrease the tooth movement rate (Krishnan and Davidovitch, 2006; Bartzela et al., 2009). However, acetaminophen (paracetamol) is an analgesic that does not interfere with tooth movement (Arias and Marquez-Orozco, 2006). Patients should therefore be instructed preferably to take acetaminophen for relief of pain, so that overall treatment time remains unaffected.

Corticosteroid treatment has an inhibitory effect on bone turnover that subsequently leads to secondary hyperparathyroidism. The effect on tooth movement will therefore depend on the duration of the drug treatment, and is enhanced in patients undergoing long-term corticosteroid treatment (Kalia et al., 2004). In the case where treatment is of short duration, the rate of tooth movement may not to be affected, but, at a tissue level, the remodelling process seems to be delayed. In clinical terms, if a patient is under active orthodontic treatment and has to undergo short-term steroid treatment, such as hay fever therapy, minimal adjustments should be made to the appliance during this period and the interval between appointments may be longer. In treatments of longer duration (about 12 months), the tooth movement rate is increased and the appliance should be checked as usual or more frequently. The effect of steroid treatment on root resorption has also been investigated, with higher rates of root resorption reported in rats administered steroids for a short amount of time (Verna et al., 2006). This is not surprising, since the slower turnover rate will lead to relatively larger amounts of bone covered by osteoid. Since osteoid cannot be resorbed by osteoclasts, the clastic activities are diverted towards the mineralized root surfaces. Once again, in such situations, activation of the appliance will not help. On the contrary, less frequent activation will protect against further root damage. In patients with a history of allergy, who are undergoing steroid treatment for a short time, it is advisable to postpone treatment until the patient has completed their pharmacological treatment and to follow the above-mentioned suggestions in case of a sudden need for steroids during the orthodontic treatment. The effect of corticosteroid treatment on tooth movement is also dose dependent, since high dosages induce osteoporosis, which means there is less bone available for resorption, and therefore the rate of tooth movement increases but with a higher degree of relapse (Ashcraft et al., 1992).

Tooth movement can also be accelerated by local mechanisms that increase the remodelling rate without use of drugs, such as the regional acceleratory phenomenon (RAP) that occurs after fracture healing, as described by Frost (Frost, 1994; Roblee et al., 2009). RAP is characterized by local increased resorption and formation activities with less mineralized bone formation, which is a sign of quick repair after an injury. RAP normally occurs following orthodontic tooth movement (Verna et al., 1999b) and its intensity is related to the intensity of the damage. Cortical perforations and corticotomies (with or without surgical flap) performed as part of the orthodontic treatment increase the tooth movement rate approximately twofold (Sanjideh et al., 2010) by enhancing the repair process locally, for example in tooth movement immediately following extraction.

In animal experiments the tissue reaction occurring during corticotomy-assisted tooth movement is characterized by transient bone resorption, followed by the deposition of fibrous tissue after 21 days and by bone after 60 days (Wang et al., 2009). After corticision (a transmucosal corticotomy technique) less hyalinization and more rapid removal of hyalinized tissue has been observed, together with extensive areas of resorption followed by a 3.5-fold higher accumulated mean apposition area of new bone than the control side (Kim et al., 2009). When cortical perforation is combined with alveolar augmentation, the original alveolar volume and any existing osseous dehiscences may no longer be a limitation for orthodontic tooth movement (Wilcko et al., 2009). Since bone density is decreased, the resulting dissipation of the physiological as well as orthodontic forces over the bone surface and the more effective blood supply may reduce root resorption risk. However, to date, no histological studies have analyzed the root status in areas with more relative osteoid formation, such as in the enhanced bone formation phase of RAP. Future studies should consider evaluating the duration of the RAP, and thus the possibility of speeding up tooth movement. Longitudinal animal studies have shown that the tooth movement rate approximates the level of non-corticotomy-assisted treatment after about 7 weeks (Sanjideh et al., 2010). It is therefore possible that procedures such as RAP will be effective in the alignment and levelling phase. Techniques aiming at reducing the stiffness of cortical bone and increasing the remodelling rate and blood supply may be promising in areas where cortical bone is particularly thick and trabecular bone is present in very small amounts, such as in the mandibular molar areas.

Systemic diseases influence the bone turnover rate and thereby the rate of tooth movement. Following the application of orthodontic tipping forces in rats with experimentally induced hyperthyroidism and hypothyroidism, faster tooth movement was observed in the rats . This occurs with high than with low and normal bone turnover rates. In addition, changes in the quality of the bone tend to relocate the centre of resistance, thus impacting on the type of tooth movement achieved (Verna et al., 2000). Clinically, patients may have high bone turnover rates, such as in untreated hyperthyroidism. An increasing number of adolescents and young adults present signs of eating disorders, such as anorexia nervosa, which result in an osteopenic condition not dissimilar to osteoporosis. In seeing teenage patients regularly for the orthodontic check, the orthodontic team may be the first to detect such psychological distress states.

The influence of bone metabolism on orthodontic tooth movement is particularly important when dealing with adult patients. In pregnant women, orthodontic tooth movement is faster (Hellsing and Hammarström, 1991). A low-calcium diet and lactation are associated with an increased rate of tooth movement, as a result of the decreased bone density (which is due to secondary hyperparathyroidism [Goldie and King, 1984] and consequent reversible bone loss [Karlsson et al., 2001]). In patients with transient osteopenia due to an increased bone turnover rate, it is of utmost importance to keep the force level as low as possible, and to distribute the stresses and the strains in the PDL uniformly, i.e. uncontrolled tipping should be avoided. Moreover, orthodontic checks should not simply focus on reactivation of the appliance but rather on the assessment of the proper line of action of the force to obtain the desired movement. Although the faster tooth movement is an advantage, the drawback is the resulting relapse, for which reason lifelong retention is recommended.

There has been an increase in the number of older people with metabolic diseases taking long-term medication. Adult patients often benefit from adjunctive orthodontic treatment as part of an interdisciplinary treatment approach, given that they have an adequate residual dentition and the health of the periodontium can be maintained. In such patients, bone metabolism should be regularly assessed by their physicians (Roberts, 1997).

Adult patients may also have osteopenia/osteoporosis. In an ovariectomy-induced osteoporotic rat model, tooth movement was found to be faster, with an increase in bone remodelling markers (Yamashiro et al., 1994). Since osteoporosis is bone loss resulting from a negative calcium balance, additional mechanical perturbation should be carefully considered. It has been suggested that orthodontic treatment in osteoporotic patients can increase the risk of undesirable alveolar bone and root resorption (Miyajima et al., 1996). The degree of osteopenia can be determined by evaluating bone mineral density and serum levels of bone markers. In such patients, the cost versus benefits of orthodontic treatment should be discussed with the patient's physician, especially if the patient is under pharmacological treatment.

Pharmacological treatment of osteoporosis may also influence tooth movement rates. Topical (Adachi et al., 1994; Igarashi et al., 1994; 1996) as well as systemic (Karras et al., 2009) administration of bisphosphonates in rats has been shown to result in a decrease in both the rate of tooth movement and relapse. Osteoporotic patients undergoing treatment with bisphosphonates can thus be expected to exhibit delayed orthodontic tooth movement. These findings, together with the osteonecrosis of the jaws found in a small percentage of patients undergoing bisphosphonate treatment for osteoporosis (Yoneda et al., 2010), indicate that orthodontic treatment in such patients should be cautiously performed. It has recently been suggested that the appropriateness of a 'drug holiday' should be discussed with the patient's physician to minimize adverse effects and optimize orthodontic treatment (Zahrowski, 2009). However, due to the extremely long duration of storage of bisphosphonates in bone, the usefulness of this approach in reducing the risk of potential complications is questionable.

Besides the rate of tooth movement, the risk of root resorption is also influenced by the general status of the skeleton. Osteoclasts resorb only mineralized surfaces. In diseases in which there is an increase in the relative amount of osteoid-covered surfaces, such as in Paget's disease, it is more likely that osteoclasts/odontoclasts will resorb the nearest mineralized areas instead, i.e. the root surface. This has been confirmed by the finding that rats with low bone remodelling rates show an increased amount of root resorption compared with those with high and normal turnover rates. However, application of an orthodontic force can cancel out these baseline differences (Verna et al., 2003). The presence of osteoid is also relatively increased in cases of fracture healing, and thus the callus requires an increase in the activation frequency of BMUs. It is not surprising that root resorption has been demonstrated in beagle dogs when teeth are actively moved into the regenerate immediately after distraction osteogenesis (Nakamoto et al., 2002). This is why it is advised not to commence orthodontic tooth movement straight after the active phase of rapid palatal expansion.

The impact of general bone turnover on the local tissue reaction to orthodontic forces emphasizes the importance of taking a thorough general history at the patient's first visit. In patients with a history of bone metabolic problems, the patient's physician should be contacted in order to evaluate the degree of medical control of the condition. These patients are mostly under medical control but, depending on the specific pathology, sufficient diagnostic data, such as serum or urine bone markers and bone mineral density, should be acquired from the physician. However, as previously mentioned, bone remodelling seems to be site specific, and general whole-body data may not reflect the local condition in the jaws. In the case of osteoporosis, a clear association between systemic osteoporosis and bone loss in the jaws has not been established, probably due to individual variations in loading, jaw anatomy, dental health status, and methodological differences among studies (Ejiri et al., 2008). Recently, cortical erosion and/or thickness noted at the inferior mandibular border on dental panoramic radiographs has been shown to be associated with low vertebral bone mineral density or osteoporosis (Taguchi et al., 2008). Dental practitioners could therefore be in a position to screen for osteoporosis at no additional expense.

Basic research in bone biology is increasingly focusing on the genetic markers that characterize the clinically observed individual variability. The field of orthodontics is also taking advantage of recent findings in attempts to identify individuals who will react differently to identical biomechanical systems, or to identify patients at risk for developing root resorption. The presence of one or more

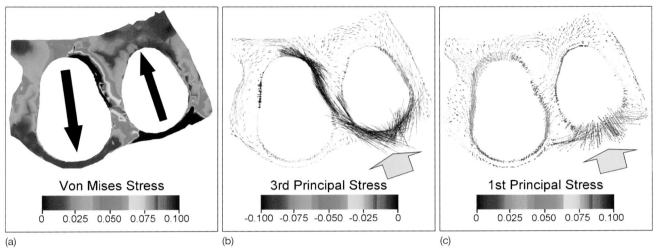

Figure 10.6 Finite element study of a canine and a premolar showing a coronal section of the alveolar bone when a tipping movement is simulated in the direction of the arrow, with material properties assumed to be non-linear. (a) Stress concentration, described by Von Mises stresses, show the lowest values in the direction of the force, while the contrary is observed on the opposite side. Compressive stresses are the lowest in the direction of the force (b), and tensile stresses (c) show an opposite trend. Note that compressive and tensile stresses are simultaneously present in the same area (yellow arrow). (From Cattaneo et al. [2005] with permission from SAGE.)

copies of allele 2 of interleukin (IL)1-β, collected from human cheek-wipe samples, has been associated with faster tooth movement (Iwasaki et al., 2009). The presence of allele 2 allows for greater production of IL1-β and for increased bone resorption, and therefore faster rates of tooth movement. The increase in bone resorption decreases the risk of root resorption in these patients (Al Qawasmi et al., 2003). According to Hartsfield (2009), around one-half to two-thirds of the variation observed among orthodontic patients with external apical root resorption is related to genetic factors.

Pressure and tension

Another lexical inconsistency in the description of the mechanical reaction to orthodontic force involves the terms pressure and tension. According to orthopaedists, the change in shape observed subsequent to loading in long bones is a result of apposition on the compressed side and resorption on the side on which tension prevails (Casagrande and Frost, 1953), as loading leads to positive bone balance, as is well known. It therefore seems contentious that the orthodontists associate compression with resorption, as postulated in the traditional pressure–tension theory. However, since the mechanical load is transferred to the alveolar bone through the PDL, it is, not appropriate to extrapolate the effects of the tensile and compressive strains in long bones to those occurring in the PDL.

A finite element (FE) study has also demonstrated that the transfer mechanism of orthodontic loads through the alveolar supporting structures cannot be explained in terms of compression and tension. Based on the low forces

used in orthodontic tooth movement and non-linear properties of the PDL, the FE model revealed that tension is by far more predominant than compression. On the 'pressure' side, the fibres of the PDL become curled up and practically no stresses are transferred onto the alveolar wall (Cattaneo et al., 2005) (Figure 10.6). Within the alveolar wall, the tensile stresses generated by the pulling of the PDL fibres are transformed into compressive hoop stresses as in a Roman arch, and tensile and compressive stresses coexist. Taking into account the findings of state-of-the-art research, orthodontists should avoid using the terms pressure and tension and relate the tissue reaction to the stress/strain distribution instead. This is, furthermore, in line with the biological fact that cells detect changes in load due to deformation, and cannot distinguish between pressure and tension. The word pressure is probably still pertinent in cases of high concentration of forces over small surfaces, where the blood pressure is overcome and the root surface is separated from alveolar bone only by hyalinized areas.

Bone adaptation to mechanical deformation and orthodontic tooth movement

A mechanical load induces a deformation, a change in shape, to which the skeleton has to adapt. The bone cells in charge of sensing the change in mechanical loading, i.e. deformation, are the osteocytes. According to the osteocyte plasticity hypothesis, the osteocyte is capable of 'normalizing' its local mechanical environment by modulating its cytoskeletal architecture, attachment to the matrix,

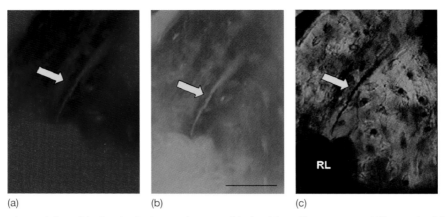

(a)   (b)   (c)

Figure 10.7 (a) A single microcrack (arrow) in the alveolar bone under green, (b) ultraviolet epifluorescence, and (c) transmitted light close to a resorption lacuna (RL) on the buccal treated side of a Danish land-race pig, at day 1. Bar = 50 μm. (From Verna et al. [2004] with permission from Oxford University Press.)

configuration of the peri-osteocytic space, and communication channels with the surrounding cells. Bonewald (2005) suggests that macroscopic strains of about 0.2% can be amplified more than 15 times at the osteocyte lacunar level. Strain patterns are highly heterogeneous, and in some locations adjacent to osteocyte lacunae they are similar to those observed in relation to microdamage. Microdamage increases with fatigue load at physiological levels and is associated with bone remodelling and osteocyte apoptosis (Verborgt et al., 2000; Noble, 2003).

Targeted bone remodelling seems to be initiated as a sign of elimination of damage, to rebuild new bone that is in equilibrium with the new mechanical demand. Since the tissue reaction induced by orthodontic loads mirrors the tissue repair to damage, the question arises whether the number of microcracks increase in the alveolar bone with orthodontic treatment. In an experimental investigation on 25 3-month-old Danish land-race pigs following a split mouth design, the lower molars were tipped buccally at different treatment time points and the development of microdamage assessed on day 1 and 2 after the application of the force (Figure 10.7). Microcracks may, therefore, be the first sites of bone damage induced by orthodontic forces to be repaired by bone remodelling (Verna et al., 2004). It therefore seems likely that the generation of microcracks by an orthodontic force is induced by overloading of bone, as the surface on which the forces are distributed is characterized by many small bony spicules. Osteocyte apoptosis following orthodontic force application has been described (Hamaya et al., 2002), but at present no studies have related it to the microcracks in the alveolar bone.

Orthopaedists associate bone strain with a change in cellular activities (effectiveness). The strain history of a bone is therefore the 'rheostat' modulating the occurrence of resorption and formation activities. In describing the response to mechanical usage of bone, Frost (2003)

defined four 'windows' according to the magnitude of bone strain.

- The acute disuse window, where remodelling increases up to five times and no modelling or RAP activities are present, for example the cases of resorption in edentulous crests.
- The adapted window, where BMUs equalize resorption and formation, and no modelling or RAP occurs. This mode tends to conserve bone and its strength, and occurs during normal mechanical usage. In dental terms, an example may be bone loading via the teeth during mastication.
- The mild overuse window, where lamellar drift usually occur with normal formation of BMUs, no RAP, and little microdamage. It is the usual mode of adaptation of bones to growth and to strain changes due to some dental implants.
- The pathological overload window, where microdamage occurs and BMUs increase in the repair process. Following fractures, surgical procedures, tooth extractions, implant positioning and periodontal disease, a RAP takes place.

If we apply this hypothesis to the reaction of the alveolar bone following the application of an orthodontic force, the direct resorption can be perceived as remodelling. With the curling of the PDL fibres during the frontal, direct resorption, no strain will be transferred to the alveolar bone when occlusal forces are applied to the teeth and the strain will be below the minimum effective strain (MES). The alveolar wall, therefore, senses a decreased mechanical load, as in the disuse window.

The orthodontic movement 'with bone' occurs when the strains are in the adapted and mild overload windows, with lamellar bone formation, and there is balance between bone resorption and formation. The woven bone commonly observed ahead of the tooth and on the periosteal surface (Reitan, 1967; Melsen, 1999; Verna et al., 1999b) can be considered as a RAP phenomenon, i.e. a healing process, occurring as a consequence of strain in the range of the overload window. Hyalinization of the PDL, ischaemia-induced necrosis of the lining cells, and micro-damage of the bone in the direction of the force frequently lead to increased BMU activation. In the light of the mechanical adaptation window, orthodontic tooth movement can be perceived as a bone adaptation to mechanical deformation that will result in different biological reactions, depending on the strain induced in the alveolar bone.

Bone reaction to skeletal anchorage

In orthopaedic surgery, screws are used to obtain mutual stability between different parts of a bone separated either due to a fracture or as part of a surgically planned correction. The rigid fixation allows for immediate function and thereby loading of the screws with controlled forces (Van Sickels and Richardson, 1996). The surgical screws are frequently connected by a mini-plate, whereby the loads acting on the screws are coordinated. This principle has also been applied within orthodontics, where transmucosal extensions of mini-plates fixed to the infrazygomatic crest or the basal bone of the mandible have been used as anchorage for both orthodontic tooth movement and in attempts to alter growth direction (De Clerck et al., 2002). The initial tissue reaction following insertion of single surgical screws or temporary anchorage devices (TADs) resembles that in permanent implant cases, as the primary stability is dependent on the design of the intraosseous part of the screw and on the type and quality of the bone into which the screw is inserted.

Like surgical screws, TADs are loaded directly or indirectly immediately following insertion. The loading generates a strain in the bone of the insertion site, which is dependent not only on the local bone, the cortical thickness and the trabecular bone density, but also on the morphology of the intraosseous part of the TAD and the applied load. According to Frost (1994), the strain will lead to a positive or a negative balance, which, in the first case, will lead to increased stability (so-called secondary stability) or, in the latter case, to loosening and loss of the screw. Dalstra et al. (2004) analyzed the relationship between strain values and different amounts of cortical thickness and trabecular density and found that in the case of cortical thickness of 1 mm or more, loosening of the mini-implants should not occur if the loading is perpendicular to the long axis. These calculations are based on an FE model of a segment of human jaw removed at autopsy and a 10 mm cylindrical implant with a 2 mm outer and a 1.2 mm inner diameter loaded with 50 cN perpendicular to the long axis (Figure 10.8). The morphology and the cut of the threading do, however, have a certain influence on these results, as shown in Figure 10.9.

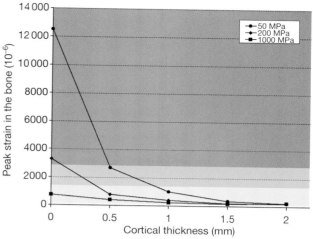

Figure 10.8 Relationship between cortical thickness, trabecular bone density expressed in megapascals, and strain values developed, when the head of the mini-implant was loaded with a 50 cN force perpendicular to the long axis. (From Dalstra et al. [2004] with permission of Quintessence.)

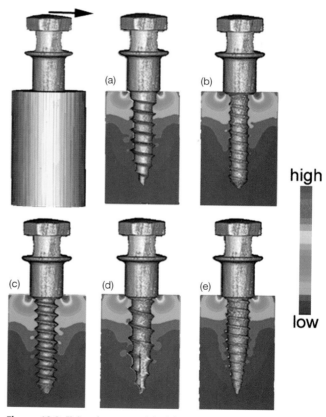

Figure 10.9 Finite element model of five different temporary anchorage devices loaded perpendicular to the long axis. Comparison of the stress intensity (von Mises stresses) distribution in the surrounding bone under force flexure loading for the Aarhus mini-screw ((Medicon, Germany) (a) and four hypothetical designs in which the threaded body was based on the Abso-Anchor (DENTOS, Daegu, Korea) (b), the MAS (Micerium S.p.A, Italy) (c), the Tomas (Dentaurum Group, Germany) (d). and the Vector (Ormco Corporation, California, USA) (e) mini-screws. Peak stresses are lowest in designs (a) and (d), suggesting that these devices can withstand the highest loading. (Courtesy of M Dalstra.)

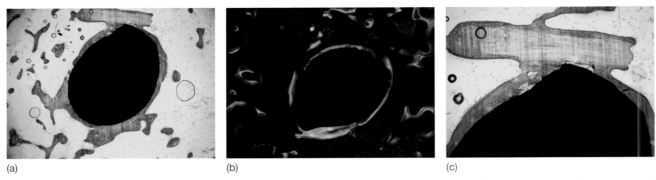

(a) (b) (c)

Figure 10.10 (a) Osseointegration of Aarhus mini-implant (a) 40× magnification. The bone adjacent to the mini-implant is composed of old lamellar bone and new woven bone. (b) The remodelling of the bone in contact with the mini-implant is reflected in the tetracycline labelling close to the mini-implant. (c) 100× magnification. Note the close contact between bone and implant.

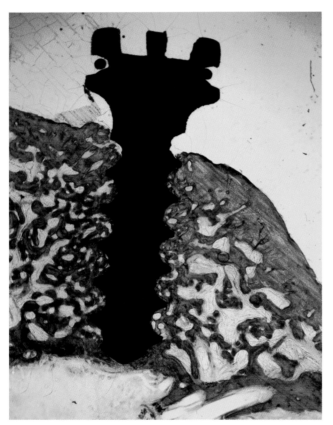

Figure 10.11 Mini-implant inserted into the infrazygomatic crest of a macaca rhesus monkey. Note the increased density of the bone 3 months after insertion.

Surgical screws and dental implants differ with regard to morphology and the preparation of the surface. Dental implants are intended to stay permanently in the alveolus and the surface treatment serves that purpose, as it increases the absolute surface and enhances the interaction of the cells and the surface (Elias and Meirelles, 2010). Surgical screws are machine polished and most frequently self-drilling. Dental implants are traditionally left unloaded

during the healing phase, although recent research has demonstrated that controlled loading can be applied in this period (Quinlan et al., 2005). In addition to the increase in osseointegration, a time-related significant increase in bone density was also observed during the first 3 months of loading (Figure 10.10) (Melsen and Costa, 2000).

Surgical screws are easy to remove but this does not mean that the screws are not osseointegrated. A certain percentage of the screw surface is in contact with bone even at magnifications of 100× (Figure 10.11). Whereas the bone to implant contact present immediately following insertion is the basis of the primary stability of the screw, secondary stability is a product of the strain generated adjacent to the screw. Over time the relative surface in contact with bone has been reported to be both unaltered and increased, which can be explained by differences in assessment techniques used or in data processing. When evaluating data on dogs and monkeys separately in each individual animal, Zhang et al. (2010) noted a strong tendency towards a time-related increase in osseointegration. Orthodontic loading does not seem to have an impact on the degree of osseointegration, as replacement of the bone supplying primary stability with newly formed, well-organized bone has been demonstrated in relation to both loaded and unloaded screws (Serra et al., 2010).

Histomorphometric analyses of the bone dynamics adjacent to the intraosseous parts of mini-implants have demonstrated a continuous increase in bone turnover identical to what has been described by Roberts et al. (1990) in relation to custom-made titanium implants in humans. This constant remodelling most likely reflects an adaptation of the differences in physical property of the bone and the implants. Osseointegration implies that screws cannot be used as temporary implants. They would submerge and cause periodontal damage to the adjacent teeth (Thilander et al., 2001). TADs, on the other hand, can be used to maintain the width and the density of the alveolar bone while waiting for cessation of growth (Figures 10.12 and 10.13). For such purposes, it is important to place the TADs

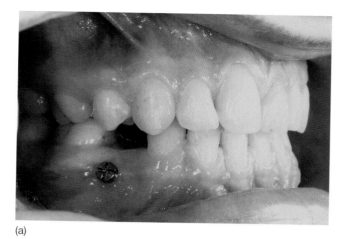

(a)

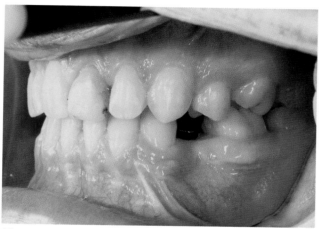

(b)

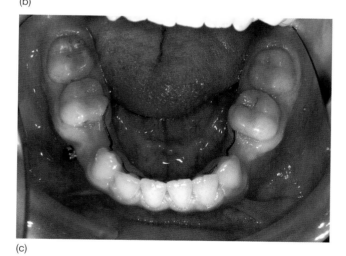

(c)

Figure 10.12 (a–c) Intraoral views in a patient with agenesis of all four lower and two upper premolars. On the right side of the lower arch the transcortical mini-implant that was used as anchorage for the mesial movement of the molar was left in place. Note that the thickness and the height of the alveolar bone has been maintained.

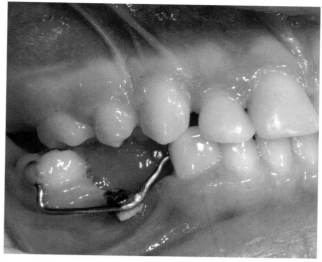

Figure 10.13 Intraoral view of another patient with agenesis of all four lower and two upper premolars. On the right side of the lower arch, a mini-implant, which was placed on the top of the alveolar process and used as anchorage for the mesial movement of the molar, was left in place. It can be seen that the eruption of molar was impeded whereas the adjacent teeth continued to erupt.

transcortically and not on top of the alveolar process as suggested by Schefler in an interview with Cacciafesta and colleagues (Cacciafesta et al., 2009).

Conclusions

So what can we learn from orthopaedists engaged in basic research?

- The tissue reaction in the jaws mirrors that of other parts of the skeleton when submitted to a variety of orthodontic forces.
- The modelling induced by tooth movement permits generation of alveolar bone thereby changing the outline of the alveolar process and allowing better conditions for occlusal rehabilitation.
- The general status of bone metabolism influences the rate and quality of tooth movement. The general health of the patient must be taken into consideration.
- As bone remodelling is patient and site related, the rate of tooth movement may differ between patients, even with the use of the same biomechanical systems.
- The strain in bone should be kept as low as possible to maintain the bone balance. The RAP phenomenon can be orthodontically induced and used to enhance bone formation.
- Skeletal anchorage units can be used as absolute anchorage and as a mean for the maintenance of alveolar bone width and density.

References

Adachi H, Igarashi K, Mitani H, et al. (1994) Effects of topical administration of a bisphosphonate (risedronate) on orthodontic tooth movements in rats. *Journal of Dental Research* 73: 1478–86.

Al Qawasmi RA, Hartsfield JK Jr, Everett ET, et al. (2003) Genetic predisposition to external apical root resorption in orthodontic patients: linkage of chromosome-18 marker. *Journal of Dental Research* 82: 356–60.

Arias OR, Marquez-Orozco MC (2006) Aspirin, acetaminophen, and ibuprofen: their effects on orthodontic tooth movement. *American Journal of Orthodontics and Dentofacial Orthopedics* 130: 364–70.

Ashcraft MB, Southard KA, Tolley EA (1992) The effect of corticosteroid-induced osteoporosis on orthodontic tooth movement. *American Journal of Orthodontics and Dentofacial Orthopedics* 102: 310–19.

Baron R (1975) Histophysiologie des reaction tissulaires au cours du deplacement orthodontique. In: M Chateau (ed.) *Orthopedie Dento-Faciale. Bases Fondamentales.* Paris: J Prelat.

Bartzela T, Turp JC, Motschall E, et al. (2009) Medication effects on the rate of orthodontic tooth movement: a systematic literature review. *American Journal of Orthodontics and Dentofacial Orthopedics* 135: 16–26.

Burr DB (1993) Remodeling and the repair of fatigue damage. *Calcified Tissue International* 53(Suppl 1): S75–S80.

Cacciafesta V, Bumann A, Cho HJ, et al. (2009) JCO Roundtable. Skeletal anchorage, part 2. *Journal of Clinical Orthodontics* 43: 365–78.

Casagrande PA, Frost HM (1953) *Fundamental of Clinical Orthopaedics.* New York, NY: Grune and Stratton.

Cattaneo PM, Dalstra M, Melsen B (2005) The finite element method: a tool to study orthodontic tooth movement. *Journal of Dental Research* 84: 428–33.

Chandler KB, Rongey WF (2005) Forced eruption: review and case reports. *General Dentistry* 53: 274–7.

Dalstra M, Cattaneo PM, Melsen B (2004) Load transfer of miniscrews for orthodontic anchorage. *Orthodontics* 1: 53–62.

Dalstra M, Cattaneo PM, Beckmann F (2006) Synchrotron radiation-based microtomography of alveolar support tissues. *Orthodontics and Craniofacial Research* 9: 199–205.

De Clerck H, Geerinckx V, Siciliano S (2002) The zygoma anchorage system. *Journal of Clinical Orthodontics* 36: 455–9.

Deguchi T, Takano-Yamamoto T, Yabuuchi T, et al. (2008) Histomorphometric evaluation of alveolar bone turnover between the maxilla and the mandible during experimental tooth movement in dogs. *American Journal of Orthodontics and Dentofacial Orthopedics* 133: 889–97.

Ejiri S, Tanaka M, Watanabe N, et al. (2008) Estrogen deficiency and its effect on the jaw bones. *Journal of Bone and Mineral Metabolism* 26: 409–15.

Elias CN, Meirelles L (2010) Improving osseointegration of dental implants. *Expert Review of Medical Devices* 7: 241–56.

Eriksen EF, Gundersen HJ, Melsen F, et al. (1984) Reconstruction of the formative site in iliac trabecular bone in 20 normal individuals employing a kinetic model for matrix and mineral apposition. *Metabolic Bone Diseases and Related Research* 5: 243–52.

Frost HM (1986) *Intermediary Organization of the Skeleton*, vol I, II. Boca Raton, FL: CRC Press.

Frost HM (1990) Skeletal structural adaptations to mechanical usage (SATMU): 1. Redefining Wolff's law: the bone modeling problem. *Anatomical Records* 226: 403–13.

Frost HM (1994) Wolff's Law and bone's structural adaptations to mechanical usage: an overview for clinicians. *Angle Orthodontist* 64: 175–88.

Frost HM (1998) A brief review for orthopedic surgeons: fatigue damage (microdamage) in bone (its determinants and clinical implications). *Journal of Orthopaedic Science* 3: 272–81.

Frost HM (2003) Bone's mechanostat: a 2003 update. *Anatomical Record. Part A, Discoveries in Molecular, Cellular, and Evolutionary Biology* 275: 1081–101.

Goldie RS, King GJ (1984) Root resorption and tooth movement in orthodontically treated, calcium-deficient, and lactating rats. *American Journal of Orthodontics* 85: 424–30.

Hamaya M, Mizoguchi I, Sakakura Y, et al. (2002) Cell death of osteocytes occurs in rat alveolar bone during experimental tooth movement. *Calcified Tissue International* 70: 117–26.

Hartsfield JK Jr (2009) Pathways in external apical root resorption associated with orthodontia. *Orthodontics and Craniofacial Research* 12: 236–42.

Hellsing E, Hammarström L (1991) The effects of pregnancy and fluoride on orthodontic tooth movements in rats. *European Journal of Orthodontics* 13: 223–30.

Igarashi K, Mitani H, Adachi H, et al. (1994) Anchorage and retentive effects of a bisphosphonate (AHBuBP) on tooth movements in rats. *American Journal of Orthodontics and Dentofacial Orthopedics* 106: 279–89.

Igarashi K, Adachi H, Mitani H, et al. (1996) Inhibitory effect of the topical administration of a bisphosphonate (risedronate) on root resorption incident to orthodontic tooth movement in rats. *Journal of Dental Research* 75: 1644–9.

Iwasaki LR, Chandler JR, Marx DB, et al. (2009) IL-1 gene polymorphisms, secretion in gingival crevicular fluid, and speed of human orthodontic tooth movement. *Orthodontics and Craniofacial Research* 12: 129–40.

Kalia S, Melsen B, Verna C (2004) Tissue reaction to orthodontic tooth movement in acute and chronic corticosteroid treatment. *Orthodontics and Craniofacial Research* 7: 26–34.

Kanzaki H, Chiba M, Shimizu Y, et al. (2002) Periodontal ligament cells under mechanical stress induce osteoclastogenesis by receptor activator of nuclear factor kappaB ligand up-regulation via prostaglandin E2 synthesis. *Journal of Bone and Mineral Research* 17: 210–20.

Kanzaki H, Chiba M, Takahashi I, et al. (2004) Local OPG gene transfer to periodontal tissue inhibits orthodontic tooth movement. *Journal of Dental Research* 83: 920–5.

Kanzaki H, Chiba M, Arai K, et al. (2006) Local RANKL gene transfer to the periodontal tissue accelerates orthodontic tooth movement. *Gene Therapy* 13: 678–85.

Karlsson C, Obrant KJ, Karlsson M (2001) Pregnancy and lactation confer reversible bone loss in humans. *Osteoporosis International* 12: 828–34.

Karras JC, Miller JR, Hodges JS, et al. (2009) Effect of alendronate on orthodontic tooth movement in rats. *American Journal of Orthodontics and Dentofacial Orthopedics* 136: 843–7.

Kim SJ, Park YG, Kang SG (2009) Effects of corticision on paradental remodeling in orthodontic tooth movement. *Angle Orthodontist* 79: 284–91.

King GJ, Keeling SD, Wronski TJ (1992) Histomorphological and chemical study of alveolar bone turnover in response to orthodontic tipping. In: DS Carlson, SA Goldstein (eds.) *Bone Biodynamics in Orthodontic and Orthopedic Treatment.* Ann Arbor, MI: Center for Human Growth and Development.

Krishnan V, Davidovitch Z (2006) The effect of drugs on orthodontic tooth movement. *Orthodontics and Craniofacial Research* 9: 163–71.

Mantzikos T, Shamus I (1999) Forced eruption and implant site development: an osteophysiologic response. *American Journal of Orthodontics and Dentofacial Orthopedics* 115: 583–91.

Melsen B (1999) Biological reaction of alveolar bone to orthodontic tooth movement. *Angle Orthodontist* 69: 131–8.

Melsen B, Costa A (2000) Immediate loading of implants used for orthodontic anchorage. *Clinical Orthodontics and Research* 3: 23–8.

Melsen B, Verna C (2000) A rational approach to orthodontic anchorage. *Progress in Orthodontics* 1: 10–22.

Melsen B, Garbo D (2004) Treating the 'impossible case' with the use of the Aarhus Anchorage System. *Journal of Orthodontics* 1: 13–20.

Miyajima K, Nagahara K, Iizuka T (1996) Orthodontic treatment for a patient after menopause. *Angle Orthodontist* 66: 173–8.

Mohri T, Hanada K, Osawa H (1991) Coupling of resorption and formation on bone remodeling sequence in orthodontic tooth movement: a histochemical study. *Journal of Bone and Mineral Metabolism* 9: 57–69.

Mori S, Burr DB (1993) Increased intracortical remodeling following fatigue damage. *Bone* 14: 103–9.

Nakamoto N, Nagasaka H, Daimaruya T, et al. (2002) Experimental tooth movement through mature and immature bone regenerates after distraction osteogenesis in dogs. *American Journal of Orthodontics and Dentofacial Orthopedics* 121: 385–95.

Noble B (2003) Bone microdamage and cell apoptosis. *European Cells and Materials* 6: 46–55.

Ogasawara T, Yoshimine Y, Kiyoshima T, et al. (2004) In situ expression of RANKL, RANK, osteoprotegerin and cytokines in osteoclasts of rat periodontal tissue. *Journal of Periodontal Research* 39: 42–9.

Oshiro T, Shiotani A, Shibasaki Y, et al. (2002) Osteoclast induction in periodontal tissue during experimental movement of incisors in osteoprotegerin-deficient mice. *Anatomical Records* 266: 218–25.

Quinlan P, Nummikoski P, Schenk R, et al. (2005) Immediate and early loading of SLA ITI single-tooth implants: an in vivo study. *International Journal of Oral and Maxillofacial Implants* 20: 360–70.

Reitan K (1967) Clinical and histologic observations on tooth movement during and after orthodontic treatment. *American Journal of Orthodontics* 53: 721–45.

Ricketts RM (1998) The wisdom of the bioprogressive philosophy. *Seminars in Orthodontics* 4: 201–9.

Roberts WE (1997) Adjunctive orthodontic therapy in adults over 50 years of age. Clinical management of compensated, partially edentulous malocclusion. *Journal of the Indiana Dental Association* 76: 33–8, 40.

Roberts WE, Helm FR, Marshall KJ, Gongloff RK (1990) Rigid endosseous implants for orthodontic and orthopaedic anchorage. *Angle Orthodontist* 59: 247–56.

Roblee RD, Bolding SL, Landers JM (2009) Surgically facilitated orthodontic therapy: a new tool for optimal interdisciplinary results. *Compendium of Continuing Education in Dentistry* 30: 264–75.

Sanjideh PA, Rossouw PE, Campbell PM, et al. (2010) Tooth movements in foxhounds after one or two alveolar corticotomies. *European Journal of Orthodontics* 32: 106–13.

Serra G, Morais LS, Elias CN, et al. (2010) Sequential bone healing of immediately loaded mini-implants: histomorphometric and fluorescence analysis. *American Journal of Orthodontics and Dentofacial Orthopedics* 137: 80–90.

Steineche T, Hauge E (2003) Normal structure and function of bone. In: HA Yuehuei, ML Kylie (eds) *Handbook of Histology Methods for Bone and Cartilage*. Totowa: Humana Press.

Taguchi A, Asano A, Ohtsuka M, et al. (2008) Observer performance in diagnosing osteoporosis by dental panoramic radiographs: results from the osteoporosis screening project in dentistry (OSPD). *Bone* 43: 209–13.

Tanne K, Nagataki T, Matsubara S, et al. (1990) Association between mechanical stress and bone remodeling. *Journal of the Osaka University Dental School* 30: 64–71.

Thilander B, Odman J, Lekholm U (2001) Orthodontic aspects of the use of oral implants in adolescents: a 10-year follow-up study. *European Journal of Orthodontics* 23: 715–31.

Van Sickels JE, Richardson DA (1996) Stability of orthognathic surgery: a review of rigid fixation. *British Journal of Maxillofacial Surgery* 34: 279–85.

Verborgt O, Gibson GJ, Schaffler MB (2000) Loss of osteocyte integrity in association with microdamage and bone remodeling after fatigue in vivo. *Journal of Bone and Mineral Research* 15: 60–7.

Verna C, Melsen B (2002) The biology of tooth movement. In: G Fiorelli, B Melsen (eds) *Biomechanics in orthodontics – Rel.1 on CD ROM*. Arezzo, Italy: Libra Ortodonzia.

Verna C, Melsen B, Melsen F (1999a) Differences in static cortical bone remodeling parameters in human mandible and iliac crest. *Bone* 25: 577–83.

Verna C, Zaffe D, Siciliani G (1999b) Histomorphometric study of bone reactions during orthodontic tooth movement in rats. *Bone* 24: 371–9.

Verna C, Dalstra M, Melsen B (2000) The rate and the type of orthodontic tooth movement is influenced by bone turnover in a rat model. *European Journal of Orthodontics* 22: 343–52.

Verna C, Dalstra M, Melsen B (2003) Bone turnover rate in rats does not influence root resorption induced by orthodontic treatment. *European Journal of Orthodontics* 25: 359–63.

Verna C, Dalstra M, Lee TC, et al. (2004) Microcracks in the alveolar bone following orthodontic tooth movement: a morphological and morphometric study. *European Journal of Orthodontics* 26: 459–67.

Verna C, Hartig L, Kalia S, et al. (2006) Influence of steroid drugs on orthodontically induced root resorption. *Orthodontics and Craniofacial Research* 9: 57–62.

von Bohl M, Maltha JC, Von Den Hoff JW, et al. (2004) Focal hyalinization during experimental tooth movement in beagle dogs. *American Journal of Orthodontics and Dentofacial Orthopedics* 125: 615–23.

Wang L, Lee W, Lei DL, et al. (2009) Tissue responses in corticotomy- and osteotomy-assisted tooth movements in rats: histology and immunostaining. *American Journal of Orthodontics and Dentofacial Orthopedics* 136: 770–1.

Wilcko MT, Wilcko WM, Pulver JJ, et al. (2009) Accelerated osteogenic orthodontics technique: a 1-stage surgically facilitated rapid orthodontic technique with alveolar augmentation. *Journal of Oral and Maxillofacial Surgery* 67: 2149–59.

Winkler DG, Sutherland MK, Geoghegan JC, et al. (2003) Osteocyte control of bone formation via sclerostin, a novel BMP antagonist. *EMBO Journal* 22: 6267–76.

Yamaguchi M (2009) RANK/RANKL/OPG during orthodontic tooth movement. *Orthodontics and Craniofacial Research* 12: 113–19.

Yamashiro T, Sakuda M, Takano-Yamamoto T (1994) Experimental tooth movement in ovariectomozed rats. *Journal of Dental Research* 73: 148.

Yoneda T, Hagino H, Sugimoto T, et al. (2010) Bisphosphonate-related osteonecrosis of the jaw: position paper from the Allied Task Force Committee of Japanese Society for Bone and Mineral Research, Japan Osteoporosis Society, Japanese Society of Periodontology, Japanese Society for Oral and Maxillofacial Radiology, and Japanese Society of Oral and Maxillofacial Surgeons. *Journal of Bone and Mineral Metabolism* 28: 365–83.

Zaffe D, Verna C (1995) Acid and alkaline phosphatase activities in rat's alveolar bone experimentally loaded by orthodontic forces. *Italian Journal of Mineral and Electrolyte Metabolism* 9(Suppl 1): 11.

Zahrowski JJ (2009) Optimizing orthodontic treatment in patients taking bisphosphonates for osteoporosis. *American Journal of Orthodontics and Dentofacial Orthopedics* 135: 361–74.

Zhang L, Zhao Z, Li Y, et al. (2010) Osseointegration of orthodontic micro-screws after immediate and early loading. *Angle Orthodontist* 80: 354–60.

11

When Should an Orthodontist Seek the Advice of an Endocrinologist?

Nadine G Haddad, Linda A DiMeglio

Summary

A variety of dental abnormalities should prompt referral to an endocrinologist. A single central incisor and/or delayed dentition and a small chin are suggestive of possible growth hormone deficiency and accompanying hypopituitarism. Alternatively, widely spaced teeth, an enlarged tongue, and a prominent lower jaw (which may be associated with significant tall stature) may indicate acromegaly/gigantism due to growth hormone excess. Delayed or premature eruption of teeth in association with symptoms of hypo- or hyperthyroidism, with or without an enlarged thyroid gland, should prompt an endocrine referral. A diagnosis of ossifying fibroma of the mandible or maxilla with hypercalcemia raises concerns for hyperparathyroidism-jaw tumor syndrome. Consultation with an endocrinologist should also be obtained if deciduous teeth are lost prematurely with the root of the tooth still intact, since this may be indicative of hypophosphatasia. Dental abscesses in association with rickets raise concerns about X-linked hypophosphatemic rickets, whereas radiodensity of the maxilla and/or mandible may be suggestive of osteopetrosis. Fibrous dysplasia of the maxilla or mandible may be a component of McCune–Albright syndrome. Patients with diabetes should be monitored closely for periodontal disease. Maintaining contact with an endocrinologist is important to optimize diabetes control as an important step in preventing gum disease. When a high-arched palate and crowded teeth are noted in a young girl with short stature and any other clinical characteristics of Turner syndrome, a referral to an endocrinologist should be made. In addition, hyperpigmented gingivae in a patient with unusual skin hyperpigmentation may be a sign of primary adrenal insufficiency.

Introduction

Much is now known about the influence of hormones on orthodontic treatment. Hormones exert their influences in a variety of ways: endocrine (hormones acting on remote tissues), paracrine (hormones acting on nearby tissues), and autocrine (hormones acting on the tissues that secrete them). Orthodontic tooth movement and bone remodeling are closely linked and depend on both systemic and local hormone actions. The modeling and remodeling necessary for orthodontic tooth movements are part of a continuous process where mature bone is removed (bone resorption) and new bone is formed (bone formation). Bone resorption and formation are dependent on hormones including parathyroid hormone (PTH), 1,25 (OH)$_2$ vitamin D, insulin-like growth factor 1 (IGF-1), and thyroid hormones.

Many endocrinological disorders have dental and oral manifestations as characteristic features. Recognizing these disorders is important in order to facilitate proper diagnosis and orthodontic therapy. This chapter is aimed at promoting communication between endocrinologists and orthodontists in the identification and management of growth- and bone metabolism-related endocrinopathies, and details the most common endocrine disorders with orthodontic or oral manifestations. Table 11.1 provides an overview of the conditions discussed in the chapter, their etiologies, and their main oral/dental manifestations.

Growth hormone deficiency

Growth hormone deficiency (GHD) can either be isolated or seen in conjunction with other pituitary hormone abnormalities. Growth hormone, which is produced by the pituitary gland under regulation by the hypothalamus, is necessary for normal growth and development in children and for maintaining proper body fat distribution, muscle and bone health in adults. GHD can be either congenital or

Table 11.1 Endocrine disorders with dental/oral manifestations

Condition	Etiology	Dental/oral manifestations
Growth hormone deficiency	Variable genetic etiology, most idiopathic	Delayed dentition, small mandible, midfacial hypoplasia, single central incisor
Acromegaly/gigantism	Most commonly due to a pituitary adenoma, can be seen in association with McCune–Albright syndrome and neurofibromatosis type 1	Widely spaced teeth, prominent lower jaw, crossbite, coarse facial features
Thyroid disease	Variable, congenital versus acquired	Delayed or premature eruption of teeth, gum disease, large tongue
Hyperparathyroidism-jaw tumor syndrome	HRPT2 gene mutations	Ossifying fibroma of the mandible or maxilla
Hypophosphatasia	ALPL gene mutations	Premature loss of primary teeth
Nutritional rickets	Associated with calcium, phosphate, or vitamin D deficiency	Enamel hypoplasia Delayed dentition Increased susceptibility for caries
1-α hydroxylase deficiency rickets	CYP27B1 mutations	Hypoplastic enamel with yellowish to brownish discoloration Large pulp chambers and short roots
X-linked hypophosphatemic rickets	PHEX gene mutations	Defective dentin leading to recurrent dental abscesses
Fibrous dysplasia	GNAS1 gene mutations	Well-defined radiolucent bony lesions with ground-glass appearance in maxilla or mandible
Diabetes	Type 1 diabetes is autoimmune mediated and polygenic, type 2 diabetes is associated with obesity and is polygenic; most genetic mechanisms responsible for both type 1 and type 2 diabetes are unknown	Gingivitis and periodontitis; the latter can lead to early tooth loss
Primary adrenal insufficiency	Variable, congenital versus acquired	Hyperpigmented gingivae
Turner syndrome	Complete or partial loss of one of the X chromosomes	High-arched palate, crowding of teeth, mandibular retrognathia

acquired. Although most instances of GHD are idiopathic, other causes include central nervous system (CNS) anatomical abnormalities involving the hypothalamic–pituitary axis, brain tumors, CNS surgery, trauma and infection, and radiation therapy to the brain.

Clinical and biochemical findings

GHD is commonly accompanied by delayed eruption of both primary and permanent teeth. Children with untreated GHD tend to have smaller facial heights and widths and smaller head circumferences than their age-matched peers (Segal et al., 2004). Growth hormone is necessary for both maxillary and mandibular growth, especially mandibular growth. Children with GHD tend to have a disparity in size between the mandible and maxilla and often exhibit a retrognathic mandible and crowding of teeth. The characteristic feature of GHD is linear growth delay. Laboratory findings include low insulin-like growth factor 1 (IGF-1 or somatomedin-C) level and low growth hormone levels on pharmacological stimulation testing. A referral to an endo-crinologist should be considered in a child with delayed dentition, a small jaw, or a single central incisor, especially if slow growth or short stature is noted.

Diagnosis

The diagnosis of GHD relies on clinical and biochemical features. When a diagnosis of GHD is made, brain magnetic resonance imaging (MRI) is usually performed to assess the pituitary gland and rule out an underlying CNS abnormality.

Management

Treatment of GHD is with growth hormone therapy given in the form of daily subcutaneous injections. Although this therapy does not affect tooth formation (Ito et al., 1993), it will impact the timing of orthodontic interventions. Therefore, it is important for the treating endocrinologist and orthodontist to maintain good communication. Growth hormone therapy increases facial height, with a lesser effect on facial width, and may affect jaw alignment

(Segal et al., 2004). Overtreatment with growth hormone can cause mandibular overgrowth. Orthodontic intervention when done in conjunction with growth hormone replacement therapy can resolve micrognathia associated with GHD to an extent. In a case report, Tsuboi et al. (2008) suggested that catch-up growth in the craniofacial structures (with increases in Z-scores) occurs alongside increases in stature during orthodontic treatment carried out concurrently with growth hormone therapy.

A single central incisor has also been described in isolated GHD and GHD in association with additional pituitary hormone deficiencies (Artman and Boyden, 1990; Hamilton et al., 1998). It is also the hallmark of the solitary median maxillary central incisor (SMMCI) syndrome (Hall, 2006), which is described in detail in Chapter 7. Thus, when a single central incisor is detected on examination, the treating dentist should elicit a history of short stature or growth delay and a referral to an endocrine clinic and craniofacial center should be considered for further investigations and management.

Growth hormone excess

Excessive pituitary production of growth hormone results in characteristic clinical features. In a growing child, the condition is referred to as gigantism and is associated with abnormally tall stature. When growth hormone excess develops in adulthood, the term acromegaly is used. The most common cause of gigantism and acromegaly is a pituitary adenoma, a benign tumor of the pituitary gland (Eugster and Pescovitz, 1999). Patients with suspected acromegaly, based on clinical features, should be referred to an endocrinologist.

Clinical features

Common facial features of acromegaly include a protruding lower jaw (prognathism) due to mandibular bone overgrowth, an enlarged tongue, coarse facial features with a prominent forehead, widening of the maxilla, widely spaced teeth and a skeletal Class III relationship (Figure 11.1). Additional features include significant tall stature, especially when the disease onset is in childhood, large hands and feet, excessive sweating, muscle weakness, and thick skin. When the tumor is large, compressive symptoms can result in headaches and visual disturbances.

Diagnosis

The diagnosis of growth hormone excess is made using a combination of baseline IGF-1 levels, the response of growth hormone levels to an oral glucose tolerance test, and pituitary imaging. Occasionally, enlargement of the sella turcica may be seen on skull films. Chang et al. (2005) described the case of a patient with gigantism due to a pituitary adenoma who presented to an orthodontic office for correction of anterior crossbite due to mandibular

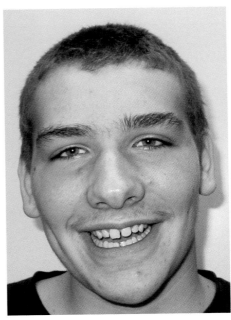

Figure 11.1 Widely spaced teeth, prominent lower jaw, and coarse facial features in a child with gigantism.

prognathism. Skull films demonstrated an enlarged sella turcica in all dimensions along with deepening of its floor in routine cephalometric analysis. Generally, however, diagnosis of pituitary tumor is based on MRI rather than plain X-ray analysis.

Treatment

Treatment may consist of resection of the pituitary lesion and/or therapy with somatostatin analogs. After the condition is under control, orthognathic surgery can be considered for correction of occlusion and profile. Patients need to be monitored for recurrence. Yagi et al. (2004) described a case of an acromegalic patient who had surgical–orthodontic correction after his acromegaly had been controlled with drugs for 5 years following a transsphenoidal hypophysectomy. Unfortunately, during the retention period, an MRI revealed recurrence of the lesion, resulting in higher IGF-1 levels and slight mandibular prognathic changes.

Thyroid disease

The thyroid gland produces two hormones, calcitonin and thyroxine. Calcitonin is a minor hormone in bone metabolism, which works opposite to PTH and decreases serum calcium levels. Calcitonin therapy has been reported to be useful for osteoporosis and giant cell granulomas of the jaw. However, its utility is limited due to possible allergic reactions and tachyphylaxis with multiple doses. No disease related to calcitonin excess or deficiency in humans has yet

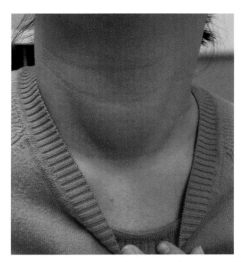

Figure 11.2 Enlarged thyroid gland (goiter) in a child with hyperthyroidism.

been described. Therefore, the remainder of this discussion will be about thyroid hormones.

Thyroxine (T_4) is a prohormone that is converted to its active form triiodothyronine (T_3). This active hormone influences the activity and metabolism of all cells, and it plays an important role in physical development and growth. Thyroid disease can be congenital or acquired. Most common etiology for acquired thyroid disease is autoimmune. Hashimoto thyroiditis is most commonly associated with hypothyroidism, whereas Graves disease is the most common cause of hyperthyroidism.

Both hypothyroidism and hyperthyroidism can affect dental health, as can the treatment for thyroid cancer. Persons with either hypo- or hyperhyroidism may also have a goiter (enlarged thyroid gland) palpable on examination (Figure 11.2), which should prompt a referral to an endocrinologist. Premature or delayed tooth eruption in a child should also alert the treating dentist to the possibility of thyroid disease.

Clinical findings

Common symptoms of hypothyroidism are fatigue, increased sleepiness, dry skin and brittle hair, cold intolerance, mild weight gain, and constipation. In children, growth may be slowed, depending on severity of hypothyroidism. Children with hypothyroidism may have a wide variety of dental problems, including malocclusion, delayed eruption of primary and permanent teeth, a prominent tongue and swollen gingivae, and an increased risk of caries and gingival disease. Adults with hypothyroidism may have an enlarged tongue, delayed postoperative wound healing, and defects in taste and smell.

Hyperthyroidism is associated with symptoms of weight loss, difficulty in sleeping, and a decline in school or work

performance. Bulging of the eyes (exophthalmos) is characteristic of Graves disease. Children with hyperthyroidism may experience premature tooth eruption. The most common forms of thyroid cancers are treated with high doses of radioactive iodine. This treatment can cause gingival pain and swelling, and increased salivation.

Diagnosis

The diagnosis of thyroid disease is made based on clinical and laboratory findings. The presence of a goiter, particularly with palpable nodularity, should prompt thyroid function testing (usually measurement of thyroid-stimulating hormone (TSH) and thyroxine levels [T_4 or free T_4]) and referral for endocrine evaluation. An elevated TSH level in association with low thyroxine levels is diagnostic of primary hypothyroidism whereas a low TSH level in association with an elevated thyroxine level usually indicates primary hyperthyroidism.

Management

Treatment of hypothyroidism is with thyroid hormone replacement. Treatment of hyperthyroidism depends on the etiology and may include radioactive iodine, antithyroid medications, and/or surgery. High levels of thyroxine (either from primary hyperthyroidism or from ingestion of too much thyroxine) may result in increases in osteoclastic activity and faster tooth movement rates (Shirazi et al., 1999). Close collaboration with an endocrinologist is preferred so that the thyroid hormone levels are monitored and controlled while orthodontic forces are applied for achieving optimal results.

Hyperparathyroidism-jaw tumor syndrome

Parathyroid hormone is secreted by the parathyroid glands and stimulates bone resorption, primarily through its effects on vitamin D metabolism. PTH also reduces renal clearance of calcium and increases intestinal calcium absorption. In primary hyperparathyroidism, autonomous production of PTH from the parathyroid glands leads to increased serum calcium levels. Secondary hyperparathyroidism is seen when PTH secretion is increased because of hypocalcemia. Orthodontic tooth movement can be stimulated by exogenous PTH in a dose-dependent manner when the jaw is exposed to continuous PTH, either by systemic infusion or by local delivery every other day in a slow-release formulation (Soma et al., 1999). Rarely, hyperparathyroidism can be associated with ossifying fibromas as part of the hyperparathyroidism-jaw tumor syndrome.

A painless mass in the mandible or maxilla could represent an ossifying fibroma, a benign fibrous tumor with local aggressive behavior. As mentioned above, ossifying fibromas are associated with the hyperparathyroidism-jaw tumor syndrome. This is a rare autosomal dominant syndrome caused by inactivating mutations of the tumor suppressor gene *HRPT2* (Carpten et al., 2002). It is characterized by multiple parathyroid tumors occurring at an early age. These tumors lead to development of hyperparathyroidism, and also ossifying fibromas of the mandible and/or maxilla, and less frequently, a variety of renal lesions and uterine tumors. When ossifying fibromas are suspected, a careful family history should be taken, focusing on history of hypercalcemia and hyperparathyroidism, which is important in making decisions regarding further investigations and management.

Clinical and biochemical findings

Symptoms of hypercalcemia are often subtle but include increased thirst and urination, nausea, vomiting, constipation, weakness, restlessness, confusion, and altered mental status. In hyperparathyroidism, serum calcium levels are elevated in association with low serum phosphorus levels. An ossifying fibroma presents as a bony, hard, non-tender mandibular swelling.

Diagnosis

Diagnosis is based on clinical, biochemical, radiological and histological findings. Radiographically, the lesions are either completely radiolucent or mixed, depending on the amount of calcification, or are completely radiopaque and surrounded by a radiolucent rim. In each type, there is a sclerotic border around the lesion. Histologically, the tumor consists of cementum-like or bony masses distributed in a highly cellular fibrous stroma.

Treatment

Ossifying fibromas are treated surgically. Large lesions, particularly of the maxilla, are often aggressive and require radical surgery. Small lesions can be treated with conservative excision. After curettage, nearly a third of mandibular lesions will recur. To minimize the likelihood of recurrence, en bloc or partial jaw resections are preferred. Gurol et al. (2001) reported successful orthognathic surgery following presurgical orthodontic treatment for correction of a retrognathic mandible in a 17-year-old girl with an ossifying fibroma.

Hypophosphatasia

Hypophosphatasia is a rare metabolic disease, with an estimated incidence of 1:100 000 (Mulivor et al., 1978). A history of premature tooth exfoliation should raise concerns for hypophosphatasia, which results from a mutation in the *ALPL* (alkaline phosphatase, liver/bone/kidney) gene encoding the tissue-nonspecific alkaline phosphatase enzyme (TNSALP) (Mornet and Simon-Bouy, 2004). TNSALP is important for normal bone and tooth mineralization. Five clinical forms are described: perinatal (lethal), infantile, childhood, adult, and odontohypophosphatasia. Children with the perinatal, infantile, and childhood forms can present with severe skeletal manifestations of under-mineralized bone, including frequent fractures. In odonto-hypophosphatasia, clinical manifestations are limited to the teeth. In a child with suspected hypophosphatasia, it is important for the dentist to inquire about a history of bone fractures or deformities and make an appropriate referral to an endocrinologist.

Clinical, radiological, and biochemical findings

Premature loss of deciduous teeth is a characteristic finding in the various forms of hypophosphatasia. The incisors tend to be the most commonly affected (Beumer et al., 1973). Premature tooth loss may result from quantitative and qualitative defects in cementum formation. Root resorption and enamel hypoplasia may also occur (Bruckner et al., 1962). Radiographic studies show enlarged pulp chambers and root canals with reduced cortical bone thickness of the mandible. Decreased cementum, varying with severity of the disease, is apparent on histological examination of the teeth. The deficiency of serum and bone alkaline phosphatase (ALP) activity leads to rickets and osteomalacia. Babies with the perinatal form are usually stillborn or die within few days of life. Patients with the infantile form develop clinical signs of hypophosphatasia during the first 6 months of life, including hypercalcemia with hypercalciuria. Premature craniosynostosis and respiratory problems due to rib fractures and rachitic deformities of the chest are common. Approximately 50% of those with the infantile form of hypophosphatasia will have spontaneous improvement in bone and dental symptoms with advancing age.

Childhood hypophosphatasia is the form that most commonly presents to the dentist due to premature loss of deciduous teeth (Chapple, 1993). Affected children present with skeletal deformities such as a dolichocephalic skull, widely opened fontanels, and rachitic skeletal changes. Delayed motor milestones, failure to thrive, and short stature are common. Hypercalcemia may not be present.

The adult form is rare and tends to be diagnosed in middle age. This milder form of hypophosphatasia needs to be distinguished from odontohypophosphatasia, since both can present with premature loss of teeth and have indistinguishable biochemical findings. Clinically, patients with the adult form present with recurrent and multiple long bone fractures and pseudofractures.

Diagnosis

Although formal diagnostic criteria are not established, all forms of hypophosphatasia share in common reduced activity of serum ALP and presence of mutations in the *ALPL* gene. The circulating concentration of pyridoxal-5'-phosphate (a substrate of the ALP enzyme) is increased and can be used as a marker of the disease (Whyte et al., 1985). The diagnosis is often made on the basis of clinical suspicion, relying on history, physical examination, and radiographic findings, in addition to demonstrating low serum ALP activity.

Management

Management of hypophosphatasia relies on supportive measures to minimize disease-related complications. There are currently no medical treatments for hypophosphatasia, although bone marrow transplants have been tried for the infantile forms and enzyme replacement trials are underway for the severe types. Dental interventions alone may be all that is needed and limited to the primary teeth. There has been one case report of a pediatric patient with hypophosphatasia and a posterior crossbite requiring palatal expansion along with total dentures, demonstrating a role for orthodontists in the management of anodontia due to hypophosphatasia (Altay et al., 1995).

Rachitic disorders

Vitamin D synthesis is a multistep process that starts both with the formation of cholecalciferol (vitamin D_3) in the skin from cholesterol, under the stimulus of ultraviolet B light, and with the absorption of vitamin D_2 and vitamin D_3 from plant and animal dietary sources or nutritional supplements. In the liver, vitamin D_2 and D_3 undergo 25-hydroxylation, producing 25(OH) vitamin D. A second hydroxylation occurs in the kidney at position 1 (via 1-α hydroxylase), forming the active metabolite $1,25(OH)_2$ vitamin D, which promotes intestinal absorption of calcium and phosphorus, increases renal phosphate reabsorption, and acts on bone to release calcium and phosphate. Deficiency states produce rickets and osteomalacia in children and adolescents, and osteomalacia in adults. Rickets and osteomalacia lead to softening and deformity of bones.

Rickets is the failure of osteoid to mineralize during the process of bony modeling when new bone forms at growth plates. Osteomalacia is the failure of bone to remineralize during bone remodeling. A child with rickets may present to the orthodontist with delayed development and emergence of the dentition, and enamel hypoplasia, particularly in association with poor weight gain or linear growth, and skeletal findings such as frontal bossing or bowing of the legs. If these findings are present, nutritional and genetic forms of rickets should be considered. In patients with recurrent unexplained dental abscesses, X-linked hypophosphatemic rickets should be a consideration. Affected patients have additional clinical and laboratory findings that help confirm this diagnosis. When rickets is suspected based on clinical findings, a referral to an endocrinologist should be made. The treating orthodontist should be aware of the effect of medical therapy on tooth development.

Clinical, radiological, and biochemical findings

Rickets can be associated with delayed tooth eruption, with deciduous incisors not appearing until 9 months of age and first molars not appearing before 14 months. The enamel

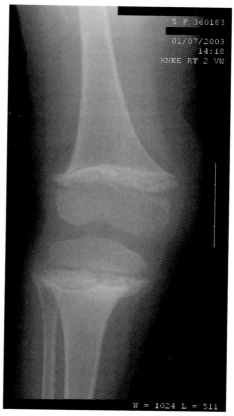

Figure 11.3 Radiographic findings in rickets: note the wide metaphyses with fraying of the bone.

may be hypoplastic, leading to greater susceptibility to caries (Wharton and Bishop, 2003). Clinical features of rickets include hypotonia, craniotabes (softening and thinning of the infant skull), frontal bossing, costochondral junction swelling (rachitic rosary), scoliosis, and bowing of the legs due to weight-bearing. Often the infant will have darker skin tone, a history of prolonged breastfeeding, and/or little cutaneous sun exposure. Characteristic X-ray findings include cupping, flaring, and splaying of the metaphyses (Figure 11.3). Nutritional rickets due to vitamin D deficiency is associated with low 25(OH) vitamin D levels, and elevated serum ALP and PTH levels. Low calcium and phosphate levels are also often seen. Similar laboratory findings are present in rickets due to calcium and phosphate deficiencies. However, 25(OH) vitamin D levels are normal in these states.

Diagnosis

The diagnosis of nutritional rickets due to vitamin D deficiency relies on clinical and biochemical findings, as detailed above.

Management

Depending on the form of rickets, medical therapy usually involves administration of vitamin D or one of its metabolites, which affect tooth development and orthodontic tooth movement. Kawakami and Takano-Yamamoto (2004) found that local application of 1,25 $(OH)_2$ vitamin D_3 to molar roots of rats increased mineral appositional rate on alveolar bone after orthodontic force application.

Nutritional rickets

Dietary deficiencies in calcium, phosphate, and/or vitamin D can result in rickets and osteomalacia. Treatment of nutritional rickets consists of replacement of the missing dietary components (Wharton and Bishop, 2003).

1-α hydroxylase deficiency

1-α hydroxylase deficiency is an autosomal recessive disease of vitamin D metabolism caused by mutations in the gene coding for p450c1α (Wang et al., 2002), the enzyme necessary for conversion of 25(OH) vitamin D to 1,25$(OH)_2$ vitamin D. Dental manifestations of 1-α hydroxylase deficiency include hypoplastic enamel that has a yellow to brown discoloration (Zambrano et al., 2003). Malocclusion, gingivitis, and periodontitis can be present. Radiographic findings include large tooth pulp chambers and short roots. Histological features include abnormal enamel matrix and dysplastic dentin. Laboratory findings include hypocalcemia with elevated PTH and ALP levels (Thomas and Demay, 2000). 25(OH) vitamin D concentrations are normal or high, while the concentrations of 1,25$(OH)_2$ vitamin D are low or undetectable.

In addition to features of rickets, patients with 1-α hydroxylase deficiency can have muscle weakness, seizures and tetany due to associated hypocalcemia. Diagnosis is made on the basis of clinical, laboratory, and radiological findings. Early diagnosis of 1-α hydroxylase deficiency is important to prevent major bone deformities and address dental abnormalities early. Treatment is with 1,25$(OH)_2$ vitamin D (calcitriol) replacement in physiological replacement doses.

X-linked hypophosphatemic rickets

X-linked hypophosphatemic rickets (XLH, formerly known as vitamin D-resistant rickets) is an X-linked dominant disease resulting from a mutation in *PHEX* (phosphate regulating gene with homologies to endopeptidases on the X-chromosome) (Dixon et al., 1998). XLH is one of the most common forms of rickets in developed countries, with an incidence of 1 in 20 000 persons (Tenenhouse and Scriver, 1992). XLH should be considered in the differential diagnosis of unusual dental abscesses (Seow, 2003).

In persons with XLH, chronic hypophosphatemia leads to defective mineralization of bone and teeth. Dental manifestations result from the defect in dentin mineralization. A large pulp chamber is common on dental radiographs. However, channels may form between the pulp chamber and dentinoenamel junction, which allow microorganisms to enter the pulp, with consequent formation of abscesses, particularly when the enamel is lost through attrition or caries.

Clinical manifestations of XLH include poor linear growth and lower extremity bowing that become more apparent at the time of weight-bearing and progress over time, leading to significant short stature. Frontal bossing and dolichocephaly can be present. Laboratory findings include hypophosphatemia, increased serum ALP, normal to low normal serum calcium, inappropriately normal to low normal 1,25$(OH)_2$ vitamin D, and normal to mildly increased PTH. The diagnosis of XLH is based on clinical and laboratory findings, and should be suspected in persons with a history of recurrent spontaneous idiopathic dental abscesses.

Medical management of XLH includes phosphate replacement and 1,25$(OH)_2$ vitamin D therapy to enhance calcium and phosphorus absorption. Treatment with phosphate and calcitriol helps to restore normal growth and to prevent or ameliorate deformities. Even with good compliance, many children and adults with XLH require orthopedic procedures to address limb deformities. The best treatment strategy for the dental manifestations of XLH is prevention of abscess formation. Good dental hygiene is recommended and prophylactic coverage of teeth with crowns may be advisable. Early treatment with 1,25 $(OH)_2$ vitamin D_3 has been shown to improve the dental status of children with XLH (Chaussain-Miller et al., 2003).

Osteopetrosis

The observation of radiodense bone on plain radiographs should raise suspicion of osteopetrosis, a rare, inherited bone disease with an overall incidence of 1 in 100 000–500 000 (Stark and Savarirayan, 2009). Osteopetrosis encompasses a group of heterogeneous conditions, ranging in severity from being fatal in infancy to asymptomatic. The more severe forms tend to have an autosomal recessive inheritance, while the milder forms are inherited in an autosomal dominant manner. Table 11.2 lists the different forms of osteopetrosis. Osteopetrosis results from defects in osteoclast function that leads to a decrease in bone resorption. The defect in bone turnover characteristically results in skeletal fragility despite increased bone mass.

Lack of osteoclastic activity and thereby bone remodeling is of concern in orthodontics. Children with the infantile forms of osteopetrosis have been reported to have dental issues including delays in tooth eruption, missing and malformed teeth, enamel hypoplasia, problems with dentinogenesis, mandibular protrusion, and odontomas (Luzzi et al., 2006). Those with dominant osteopetrosis have normal tooth eruption. Tooth removal in either condition should be handled conservatively, as such procedures can result in bony fractures and osteomyelitis.

Table 11.2 Clinical manifestations and genetic bases of the different forms of osteopetrosis

Osteopetrosis type	Mode of inheritance	Clinical features	Oral manifestations
Infantile	Autosomal recessive	Diagnosed in infancy. Presenting features include failure to thrive, growth retardation, and nasal stuffiness due to sinus malformation. Pancytopenia due to bone marrow failure is present. Cranial nerve entrapment may lead to deafness and blindness. Hydrocephalus may be present	Delayed dentition, osteomyelitis of the mandible, increased bone density on plain X-ray
intermediate	Autosomal recessive	Clinical features appear before age 10 years. Features are similar to the infantile form but are less severe.	Same as infantile form
Adult onset Type 1	Autosomal dominant	Diagnosed in late adolescence or adulthood. Characterized by marked sclerosis of cranial vault, normal serum acid phosphatase level, and low risk of fractures	None other than bony sclerosis
Adult onset Type 2	Autosomal dominant	Diagnosed in late adolescence or adulthood. Many obligate carriers are asymptomatic. Those affected may have the following: – Sclerosis of the cranial base – Endobones (see Figure 11.4) – High risk of fractures – Neuropathies due to cranial nerve entrapment – Compromised bone marrow function – Elevated serum tartrate-resistant acid phosphatase (TRAP) and creatine kinase (CK)-BB	Osteomyelitis of the mandible in 10% of patients, increased bone density on plain X-ray

Clinical, radiological, and biochemical findings

Oral and facial manifestations of osteopetrosis include facial growth anomalies, altered mineralization of bone, increased radiodensity of the maxilla and mandible, malformed teeth, unerupted teeth, delayed development of the dentition, early tooth exfoliation, and ankylosed teeth. Recurrent osteomyelitis of the mandible is a serious complication that commonly occurs in patients with the autosomal recessive form and in approximately 10% of patients with the autosomal dominant form. It results from an abnormal blood supply to the bones. Affected infants with recessive osteopetrosis fail to grow and gain weight. Nasal stuffiness due to sinus malformation is often the presenting feature. Neuropathies related to cranial nerve entrapment occur due to failure of skull foramina to widen completely. These entrapments may result in deafness and visual loss. Defective bone tissue tends to replace bone marrow, causing bone marrow failure. As a result, patients develop anemia, thrombocytopenia with resultant easy bruising and bleeding, and leukopenia with recurrent infections. Bone pain and fractures are common. Osteomyelitis of the maxilla or mandible typically occurs in older adults (Waguespack et al., 2007).

Radiographic findings in osteopetrosis include osteosclerosis. Bones may be uniformly sclerotic, or sclerotic areas may alternate with lucent bands. Sometimes 'endobones' (bones within bones) are seen (Figure 11.4). In the autosomal dominant form, only two-thirds of persons with *CLCN-7* mutations express any manifestations of the disease. Of those who are affected, severity ranges widely from severely affected individuals to those in whom the diagnosis is made incidentally because of radiological abnormalities. High serum levels of tartrate-resistant acid

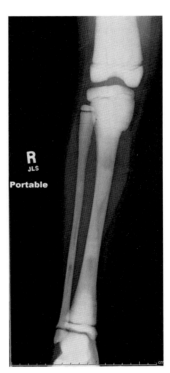

Figure 11.4 Tibial X-ray of a 10-year-old girl with osteopetrosis demonstrating extensive cortical sclerosis, endobones, and Erlenmeyer flask deformities of metaphyses.

phosphatase (TRAP) and the BB isoenzyme of creatine kinase (CK-BB) are detected in patients with osteopetrosis, and can differentiate carriers from affected individuals (Waguespack et al., 2002).

Diagnosis

The diagnosis of osteopetrosis is based on clinical, laboratory, and radiographic findings. Family history is also informative in dominant cases.

Management

Treatment for infantile osteopetrosis is primarily supportive of hypercalcemia and anemia followed by bone marrow transplantation at an experienced center (Mazzolari et al., 2009). Treatment of dominant osteopetrosis is generally supportive, and consists of orthopedic management of fractures, neurosurgical intervention for cranial nerve entrapments, and iron supplementation and/or transfusions, if needed for anemia. Other therapies have been tried but remain experimental. Large doses of $1,25(OH)_2$ vitamin D, along with restricted calcium intake, have been reported to improve osteopetrosis in a few selected cases (Key et al., 1984). $1,25(OH)_2$ vitamin D may help by stimulating osteoclastic bone resorption. However, clinical improvement is not sustained after therapy is discontinued. Treatment with gamma interferon, which improves white blood cell function and thereby decreases the incidence of new infections, has also been reported to produce long-term benefits. Bone marrow transplantation has also been performed for severe cases, and is the treatment of choice for the recessive, infantile forms.

Fibrous dysplasia

Fibrous dysplasia is a skeletal developmental anomaly of the bone-forming mesenchyme that manifests as a defect in osteoblastic differentiation and maturation, resulting in destruction and replacement of normal bone with fibrous bone tissue (Whyte, 1999). Gingival swelling and/or facial asymmetry may be representative of craniofacial fibrous dysplasia. Fibrous dysplasia generally presents in childhood, usually between the ages of 3 and 15 years. When this diagnosis is made, a referral to the endocrine clinic should be undertaken to evaluate for possible associated endocrinopathies as part of the McCune–Albright syndrome, which classically is a triad of polyostotic fibrous dysplasia, hyperpigmented skin patches called café-au-lait macules, and hyperfunction of one or more endocrine systems. Recognizing other clinical features of the McCune–Albright syndrome in persons with craniofacial fibrous dysplasia is important for making the correct diagnosis and targeting therapy.

Fibrous dysplasia and the McCune–Albright syndrome are caused by post-zygotically acquired activating mutations of *GNAS1*, the gene encoding the α subunit of the stimulatory G-protein, a major mediator of several hormone receptors (Shenker et al., 1994). The mutations lead to constitutive activation of receptors in affected tissues, independent of ligand binding, resulting in bony lesions and endocrine hyperfunction. The extent of clinical manifestations depends on the onset and extent of tissue distribution of the mutations during embryogenesis.

Clinical, radiological, and biochemical findings

Fibrous lesions in bones often result in pain, fracture, and/or deformity. Lesions can be limited to one bone (monostotic) or can be multifocal (involving multiple bones – polyostotic). The long bones and ribs are typically involved. Craniofacial fibrous dysplasia of the skull most commonly affects the mandible and maxilla, with an equal likelihood of disease in either location (Dhiravai-Angkura et al., 1994).

Radiologically, fibrous dysplasia lesions are well defined and are characterized by thin cortices and a ground-glass appearance resulting from calcification of fibrous tissue and bone formation. Occasionally, these lesions are lobulated with trabeculated areas of radiolucency. Painless bone swelling is the most common presenting symptom, with approximately a quarter of patients presenting with painful lesions. Lesions can slowly expand and cause facial asymmetry (Figure 11.5). In children, fibrous dysplasia lesions can affect tooth eruption by direct destruction of tooth buds. Tooth rotation and displacement may also be seen, depending on the location and extension of the lesion. Lesions affecting the maxilla often infiltrate and can obliterate the maxillary sinus and cause the line of the floor of the maxillary sinus to disappear on cephalometric radiographs (Araki et al., 1995). Mandibular lesions commonly invade the buccal and buccolingual areas (Dhiravai-Angkura et al., 1994).

Serum bone markers in fibrous dysplasia are usually unremarkable. ALP activity and markers of bone remodeling may be sometimes elevated (Chapurlat et al., 1997)

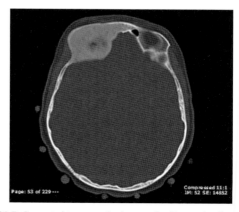

Figure 11.5 Computed tomography image of a fibrous dysplasia lesion of the maxilla presenting as a periorbital protuberance in an 8-year-old child.

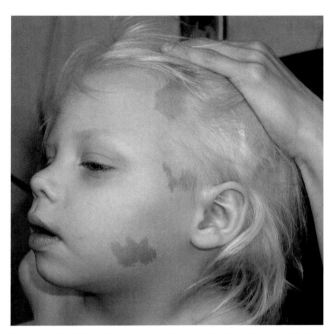

Figure 11.6 Café-au-lait macules in McCune–Albright syndrome with characteristic irregular borders.

although calcium and phosphorus levels tend to be normal. Endocrine testing might show endocrine hyperfunction such as hyperparathyroidism, growth hormone and cortisol excess, and hyperprolactinemia. Hyperthyroidism may be present and a multinodular goiter can be visualized on ultrasonography. A low serum phosphorus level in association with phosphaturia may also be present.

Precocious puberty is common in girls with McCune–Albright syndrome, resulting from development of estrogen-secreting ovarian cysts. Less commonly, hyperthyroidism, cortisol and growth hormone excess, and hyperprolactinemia may be present. The café-au-lait macules associated with McCune–Albright syndrome have a typical appearance and distribution. Lesions have irregular borders, follow dermatomal distributions and, generally, do not cross the midline (Figure 11.6).

Diagnosis

When fibrous dysplasia is diagnosed, the treating physician should have a high level of suspicion for associated McCune–Albright syndrome. Thus, a careful examination of the skin for café-au-lait macules and endocrine testing is recommended for all patients with fibrous dysplasia since McCune–Albright syndrome can be overlooked. In a study of nine patients with fibrous dysplasia, five were found to have café-au-lait pigmentation and three had abnormal thyroid levels. One patient had hyperthyroidism requiring thyroidectomy (Hannon et al., 2003). Routine diagnostic aids used by orthodontists are very valuable in diagnosis of the lesions. The panoramic radiograph will show the asym-

metry and heterogenic structure of the bone with areas of 'ground glass'.

Management

There is no established medical treatment for the skeletal disease of fibrous dysplasia. In patients with mild disease, lesions tend to remain unchanged over time. In those with severe disease, lesions may progress and new lesions may develop. Patients with progressive bone lesions tend to develop significant deformities of the long bones and skull and have recurrent fractures. Bisphosphonates may decrease bone pain in some patients, but do not affect the natural history of the bony lesions (DiMeglio, 2007). Treatment of endocrine manifestations depends on the endocrine system involved and extent of clinical findings.

A diagnosis of fibrous dysplasia of the skull commands periodic observation. In general, orthodontic treatments should be postponed until after puberty, since lesions are less likely to change much during adulthood. Occasionally, when lesion overgrowth impairs function, earlier surgical excision may be warranted. Most patients who undergo orthodontic therapy do not experience satisfactory results, with frequent relapses requiring subsequent re-treatments (Akintoye et al., 2003). Close collaboration with an endocrinologist is warranted to decide when to intervene for orthodontic problems in children and adults with fibrous dysplasia.

Diabetes

Diabetes is defined by high blood glucose levels due to either insulin deficiency or resistance to insulin action. Signs and symptoms of diabetes include polydipsia, polyuria, and weight loss. The two most common forms are type 1 and type 2 diabetes. Type 1 diabetes, formerly known as juvenile diabetes results from autoimmune destruction of insulin-producing islet cells of the pancreas. The onset of type 1 diabetes is usually in childhood and treatment is with insulin and nutritional therapy. Type 2 diabetes is characterized by insulin resistance and relative insulin deficiency, and is the form of diabetes linked to obesity. The incidence of both type 1 and type 2 diabetes is increasing, and with the rise in obesity in children, type 2 diabetes in particular is increasing in prevalence in children and adolescents. Poor vascular circulation, decreased immunity, and high glucose levels in saliva, all in association with poorly controlled diabetes, can increase susceptibility to gingival as well as periodontal infections (Iacopino, 2001). This risk may be further increased in the presence of smoking and poor dental hygiene.

Clinical findings

Individuals with uncontrolled diabetes are prone to develop periodontal disease. Gingivitis is an initial presentation, manifesting as erythematous and swollen gingivae that tend to bleed easily and separate from the teeth. If left untreated, this can progress to periodontitis and can lead to tooth loss.

Management

Maintenance of good diabetes control is important to prevent periodontal disease. Good oral hygiene, avoiding smoking and frequent dental check-ups are essential for preventing gingival disease. Type 2 diabetes is generally initially managed with increasing exercise and dietary modification if the hyperglycemia is mild but as the condition progresses medical intervention in the form of oral hypoglycemic agents or insulin therapy is generally necessary. Poorly controlled diabetic patients are poor candidates for orthodontic treatment as the mechanical force applied might lead to exaggerated tissue response and tooth mobility. Moreover, periodontal support in these patients is always compromised. Close collaboration with endocrinologists is warranted in these situations, so that the disease is under control throughout the course of orthodontic treatment.

Adrenal disorders

Primary adrenal insufficiency (PAI) results when the adrenal gland is not able to produce cortisol and aldosterone. The most common cause is autoimmune adrenal gland destruction (Addison disease) followed by tuberculosis infection (Ten et al., 2001). The presence of hyperpigmented oral mucosa in combination with unusual skin hyperpigmentation should alert the treating dentist to the possibility of PAI.

Clinical and biochemical findings

Persons with chronic adrenal insufficiency have a variety of symptoms, including fatigue, anorexia, weight loss, abdominal pain, nausea, vomiting, and/or weakness. Patients have increased skin pigmentation, particularly within scars (Figure 11.7) and areas unexposed to the sun, such as the areolae, palmar creases, and axillae. Pigmentary lines in the gingiva are also present. Symptoms of hypoglycemia and hypotension may be present. Laboratory findings include hyponatremia and hyperkalemia, due to mineralocorticoid deficiency. Characteristic laboratory findings include low serum sodium and high potassium in combination with a low cortisol and elevated adrenocorticotropic hormone (ACTH) levels.

Diagnosis

Diagnosis of PAI is based on clinical and biochemical findings.

Treatment

Treatment of PAI is with oral glucocorticoid and mineralocorticoid replacement. Of note, special care should be pro-

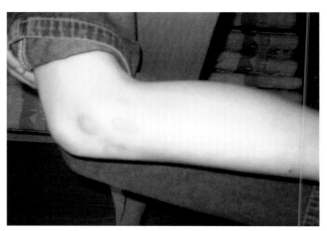

Figure 11.7 Hyperpigmented scars in a child with primary adrenal insufficiency.

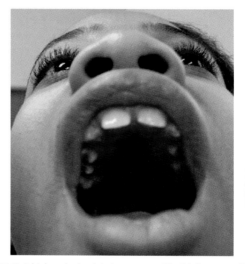

Figure 11.8 A high-arched palate in a young girl with Turner syndrome.

vided to patients with established adrenal insufficiency requiring orthodontic treatment since in times of stress or illness they must increase their glucocorticoid replacement dosage to mimic normal physiological responses. Again, consulting with an endocrinologist prior to surgery is an essential part of management of these individuals, since surgical procedures (and other stresses) require an increase in glucocorticoid dosage.

Turner syndrome

Turner syndrome is the result of complete or partial loss of one of the X chromosomes and should be suspected in girls and women with high-arched palates and crowding of the teeth (Figure 11.8). The presence of additional facial features such as epicanthal folds, low-set ears, proptosis, a webbed neck or a short neck with a low posterior hair line should prompt confirmatory evaluation. Since nearly all untreated girls and women with Turner syndrome have short stature, assessment of height and growth patterns is also important in establishing the diagnosis (Sybert and McCauley, 2004).

Clinical and radiological findings

In addition to short stature, girls with Turner syndrome also usually have premature ovarian failure, leading initially to failure to go through normal puberty and later infertility. Premature ovarian failure results from rapid oocyte apoptosis and fibrosis of the ovaries. Short stature is partially due to the loss of one copy of the *SHOX* (short stature homeobox gene) gene on the X chromosome. This particular gene is important for long-bone growth. Linear growth is slow during childhood and adolescence, resulting in adult heights of 143–145 cm (approximately 4 feet 8 inches). Additional clinical features that may be present include a wide carrying angle (cubitus valgus), short fourth and fifth metacarpals, Madelung deformity of the wrist, and a shield chest with widely spaced nipples. Some of these skeletal manifestations are due to loss of *SHOX*. Congenital heart defects (specifically coarctation of the aorta and aortic stenosis) and kidney abnormalities (such as horseshoe kidney) are common findings.

Girls with Turner syndrome often have a high-arched palate as well as cephalometric features that differ from those of other family members (mothers and sisters). These features include: shortened posterior cranial base length; shorter distance between the sella and the palate, glenoid fossa, and gonion; and shorter mandibular length and the presence of mandibular retrognathia (Perkiömäki et al., 2005).

Diagnosis

The diagnosis of Turner syndrome is based on clinical findings and chromosomal analysis.

Management

Height is improved with growth hormone therapy. Final adult height can be increased by several inches if growth hormone treatment is given relatively early in childhood. Most girls require estrogen replacement at the time of puberty to induce or complete pubertal development.

Orthodontic treatment for girls with Turner syndrome is influenced by the craniofacial characteristics of the syndrome as well as the rate and timing of craniofacial growth. Orthodontic treatment plans may need to incorporate: antibiotic prophylaxis if the patient has associated cardiac anomalies; occlusal adjustments for altered dental morphology; changes in timing of therapies in order to accommodate differences in growth and progress towards puberty;

and consideration of effects of growth hormone therapy (Russell, 2001). Close collaboration with the treating endocrinologist, cardiologist, and geneticist is warranted to prevent any untoward effects during the course of treatment.

Conclusions

The initial step in collaboration with endocrinologists starts with understanding basic concepts of hormonal actions and their effects on dental development. This will enable dentists and orthodontists to diagnose and co-manage several endocrine and metabolic bone diseases in which dental findings can be a presenting sign. Making a correct diagnosis is important to target therapy and prevent long-term sequelae of untreated endocrine and metabolic bone disease. If a disorder is suspected, referral to an endocrinologist can help confirm or refute the diagnosis. Once the endocrine disorder is under control, generally orthodontic treatment can proceed, with continued close collaboration with the treating endocrinologist for maximizing treatment effectiveness and preventing any untoward effects.

References

Akintoye SO, Lee JS, Feimster T, et al. (2003) Dental characteristics of fibrous dysplasia and McCune-Albright syndrome. *Oral Surgery, Oral Medicine, Oral Pathology, Oral Radiology and Endodontics* 96: 275–82.

Altay AN, Kocadereli I, Atar G (1995) Palatal expansion with a total denture. *Journal of Clinical Pediatric Dentistry* 19: 251–3.

Araki M, Hashimoto K, Sawada K, et al. (1995) Radiographic appearance of fibrous dysplasia associated with the maxillary sinus. *Oral Radiology* 11: 23–30.

Artman HG, Boyden E (1990) Microphthalmia with single central incisor and hypopituitarism. *Journal of Medical Genetics* 27: 192–3.

Beumer J, Trowbridge HO, Silverman S Jr, et al. (1973) Childhood hypophosphatasia and the premature loss of teeth. A clinical and laboratory study of seven cases. *Oral Surgery, Oral Medicine, Oral Pathology* 35: 631–40.

Bruckner RJ, Rickles NH, Porter DR (1962) Hypophosphatasia with premature shedding of teeth and aplasia of cementum. *Oral Surgery, Oral Medicine, Oral Pathology* 15: 1351–69.

Carpten JD, Robbins CM, Villablanca A, et al. (2002) HRPT2, encoding parafibromin, is mutated in hyperparathyroidism-jaw tumor syndrome. *Nature Genetics* 32: 676–80.

Chang H, Tseng Y, Chou T (2005) An enlarged sella turcica on cephalometric radiograph. *Dentomaxillofacial Radiology* 34: 308–12.

Chapple IL (1993) Hypophosphatasia: dental aspects and mode of inheritance. *Journal of Clinical Periodontology* 20: 615–22.

Chapurlat RD, Delmas PD, Liens D, et al. (1997) Long-term effects of intravenous pamidronate in fibrous dysplasia of bone. *Journal of Bone and Mineral Research* 12: 1746–52.

Chaussain-Miller C, Sinding C, Wolikow M, et al. (2003) Dental abnormalities in patients with familial hypophosphatemic vitamin D-resistant rickets: prevention by early treatment with 1-hydroxyvitamin D. *Journal of Pediatrics* 142: 324–31.

Dhiravai-Angkura P, Cholitgul W, Chai-U-Dom O (1994) Clinieo-radiological study of fifty cases of fibrous dysplasia in the jaw bones. *Oral Radiology* 2: 95–102.

DiMeglio LA (2007) Bisphosphonate therapy for fibrous dysplasia. *Pediatric Endocrinology Reviews* 4(Suppl 4): 440–5.

Dixon PH, Christie PT, Wooding C, et al. (1998) Mutational analysis of PHEX gene in X-linked hypophosphatemia. *Journal of Clinical Endocrinology and Metabolism* 83: 3615–23.

Eugster EA, Pescovitz OH (1999) Gigantism. *Journal of Clinical Endocrinology and Metabolism* 84: 4379–84.

Gurol M, Uckan S, Guler N, et al. (2001) Surgical and reconstructive treatment of a large ossifying fibroma of the mandible in a retrognathic patient. *Journal of Oral and Maxillofacial Surgery* 59: 1097–100.

Hall R (2006) Solitary median maxillary central incisor (SMMCI) syndrome. *Orphanet Journal of Rare Diseases* 1: 12.

Hamilton J, Blaser S, Daneman D (1998) MR imaging in idiopathic growth hormone deficiency. *American Journal of Neuroradiology* 19: 1609–15.

Hannon TS, Noonan K, Steinmetz R, et al. (2003) Is McCune-Albright syndrome overlooked in subjects with fibrous dysplasia of bone? *Journal of Pediatrics* 142: 532–8.

Iacopino AM (2001) Periodontitis and diabetes interrelationships: role of inflammation. *Annals of Peridontology* 6: 125–37.

Ito RK, Vig KW, Garn SM, et al. (1993) The influence of growth hormone (rhGH) therapy on tooth formation in idiopathic short statured children. *American Journal of Orthodontics and Dentofacial Orthopedics* 103: 358–64.

Kawakami M, Takano-Yamamoto T (2004) Local injection of 1,25-dihydroxyvitamin D3 enhanced bone formation for tooth stabilization after experimental tooth movement in rats. *Journal of Bone and Mineral Metabolism* 22: 541–6.

Key L, Carnes D, Cole S, et al. (1984) Treatment of congenital osteopetrosis with high-dose calcitriol. *New England Journal of Medicine* 310: 409–15.

Luzzi V, Consoli G, Daryanaani V, et al. (2006) Malignant infantile osteopetrosis: dental effects in paediatric patients. Case reports. *European Journal of Pediatric Dentistry* 7: 39–44.

Mazzolari E, Forino C, Razza A, et al. (2009) A single-center experience in 20 patients with infantile malignant osteopetrosis. *American Journal of Hematology* 84: 473–9.

Mornet E, Simon-Bouy B (2004) Genetique de l'hypophosphatasie. *Archives de Pediatrie* 11: 444–8.

Mulivor RA, Mennuti M, Zackai EH, et al. (1978) Prenatal diagnosis of hypophosphatasia; genetic, biochemical, and clinical studies. *American Journal of Human Genetics* 30: 271–82.

Perkiömäki MR, Kyrkanides S, Niinimaa A, et al. (2005) The relationship of distinct craniofacial features between Turner syndrome females and their parents. *European Journal of Orthodontics* 27: 48–52.

Russell KA (2001) Orthodontic treatment for patients with Turner syndrome. *American Journal of Orthodontics and Dentofacial Orthopedics* 120: 314–22.

Segal DG, Pescovitz OH, Schaefer GB, et al. (2004) Craniofacial and acral growth responses in growth hormone-deficient children treated with growth hormone. *Journal of Pediatrics* 144: 437–43.

Seow WK (2003) Diagnosis and management of unusual dental abscesses in children. *Australian Dental Journal* 48: 156–68.

Shenker A, Weinstein LS, Sweet DE, et al. (1994) An activating Gs alpha mutation is present in fibrous dysplasia of bone in the McCune-Albright syndrome. *Journal of Clinical Endocrinology and Metabolism* 79: 750–5.

Shirazi M, Dehpour AR, Jafari F (1999) The effect of thyroid hormone on orthodontic tooth movement in rats. *Journal of Clinical Pediatric Dentistry* 23: 259–64.

Soma S, Iwamoto M, Higuchi Y, et al. (1999) Effects of continuous infusion of PTH on experimental tooth movement in rats. *Journal of Bone and Mineral Research* 14: 546–54.

Stark Z, Savarirayan R (2009) Osteopetrosis. *Orphanet Journal of Rare Diseases* 4: 5.

Sybert VP, McCauley E (2004) Turner's syndrome. *New England Journal of Medicine* 351: 1227–38.

Ten S, New M, Maclaren N (2001) Clinical review 130: Addison's disease 2001. *Journal of Clinical Endocrinology and Metabolism* 86: 2909–22.

Tenenhouse HS, Scriver CR (1992) X-linked hypophosphatemia. A phenotype in search of a cause. *International Journal of Biochemistry* 24: 685–91.

Thomas MK, Demay MB (2000) Vitamin D deficiency and disorders of vitamin D metabolism. *Endocrinology and Metabolism Clinics of North America* 29: 611–27.

Tsuboi Y, Yamashiro T, Ando R, et al. (2008) Evaluation of catch-up growth from orthodontic treatment and supplemental growth hormone therapy by using Z-scores. *American Journal of Orthodontics and Dentofacial Orthopedics* 133: 450–8.

Waguespack SG, Hui SL, White KE, et al. (2002) Measurement of tartrate-resistant acid phosphatase and the brain isoenzyme of creatine kinase accurately diagnoses type II autosomal dominant osteopetrosis but does not identify gene carriers. *Journal of Clinical Endocrinology and Metabolism* 87: 2212–17.

Waguespack SG, Hui SL, DiMeglio LA, et al. (2007) Autosomal dominant osteopetrosis: clinical severity and natural history of 94 subjects with a chloride channel 7 gene mutation. *Journal of Clinical Endocrinology and Metabolism* 92: 771–8.

Wang X, Zhang MY, Miller WL, et al. (2002) Novel gene mutations in patients with 1alpha-hydroxylase deficiency that confer partial enzyme activity in vitro. *Journal of Clinical Endocrinology and Metabolism* 87: 2424–30.

Wharton B, Bishop N (2003) Rickets. *Lancet* 362: 1389–400.

Whyte MP (1999) Fibrous dysplasia. In: MJ Favus (ed.) *Primer on the Metabolic Bone Diseases and Disorders of Mineral Metabolism*, 4th edn. Philadelphia, PA: Lippincott Williams & Wilkins, pp. 384–6.

Whyte MP, Mahuren JD, Vrabel LA, et al. (1985) Markedly increased circulating pyridoxal-5′-phosphate levels in hypophosphatasia. Alkaline phosphatase acts in vitamin B6 metabolism. *Journal of Clinical Investigation* 76: 752–6.

Yagi T, Kawakami M, Takada K (2004) Surgical orthodontic correction of acromegaly with mandibular prognathism. *Angle Orthodontist* 74: 125–31.

Zambrano M, Nikitakis NG, Sanchez-Quevedo MC, et al. (2003) Oral and dental manifestations of vitamin D-dependent rickets type I: report of a pediatric case. *Oral Surgery Oral Medicine Oral Pathology Oral Radiology and Endodontics* 95: 705–9.

12

The Benefits of Consulting with an Ear, Nose, and Throat (ENT) Specialist Before and During Orthodontic Treatment

Joseph G Ghafari, Anthony T Macari

Summary

The mouth is anatomically at the center of the region in which the otolaryngologist/head and neck surgeon operates. Thus, many interactions between the ear, nose, and throat (ENT) specialist and the orthodontist become natural and often necessary. In this chapter, the anatomical relations between the mouth, nose, ear, and throat are reviewed. The areas of interaction include conditions that usually involve only the orthodontist and the ENT specialist (such as airway obstruction, temporomandibular dysfunction, and possibly conductive hearing loss), or both of them in the context of a cooperative team in the treatment of craniofacial anomalies. Most prominent among conditions requiring interaction is airway obstruction and its consequent effects on facial morphology and function. The evidence for early adenoidectomy and/or tonsillectomy is emerging from recent studies; however, specific guidelines are yet to be formulated. Conductive hearing loss may be improved by maxillary expansion but focused research should validate this potential. Ear pain is a ground for cooperation, particularly when the temporomandibular joint is affected. In the context of a working team, treatment of cleft lip/palate and other craniofacial anomalies engages both specialists at various stages of interventions that usually span the growing years of the patient.

Introduction

The obvious reason for the important interaction between the orthodontist and the otolaryngologist is the critical position of the mouth between the nose and throat. In as much as the jaws extend laterally, the connection extends to the areas of the ears. The scope of interaction between dentists in general and ENT specialists is summarized with respect to each of these anatomical entities in Box 12.1, with the more focused interface with the orthodontists specifically indicated. Certain problems benefit from consultation with the ENT specialist before orthodontic treatment (malocclusions associated with mouth breathing), while others would require consultation before and during treatment (cleft lip/palate).

The anatomical connection: the mouth in its relation with the nose, throat, and ear

Normal anatomy

The posterior boundary of the oral cavity comprises two pairs of folds of mucous membrane that cover two palatal muscles, the palatoglossus and the palatopharyngeus (Figure 12.1a). The tonsil lies between these folds, which provide the contour of an opening, the exit from the oral cavity (fauces) to the pharyngeal area. The nasal cavity, extending from the nostrils anteriorly to the choanae posteriorly, is divided into halves by the septum, which is formed by the perpendicular plate of the ethmoid bone above, the vomer bone posteriorly, and by an extensive cartilage anteriorly (Figure 12.1b). The roof of each nasal cavity is formed by the cribriform plate of the ethmoid bone, through which olfactory nerves enter the nasal cavity. The most important features of the lateral walls are the three bony shelf-like conchae or turbinates, which are covered with highly vascular mucous membranes (Figure 12.1c). Air is heated and humidified past the conchae during breathing. Beneath each concha is a meatus that

Integrated Clinical Orthodontics, First Edition. Edited by Vinod Krishnan, Ze'ev Davidovitch.
© 2012 Blackwell Publishing Ltd. Published 2012 by Blackwell Publishing Ltd.

Box 12.1 Conditions of potential interaction between ENT specialist and dentists in head and neck areas

Mouth and jaws
Related to function and facial esthetics
- Cleft palate and cleft lip[a]

Not related to facial esthetics
- Cold sores
- Periodontal (gum) disease
- Oral ulcers
- Tongue problems
- Halitosis or bad breath
- Temporomandibular dysfunction (TMD)

Nose
Related to breathing
- Adenoids[a]
- Turbinates[a]
- Septum[a]
- Hay fever
- Polyps
- Sinusitis

Not related to breathing
- Cosmetic surgery-rhinoplasty

Ear
Related to potential effect of maxillary expansion on Eustachian tube
- Conductive hearing

Related to pain and oral function
- Ear ache (possibly from TMD)

Throat
Related to breathing
- Tonsils[a]
- Infections

[a]Most common areas of interaction between orthodontist and otolaryngologist.

opens the nasal cavity to the paranasal sinuses and the nasolacrimal duct.

The paranasal sinuses are membrane-lined cavities within the frontal, maxillary, ethmoid, and sphenoid bones (Figure 12.1d). The ethmoid sinus comprises a series of small, interconnected air cells instead of a single hollow space. The sinuses communicate with the nasal cavity at the level of the superior and middle meatuses and lateral walls of the cavity, but not through the inferior meatus in which the nasolacrimal duct opens. Thus tears produced in the eye by the lacrimal (and other) glands are collected into this duct and enter the nasal cavities. Not well known, the function of the paranasal sinuses has been subject to various hypotheses: lightening the housing bones, acting as resonance chambers during speaking (increasing voice resonance), buffering against blows to the face, humidifying and heating the inhaled air, or as we suggest, being part of the oropharyngeal capsular matrix (as defined by Moss, 1969, 1997a,b) to which the adjacent structures adapt to

maintain the functional primacy of the matrix (see section on Growth concepts below).

Common sources of anomalies in the oronasal area

Particularly in children, hypertrophy of the adenoids and tonsils is a primary cause of nasal airway obstruction, leading to mouth breathing, which, in turn, may affect facial morphology. Located in the roof of the nasopharynx, anterior to the basiocciput and inferior to the sphenoid, the adenoids are a mass of lymphoid tissue that merges with the lymphoid tissue of the fossa of Rosenmuller near the opening of the Eustachian tube, which connects to the ear. Development of the adenoids is unique among major tissues of the body: they increase in size to a peak of approximately 200% the adult size around puberty then decrease to near-total regression in most adults (Scammon et al., 1930; Linder-Aronson and Leighton, 1983). The nasopharynx enlarges to accommodate the growing adenoids, thus maintaining a patent nasopharyngeal airway (Diamond, 1980) but any imbalance between the developing airway and the concomitant adenoid growth may result in nasopharyngeal obstruction or reduced potency (Diamond, 1980). Also, some reports indicate that the lymphoid tissues do not follow a specific growth curve, but respond individually to different environmental factors (Pruzansky, 1975). Given their critical anatomical position, hypertrophied adenoids may affect nasal function as well as obstruct the Eustachian tubes, participating in the formation of middle ear effusions. Tonsillar hypertrophy may also lead to airway obstruction. In the rare condition when tonsils touch or meet in the midline, they are called 'kissing tonsils'.

The tonsils (palatine or faucial tonsils) and the adenoids (pharyngeal tonsils) are part of Waldeyer's tonsillar ring (or pharyngeal lymphoid ring), named after a nineteenth-century German anatomist. The ring also includes the tubal tonsil, where the Eustachian tube opens in the nasopharynx and the lingual tonsils. As the tonsils and adenoids are located at the gate of the upper respiratory and alimentary tracts, where they are constantly exposed to antigens, they are mostly composed of immunologically reactive lymphoid tissue containing antibody-producing lymphocytes. A number of observations and findings may be noted regarding the associated immunological role (Hata et al., 1996; Valtonen et al., 2000; Kaygusuz et al., 2009):

- Adenoids and tonsils are related to a sounder immune status and general health of patients, carrying out the functions of humoral and cellular immunity.
- Inflammation and/or hypertrophy of adenoids and tonsils are caused by hypofunction of local and systemic immunity.
- There is not enough evidence to corroborate the suggestion that the adenoids and tonsils become a health liabil-

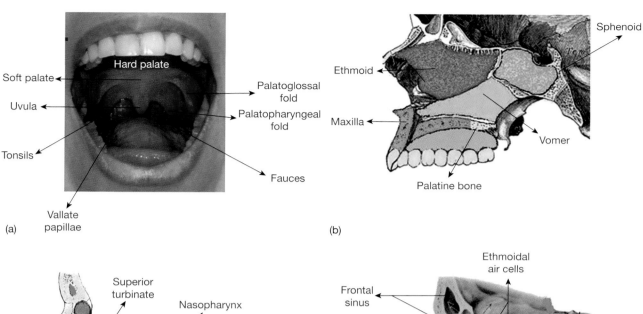

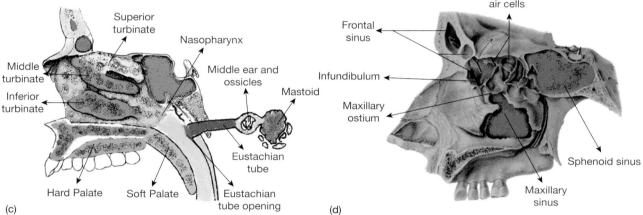

Figure 12.1 Anatomical structures in mouth and face: (a) oral and pharyngeal soft tissues; (b–d) sagittal cross-sections through oral and nasal hard tissues near-midline (b), lateral (c) and through nasal and paranasal sinuses (d). (Figure d is adapted from Moore K (1992) Chapter 7, 'The Head', Figure 7, in Clinically Oriented Anatomy, 3rd edn. Courtesy of Lippincott, Williams & Wilkins.)

ity because they may not be able to cope with the various viral infections attacking children in urban areas.

• Though still debated, particularly regarding the timing of surgery relative to patient's age, more recent findings indicate that removal of the lymphoid tissues has no adverse effect on immunity.

As alluded to in the list above, tonsils and/or adenoids present a health problem when they become the nest of continuous infections and cause airway obstruction. Not only does the blockage induce mouth breathing, but also a nasal twang to the voice, snoring, restless sleep (and associated learning problems if chronic), and facial dysmorphology. Hence, reasons for adenoidectomy often include chronic and recurrent fluid or infections of the ears, chronic or recurrent sinus infections or 'rhinosinusitis', and nasopharyngeal blockage. Because tonsillar infection is rarely associated with ear infections, tonsillectomy is usually indicated when tonsils are enlarged.

Often conducted with the assistance of a small mirror and completed on average within 15–20 minutes, adenoid-ectomy involves 'shaving' or curetting the adenoid tissue from the back of the nose. Usually low-grade bleeding is eliminated by cauterization. Though rare, surgical complications include infection of the surgical site (a source of bad breath), minor bleeding, and infrequently velopharyngeal insufficiency, possibly related to neglect of anatomical considerations. Postsurgical pain is more pronounced with tonsillectomy.

Areas of interaction

Airway obstruction

Effect on facial and occlusal morphology

The impact of airway impairment on dentofacial morphology has been evaluated extensively (Emslie et al., 1952; Linder-Aronson, 1970; Subtelny, 1975; Linder-Aronson et al., 1986; Behlfelt et al., 1989a,b, 1990; Kerr et al., 1989; Warren, 1990; Tourné, 1991; Woodside et al., 1991a,b; Linder-Aronson et al., 1993; Oulis et al., 1994; Valera et al., 2003; Mattar et al., 2004). In his pioneering work on definition of malocclusion, Edward Angle (1907) emphasized the consideration of not only the 'peculiarities' of the occlusion, and the relations of the jaws, but also the 'condition of the throat and nose [and] habits of the patient'. In a revealing way, Angle accounted for mouth breathing in his classification of two opposite malocclusions. He described the Class II division 1 malocclusion as 'always accompanied and, at least in its early stages, aggravated, if not indeed caused by mouth breathing due to some form of nasal obstruction'. Also, regarding the etiology of Class III, his only explanation was that: 'deformities under this class begin at about the age of the eruption of the first permanent molars, or even much earlier, and are always associated at this age with enlarged tonsils and the habit of protruding the mandible, the latter probably affording relief in breathing'.

Though Angle's specific premises, formulated before the advent of cephalometrics, still require focused study, the prevailing theory regarding the effects of nasal obstruction stipulates that ensuing chronic oral respiration becomes the etiology of occlusal and skeletal deformities. Children with chronic mouth breathing have often been found to have narrow maxillary dental arches (Subtelny, 1975; Oulis et al., 1994), anterior open bite, usually through excessive eruption of posterior teeth and a hyperdivergent skeletal pattern (Subtelny, 1975). Development of malocclusion seems to be related primarily to low posturing of the tongue (and the subsequent adaptation of other facial muscles) that may influence growth of the jaws and the occlusion. The lips, in repose, have been described to part (Subtelny, 1975), although nasal breathing is possible with incompetent lips when the tongue provides an anterior seal (Hepper et al., 1990).

Airway obstruction has been mostly associated with adenoid hypertrophy, and thus the use of the term 'adenoid facies' (apparently coined over 100 years ago (Proffit, 2007), synonymous with 'long face syndrome' (Tomes, 1872; Angle, 1907; Hershey et al., 1976) and 'high-angle' facial pattern. Children who need adenoidectomy have been reported to have longer facial height, steeper mandibular plane angles, and a more retrognathic mandible than corresponding controls (Linder-Aronson, 1970; Linder-Aronson et al., 1986, 1993; Kerr et al., 1989; Woodside et al., 1991a,b). Likewise, children with enlarged tonsils have been reported with more retrognathic and posterosuperiorly inclined mandibles, greater anterior total and lower facial heights, and increased mandibular plane angles (Behlfelt et al., 1989a).

Methods of evaluating airway obstruction

Tonsillar hypertrophy is more readily diagnosed clinically and its cephalometric determination is mostly corroborative (Figure 12.2a). Cephalometric imaging and the more

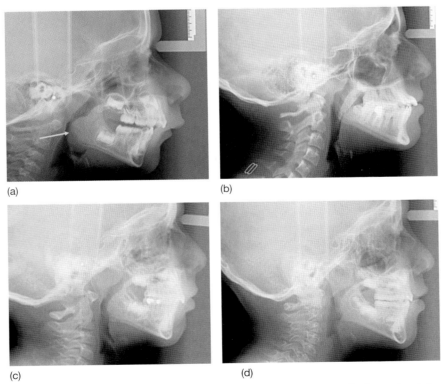

(a)

(b)

(c)

(d)

Figure 12.2 (a) Enlarged tonsils (arrow) on lateral cephalogram. The tonsil extends posteriorly and inferiorly. (b–d) Lateral cephalograms of three children with chronic mouth breathing showing different grades of airway obstruction relative to adenoid size: (b) grade 1 (less than 50% obstruction of airway) in a girl aged 12 years and 3 months; (c) grade 2 (more than 50% obstruction but less than 100% airway obstruction) in a boy aged 4 years and 4 months; and (d) grade 3 (total obstruction) in a boy aged 4 years and 9 months.

intrusive endoscopic examination are more reliable in the diagnosis of adenoid hypertrophy. Cephalometric assessment of palatal airway may be through subjective rating or direct measurement of defined distances.

- Various grading systems are available based on direct observation of the adenoid within the pharyngeal space. One such system stratifies three grades by estimating the space the adenoid occupies between the posterior cranial base and the soft palate:
  —Grade 1 – less than 50% of the airway is blocked
  —Grade 2 – more than 50% but less than 100% of airway is obstructed
  —Grade 3 – a near-total to total obstruction is observed (Figure 12.2b–d).
- The adenoids have been evaluated from a two-dimensional cephalometric record that simplifies the imaging of three-dimensional structures. Cephalometric assessment has been reported to have moderate to high correlations with the diagnosis of actual obstruction (r 0.60–0.88) by endoscopic evaluation or actual size of excised lymphoid tissue (Major et al., 2006). Measurements of the shortest distance between adenoid and soft palate (SAD), and the distance between the maximum convexity point and soft palate (CAD) have correlated best with actual size (Figure 12.3).

In a study of the correspondence among and between subjective and linear measurements of palatal airway on lateral cephalographs, Bitar et al. (2010) found a high correlation between SAD and CAD (r 0.915), and moderate to high correlations between the palatal airway grading (1–3) and SAD and CAD measurements (r −0.73 and −0.79, respectively), accounting for correspondence of evaluation in more than 50% of the population.

Developing technologies should improve imaging and appraisal of hypertrophied tissues and their proportionate relations to the nasal passages. When cephalometric adenoid rating is negative, the ENT specialist may resort to other means of assessment (endoscopy) to investigate other obstructive causes (e.g. enlarged turbinates).

The determination of mouth breathing is often based on subjective reporting by the patient or parents, usually incorporated in the health history questionnaire, with inquiry on respiratory mode during the day and at night. The high correlation observed in the aforementioned study between the subjective ratings, commonly utilized by otolaryngologists and the cephalometric measurement of airway clearance (SAD, CAD), indicates the significance of the radiographic record. Three-dimensional imaging of nasopharyngeal space and structures yields more accurate information (Grauer et al., 2009), but its potential association with mouth breathing requires quantitative assessments of respiration. Various means to generate objective evidence, such as rhinometry, nasal flow, and nasal resistance, have yet to be proven effective or practical

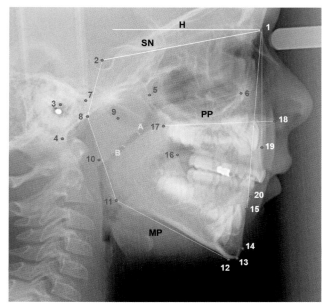

Figure 12.3 Cephalometric landmarks, planes, and measurements in study of craniofacial morphology related to adenoid hypertrophy. Linear measurements of the palatal airway (between the adenoids and soft palate). 'A' is the distance between most convex contour of the adenoid and soft palate (CAD); and 'B' is the shortest distance between adenoid and soft palate (SAD). Various hard tissue landmarks (1-20) were used for linear and angular measurements. Key findings included the increased posteroinferior inclination of the palatal plane (PP) relative to the horizontal (H) oriented on natural head position, augmented hyperdivergence between PP and MP (mandibular plane through Me and Go), as well as increased angle between MP and SN.

for determining or predicting mouth breathing. New devices need additional validation (Fujimoto et al., 2009; Ovsenik, 2009). The variety in frequency, duration, and intensity of mouth breathing is probably the reason for variation in outcome of these quantitative measurements. Yet, objective measures are preferable to simply subjective reports or assessments.

Time and sequence of the effect of obstruction on facial alterations

In a recent study (Bitar et al., 2010), we analyzed the cephalographs of 200 Caucasian children (ages 1.71–12.62 years, nearly 50% of them <5 years). They were diagnosed as chronic mouth breathers by the pediatric otolaryngologist who referred them for cephalometric appraisal of adenoid hypertrophy. Facial dysmorphology was observed as early as the second year of life in the youngest patient evaluated (1.71 years). Posteroinferior tilt of the maxilla (average inclination of palatal plane to horizontal: −7.68° ± 3.44°; norm: 0° ± 2.5° (Ricketts, 1981), possibly the initial response to functional alteration, occurred separately or together with one or all of the following modifications, compatible with a hyperdivergent vertical pattern: increased palatal

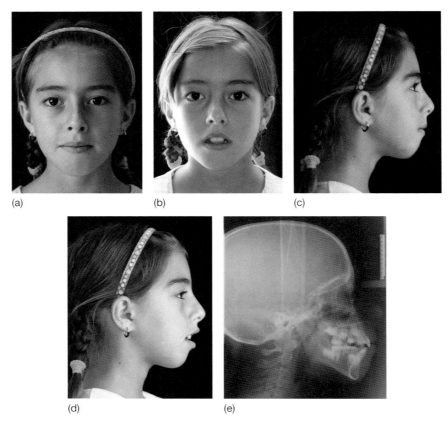

(a) (b) (c)

(d) (e)

Figure 12.4 Morphological characteristics of the 'long face' syndrome in a 10 years and 10 months old girl with chronic mouth breathing. Extraoral photographs (a–d) reveal lip incompetency, increased lower facial height, narrow nose base width and shadows under the eyes from chronic venous congestion. (e) Lateral cephalograph of the same patient shows characteristic findings of adenoid facies: palatal plane (ANS-PNS) tipped posteroinferiorly, steep mandibular plane (MP: menton-gonion), angular notching, reduced inclination of anterior slope of chin, increased lower face height.

to mandibular plane angle; increased lower face height, steep mandibular plane, mandibular antegonial notching, increased gonial angle, and elongated and thinner symphysis (Figures 12.3 and 12.4). The palatal tilt reached severe levels (8–9°) between ages 4 and 5 years. The occlusion ranged from normal with adequate overjet/overbite to malocclusions that contained one or more of these characteristics: posterior crossbite, increased overjet, Class II molar relationship, open bite, and anterior crossbite.

The research suggests formulations regarding the association between airway status and craniofacial morphology and growth, as well as clinical implications that require additional research for validation.

Growth concepts revisited

Facial dysmorphology related to nasal obstruction apparently starts in structures closest to the obstruction: a posteroinferior tilt of the maxilla.

Occlusal variations among the investigated children (Bitar et al., 2010) are similar to the experimental findings of Harvold et al. (1972, 1973, 1981) in monkeys at comparable ages. Harvold et al. obstructed inspiration but allowed slight air escape during expiration in growing monkeys between ages 2 and 6 years, most of them (34/42) in the late deciduous and mixed dentitions (ages 2–4 years). The response differed considerably, each animal finding its 'own most convenient way to secure the oral flow, and then develop a dental occlusion in accordance with this new function' (Harvold et al., 1981). Therefore, oral respiration induced mesioclusion, maxillary protrusion with distocclusion, open bite, dual bite and some common cephalometric traits: increased face height, steeper mandibular inclination, and a larger gonial angle. The array of occlusal and cephalometric changes was similar in these animals and the investigated children, whose various malocclusions were also probably related to individual adjustments in respiration.

Our findings qualify the variable relation between nasal obstruction and facial growth in line with Moss's functional matrix theory, which stipulates that facial growth is related to the function of the various components in the head and neck region (Moss, 1969, 1997a,b). The oropharyngeal space is a primary entity (capsular matrix related to respiration) that influences the position and behavior of the surrounding soft tissues, which in turn shape the associated skeletal units. Impingement on the oropharyngeal space leads to adaptive reorganization of the latter. Thus, the adaptation begins with and may be restricted to the posteroinferior maxillary tilt, probably because of its proximity to the obstructed pharynx.

The greater amplitude of adaptation in younger ages suggests that growth at early ages (≤5 years) is affected with more deviation from the norm. The adjustment may also start with mandibular remodeling favoring an increase in the gonial angle and mandibular plane inclination. Additional or more severe morphological changes would be associated with more severe airway blockage, the long face syndrome representing the extreme expression of sustained functional disturbance. Conversely, any degree of adaptive morphological change may result in a level of restoration of nasal breathing. Accordingly, as airway obstruction ranges from total to partial, and adaptation to either is an individual response to preserve the oropharyngeal matrix, the variation in malocclusions is not surprising. The association between *amount* of blockage and *specific signs* of malocclusion remains unknown. The severity and extent of dysmorphology would depend on the timing, duration, and rate of oral breathing and associated functional changes, given that a percentage of nasal breathing may coexist with mouth breathing (Fields et al., 1991).

As suggested by Angle, and also observed in a number of patients, a forward positioning of the mandible enlarges the airway and enhances breathing through the consequent increase of airflow, in a manner akin to mandibular manipulation in the treatment of sleep apnea (Liu et al., 2000). If sustained, the ensuing anterior crossbite may induce maxillary retrognathism that otherwise would not exist. This phenomenon reflects intra-growth orthopedics (maxillary retrognathism) generated by the transfer of functional forces through a non-therapeutic occlusal 'environmental induction' (anterior crossbite) (Ghafari, 2004).

Clinical implications

The critical clinical issue is determining the optimal time of lymphoid tissue removal to enhance nose breathing and prevent potential, or reverse existing, abnormal facial growth. The above findings emphasize the need for pediatricians and pediatric otolaryngologists to examine children for impaired nasal respiration early in childhood, and ascertain their breathing mode at night from the parents. Otolaryngologists and orthodontists should appreciate the early impact of enlarged adenoids and tonsils, the most common obstructive agents of the posterior pharyngeal airway. Other causes that raise nasal resistance may involve the hard tissues such as a deviated septum, turbinate irregularities and congenital or traumatic asymmetries of the nasal cavity, or the soft tissues such as catarrhal and allergic rhinitis and nasal polyps (Figure 12.5) (Timms, 1981).

Otolaryngology

The prevailing practice among otolaryngologists is to delay removal of the pharyngeal lymphoid tissues because of their role in immunological defenses, and the peculiar adenoid growth between ages 3 and 16 years, that is, the increase in size in preschool and primary grade years followed by a decrease during pre- and early adolescence (Linder-Aronson and Leighton, 1983). Commonly, otolaryngologists follow the guidelines for adenotonsillectomy, in general as supported by the American Academy of Otolaryngology. The indications include:

- Hypertrophy causing upper airway obstruction (sleep apnea), severe dysphagia, sleep disorders, or cardiopulmonary complications
- Peritonsillar abscess unresponsive to medical management and drainage documented by the surgeon, unless surgery is performed during an acute stage
- Patients having three or more infectious episodes related to the tonsils and/or adenoids per year despite adequate medical therapy
- Recurrent acute otitis media or chronic serous otitis media. Adenoidectomy should not be performed with the insertion of the first set of myringotomy (ear) tubes unless there is another indication for adenoidectomy besides chronic otitis media. However, repeat surgery for chronic otitis media should consist of adenoidectomy with myringotomy (with or without tube placement). Adenoidectomy for the treatment of otitis media in children under the age of 2 years has not been found to be beneficial (Mattila, 2006).
- Unilateral tonsil hypertrophy presumed euplastic. Most asymmetries can be followed conservatively without other indications for potential surgery such as abnormal appearance, symptoms, or history
- Hypertrophy causing malocclusion or adversely affecting orofacial growth, documented by the orthodontist
- Chronic or recurrent tonsillitis associated with the streptococcal carrier state and not responding to β-lactamase-resistant antibiotics.
- Persistent foul taste or breath caused by chronic tonsillitis and not responsive to medication.

Development of long-face features may be minimized or reversed through resumption of normal breathing, possibly aided by orthodontic/orthopedic treatment. Post-treatment studies of adenoidectomy (Linder-Aronson et al., 1986; Woodside et al., 1991a; Bahadir et al., 2006) record a more anterior direction of symphyseal growth, reversal of the tendency to posterior mandibular rotation, increased amount of mandibular growth, and no difference in direction of maxillary growth. Yet, individual growth direction after adenoidectomy has been shown to be more variable than in control children with clear airways matched for age and gender (Linder-Aronson et al., 1986). When Harvold et al. removed the nose plugs in their experimental animals

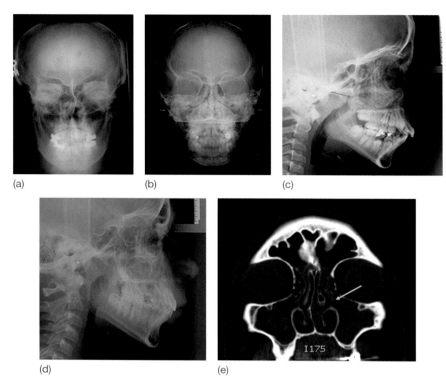

(a)   (b)   (c)

(d)   (e)

Figure 12.5 (a) Septal deviation: S-shaped deviation of nasal septum shown on a posteroanterior cephalograph. (b) Bilateral obstruction of the airway in a patient aged 10 years and 7 months, by the hypertrophied inferior turbinates (right and left, arrows) shown on a posteroanterior cephalograph. (c) The lateral cephalometric radiograph of the same patient shows the posterior extension of the inferior turbinate toward the posterior wall of the nasopharynx (arrow), causing the obstruction of the airway. On endoscopic otolaryngological examination, the diagnosis of inferior turbinate hypertrophy was confirmed, and medication (nasal topical steroids) improved breathing. (d) Cephalometric radiograph of a 14-year-old chronic mouth-breathing patient with hyperdivergent vertical pattern but positive clinical overbite (30%). Note the hypertrophic adenoids, and a unilateral nasal polyp (yellow circle) that contributed to nasal obstruction. (e) The computed tomography (CT) scan shows the extension of the polyp (arrow) from the sinus.

2 years after nasal obstruction, nasal breathing returned, and some of the dentofacial changes were undone, but facial features and malocclusion were often retained (Harvold et al., 1973, 1981; Hepper et al., 1990). More research is needed on the extent of orofacial counteradaptation in relation to age.

The early morphological changes observed with nasal airway obstruction support early surgical intervention to avoid a permanent setting of one or more characteristics of the long-face syndrome that would be difficult to control orthodontically. However, intervention at an early age (<5 years) to avoid irreversible morphological changes may not be advisable in general for several reasons.

- If compensation occurs within the dentition (absence of crossbite, open bite, or gummy smile) and morphological changes do not get worse at a later follow-up, early surgery may not be needed.
- With increasing age, the airway is less obstructed (Figure 12.6) and the effects on the palatal plane (Figure 12.7) and other morphological features decrease in intensity, indicating a gradual adjustment to growth of the nasopharyngeal airway and face.

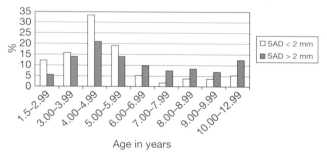

Figure 12.6 Percentage of children by age with the shortest distance between the adenoid and soft palate (SAD) less than and greater than 2 mm.

- In about 10% of children after 5 years (n = 22) in the aforementioned study (Bitar et al., 2010), obstruction was nearly complete (SAD <2 mm or grade 3), possibly related to sustained mouth breathing, with probably irreversible facial morphological changes (Güray and Karaman, 2002). When the data were computed for all patients with SAD <2 mm (Table 12.1), features relating to hyperdivergence (palatal and mandibular plane incli-

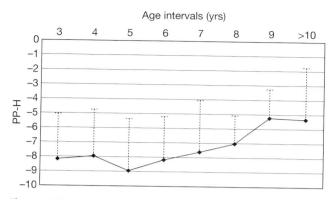

Figure 12.7 The palatal plane tip to the horizontal plane (PP-H) with age. The inferosuperior inclination decreases in older children, progressing from −8.2° to −5.3° in the age brackets 1.7–2.9 years to 10–12.9 years.

Table 12.1 Selected measurements for all patients with the shortest distance between the adenoid and the soft palate (SAD) ≤2 mm

Age (mean)	SAD	N	PP-H	MP-SN	PP-MP	LFH
<5 yrs (3.88)	0.99	35	−8.54	40.45	32.60	0.61
5–7 yrs (5.64)	1.46	14	−8.74	39.49	32.53	0.60
7–13 yrs (9.66)	0.58	8	−8.01	44.81	35.99	0.58

H, horizontal; MP, mandibular plane; PP, palatal plane. Angular measurements between planes in degrees. LFH, lower face height as percentage of total face height.

nations) and other long-face syndrome (LFS) characteristics (increased lower face height) were at least equally present across ages.

These data not only favor intervention when SAD is less than 2 mm but also indicate that a minority of a 'mouth-breathing' population fits this description. Actually, the very description of long-face syndrome is controversial, commonly involving increased anterior total and lower face height across ages, with vertical maxillary excess in adults (Schendel et al., 1976). Yet, the potential environmental influence on and lower genetic components of craniofacial size and form would point to the possibility of minimizing or avoiding the full expression of long-face syndrome (King et al., 1993). Therefore, there is a need to develop guidelines for early adenoidectomy and/or tonsillectomy that account for the varied response to the obstruction and normal growth changes. Indications for early adenoidectomy might include a combination of:

- An existing skeletal dysmorphology (palatal plane tip, steep mandibular plane, or increased lower face height) probably beyond 1 SD from the norm
- Persistent nasopharyngeal airway obstruction (SAD <2 mm or grade 3), or evidence of mouth breathing, preferably supported by objective testing, particularly because mouth breathing may be a habit
- Signs of malocclusion (constricted maxillary arch, anterior open bite or crossbite).

The complexity of the issue accentuates the need for prediction equations, based on longitudinal investigation to sort out at least the potential long-face syndrome (described with and without anterior open bite [Schendel et al., 1976]). Adenoidectomy may then be recommended in patients found at risk of long-face syndrome or perhaps some of its characteristics least affected by orthodontic treatment. Linder-Aronson advocates adenoidectomy in mouth breathers with a small nasopharynx (Linder-Aronson, 1970; Linder-Aronson et al., 1986, 1993; Kerr et al., 1989; Woodside et al., 1991a,b), but this recommendation is not supported by objective measures.

Orthodontics

Orthodontic intervention is confounded by several facts:

- A direct relation between mouth breathing and malocclusion is not established for all mouth breathers (Leiter and Baker, 1989), some of whom may exhibit normal occlusion, possibly because total nasal obstruction is seldom total or, as suggested earlier, because the functional balance is reached at various individual levels
- The type and severity of malocclusion are determined by the individual pattern of adaptation to nasal obstruction
- Clearing the nasal airway does not necessarily improve dentofacial relationships.

Thus, orthodontic correction may be needed to foster adequate tongue posture (e.g. widening the maxillary arch to favor and maintain an upward position of the tongue at rest). Sometimes, palatal splitting improves respiration and helps reverse mouth breathing (habitual or from anterior obstruction) to nose breathing, or may even ameliorate hearing (Kilic et al., 2008a,b). However, these responses cannot be predicted. When the mandible is thrust forward for better breathing, and an anterior crossbite follows possibly inducing maxillary retrognathism, early correction of the latter is recommended (Ghafari, 2004), along with the medical/surgical management of the respiratory problem.

Interestingly, in patients with the long-face syndrome who are treated with a combination of orthodontics and orthognathic surgery, the surgery reverses the characteristics observed in conjunction with sustained chronic mouth breathing during growth namely, posterior impaction of the maxilla, mandibular advancement and genioplasty (Figure 12.8).

Interaction between specialists (orthodontist, ENT, pediatrician) involves a process of reciprocal education on evidence-based practice. Accordingly, parents become more receptive to surgical intervention to correct nasal

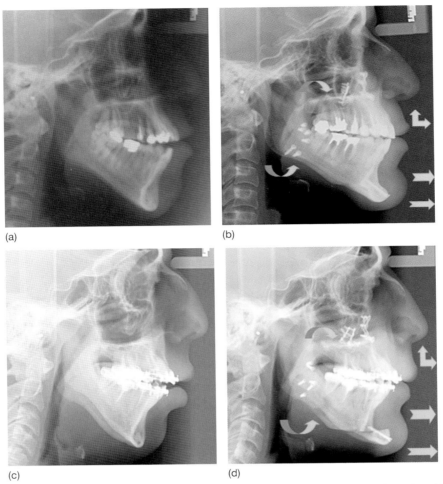

(a)

(b)

(c)

(d)

Figure 12.8 Process of rectification of long-face syndrome involves surgical movements in a direction opposite the description of its development following nasal obstruction and chronic mouth breathing. (a,b) Pretreatment and postsurgical cephalographs of adult female with long-face syndrome treated with a combination of orthodontics and orthognathic surgery. The surgical movements (arrows) reversed the dentoskeletal dysmorphology through compensatory movements of the incisors, maxillary impaction, posterior rotation and advancement, mandibular anterior autorotation, mandibular advancement osteotomy, and further chin advancement genioplasty. (c,d) Presurgical and postsurgical cephalograms of adult male with the same syndrome. A similar approach (arrows) and surgical osteotomies were performed as for the patient in Figure 12.8a,b.

respiratory impairment when indicated in younger children. Bahadir et al. (2006) related a high rate of parent satisfaction following reported improvement of preoperative symptoms in children post-adenoidectomy.

Difficulties in research of nasopharyngeal obstruction and mouth breathing include:

- Taking radiographs using the cephalostat in children, as they need to remain still during the exposure and keep the teeth in contact
- The inclusion of control groups is problematic for several reasons: difficulty to properly define the absence of mouth breathing until objective measures are correlated with various respiratory modes that would preclude overlapping groups; a general description of 'nasal' or normal breather would need objective assessment of airflow or nasal resistance, albeit they do not always reflect the mode of breathing (Leiter and Baker, 1989); the variability of malocclusion and underlying morphology may restrict the attainment of adequate sample numbers

- The need for long-term follow-up post-treatment and sorting out the various sources of airway blockage that may coexist (e.g. adenoid and inferior turbinate hypertrophy).

Conductive hearing loss

Otitis media

Pathogenesis

Otitis media is a frequently occurring disease in childhood, characterized by middle ear inflammation. It is one of the most prevailing causes of medical visits (Freid et al., 1998) and the most common reason for antibiotic consumption and surgical intervention in children (Alsarraf et al., 1999; Bondy et al., 2000). The condition results, mainly, from the rupture of equilibrium between microbial (viral and bacterial) load and immune response (Rovers et al., 2004). Accumulation of fluid in the middle ear can follow because of the negative pressure produced by altered Eustachian tube function. If untreated, this fluid can induce conductive hearing impairment.

Several mechanisms have been reported to cause otitis media, with possible multifactorial contributions.

Microbiological and immunological interaction

Bacterial pathogens and respiratory viruses (cold viruses) can cause otitis media. The most common bacterial pathogens in children are *Streptococcus pneumoniae*, *Moraxella catarrhalis*, and nontypeable *Haemophilus influenzae* (Rovers et al., 2004), the latter being the predominant pathogen among adolescents and young adults. The resulting congestion and ensuing malfunctioning of the Eustachian tube disturb the pressure regulation of the middle ear, which in turn can be followed by aspiration of more pathogens from the oropharyngeal space into the middle ear, aggravating the original problem (Bluestone, 1996).

The adenoids are not only providers of local immune defenses against pathogen invasion through the upper respiratory tract but also produce effector and memory lymphocytes that migrate to adjacent mucosal structures, strengthening local immune competence (Van Kempen et al., 2000). In addition, secretory IgA, produced by the nasopharyngeal mucosa, reinforces the defense mechanism by restraining bacterial and viral adherence and reducing bacterial colonization (Kurono et al., 1991; Lim and Mogi, 1994). Children with recurrent otitis media showed lack of IgA (Stenfors and Raisanen, 1993) and specific IgG2 antibodies (Sanders et al., 1995).

Environmental and genetic influences

Environmental risk factors include history of otitis media in the family, parental smoking, pacifier usage, and outside day care, which is related to the number of children in the facility (Uhari et al., 1996; Dewey et al., 2000). Findings are anecdotal on the effect of breastfeeding on decreasing the risk of otitis media (Uhari et al., 1996).

In a longitudinal study conducted on 1373 twin pairs, Kelly (1993) showed a strong genetic component of otitis media with higher concordance in monozygotic versus dizygotic twins. Moreover, recurrent otitis media is associated with genetically determined immunoglobulin markers (Kelly, 1993).

Eustachian tube dysfunction

The Eustachian tube (also known by its medical designations of auditory or pharyngotympanic tube) is named

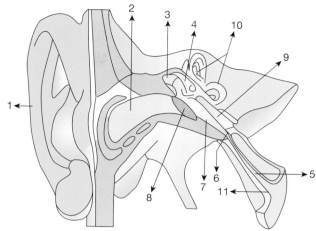

Figure 12.9 Schematic representation of the human ear. The ear is divided into three parts: external, middle, and internal. The external ear comprises: 1 – the auricle; 2 – the external acoustic meatus. The middle ear includes: 3 – the epitympanic recess; 4 – the tympanic cavity; 5 – the Eustachian tube; 6 – the isthmus of the tube, where the bony and the cartilaginous parts of the Eustachian tube merge; 7 – the bony part of the Eustachian tube heading towards the tympanic cavity; 8 – the tympanic membrane; 9 – the tensor tympani muscle. The inner ear has: 10 – the bony labyrinth. Note: 11 – the pharyngeal opening of the Eustachian tube (based on Kahle, 1993).

after Bartolomeus Eustachius, a famous sixteenth-century anatomist. The tube connects the middle ear with the nasopharynx at the level of the inferior turbinate and measures 3–4 cm in adults. Narrow and formed by bone at its upper end, it becomes wider and cartilagenous at the pharyngeal end (Figure 12.9).

The Eustachian tube has an essential function in preserving a healthy middle ear; its opening and closing are physiologically and pathologically important. Normally it is closed in adults, but it opens during yawning, chewing, and swallowing, allowing air flow in the middle ear. Many functions have been attributed to the Eustachian tube (Lim et al., 2000):

- Ventilation: the opening of the tube equilibrates the pressure between the middle ear and ambient air
- Protection: the closure of the tube protects the middle ear against nasopharyngeal pressure fluctuations and ascending secretions or pathogens (Rovers et al., 2004)
- Clearance: the mucus is drained away from the middle ear into the nasopharynx, thus preventing infection from ascending to the middle ear.

Relative to the Frankfort plane, the position of the Eustachian tube is more horizontal in children (10°) than in adults (45°), and the tube is relatively shorter and wider (Cummings et al., 1998). Many researchers related this topography to the higher occurrence of otitis media in children because the flatter inclination hinders mucus drainage (Seibert and Danner, 2006). However, some authors have also ascribed Eustachian tube dysfunction to muscular problems (Bylander and Tjernstrom, 1983; Bylander, 1984). The tensor veli palatini, levator veli palatini, salpingopharyngeus, and the tensor tympani are the muscles responsible for opening and closing the Eustachian tube (Seibert and Danner, 2006). Through finite element analysis, Ghadiali et al. (2004) found that muscle forces play a more sensitive role in the tube's opening and closure than cartilage elasticity. In children, the tensor palatini muscle operates less efficiently. In children with otitis media, contraction of the levator veli palatini muscles closes the pharyngeal orifices and restrains the tensor veli palatini muscle from opening the Eustachian tube (Cozza et al., 2007). These factors increase the chance for Eustachian tube dysfunction and middle ear disease among infants and young children.

When sounds in the environment reach the ear, they propagate through the ear canal and impinge on the tympanic membrane, causing it to vibrate. The vibrations are transmitted through the middle ear via the ossicular chain (malleus, incus, and stapes) to the fluid-filled cochlea. The cochlea transduces the vibrations into nerve impulses. The cochlear division of the vestibulocochlear nerve carries information into the brain where it undergoes further processing in both the brainstem and thalamus before reaching the cerebral cortex.

When the Eustachian tube malfunctions, proper ventilation of the middle ear does not occur and air within the middle ear cavity stagnates. Part of the stagnant air is then absorbed by the tissues of the middle ear. As a result, the outer pressure at the level of the tympanic membrane becomes greater than the air pressure in the middle ear, thus the membrane is pushed and restrained from proper vibration when hit by sound waves. Over a period of time, the absorbed air from the middle ear is replaced with an accumulation of fluid, called effusion. The chronic presence of this fluid induces muffled or dulled hearing because sound is not conducted efficiently through the middle ear system. When a disease or condition involves the outer or middle ear, as in the case of otitis media, any decrease in hearing sensitivity is called conductive hearing loss.

Diagnosis

Audiological tests are mandatory to confirm the presence of conductive hearing loss.

Audiometry

Audiological test protocols vary according to the age of the child and often include a combination of behavioral and physiological tests. For children under the age of 6 months, behavioral observation audiometry (BOA), visual reinforcement audiometry (VRA), evoked otoacoustic emissions (EOAE), and auditory brainstem response (ABR) are often used. BOA involves watching an infant's response to sudden and relatively intense sounds with different frequency and intensity composition. VRA, which is another behavioral test, involves the use of a conditioned localization response from the child and a visual reinforcer. Specifically, sounds of varying frequencies and intensities are presented through loudspeakers located off to the side of the child, in a test room. When a sound is presented through a loudspeaker, the child is conditioned to turn his or her head toward the source of the sound. When the child turns to the source, this response is followed by the illumination of a visually appealing object (e.g. animated stuffed animal), which serves as a reward or reinforcement. The reinforcer increases the chances that the child will continue responding to subsequent sound presentations.

Otoacoustic emissions are sounds emitted from the inner ear as a result of microscopic biomechanical activity associated with healthy cochlear outer hair cells. The EOAE is a physiological test that measures this biomechanical activity via a sensitive microphone seated in the ear canal, in response to an acoustic stimulus presented to the ear. EOAEs are present in 99+ percent of individuals with normal hearing sensitivity; absence of EOAEs suggests the presence of hearing loss. The ABR is another physiological test that measures a change in the electrical activity of the nervous system when it reacts to a sound stimulus presented through earphones to an ear. This change in electrical activity can be picked up by electrodes placed on a child's head and then displayed as waves on the screen of a recording device. Sound levels presented to the ear are progressively lowered until a level is reached where a replicable waveform is no longer observed. This level indirectly suggests the child's threshold of hearing.

For children aged 6–24 months, VRA and EOAE are often used to assess hearing. Above the age of 24 months, play audiometry can be used. Play audiometry involves training the child to listen for sounds and then make a specific motor response (e.g. throw a ball in a bucket, add a block to a stack of blocks, or place a peg into a pegboard). When a child hears a sound presented, he or she makes the motor response. Sounds (pure tones and speech) are presented to the child via earphones (known as air conduction) and through a bone vibrator positioned behind the child's ear on the mastoid process (known as bone conduction). Testing by air conduction assesses the entire auditory system, whereas testing by bone conduction assesses the auditory system at the level of the cochlear and beyond (i.e. the status of the sensorineural component of the hearing is assessed). A comparison of hearing sensitivity, as measured by air conduction and bone conduction, assists in determining the nature of the hearing impairment: conductive, sensorineural or mixed (Figure 12.10) (Kutz et al., 2010). An 'air bone gap' (i.e. hearing sensitivity is better by bone conduction compared with sensitivity by air conduction) suggests conductive or mixed hearing loss.

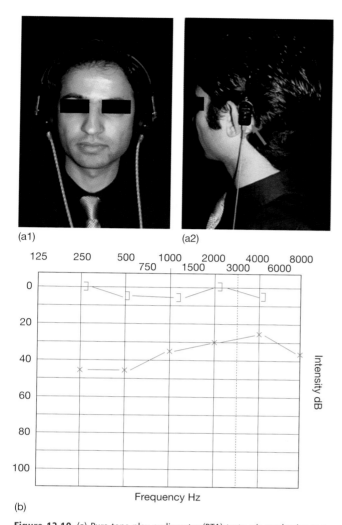

(a1)   (a2)

(b)

Figure 12.10 (a) Pure tone play audiometry (PTA) tests: air conduction test performed with headphones at the level of the outer ears (a1) and bone conduction test done with earphones behind the ears over the mastoid bones (a2). (b) Audiogram depicting a normal bone conduction hearing (top graph) with a moderate rising (40 decibels) conductive hearing loss depicted by air conduction test (bottom graph). Note that severe hearing loss is present when the threshold moves to more than 70 decibels (based on Kutz et al., 2010).

Tympanometry

Tympanometry involves measuring the acoustic admittance of the ear using varying amounts of air pressure in a hermetically sealed ear canal. During tympanometry, a probe is seated in the child's ear canal. The probe introduces positive and negative air pressure on the tympanic membrane. The resulting movement of the eardrum is measured and depicted on a diagram called a tympanogram. In the presence of fluid in the middle ear, the tympanic membrane does not vibrate properly and the tympanogram is flat (Figure 12.11). Used in conjunction with the audiogram, tympanometry helps detect the presence of conductive hearing loss.

Treatment

Treatment of otitis media ranges from watchful waiting to antibiotics prescription and surgical intervention aiming to restore pressure equilibrium between the middle ear and the nasopharynx. Treatment modalities are related to the severity of the condition and timing of the intervention in relation to the original onset period. Guidelines on antibacterial treatment have been produced by the American Academy of Pediatrics and American Academy of Family Physicians (2004) and recommend an observation period of 48 hours after initial diagnosis, without use of antibiotics. Prescription of antibacterial agent is recommended (amoxicillin 80–90 mg/kg per day) if initial management fails.

Conductive hearing loss and maxillary expansion

Rapid maxillary expansion (RME) was first introduced in the nineteenth century by Angell (1860) to correct maxillary constriction and open space for the canines to erupt. The method consists of orthopedic separation of the mid-palatal suture through the activation of a jackscrew embedded in mostly fixed expanders but possibly removable appliances in younger children (generally less than 6 years old). Mesnard (1929) demonstrated that bone fills the middle space between the palatal bones at around 4–6 weeks post expansion. Currently, RME is commonly used by orthodontists for the correction of posterior crossbites, gaining space to correct crowding, and improvement of smile esthetics by reducing the space between the maxillary buccal teeth and commissure, also known as the black corridor or 'negative' space (Huertas and Ghafari, 2001). RME has also been advocated in the treatment of cleft palate (Isaacson and Murphy, 1964). RME can be used during the primary, mixed, or permanent dentition periods, but splitting the palate becomes difficult to achieve once the adolescent growth spurt has passed, presumably because of the increased resistance of the buttressing bones.

RME generates lateral movement of the walls of the nasal cavity, typically more anteriorly than posteriorly because of less resistance from the buttressing bones anteriorly. Consequently, the width of the cavity is increased (Haas, 1961; Wertz, 1968; Warren et al., 1987). This enlargement does not translate necessarily into improved respiration and it is not predictive of normalizing the mode of breathing related to nasal obstruction (Hershey et al., 1976). Improvement in nocturnal enuresis, also associated with mode of breathing, has been observed after palatal splitting (Timms, 1990; Kurol et al., 1998; Usumez et al., 2003; Schütz-Fransson and Kurol, 2008).

In an initial report correlating RME and conductive hearing loss, Laptook (1981) described maxillary constriction concomitant with a high palatal vault as part of a 'skeletal development syndrome' that includes certain rhinological and dental characteristics. Earlier, Rudolph (1977) had related Eustachian tube dysfunction to a malfunction

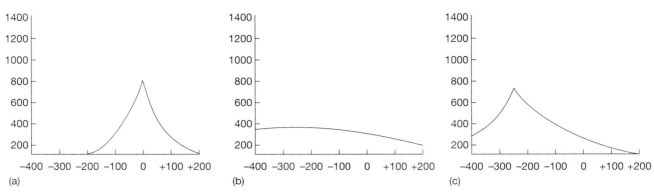

Figure 12.11 Three different types of tympanograms, plotting the pressure measured in decaPascals (daPa; x-axis) relative to the conductivity of sounds in millimho (mmho; (y-axis) (a) A type A tympanogram indicates a normal middle ear system, free of fluid or physiological anomalies that would prevent the admittance of sound from the middle ear into the cochlea. (b) The type B tympanogram is consistent with middle ear pathology, such as fluid or infection behind the ear drum. (c) The type C tympanogram indicates negative pressure (below 0) in the middle ear space, often consistent with sinus or allergy congestion, or the end-stages of a cold or ear infection.

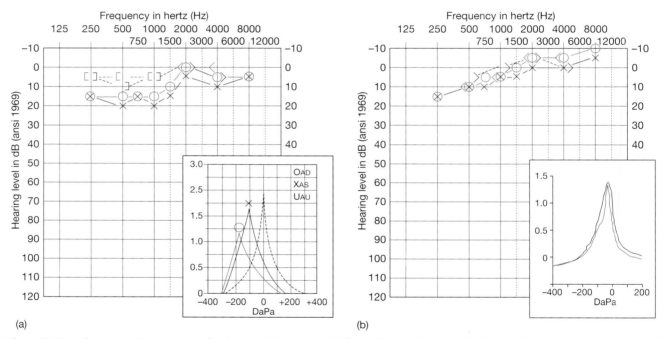

Figure 12.12 Audiograms and tympanograms of an 11-year-old boy before and after maxillary rapid expansion. (a) Pre-expansion audiometric tests show mild conductive hearing loss and a type C tympanogram (see Figure 12.11c) denoting negative middle ear pressure bilaterally. (b) The postexpansion audiogram and tympanogram are within the normal limits.

of the tensor and levator palatini muscles that results in the inability of the tube to open in response to negative pressure in the middle ear. Observing that this malfunction was more frequent in the presence of high palatal vault, Rudolph considered the combination of these two anatomical variations as predisposing factors for otitis media. In 310 patients treated with RME to correct maxillary constriction, Gray (1975) found a remarkable decrease of recurrent serous otitis media. The results of subsequent studies are indicative of improvement in hearing a few weeks after palatal expansion (Fingeroth, 1991; Ceylan et al., 1996; Villano et al., 2006; Cozza et al., 2007). Figure 12.12 illustrates improvement in pure tone audiometry and tympanometry measurements, reflecting amelioration in hearing sensitivity and middle ear function, 1 week after palatal expansion in a boy we enrolled in a pilot study on the relation between maxillary distraction and conductive hearing loss.

Later studies with longer-term assessments support the initial findings. Taspinar et al. (2003) reported the effects of expansion in 35 subjects on hearing levels to be positive in nearly 75% of the patients; the results remained stable over 2 years of observation. In a more recent study, Kilic et al. (2008a) evaluated the long-term effects of semi-rapid maxillary expansion with an acrylic bonded appliance on conductive hearing loss in 19 patients (age 13 years 5 months ± 1 year). Hearing tests included pure tone audiometry and tympanometry before expansion and at three subsequent time points up to 2 years later. The improvement in hearing levels and decrease in the air bone gap during the active expansion period remained stable. The results of another study using a fixed RME appliance but similar design were comparable (Kilic et al. 2008b).

The available long-term evidence is not definitive because of shortcomings in the hearing and otological examinations used, including failure in reporting the status of the tympanic membrane by simple otoscopy and the reporting modality of tympanometric measurements. The significance of more controlled long-term studies is the potential determination of whether RME may be an alternative treatment to surgical otologic options or at least it may be tried before surgery in children with conductive hearing loss who also require palatal expansion.

One possible explanation of the improvement in conductive hearing loss after maxillary expansion is the stretching of the tensor veli muscle, which opens the pharyngeal orifice of the Eustachian tube and allows air to enter and exit the middle ear. Thus, the pressures on either side of the tympanic membrane are balanced and the vibration of the ossicular bones is normalized, resulting in hearing improvement.

Craniofacial anomalies

Craniofacial anomalies include mostly congenital conditions, such as syndromic and nonsyndromic cleft lip and/or plate, hemifacial microsomia, and plagiocephaly. Typically, comprehensive treatment of these problems requires a multidisciplinary approach by a team of specialists capable of managing various structures and functions in the craniofacial complex: pediatrician, pediatric dentist, nurse practitioner, otolaryngologist, geneticist, speech pathologist, orthodontist, maxillofacial surgeon, plastic surgeon, prosthodontist, social worker, and psychologist. Planning and execution of treatment require judicious coordination and proper timing because of the developmental nature of these conditions. Intervention is needed from birth to the time when growth of the facial skeleton has ceased. If the intervention does not accompany key growth events (e.g. dental development, adolescent growth spurt), opportunities are lost and the outcome is at best the result of a series of compromises instead of optimal function of the orofacial structures and esthetics of the facial structures, as well as optimal hearing and intelligible speech

for some of the anomalies. The epidemiology, diagnosis and management of these anomalies are discussed in Chapters 7–9. A brief summary is presented within the context of interaction between orthodontist and ENT specialist.

Cleft lip/palate

Clefting of the lip, alveolus, and palate is the most common craniofacial congenital malformation of the head and neck, and the second most common congenital malformation of the entire body after clubfoot deformity (Bailey, 1998). Treatment timing, sequence and modalities employed in these patients depend on key growth events. Treatment periods are usually determined in reference to the average ages of dental development, from the primary, through the mixed, to the full permanent dentitions (Haddad et al., 2006). Soon after the birth of an infant with orofacial cleft, the various specialists in a cleft palate or craniofacial center will evaluate the newborn. They delineate the best management options, institute a treatment plan, and then continuously review progress and carry out revisions of individual procedures and treatments when needed over the follow-up period.

Typically, and in the absence of a universal approach to treatment, the sequence, timing and modalities of cleft treatment are specific to teams and centers. The general sequence of procedures is comparable in different centers and between different specialists, but the timing is more variable. Treatment stages commonly include intervention in the neonatal period, the toddler years, grade school years, and ideally ends in the later teenage years. The timing of certain procedures might overlap between one and another period, particularly those defined as adjunctive procedures (i.e. speech therapy, psychotherapy) (See Chapter 10 for more details.)

Other craniofacial anomalies

The interaction between the orthodontist and ENT specialist is maintained within the team approach as defined within specific centers. Accordingly, in those anomalies where hearing and breathing may be impaired, the ENT specialist may also assume the role of the otolaryngologist and/or maxillofacial or plastic surgeon.

Nonspecific conditions

These conditions are included in this chapter for completeness, because the ENT specialist may be involved in the course of their management. The main condition is otalgia, or ear pain, because it may relate to temporomandibular dysfunction (TMD).

Ear pain

Otalgia is a condition commonly seen by the dentist and/or the otolaryngologist because of the proximity and similar innervation of the ear and oromaxillary structures. The patient may also be referred from one specialist to another depending on the results of the initial evaluation.

The sensory innervation of the ear derives from branches of cranial nerves V, VII, IX, and X. Primary otalgia results from pathologies affecting the ear itself, encompassing local inflammation or infection such as in otitis externa or otitis media, Eustachian tube problems with pressure gradient disparities on both sides of the tympanic membrane, infections of the skull base (such as in necrotizing otitis externa) or, less commonly, primary malignancies involving the ear. Associated symptoms of hearing loss, aural fullness, otorrhea (or drainage of pus to outside the ear), and dizziness may occur variably.

Secondary or referred otalgia originates from pathologies affecting any of the structures innervated by the above mentioned nerves: the temporomandibular joint (TMJ), mandible, teeth, gingiva, nose, paranasal sinuses, nasopharynx, oropharynx (including tonsils and tongue), parotid gland, larynx, and esophagus.

Evaluation

The history is an important element in the evaluation of the patient with otalgia. The character and duration of the pain must be assessed. Otalgia can present as a sharp, dull, or burning pain. It can be acute or chronic, constant or intermittent. The pain can involve only the ear or radiate to surrounding structures. The diurnal pattern of the pain is noted, along with any association with chewing or swallowing, hearing loss, discharge, or dizziness. Difficulties or pain with swallowing, changes in voice or breathing and blood in the sputum are serious symptoms as they may relate to a malignancy of the head and neck. The patient is asked about any obvious precipitating factors such as trauma to the head or local trauma to the ear. A history of smoking and/or alcohol intake increases the suspicion for malignancies.

On examination, the ear is carefully evaluated to rule out any primary otologic etiology. More specifically, the ENT examination focuses on the ears and adjacent areas in the head and neck region, including the areas of the pinna and over the mastoid process for redness and swelling; the ear canal for redness, discharge, cerumen, foreign body, and lesions; the tympanic membrane for redness, perforation, and signs of middle ear fluid collection such as bulging, distortion, or change in normal light reflex, and hearing (through a brief bedside test (see section on Conductive hearing loss p.204). It is often helpful to ask the patient to point to the origin of the pain with one finger. A full head and neck examination is important, including flexible endoscopy to evaluate the pharynx and larynx. Clicking or grinding of the TMJs along with point tenderness and trismus may indicate a non-otological etiology.

Most problems are properly diagnosed after taking the history and conducting a physical examination. Non-

otological causes, such as TMD, are considered when examination of the ear yields normal results. Depending on clinical findings, non-otological causes may require further testing, such as computed tomography (CT) or magnetic resonance imaging (MRI). Treatment is targeted to the underlying disorder, including oral analgesics, topical analgesics, local manipulation (e.g. suction of debris, ear drops), and surgery.

Key to the differential diagnosis on TMJ involvement is the ear examination findings: absence of middle and external ear problems; absence of oropharyngeal cause (tonsillitis, peritonsillar abscess); and absence of potential red flags such as redness over the mastoid, immunocompromised condition, or chronic pain concomitant with other symptoms of the head and neck region. While in case of neuralgia sharp pain occurs in brief severe episodes (seconds up to 2 minutes), TMD might be accompanied with chronic otalgia.

Temporomandibular dysfunction

When the ears appear to be normal and an earache is traced to TMJ function, the orthodontist or dentist concerned with the treatment should conduct a thorough examination to differentiate structural TMJ problems from neuromuscular conditions.

TMJ-related symptoms are caused by degeneration of joint structures (arthritis, fractures, congenital) or the effects of physical stress on the structures around the joint. The etiology is multifactorial. Though the disorders have been related to stress, tooth clenching or bruxism, malocclusion, orthodontic treatment, and even muscular strain from poor posture, there is no evidence to prove a definitive relation between occlusion and TMD.

TMD symptoms include clicking, 'cracking', popping, fremitus, difficulty, or discomfort when biting or chewing, pain in the jaw, ear, face, or head, limitation in mouth opening, and tenderness on palpation of cheek or temple areas. Depending on the symptoms, the patient may seek the dentist or ENT specialist first, whose examination to determine any TMJ disorder would include palpation of the joint area, oral examination covering static and functional occlusion, and radiographs if needed.

The approach to treatment has ranged from prior emphasis on occlusal associations with TMD, and treatment of minor clicking to minimizing the occlusal impact and treatment of the disorder when pain is involved. Details on pathogenesis, diagnosis, and controversies related to the treatment of TMDs are presented in Chapter 24. When TMD is confirmed, ideally it should be addressed before the start or resumption of orthodontic treatment.

Accidental conditions

The ENT surgeon may be consulted for management of iatrogenic complications of dental treatment. These include forcing of impacted third molars in the maxillary sinus during extraction, which may occur if the position of maxillary molar is 'high'(cephalad). Various methods have been described for retrieval of the teeth from the sinus (Hasbini et al., 2001). Sinus perforation may also occur during other dental procedures.

Conclusion

Unlike general dentists or other dental specialists, the orthodontist may be the dental practitioner with the least need to interact with physicians during regular treatment of patients. Perhaps the most common dealings of an orthodontist are with the maxillofacial or other facial surgeon in patients requiring orthognathic surgery and, to a lesser extent, in the treatment of craniofacial anomalies. Research and developing practice trends indicate that more regular communication between orthodontist and otolaryngologist should take place in specific although various conditions. Based on the above discussion, the following conclusions may be formulated on such interaction:

- Chronic mouth breathing is probably the most significant ground for sustained collaboration as the condition may impact facial morphology irreversibly. Children with chronic mouth breathing must be examined by an ENT specialist at an early age because of the potential for progressive impact on craniofacial morphology. The orthodontist and pediatric ENT specialist must engage in a process of reciprocal education on evidence-based removal of lymphoid tissues obstructing, or medical clearance of obstacles, to nasal respiration. Common practice may be at a misstep from current knowledge in this area and much collaborative work is still needed to avoid mismanagement of genuine nasal obstruction or performing unnecessary excision of adenoids or tonsils.
- Diagnosis of hypertrophic adenoids is helpful and less invasive on a cephalogram, the most common orthodontic radiographic record. The orthodontist (and ENT specialist) should be familiar with the radiographic appearances of the adenoids and other structures (hypertrophied inferior turbinate, tonsils, septal deviation) on lateral and posteroanterior cephalograms, even if definitive diagnosis is confirmed with other tests (e.g. endoscopy for enlarged turbinates).
- The potential of RME to improve conductive hearing loss should be further explored for possible beneficial applications.
- The role of the ENT specialist both as an otolaryngologist and/or facial surgeon in the treatment of cleft lip/palate and other craniofacial anomalies is asserted as part of the team handling these conditions.
- Collaboration is needed in the evaluation of otalgia thought to be caused by TMD to rule out the possibility of otologic origins.

Acknowledgments

We thank Dr Kim Smith Abouchacra, Associate Professor and Director, Audiology, and Dr Marc Bassim, Assistant Professor of Otolaryngology-Head and Neck Surgery, American University of Beirut Medical Center, for their critical review of the material related to their respective specialties.

References

Alsarraf R, Jung CJ, Perkins J, et al. (1999) Measuring the indirect and direct costs of acute otitis media. *Archives of Otolaryngology-Head and Neck Surgery* 125: 12–18.

American Academy of Pediatrics and American Academy of Family Physicians, Clinical Practice Guideline (2004) Diagnosis and management of acute otitis media. *Pediatrics* 113: 1451–65.

Angell EC (1860) Treatment of irregularities of the permanent or adult teeth. *Dental Cosmos* 1: 540–4.

Angle EH (1907) *Treatment of Malocclusion of the Teeth*, 7th edn. Philadelphia, PA: SS White, pp. 52–4.

Bahadir O, Caylan R, Bektas D, et al. (2006) Effects of adenoidectomy in children with symptoms of adenoidal hypertrophy. *European Archives of Oto-Rhino-Laryngology* 263: 156–9.

Bailey BJ (1998) *Head and Neck Surgery – Otolaryngology*, 2nd edn. New York, NY: Lippincott Williams & Wilkins/Raven.

Behlfelt K, Linder-Aronson S, McWilliam J, et al. (1989a) Dentition in children with enlarged tonsils compared to control children. *European Journal of Orthodontics* 11: 416–29.

Behlfelt K, Linder-Aronson S, Neander P (1989b) Posture of the head, the hyoid bone, and the tongue in children with and without enlarged tonsils. *European Journal of Orthodontics* 12: 458–67.

Behlfelt K, Linder-Aronson S, McWilliam J, et al. (1990) Craniofacial morphology in children with and without enlarged tonsils. *European Journal of Orthodontics* 12: 233–43.

Bitar MA, Macari AT, Ghafari JG (2010) Correspondence between subjective and linear measurements of the palatal airway on lateral cephalometric radiographs. *Archives of Otolaryngology-Head and Neck Surgery* 136: 43–7.

Bluestone CD (1996) Pathogenesis of otitis media: role of Eustachian tube. *Pediatric Infectious Disease Journal* 15: 281–91.

Bondy J, Berman S, Glazner J, et al. (2000) Direct expenditures related to otitis media diagnosis: extrapolations from a pediatric Medicaid cohort. *Pediatrics* 105: e72.

Bylander A (1984) Function and dysfunction of the Eustachian tube in children. *Acta Oto-Rhino-Laryngologica Belgica* 38: 238–45.

Bylander A, Tjernstrom O (1983) Changes in Eustachian tube function with age in children with normal ears: A longitudinal study. *Acta Oto-Laryngologica* 96: 467–77.

Ceylan I, Oktay H, Demicri M (1996) The effect of rapid maxillary expansion on conductive hearing loss. *Angle Orthodontist* 66: 301–8.

Cozza P, Di Girolamo S, Ballanti F, et al. (2007) Orthodontist-otorhinolaryngologist: an interdisciplinary approach to solve otitis media. *European Journal of Paediatric Dentistry* 8: 83–8.

Cummings BJ, Fredrickson JM, Harker LA, et al. (1998) *Anatomy and Physiology of the Eustachian Tube*, 3rd edn. St. Louis, MO: Mosby-Year Book, Inc.

Dewey C, Midgeley E, Maw R (2000) The relationship between otitis media with effusion and contact with other children in a British cohort studied from 8 months to 3 1/2 years: Avon longitudinal study of pregnancy and childhood. *International Journal of Pediatric Otorhinolaryngology* 55: 33–45.

Diamond O (1980) Tonsils and adenoids: Why the dilemma? *American Journal of Orthodontics* 78: 495–503.

Emslie RD, Massler M, Zwemer JD (1952) Mouth breathing: Etiology and effects. *Journal of the American Dental Association* 44: 506–21.

Fields HW, Warren DW, Black K, et al. (1991) Relationship between vertical dentofacial morphology and respiration in adolescents. *American Journal of Orthodontics and Dentofacial Orthopedics* 99: 147–54.

Fingeroth AI (1991) Orthodontic-orthopedics as related to respiration and conductive hearing loss. *Journal of Clinical Pediatric Dentistry* 15: 83–9.

Freid VM, Mukuc DM, Rooks RN (1998) Ambulatory health care visits by children: principal diagnosis and place of visit. *Vital and Health Statistics* 13: 1–23.

Fujimoto S, Yamaguchi K, Gunjigake K (2009) Clinical estimation of mouth breathing. *American Journal of Orthodontics and Dentofacial Orthopedics* 136: 630.e1–7; discussion 630–1.

Ghadiali SN, Banks J, Swarts JD (2004) Finite element analysis of active Eustachian tube function. *Journal of Applied Physiology* 97: 648–54.

Ghafari J (2004) Therapeutic and developmental maxillary orthopedics: Evaluation of effects and limitations. In: Z Davidovitch, J Mah (eds) *Biological Mechanisms of Tooth Movement and Craniofacial Adaptation.* Boston, MA: Harvard Society for the Advancement of Orthodontics, pp. 167–81.

Grauer D, Cevidanes LS, Styner MA, et al. (2009) Pharyngeal airway volume and shape from cone-beam computed tomography: relationship to facial morphology. *American Journal of Orthodontics and Dentofacial Orthopedics* 136: 805–14.

Gray LP (1975) Results of 310 cases of rapid maxillary expansion. *Journal of Laryngology and Otology* 89: 601–14.

Güray E, Karaman AI (2002) Effects of adenoidectomy on dentofacial structures: A 6-year longitudinal study. *World Journal of Orthodontics* 3: 73–81.

Haas AJ (1961) Rapid expansion of the maxillary dental arch and nasal cavity by opening the midpalatal suture. *Angle Orthodontist* 31: 73–90.

Haddad RV, Abou Chebel N, Ghafari JG (2006) Sequencing cleft lip and palate treatment. *Journal of the Lebanese Dental Association* 43: 9–20.

Harvold EP, Chierici G, Vargervik K (1972) Experiments on the development of dental malocclusions. *American Journal of Orthodontics* 61: 38–44.

Harvold EP, Vargervik K, Chierici G (1973) Primate experiments on oral sensation and dental malocclusions. *American Journal of Orthodontics* 63: 494–508.

Harvold EP, Tomer BS, Vargervik K, et al. (1981) Primate experiments on oral respiration. *American Journal of Orthodontics* 79: 359–72.

Hasbini AS, Hadi U, Ghafari J (2001) Endoscopic removal of an ectopic third molar obstructing the osteomeatal complex. *Ear, Nose and Throat Journal* 80: 667–70.

Hata M, Asakura K, Saito H, et al. (1996) Profile of immunoglobulin production in adenoids and tonsil lymphocytes. *Acta Oto-Laryngologica* 523: 84–6.

Hepper PG, Shahidullah S, White R (1990) Origins of fetal handedness. *Nature* 347: 431.

Hershey HG, Stewart BL, Warren DW (1976) Changes in nasal airway resistance associated with rapid maxillary expansion. *American Journal of Orthodontics* 69: 274–84.

Huertas D, Ghafari J (2001) New posteroanterior cephalometric norms: a comparison with craniofacial measures of children treated with palatal expansion. *Angle Orthodontist* 71: 285–92.

Isaacson RJ, Murphy TD (1964) Some effects of rapid maxillary- Expansion in cleft lip and palate patients. *Angle Orthodontist* 34: 143–54.

Kahle W (1993) *Nervous System and Sensory Organs.* 3rd ed., Vol. 3. New York: Thieme Medical Publishers.

Kaygusuz I, Alpay HC, Godekmerdan A, et al. (2009) Evaluation of long-term impacts of tonsillectomy on immune functions of children: A follow-up study. *International Journal of Pediatric Otorhinolaryngology* 73: 445–9.

Kelly KM (1993) Recurrent otitis media: genetic immunoglobulin markers in children and their parents. *International Journal of Pediatric Otorhinolaryngology* 25: 279–80.

Kerr WJ, McWilliam JS, Linder-Aronson S (1989) Mandibular form and position related to changed mode of breathing- a 5-year longitudinal study. *Angle Orthodontist* 59: 91–6.

Kilic N, Husamettin O, Selimoglu E, et al. (2008a) Effects of semirapid maxillary expansion on conductive hearing loss. *American Journal of Orthodontics and Dentofacial Orthopedics* 133: 846–51.

Kilic N, Kiki A, Husamettin O, et al. (2008b) Effects of rapid maxillary expansion on conductive hearing loss. *Angle Orthodontist* 78: 409–14.

King L, Harris EF, Tolley EA (1993) Heritability of cephalometric and occlusal variables as assessed from siblings with overt malocclusions. *American Journal of Orthodontics and Dentofacial Orthopedics* 104: 121–31.

Kurol J, Modin H, Bjerkhoel A (1998) Orthodontic maxillary expansion and its effect on nocturnal enuresis. *Angle Orthodontist* 68: 225–32.

Kurono Y, Shimamura K, Shigemi H, et al. (1991) Inhibition of bacterial adherence by nasopharyngeal secretions. *Annals of Otology, Rhinology and Laryngology* 100: 455–8.

Kutz JW Jr, Mullin G, Campbell K (2010). Audiology, pure-tone testing. Available at: http://emedicine.medscape.com/article/1822962-media (accessed 24 June 2011).

Laptook T (1981) Conductive hearing loss and rapid maxillary expansion. *American Journal of Orthodontics* 80: 325.

Leiter JC, Baker GL (1989) Partitioning of ventilation between nose and mouth: the role of nasal resistance. *American Journal of Orthodontics and Dentofacial Orthopedics* 95: 432–8.

Lim DJ, Mogi G (1994) Mucosal immunology of the middle ear and Eustachian tube. In: PL Ogra, J Mestechy, ME Lamen, et al. (eds) *Handbook of Mucosal Immunology.* San Diego: Academic Press, pp. 599–606.

Lim DJ, Chun YM, Lee HY, et al. (2000) Cell biology of tubotympanum in relation to pathogenesis of otitis media: a review. *Vaccine* 19(Suppl 1): S17–25.

Linder-Aronson S (1970) Adenoids: their effect on mode of breathing and nasal airflow and their relationship to characteristics of the facial skeleton and the dentition. A biometric, rhino-manometric and cephalometro-radiographic study on children with and without adenoids. *Acta oto-laryngologica Supplement Stockholm* 265: 1–132.

Linder-Aronson S, Leighton BC (1983) A longitudinal study of the development of the posterior nasopharyngeal wall between 3 and 16 years of age. *European Journal of Orthodontics* 5: 47–58.

Linder-Aronson S, Woodside DG, Lundström A (1986) Mandibular growth direction following adenoidectomy. *American Journal of Orthodontics* 89: 273–84.

Linder-Aronson S, Woodside DG, Hellsing E, et al. (1993) Normalization of incisor position after adenoidectomy. *American Journal of Orthodontics and Dentofacial Orthopedics* 103: 412–27.

Liu Y, Zeng X, Fu M, et al. (2000) Effects of a mandibular repositioner on obstructive sleep apnea. *American Journal of Orthodontics and Dentofacial Orthopedics* 118: 248–56.

Major MP, Flores-Mir C, Major PW (2006) Assessment of lateral cephalometric diagnosis of adenoid hypertrophy and posterior upper airway obstruction: A systematic review. *American Journal of Orthodontics and Dentofacial Orthopedics* 130: 700–8.

Mattar SE, Anselmo-Lima WT, Valera FC, et al. (2004) Skeletal and occlusal characteristics in mouth-breathing pre-school children. *Journal of Clinical Pediatric Dentistry* 28: 315–18.

Mattila PS (2006) Adenoidectomy and tympanostomy tubes in the management of otitis media. *Current Allergy and Asthma Reports* 6: 321–6.

Mesnard L (1929) immediate separation of the maxillae as a treatment for nasal impermeability. *Dental Records* 49: 371–2.

Moss ML (1969) The primary role of functional matrices in facial growth. *American Journal of Orthodontics* 55: 566–77.

Moss ML (1997a) The functional matrix hypothesis revisited. 3. The genomic thesis. *American Journal of Orthodontics and Dentofacial Orthopedics* 112: 338–42.

Moss ML (1997b) The functional matrix hypothesis revisited. 4. The epigenetic antithesis and the resolving synthesis. *American Journal of Orthodontics and Dentofacial Orthopedics* 112: 410–17.

Oulis CJ, Vadiakas GP, Ekonomides J, et al. (1994) The effect of hypertrophic adenoids and tonsils on the development of posterior crossbite and oral habits. *Journal of Clinical Pediatric Dentistry* 18: 197–201.

Ovsenik M (2009) Incorrect orofacial functions until 5 years of age and their association with posterior crossbite. *American Journal of Orthodontics and Dentofacial Orthopedics* 136: 375–81.

Proffit WR (2007) The etiology of orthodontic problems- Respiratory pattern. In: WR Proffit, HW Fields Jr, DM Sarver (eds) *Contemporary Orthodontics,* 4th edn. St Louis, MO: Mosby, pp. 154–8.

Pruzansky S (1975) Roentgencephalometric studies of tonsils and adenoids in normal and pathological states. *Annals of Otology, Rhinology and Laryngology* 84(Suppl 19): 55–62.

Ricketts RM (1981) Perspectives in the clinical application of cephalometrics: the first 50 years. *Angle Orthodontist* 51: 115–50.

Rovers MM, Schilder AG, Zielhuis GA, et al. (2004) Otitis media. *Lancet* 363: 465–73.

Rudolph AM (1977) *Pediatrics*, 16th edn. New York, NY: Appleton-Century-Crofts, pp. 954–68.

Sanders EA, Tenbergen-Meekes AM, Voorhorst-Ogink MM, et al. (1995) Immunoglobulin isotype-specific antibody responses to pneumococcal polysaccharide vaccine in patients with recurrent respiratory tract infections. *Pediatric Research* 37: 812–19.

Scammon RE, Harris JA, Jackson CM, et al. (1930) *The Measurement of Man*. Minneapolis, MN: University of Minnesota Press.

Schendel SA, Eisenfeld J, Bell WH, et al. (1976) The long face syndrome: vertical maxillary excess. *American Journal of Orthodontics* 70: 398–408.

Schütz-Fransson U, Kurol J (2008) Rapid maxillary expansion effects on nocturnal enuresis in children: a follow-up study. *Angle Orthodontist* 78: 201–8.

Seibert JW, Danner CJ (2006) Eustachian tube function and the middle ear. *Otolaryngologic clinics of North America* 39: 1221–35.

Stenfors LE, Raisanen S (1993) Secretory IgA-, IgG- and C3b-coated bacteria in the nasopharynx of otitis-prone and non-otitis-prone children. *Acta Oto-Laryngologica* 113: 191–5.

Subtelny JD (1975) Effect of diseases of tonsils and adenoids on dentofacial morphology. *Annals of Otology, Rhinology and Laryngology* 84: 50–4.

Taspinar F, Ucuncu H, Bishara SE (2003) Rapid maxillary expansion and conductive hearing loss. *Angle Orthodontist* 73: 669–73.

Timms DJ (1981) *Rapid Maxillary Expansion*. Chicago, IL: Quintessence Publishing Co. Inc., pp. 15–121.

Timms DJ (1990) Rapid maxillary expansion in the treatment of noctural enuresis. *Angle Orthodontist* 60: 229–33.

Tomes CS (1872) On the developmental origins of the v-shaped contracted maxilla. *Monthly Review of Dental Surgery* 1: 2. Cited in: Rubin RM (1979) The orthodontist's responsibility in preventing facial deformity. In: JA McNamara Jr (ed.) *Naso-Respiratory Function and Craniofacial Growth*. Monograph 9, Craniofacial Growth Series. Ann Arbor, MI: Center for Human Growth and Development, University of Michigan, pp. 323–32.

Tourné LPM (1991) Growth of the pharynx and its physiologic implications. *American Journal of Orthodontics and Dentofacial Orthopedics* 99: 129–39.

Uhari M, Mäntysaari K, Niemelä M (1996) A meta-analytic review of the risk factors for acute otitis media. *Clinical Infectious Diseases* 22: 1079–83.

Usumez S, Işeri H, Orhan M, et al. (2003) Effect of rapid maxillary expansion on nocturnal enuresis. *Angle Orthodontist* 73: 532–8.

Valera FC, Travitzki LV, Mattar SE, et al. (2003) Muscular, functional and orthodontic changes in pre school children with enlarged adenoids and tonsils. *International Journal of Pediatric Otorhinolaryngology* 67: 761–70.

Valtonen HJ, Blomgren KE, Qvarnberg YH (2000) Consequences of adenoidectomy in conjunction with tonsillectomy in children. *International Journal of Pediatric Otorhinolaryngology* 30: 105–9.

Van Kempen MJ, Rijkers GT, Van Cauwenberge PB (2000) The immune response in adenoids and tonsils. *International Archives of Allergy and Immunology* 122: 8–19.

Villano A, Grampi B, Fiorentini R, et al. (2006) Correlations between rapid maxillary expansion (RME) and the auditory apparatus. *Angle Orthodontist* 76: 752–8.

Warren DW (1990) Effect of airway obstruction upon facial growth. *Otolaryngologic Clinics of North America* 23: 699–712.

Warren DW, Hershey HG, Turvey TA, et al. (1987) The nasal airway following maxillary expansion. *American Journal of Orthodontics* 91: 111–16.

Wertz RA (1968) Changes in nasal airflow incident to rapid maxillary expansion. *Angle Orthodontist* 38: 1–11.

Woodside DG, Linder-Aronson S, Lundström A, et al. (1991a) Mandibular and maxillary growth after changed mode of breathing. *American Journal of Orthodontics and Dentofacial Orthopedics* 100: 1–18.

Woodside DG, Linder-Aronson S, Stubbs DO (1991b) Relationship between mandibular incisor crowding and nasal mucosal swelling. *Proceedings of the Finnish Dental Society* 87: 127–38.

13

Obstructive Sleep Apnea: Orthodontic Strategies to Establish and Maintain a Patent Airway

Mimi Yow, Eric Lye Kok Weng

Summary

Obstructive sleep apnea (OSA) is a significant chronic condition that can occur in young and old patients. The etiology is complex and multifactorial in nature. Dental, medical, and surgical practitioners all have a role to play in the diagnosis and treatment planning of OSA. The responsibility of the orthodontist is to recognize patients, either at risk of or those who may already have OSA. The diagnosis and appropriate modalities of treatment are established in consultation with medical and surgical colleagues. Although the gold standard treatment of continuous positive airway pressure (CPAP) can be applied to both groups of patients, compliance with its long-term use can be challenging. Besides CPAP, there are other OSA treatment modalities that can be considered. In growing children, dentofacial orthopedic treatment for maxillary expansion and mandibular growth, in conjunction with otolaryngological management of hyperplastic lymphoid tissues, may alleviate or cure apnea. The orthodontist should always consider pre-existing narrow, posterior airway space in adult patients so that orthodontic and orthognathic treatment does not further embarrass a compromised airway. Mandibular advancement splints are efficacious in relieving mild to moderately severe OSA. Long-term follow-up is a necessary part of the interdisciplinary care of OSA patients and involves review and management of medical comorbidities and obesity.

Introduction

Apnea is derived from the Greek words, *a* (without), and *pnoia* (wind) (Lechner, 1990). There are three distinct types of sleep apnea: central, obstructive, and complex, with an estimated frequency of 0.4%, 84%, and 15%, respectively. Complex apnea is a combination of apneas with a transition of features from central to obstructive apnea (Morgenthaler et al., 2006).

Obstructive sleep apnea (OSA) is defined as interrupted airflow despite persistent respiratory effort. It occurs several times every hour during sleep. Breathing continues but the airflow is blocked. This is due to the complete or partial collapse, and/or complete or partial obstructions, of the upper airway during sleep but not during wakefulness. With reduced airflow, gaseous exchange is impaired. Sleep is fragmented due to recurrent arousals (American Academy of Sleep Medicine, 2005).

OSA is a common sleep-breathing disorder. It affects approximately 2–4% of the middle-aged American population; men are twice as likely as women to have OSA. Among habitual snorers between the ages of 30 and 60 years, approximately 25% of men and 10% of women have OSA. The gender difference diminishes with age, and by 50 years of age, the incidence of OSA is similar in both sexes.

Body mass index (BMI) is an independent factor that correlates with severe OSA. In the morbidly obese, the incidence of OSA increases by at least 12–30 times (Young et al., 1993; Kyzer and Charuzi, 1998; Resta et al., 2001). Weight gain and obesity are important factors in the development and progression of OSA in middle-aged patients. The World Health Organization (WHO) recommends cut-off points to indicate obesity at BMI $\geq 30 \, \text{kg/m}^2$ for Caucasian adults and $\geq 28 \, \text{kg/m}^2$ for Asian adults; Asians have higher body fat percentage at a lower BMI (WHO Expert Consultation, 2004). Other than age, gender, and obesity, general characteristics of OSA patients are low waist-hip ratio and high serum cholesterol concentration (Tishler et al., 2003).

The estimated prevalence of pediatric OSA is 1–3%, affecting children at around 2–6 years of age with no gender

Integrated Clinical Orthodontics, First Edition. Edited by Vinod Krishnan, Ze'ev Davidovitch.
© 2012 Blackwell Publishing Ltd. Published 2012 by Blackwell Publishing Ltd.

predilection (Rosen et al., 2004). Among the morbidly obese children between the ages of 6 and 19 years, OSA prevalence increases to 55% (Chay et al., 2000). There is evidence linking OSA with cardiovascular and metabolic diseases, affecting not only children with OSA, but also in children with primary or habitual snoring (Ali et al., 1993; Brunetti et al., 2001; Ferreira et al., 2000; Gozal and Pope, 2001; Chervin et al., 2002, 2006; Chng et al., 2004; Gottlieb et al., 2004; Kennedy et al., 2004; Montgomery-Downs and Gozal, 2006). Approximately 6–11% of children in Asian and Caucasian populations snore habitually. In a Caucasian group of 3–6-year-olds who were habitual snorers, 13% had OSA, whereas in an Asian population of 7-year-olds who were habitual snorers, 9% developed OSA after 3 years. In most children, habitual or primary snoring does not progress to OSA and resolves spontaneously (Castronovo et al., 2003; Anuntaseree et al., 2005).

Regardless of the type of sleep apnea, the patient is usually unaware of the problem. Commonly, symptoms may be present for years without recognition, and over time, the patient may become accustomed to daytime sleepiness related to respiratory-related sleep disturbances at night. Sleep apnea is more often than not reported by bedpartners who witness the patient's sleep-breathing problems or there may be suspicion of OSA when sequelae of chronic OSA are noticed by the patient or physician.

There is still much to understand about the etiology, pathogenesis, and progression of OSA, despite decades of studies into the nature of the condition and ability to view the awake and asleep airway tract with modern imaging technologies. Clinicians face many, as yet unanswered, questions:

- What is the relationship between OSA in childhood and later on in life? Does childhood OSA progress to adult OSA?
- What are the risk factors and how much time does it take for childhood OSA to progress to adult OSA?
- Does a small-sized pharyngeal airway and mandible predispose to OSA?
- Why do age-related changes in anatomy and muscle physiology lead to development of OSA in some people but not in others?
- What is best practice in orthodontic and orthognathic treatment with regard to OSA patients with malocclusions?

The spectrum of obstructive sleep-disordered breathing

The signs and symptoms of what we now know as the sleep-disordered breathing spectrum were recognised many centuries ago. They were described in literary works by William Shakespeare and Charles Dickens, in the seventeenth and nineteenth century, respectively. In Shakespeare's last play,

The Tempest, Sebastian says to Antonio as they circle the sleeping bodies, 'Thou dost snore distinctly; there is meaning in thy snores' (Shakespeare *circa* 1611). In his first novel, the *Posthumous Papers of the Pickwick Club*, Dickens (1837) described one of his characters, Joe, as 'a wonderfully fat boy – habited as a serving lad, standing upright on a mat, with his eyes closed as if in sleep'. Obesity-hypoventilation or Pickwickian Syndrome, named with reference to fat Joe, was medically recognised in the 1950's as severe obesity associated with hypoxia from OSA, hypercapnia from hypoventilation leading to excessive daytime sleepiness, fatigue and heart failure.

OSA is but one entity in a wide-ranging SDB spectrum of conditions with variable severity and overlapping symptoms (Figure 13.1). There are different grades of OSA; simple snoring without arousals or symptoms is at the lower end of the spectrum, whereas upper airway resistance syndrome (UARS) is considered more severe and is associated with multiple respiratory effort-related arousals (RERAs). Sleep hypopnea syndrome is characterized by snoring with symptoms increasing in severity but with the absence of apneas. Mild, moderate, and severe OSA increases with severity in the continuum. At the extreme end of the spectrum is the obesity-hypoventilation syndrome or the Pickwickian syndrome. The Pickwickian syndrome is classified as an extreme form of OSA and is associated with severe morbidity and very high mortality (Burwell et al., 1994; American Academy of Sleep Medicine Task, 1999; Moore, 2000).

Decoding OSA

A thorough physical examination of the patient with OSA is necessary to establish an accurate medical status.

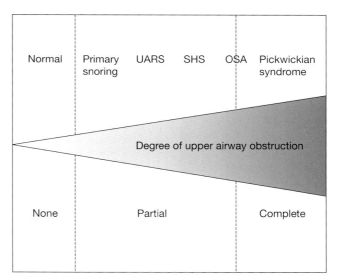

Figure 13.1 Spectrum of sleep-disordered breathing: UARS-upper airway resistance syndrome; SHS-sleep hypopnea syndrome; OSA-obstructive sleep apnea.

Coexistence of a wide range of medical conditions such as obesity, hypertension, cardiac dysfunction, chronic obstructive pulmonary disease, restrictive lung diseases, metabolic disease, muscular dystrophy, kyphoscoliosis, hypothyroidism, and pituitary tumors highlights the importance of interactive collaboration in the overall management of a patient with OSA (Davila, 1995; Mathur and Douglas, 1995).

The gold standard test for confirmation of OSA is an attended overnight polysomnography (PSG). This is a hospital-based test that records specific physiological parameters during sleep, which enables the diagnosis of OSA and other types of sleep disorders to be made. The total number of respiratory events in an hour is expressed as the apnea-hypopnea index (AHI). AHI is derived from the sum of apneas and hypopneas in an hour of sleep.

An adult apneic event is defined as complete cessation of airflow, for 10 seconds or more, despite persistent respiratory effort. Hypopnea occurs when airflow reduces, by 30% or more, in a partially obstructed airway. Each episode of reduced airflow is significant if it lasts for at least 10 seconds' with an arterial oxygen desaturation of 4% or more; or if there is a 50% or greater reduction in airflow for at least 10 seconds associated with an arousal due to hypercapnia. The criterion of apneas and hypopneas of 10 seconds duration is based on two lost breaths during normal adult respiration rates. Five to 15 apnea and/or hypopnea events per hour is classified as mild OSA, more than 15 and up to 30 events per hour is moderately severe OSA, and more than 30 events per hour is classified as severe OSA (Guilleminault et al., 1978; American Academy of Sleep Medicine Task Force, 1999).

The criteria for defining pediatric OSA differ from those of adult OSA (Table 13.1). In children, OSA consists of shorter apnea and hypopnea periods associated with pediatric respiration rates. An apneic event lasts for the duration of two lost breaths in children, about 6 seconds. Hypopnea in children refers to a drop in airflow by at least 50% and associated with an arousal or an arousal with 3% desaturation of arterial oxygen. An AHI of 1–5

events per hour is indicates very mild OSA, 5–10 events per hour is mild OSA, 10–20 events per hour is moderately severe OSA, and greater than 20 events per hour is severe OSA in children (American Academy of Sleep Medicine, 2005).

Polysomnographic values of note are the AHI and the apnea index (AI) in grading the severity of OSA. Based on positive clinical findings, even if the AHI value is low, a diagnosis of OSA with an AHI of 1 is considered to be significant in children. Clinical information is as important as AHI and AI values in determining the clinical severity and morbidity of pediatric sleep-disordered breathing (Marcus et al., 1992; American Thoracic Society, 1999; Chan et al., 2004). Affected children demonstrate behavioral problems and learning problems, hyperactivity, inattention, aggression, and neurocognitive deficits with impact on memory, learning, and executive functions. Research suggests that neurocognitive deficits are partially reversible but there may be a residual learning deficit representing a 'learning debt' (Gozal and Pope, 2001; Larkin et al., 2005). Children with AHI ≥5 have raised levels of C-reactive protein (CRP), which is known to increase the risk of cardiovascular disease. Children with OSA may also have autonomic dysfunction with increased sympathetic activity (Gozal and O'Brien, 2004). There is also evidence of systemic inflammation in OSA patients (AM Li et al., 2008). The inflammatory mediator cysteinyl leukotriene (cys-LT) has been found in exhaled breath condensates of children and is related to the severity of SDB (Goldhart et al., 2006).

OSA is complex in children and cannot be excluded on the basis of history and physical examination (Gottlieb and Young, 2009). A diagnosis of OSA based on history and physical examination has a sensitivity of 63%, and a specificity of 60%. All the studies conducted on the predictive value of the history and the clinical signs and symptoms indicate that there is no foolproof method for confirming OSA except by attended overnight polysomnography (Hoffstein and Szalai, 1993).

If there is a high index of clinical suspicion, the patient should be referred to a doctor trained to manage sleep

Table 13.1 Comparisons of childhood and adult obstructive sleep apnea

Parameter	Child	Adult
Peak age	2–6 years	30–60 years
Gender ratio (female : male)	1 : 1	1 : 2
Apnea–hypopnea index	≥1	≥5
Estimated prevalence		
– In the general population	1–3%	2–4%
– In habitual snorers	9%	10–40%
– In morbidly obese	37–55%	>50%
BMI	Failure to thrive or ≥98th percentile	≥28 Asian; ≥30 Caucasian
Common cause	Adenotonsillar hypertrophy	Obesity

disorders or a sleep disorders team for examination of all possible causes and confirmation of the diagnosis. Full night (type 1) polysomnography is the gold standard test and is recommended for the diagnosis of OSA both in adults and in children (Kushida et al., 2005).

Respiration: effect of anatomy and sleep

Effect of anatomy on respiration

The upper airway tract comprises three components: the nose, the pharynx, and the larynx. The nose, portal to the upper airway, is divided into two openings by the nasal septum; there is an alternative route should one nostril be blocked. The nasal airway is the preferred route for resting ventilation and infants are obligatory nasal breathers (Hall et al., 2000). The structures maintaining the patency of the anterior nares are the alar, procerus, compressor, and dilator naris muscles. The anterior nasal valves are responsible for much of the nasal resistance in patients with normal nasal apertures. The nose contributes to up to half of the total airway resistance in the normal awake patient (Ferris et al., 1964). The lateral nasal walls contain several protuberances, the nasal turbinates, which serve the following functions: creation of air turbulence to slow down airflow so as to prolong air contact with the highly vascularized nasal mucosa for temperature and humidity control; it contains nasal secretions with antimicrobial actions on inhaled air before it is channeled into the lungs. With increased ventilatory drives to meet physiological demands, the nasal apertures widen and nasal mucosa constricts to reduce airflow resistance. At a physiological threshold of ventilatory demand, the mouth opens for oral breathing to increase volume per breath, bypassing nasal resistance.

Inspired air passes through the nasal airway to the pharynx via the bilateral choanae. The pharynx traverses three regions: the nasopharynx which extends from the posterior nasal choanae to the hard palate; the oropharynx which comprises the retropalatal and retroglossal segments – the former extends from the level of the hard palate to the caudal margin of the soft palate and tip of the uvula, and the latter from the soft palate margins to the base of the epiglottis; the laryngopharynx, which is the segment from the base of the tongue to the larynx. Narrowing of the posterior nasal choanae occurs in patients with craniofacial abnormalities. Pharyngeal airway narrowing or collapse is common at the retropalatal and the retroglossal aspects of the pharynx, with a majority of patients having more than one site of obstruction (Hudgel, 1988; Horner et al., 1989; Launois et al., 1993; Morrison et al., 1993; Suto et al., 1993; Trudo et al., 1998; Ciscar et al., 2001).

Nasendoscopic studies describe the mechanics of pharyngeal airway narrowing as a function of sphincteric movement of the lateral pharyngeal walls together with backward movement of the anterior structures. Posterior pharyngeal wall movement is not implicated in airway narrowing (Weitzman et al., 1978).

The larynx connects the pharynx with the lower airway, the trachea. It is responsible for phonation as well as protection of the trachea. It is bounded superiorly by the epiglottis, inferiorly by the vocal chords, and laterally by the aryepiglottic folds. These structures work in synchrony to channel air into the anterior tract, the trachea, whereas food and liquids are directed into the posterior tract, the esophagus. The epiglottis acts as a valve to separate the trachea from the esophagus during deglutition and to maintain a patent airway during respiration. The posterior cricoarytenoid is the only abductor muscle that widens the glottic aperture during inspiration and expiration. The tongue and lingual tonsils, which stud the dorsum of the posterior third of the tongue, may hinder the function of the epiglottis if the lingual tissues are enlarged and encroach into the posterior airway space (Suzuki and Kirchner, 1969; Wyke, 1974).

Redundant mucosa in the arytenoid-aryepiglottic region has been associated with OSA. Vocal chord abnormalities are rarely implicated in symptomatic OSA, however, bilateral vocal chord paralysis has been reported to be associated with snoring. Rarely, congenital vallecula cysts occur between the base of the tongue and the epiglottis. When cysts are present in this region or in the larynx, they are sometimes associated with airway obstruction, stridor, pyoceles, or vocal chord paralysis (Griffith et al., 1993).

Many cephalometric studies have shown an association between certain craniofacial characteristics and OSA. These include hard and soft tissue features such as reduced mandibular body length (Miles et al., 1996), posteriorly positioned maxilla, and inferiorly positioned hyoid bone (deBerry-Borowiecki et al., 1988; Bacon et al., 1990; Pracharktam et al., 1994; Lowe et al., 1995). Other distinguishing craniofacial features of OSA patients are reduced cranial base length, mandibular or maxillomandibular retrusion, increased lower face height, an elongated soft palate, large tongue and a smaller upper airway compared with normal individuals (Horner et al., 1989; Ciscar et al., 2001).

The oropharyngeal airway is usually narrowed (Shepard and Thawley, 1989; Schwab et al., 1993, 2003) in OSA. Reduced size of the posterior airway space and increased distance of the hyoid bone to the mandible are also associated with OSA. The two cephalometric parameters that are used as indicators of OSA are: posterior airway space of less than 11 mm and a hyoid to mandible distance of greater than 15.4 mm (Riley et al., 1983). Severe respiratory disturbance indices are associated with a posterior airway space of less than 5 mm at the base of the tongue and a distance of the hyoid bone to the lower border of the mandible distance of 24 mm or greater (Partinen et al., 1988). There is low probability of OSA if the airway cross-sectional area is greater than 110 mm^2, but a high probability of severe OSA if the area measures less than 52 mm^2. Most constrictions are located in the oropharynx (Lowe et al., 1986; Avrahami and Englender, 1995; Ogawa et al., 2007).

There are also differences in the soft tissue characteristics of OSA patients compared with those without OSA; besides a larger tongue, OSA patients have thicker and longer soft palates and parapharyngeal fat pads in the lateral pharyngeal walls (Schwab, 2003; Schwab et al., 2003).

Effects of sleep on respiration

The diaphragm is the main driver of ventilation during sleep. Pharyngeal airway patency is well maintained during wakefulness but during sleep, pharyngeal and genioglossal muscle activity is reduced, which predisposes to sleep-dependent pharyngeal airway collapse (McNicholas, 2002; Jordan and White, 2008). Sleep adversely affects tonic and phasic skeletal muscle functions. There is evidence suggesting that in OSA, the intrinsic upper airway muscle function and central neural regulation of the upper airway dilator muscles and genioglossus may be impaired. Recurrent apnea during sleep induces intermittent hypoxia that alters respiratory muscle contraction, reducing muscle endurance with diminished pharyngeal electromyographic (EMG) responses to physiological changes (Bradford et al., 2005).

Sleep depresses muscular contractions, which allows the negative pressure of inspiration to pull the tongue into the pharyngeal airway (Remmers et al., 1978). The mechanical properties of the upper airway, that maintain tissue stiffness and thus airway patency, are reliant on intrinsic physiological properties. In OSA patients, there is reduced effectiveness of upper airway dilator contraction and reduced genioglossal reflex. The genioglossal negative pressure reflex declines with age, which may explain age-related increase in OSA. Current evidence suggests a biomechanical basis for OSA in patients who have an anatomical and sleep-positional predisposition to pharyngeal collapse (White et al., 1985; Sériès, 2002; Malhotra et al., 2004; Dempsey et al., 2010).

Mechanical influences on respiration

A number of mechanical influences impact the airway diameter causing it to be open, narrowed, or closed. These factors can be either static or dynamic. Static factors are surface adhesive forces, neck and jaw posture, tracheal tug, gravity, and sleep position. Dynamic factors comprise upstream resistance within the nasal airway and pharynx: the Bernoulli effect and dynamic compliance (Schwab et al., 2005).

Several studies have demonstrated a smaller upper airway width in OSA patients compared with patients without OSA. The reduction in size of the upper airway has been attributed to the enlargement of the surrounding soft tissues: lateral pharyngeal walls, parapharyngeal fat, tongue, and soft palate. Reduced airway diameter affects airway resistance the most, as described by Poiseuille's law: $R = 8nl/pr4$; the resistance (R) and the length of the tube (l) are inversely related to its radius (r) and pressure (p). By halving the size of the tube, resistance increases 16 times (Shepard and Thawley, 1989; Schwab et al., 1993; Schwab, 2003; Schwab et al., 2003).

Nasal obstruction has been implicated as a cause of OSA because nasal resistance and mouth breathing increase upper airway collapsibility. Nasal resistance, measured by posterior rhinomanometry, is reported to be higher in individuals with OSA. Nasal resistance increases upper airway pressure during inspiration, placing the pharyngeal walls at a greater risk of collapse (Isono et al., 2004). In infants, during sleep, the genioglossal activity increases when an infant switches from oral to nasal breathing. There is evidence correlating increased genioglossal EMG activity with changes in airway resistance and carbon dioxide levels (Roberts et al., 1986).

Mouth-breathing may also play a role in pharyngeal airway obstruction by changed dynamics in the airway; mouth-opening destabilizes airway patency. When the tongue is lowered, it moves away from the soft palate. Once the soft palate is no longer in contact with the tongue, it becomes free moving and obstructs the pharyngeal airway when it falls backwards. Surface adhesion forces of mucosal surfaces may also be contributory in maintaining airway patency (Issa and Sullivan, 1984; Roberts et al., 1985).

OSA in children

The clinical morbidties associated with obstructed upper airways were first reported in medical publications more than a century ago. In 1889, Ambroise Guye described 'the impairment of cerebral functions by disorders of the nose'. The obstructive effect of enlarged adenoid masses, particularly during sleep, was observed to produce 'aprosexia' – the inability to fix the attention on any abstract subject. With removal of the adenoid mass from the nasopharynx, headaches ceased and learning difficulties were prevented (Guye, 1889).

This observation was confirmed soon after by William Hill (1889) who was 'much struck by the fact that operations on children, undertaken for the relief of deafness associated with adenoid growths, enlarged tonsils, and hypertrophic catarrhal conditions of the nose, have frequently resulted in such an immediate improvement in the mental acuteness of the patients as was altogether incommensurate with the often slight immediate improvement in the sense of hearing.' He advised that the 'stupid looking lazy child who frequently suffers from headache at school, breathes through his mouth instead of his nose, snores and is restless at night, and wakes up with a dry mouth in the morning, is well worthy of the solicitous attention of the medical officer'.

Despite Hill and Guye's strikingly similar observations, the controversies over the causality of OSA and what is systematic evidence-based management of children with nasal congestion, adenotonsillar hypertrophy and OSA rage on till today (Bixler et al., 2009). Although OSA in children is largely attributed to adenotonsillar hypertrophy, there is no conclusive evidence to demonstrate a causal relationship between enlarged tonsils and/or adenoids in children with SDB. Nevertheless, magnetic resonance imaging (MRI) has revealed the region of greatest pharyngeal airway narrowing as the area where the adenoid and tonsillar masses overlap (Arens et al., 2003).

Diagnosis

Proper diagnosis forms the basis for effective treatment. All children should be screened for snoring as part of well-child visits. Habitual snoring, if present, should prompt a more detailed history for other symptoms: unusual sleeping postures, restless sleep, labored sleep-breathing, observed apneas, hyperactivity, attention deficit or behavioral problems. Hyperactivity is more likely to be present in the child with OSA rather than excessive daytime sleepiness; the latter occurs more often in adults with OSA (Leach et al., 1992; Carroll, 1996). Craniofacial anomalies and hyotonia in children are positively correlated with OSA and craniofacial morphology attributed to OSA. Down syndrome children, who have hyotonia and obesity, are more likely to develop OSA (approximately 59–79%; Dyken et al., 2003; Ng et al., 2006). Treated cleft lip and palate patients have similar craniofacial, craniocervical, and pharyngeal morphology with OSA patients; narrowing of the oropharyngeal airway at the tip of the velum and a greater distance between the hyoid and the mandibular plane (Oosterkamp et al., 2007).

There is a positive correlation between OSA and obese children without adenotonsillar hypertrophy (Verhulst et al., 2008). In children with adenotonsillar hypertrophy, the greatest narrowing of the airway is seen at the retropalatal region where the soft palate, adenoid, and tonsils overlap (Isono et al., 1998; Fregosi et al., 2003). Significant cephalometric nasopharyngeal airway measurements are as follows:

- Percentage of nasopharynx occupied by the adenoid mass compared to percentage airway norm for a 6-year-old is approximately 51% (Handelman and Osborne, 1976; Schulof, 1978).
- Reduced distance from the posterior nasal spine (PNS) to the nearest adenoid mass measured along PNS-basion;

normal distance in a 6-year-old is approximately 15–21mm (Linder-Aronson, 1970; Schulof, 1978).
- Reduced distance from PNS to the nearest adenoid mass measured along a line through PNS perpendicular to sella-basion; normal measurement in a 6-year-old is approximately 15–16mm (Schulof, 1978; Linder-Aronson and Leighton, 1983).
- Reduced distance to the nearest adenoid mass from a point on the pterygoid vertical 5mm above PNS; the normal value is approximately 7mm (Ricketts, 1954; Schulof, 1978).

Screening for OSA using questionnaires in children with adenotonsillar hypertrophy has been suggested, but it has not been proven to detect the presence or the absence of OSA (Constantin et al., 2010). Adenotonsillar hypertrophy is a common finding in children. The Scammon growth curves demonstrate accelerated growth of the lymphoid tissue from birth, reaching its maximum at 11–13 years. The total body lymphoid tissue of a 13-year-old will have attained a mass of almost 200% greater than that of an adult. Lymphoid tissue growth declines and tails off gradually between 14 and 20 years of age. Craniofacial skeletal growth follows a different timing and growth trajectory; the cranial vault and the upper face follow the neural pattern of growth which peaks between 8 and 12 years of age, with growth ceasing between 12 to 16 years of age. Growth of the lower face and mandible follows the general adolescent growth spurt, peaking between 14 to 18 years, and slows down or stops after 20 years of age (Scammon, 1930).

Selective screening of special groups of children, those with craniofacial syndromes and complex craniofacial synostosis, is effective in those with complex craniosynostosis and have fusion of at least two cranial sutures. In a study of children with Apert, Crouzon, Muenke, Pfeiffer and Saethre–Chotzen craniosynostotic syndromes, the critical clinical question that identified children without OSA was 'Has the child difficulty with breathing during sleep?' A negative response excluded clinically significant OSA (high negative predictive value of 91%, sensitivity of 64%). Snoring is a common but less specific symptom as 77% of the children with craniofacial syndromes snored due to narrow noses and midface hypoplasia. Children with craniofacial syndromes or complex craniosynostoses had a 40% chance of developing OSA from midface retrusion (Bannink et al., 2010).

Some studies recommend against the use of history to distinguish the primary snorer from the child with OSA (Carroll et al., 1995; Lamm et al., 1999). Screening pediatric patients for OSA using a combination of history taking, sleep-related symptoms questionnaire and clinical assessment misses the detection of OSA of 1 in 5 children. An unusual sleep posture, as in sitting up to sleep, has been shown to be a significant predictor of a child with OSA.

However, overnight polysomnography is still the definitive diagnostic tool for confirming the presence of OSA (Chay et al., 2000).

Certain groups of children should be targeted for OSA screening. The risks of OSA are higher in children with craniofacial anomalies, Down syndrome, cleft lip and palate after pharyngoplasty, morbid obesity, and atopic disease (Guilleminault et al., 1981; Brouillette et al., 1982; Mallory et al., 1989; Marcus et al., 1991; Silvestri et al., 1993; Chng et al., 2004). The index of suspicion for OSA is further increased in children who fail to thrive or are obese and have cardiovascular symptoms. Obesity in a child is defined as having a BMI that is above the 95th percentile in their age and gender cohort. Obesity is a primary independent factor impacting on the respiratory disturbance index (RDI) in children. Children with BMI ≥180 percent of ideal body weight are deemed to be morbidly obese, and between 37–55% of such children have OSA (Brooks et al., 1998; Chay et al., 2000; Mei et al., 2002).

As part of the well-child program, all children should be screened for sleep-breathing problems. Children at risk must be referred for a thorough evaluation and confirmation of OSA by a sleep-trained pediatrician (American Academy of Pediatrics, 2002).

Orthodontic management

In 1902, Dr Pierre Robin fabricated an 'apparatus, the monobloc', the first oral appliance to be used in airway management. He prescribed the monobloc appliance for use in children who had 'hypotrophy' of the mandible from as young as 20 months. The treatment was aimed at re-establishing the normal spatial relationship of the maxilla and mandible. Dr Robin also observed that 'the great majority of children with hypoplasia of the mandible breathed through the mouth'. Most of them, at 6–7 years of age had adenoids, and 'though the adenoids were removed once or several times they continued to breathe through the mouth and the adenoid facies persisted'.

Dr Robin explained that 'why a child who has had adenoids removed is still unable to breathe through the nose, since he still suffers from glossoptosis'. He concluded that 'adenoidism without adenoids' is a morbid entity requiring general care by a physician and placement of a monobloc in the mouth even after the removal of adenoids. Interdisciplinary management was recognized even then, as necessary, for the treatment of patients with breathing disorders. By using the monobloc to posture the mandible forward, normal mastication is achieved through the 'perfect equilibration' of the temporo-maxillodental articulation' and children with 'adenoidism' are able to breathe through the nose (Robin, 1934). The monobloc was later replaced by the activator, which used in the treatment of Class II Division 1 malocclusion. Modified forms have since been used in treatment of patients with OSA (Cozza et al., 2004).

Treatment involving the maxilla

Rapid maxillary expansion (RME) or slow maxillary expansion (SME) with maxillary protraction increases the transverse width of the maxilla and enlarges the palatal and retropalatal area. This improves the ratio of airway space relative to tonsil size. Enlargement of the dental arches, transversely and anteroposteriorly increases the intraoral space for accommodating the sublingual tissues and tongue by removing the constraints of narrow maxillary and mandibular arches (Viva et al., 1992; Defabjanis, 2003). RME or SME also enlarges the nasal cavities, and purports to reduce nasal resistance thereby promoting nasal breathing. Villa et al. (2007), reported that the majority of children (78.5%) treated with RME had significantly reduced AHI, with 85.7% of the children switching from oral to nasal breathing.

The findings on outcomes of maxillary expansion with regard to reduced nasal resistance and change to nasal respiratory mode are equivocal. Increased width of the nasal floor is associated with reduced nasal resistance in the short term but was not sustained predictably over the long term. Increased nasal airflow resistance should not be the primary indication for maxillary expansion (Berretin-Felix et al., 2006; Ceroni et al., 2006; Enoki et al., 2006; Neeley et al., 2007). Rhinomanometric studies do not support RME with predictable reduction of nasal resistance and improvement of nasal breathing (Hartgerink et al., 1987). Age and gender may be confounding factors affecting the variability of nasal resistance and nasal respiration; more data is needed to distinguish normal nasal from abnormal nasal functions (Vig, 1998).

Treatment of OSA by stimulating maxillary and mandibular growth

Correction of anteroposterior maxillomandibular deficiencies in children may improve OSA. Forward repositioning of the mandible with functional appliances are shown to enlarge the upper airway, improving respiratory function after 6 months and reducing AHI in more than 60% of patients (Villa et al., 2002). Results of studies on the effects of maxillary protraction on airway dimensions in children with Class III malocclusion are contradictory. In one study, significant favorable skeletal changes in the maxilla and mandible did not result in short-term or long-term changes in sagittal airway dimensions of the nasopharynx and oropharynx (Baccetti et al., 2010). One other study reported a favorable increase in airway dimensions with maxillary protraction. Maxillary protraction increased upper airway caliber with significant increases in anteroposterior width as well as nasopharyngeal airway area (Oktay and Ulukaya, 2008). The increased airway size was significantly stable after 4 years. The oropharyngeal airway area, however, did not remarkably increase immediately after active treatment but it increased significantly during a 4-year follow-up

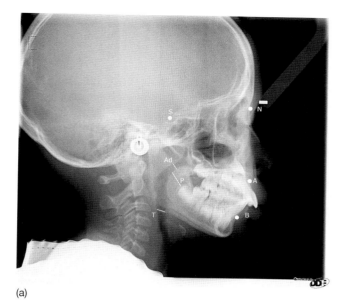

(a)

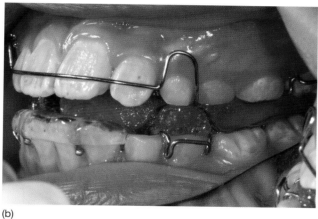

(b)

Figure 13.2 (a) Lateral cephalogram showing the significant parameters in a child with mild obstructive sleep apnea. (b) Twin-block appliance to expand the maxilla and correct the retrognathia.

period (Kaygisiz et al., 2009). The study suggested that the increase in the oropharyngeal airway after active treatment may be an effect of growth.

A randomized controlled study on non-obese 4 to 10-year-old children with OSA (AHI ≥1) reported a normalization of AHI in 50% of patients who used customized oral appliances to advance the mandible for 6 months. The use of oral appliances was associated with reduced tonsillar hypertrophy in about 67% of patients compared with 14% of children in the control group. About 74% of the patients tolerated the appliance treatment well (Villa et al., 2002) (Figure 13.2).

Long-term studies are needed to find out whether dentofacial orthopedic therapy in OSA children is curative in the long term. A review of the effects of oral and functional dentofacial orthopedic appliances indicated that they are an effective nonsurgical alternative in the management of childhood OSA in the short term. However, there is insufficient data to confirm if orthodontic and dentofacial orthopedic treatments are effective in long-term management of OSA (Carvalho et al., 2007).

Children whose OSA does not improve after adenotonsillectomy may have other underlying structural problems: narrow pharyngeal airway, hypoplastic maxilla and/or retrognathic mandible. OSA is also compounded by the coexistence of obesity, neuromuscular disorders, and craniofacial and dentofacial anomalies (Shintani et al., 1998; Chay et al., 2000; Chan et al., 2004).

OSA in adults

Many OSA patients remain undiagnosed because sleep assessments are not included in medical history taking. A thorough medical history and communication with the patient's primary physician are important to establish the patient's general medical condition. OSA is not just confined to obstructive sleep-related breathing; it is also associated with medical comorbidities such as hypertension, congestive heart failure, cardiac arrhythmia, ischemic heart disease, pulmonary hypertension, and metabolic syndrome.

Diagnosis

A thorough history and examination are important tools for identifying adult patients who require further medical evaluation. It is worth while asking the bed-partner whether the patient snores habitually or stops breathing during sleep. Hypersomnolence or excessive daytime sleepiness (EDS) is another common symptom among adults with OSA. EDS screening in adults is easily accomplished with the Epworth Sleepiness Scale (ESS), an eight-item questionnaire. The ESS is a patient-reported assessment of daytime sleepiness and drowsiness in monotonous soporific situations or during driving. ESS score ≥9 predicts a possibility of hypersomnolence (Johns, 1991, 1992).

Other than daytime sleepiness, the patient should be evaluated for hypertension. Obesity, especially upper body fat around the neck, is another reliable indicator of OSA. Routine measurement of neck circumference is recommended. If the neck measures ≥43 cm for men and ≥37 cm for women, the patient will need further evaluation for OSA (Katz et al., 1990; Kushida et al., 1997).

Loud snoring, witnessed apneas, and EDS are defining symptoms of OSA. Loud disruptive snoring has a 71% sensitivity in prediction of sleep-disordered breathing. Loud snoring coupled with witnessed apneas by the bed-partner increases the sensitivity of SBD prediction to 94%. It is important to ask family members or others who may have observed the patient's sleep behavior. Most patients are unaware of their own snoring. Other predictive symptoms are dry mouth, headache on waking, non-refreshing or restless sleep, and nocturia.

Physical examination and assessment of the dentofacial anatomy as well as the upper airway have a central role in patient evaluation for OSA. A physical feature that predisposes to OSA is obesity (BMI $\geq 30\,kg/m^2$ for Caucasian adults and $\geq 28\,kg/m^2$ for Asian adults).

Cephalometrics and imaging

Lateral cephalometry is routinely used in treatment planning of orthodontic patients presenting for treatment of malocclusions. Cephalometric studies of upright as well as supine patients reveal structural differences between apneic and nonapneic subjects. Cephalometric analysis is a two-dimensional radiographic evaluation of the craniodentofacial structures. Cephalometric features associated with OSA are: brachycephalic craniofacial configuration, short anteroposterior cranial base length, reduced nasion-sella-basion angle, inferiorly positioned hyoid, retrognathic maxilla, retrognathic and micrognathic mandible, smaller than normal values for SNA and/or SNB, increased Frankfort mandibular plane angle or maxillary-mandibular planes angle (anterior divergent face), and increased anterior lower face height.

Soft tissue features associated with OSA are narrow retropalatal and retroglossal airway spaces, thicker and longer soft palate, reduced angle between the uvula tip and posterior nasal spine, and a greater tongue mass (Miles et al., 1996; Hui et al., 2003; Ingman et al., 2004; Hsu et al., 2005) (Figure 13.3).

Airway imaging using cone-beam computed tomography (CT) and MRI improved diagnostic capabilities by providing accurate visualization of the airway and enabling volumetric airway measurements. The mean total airway volume, from the anterior nasal cavity to the epiglottic level, is found to be significantly smaller in patients with retrognathic mandibles and significantly correlated with anteroposterior and vertical cephalometric variables, notably the ANB angle and anterior face height (Kim et al., 2010). The availability of cone-beam CT has allowed acquisition of accurate three-dimensional information, which is key to understanding the biomechanical role of the craniofacial structures in the etiology of OSA (Strauss and Burgoyne, 2008; White and Pharoah, 2008) (Figure 13.4).

Examination of the tongue, soft palate, and tonsils

The oral examination of the patient focuses on the oropharynx and the tongue position. The length of the soft palate and the size of the palatine tonsils are also important features as these structures are located in the anterior boundary of the airway. Large palatine tonsils can create localized narrowing of the airway and a long soft palate can fall backwards, thereby reducing the retro-palatal airway in the supine position. These with redundant mucosal folds can

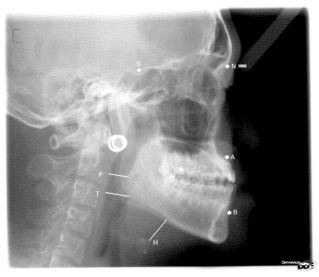

(a)

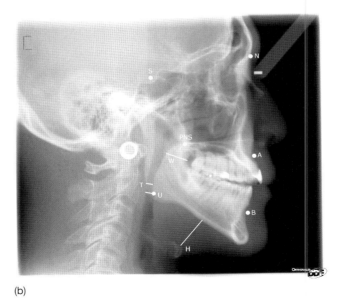

(b)

Figure 13.3 (a) Lateral cephalogram showing normal oropharyngeal airway and soft palate in an adult with no obstructive sleep apnea. (b) Lateral cephalogram showing a narrow oropharyngeal airway and a long and thickened soft palate in an adult with severe obstructive sleep apnea. S, sella; N, nasion; A, point A; B, point B; PNS, posterior nasal spine; H, hyoidale (the most anterior superior point on the body of hyoid bone; the line is drawn to mandibular plane); P, soft palate point (the most posterior point of the soft palate outline; the line is drawn to pharyngeal wall); T, tongue base airway width (the narrowest part of the airway at the base of the tongue; the line is drawn to pharyngeal wall); U, uvula (the most inferior point of the soft palate outline; the line is drawn to pharyngeal wall); W, width of the soft palate (the widest part of the soft palate).

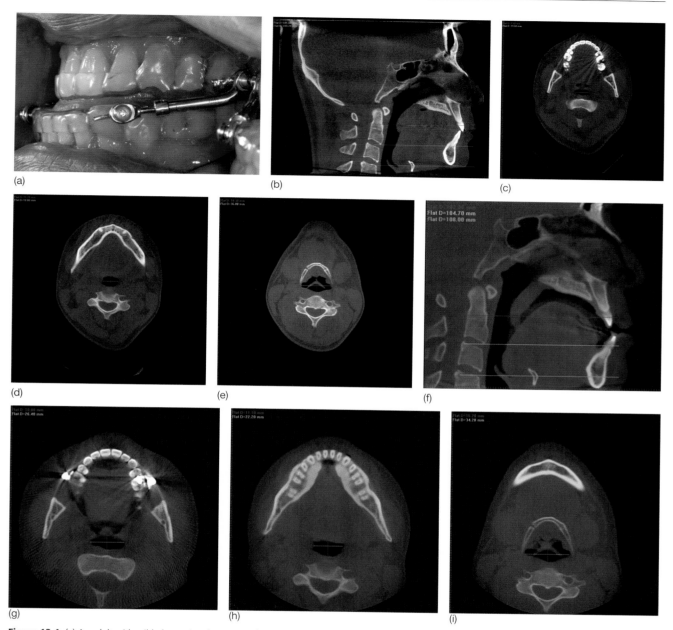

Figure 13.4 (a) An adult with mild obstructive sleep apnea (OSA) wearing a Herbst-type mandibular advancement splint (9 mm). Sagittal cone-beam computed tomography (CT) scans of the posterior airway space in the same patient (b) before the mandibular advancement, (c) at the retropalatal level, (d) at the retroglossal level, (e) at the hypopharyngeal level, (f) after 9 mm mandibular advancement using the mandibular advancement splint (MAS), (g) at the retropalatal level, showing increased anteroposterior and lateral widths, (h) at the retroglossal level showing increased lateral width, (i) but at the hypopharyngeal level the anteroposterior and lateral widths were reduced.

cause turbulence in the airflow resulting in snoring. The size of the oral cavity and the tongue are also aspects that need to be evaluated. The oral cavity size can be estimated by measuring the width of the palatal vault and dental arches and the length of the mandible.

An oral cavity that is comparatively small for the tongue will result in retro-positioning of the tongue, which results in reduced retro-lingual airway (directly) and the retro-palatal airway (by pushing the soft palate up and back). Grading scales can be used to determine the relationship of the oropharyngeal structures, such as the size of tonsils and the tongue position (Figures 13.5 and 13.6). These grading systems provide good clinical predictors of the presence of OSA (Friedman et al., 1999).

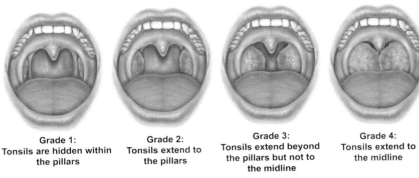

Grade 1:
Tonsils are hidden within
the pillars

Grade 2:
Tonsils extend to
the pillars

Grade 3:
Tonsils extend beyond
the pillars but not to
the midline

Grade 4:
Tonsils extend to
the midline

Figure 13.5 Tonsil size grading. (From Otolaryngology – *Head and Neck Surgery* 127(1): 13–21. Reproduced with permission from Elsevier. Copyright © by the American Academy of Otolaryngology – Head and Neck Surgery Foundation, Inc. Reproduced with permission from Elsevier.)

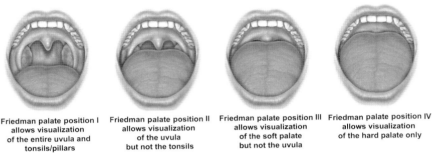

Friedman palate position I
allows visualization
of the entire uvula and
tonsils/pillars

Friedman palate position II
allows visualization
of the uvula
but not the tonsils

Friedman palate position III
allows visualization
of the soft palate
but not the uvula

Friedman palate position IV
allows visualization
of the hard palate only

Figure 13.6 Friedman palate position grading of the tongue in natural position. (From Otolaryngology – *Head and Neck Surgery* 127(1): 13–21. Reproduced with permission from Elsevier. Copyright © by the American Academy of Otolaryngology – Head and Neck Surgery Foundation, Inc. Reproduced with permission from Elsevier.)

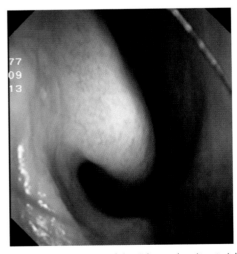

Figure 13.7 Nasendoscopic view of the right nasal cavity: straight septum, normal inferior turbinate, normal nasal mucosa.

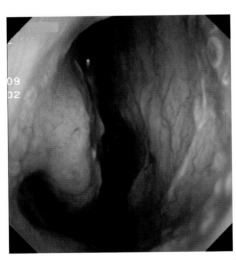

Figure 13.8 Nasendoscopic view of the right nasal cavity: straight septum, normal inferior turbinate, thick mucous discharge on nasal mucosa.

Nasendoscopic examination of the upper airway

The nasal cavity, nasopharynx, oropharynx, and hypopharynx are examined with the aid of a flexible endoscope (Figures 13.7–13.19). The examination starts from the nasal aperture. Septal deviations, internal or external valves collapse, turbinates hypertrophy, nasal polyps, chronic sinusitis with thick mucous discharge or tumor growths can contribute to reduced nasal airway diameter. This in turn leads to increased negative inspiratory pressure and a higher susceptibility of posterior airway collapse (Lavie et al., 1983).

The presence and size of any adenoid hypertrophy are noted. The retropalatal and retroglossal openings are

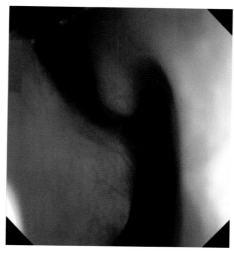

Figure 13.9 Nasendoscopic view of the left nasal cavity: severe septal deviation (in the middle, bottom part) and septal spur (in the middle, top part).

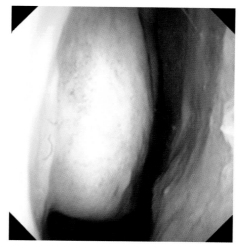

Figure 13.10 Nasendoscopic view of the right nasal cavity: hypertrophic inferior turbinate (left side of image).

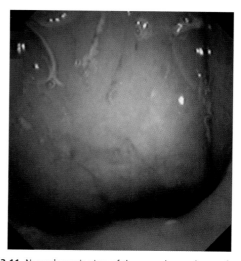

Figure 13.11 Nasendoscopic view of the normal nasopharynx from above.

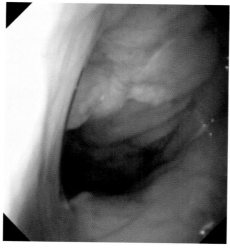

Figure 13.12 Nasendoscopic view of the nasopharynx: adenoid hypertrophy (at the top of the image).

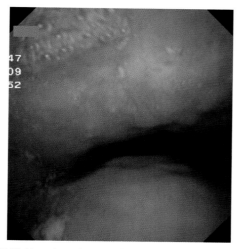

Figure 13.13 Nasendoscopic view of the oropharynx, retropalatal region: narrow airway in the anteroposterior dimension (soft palate is at the bottom of the image).

assessed. The retropalatal opening, which is formed by the soft palate and the lateral and retropharyngeal walls, is examined during normal breathing. Any constrictions in the anteroposterior or lateral dimensions are noted. A Müller maneuver is performed to ascertain the collapsibility of the surrounding soft tissues (Terris et al., 2000). The retroglossal opening is the airway at the level of the base of the tongue. The dimension at this level is affected by macroglossia or retropositioning of the tongue and mandible. The patient will be given a bite-registration wax wafer to simulate mandibular advancement for assessment of enlargement the airway. Enlarged lingual tonsils on the posterior dorsum of the tongue may also be a contributory to OSA, as lingual enlargements displace the epiglottis

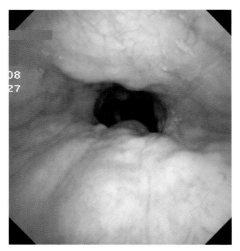

Figure 13.14 Nasendoscopic view of the oropharynx, retropalatal region: anteroposterior narrowing, lateral narrowing, mild adenoid hypertrophy (at the top of the image).

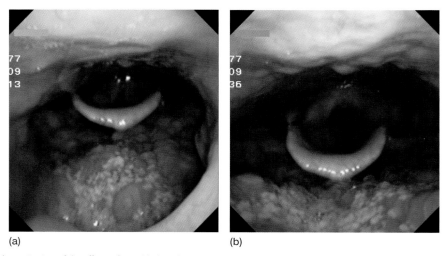

(a)   (b)

Figure 13.15 (a) Nasendoscopic view of the effects of mandibular advancement on narrow hypopharyngeal airway with enlarged lingual tonsils: pre-mandibular advancement image. (b) Nasendoscopic view of the effects of mandibular advancement on narrow hypopharyngeal airway with enlarged lingual tonsils: post-mandibular advancement image.

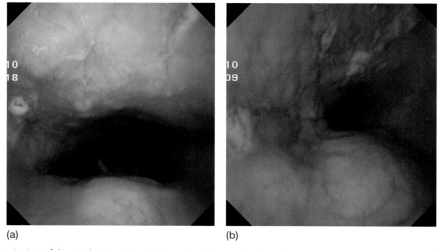

(a)   (b)

Figure 13.16 Nasendoscopic view of the oropharynx, retropalatal region: (a) normal caliber of airway with view of epiglottis, and (b) same patient with severe pharyngeal collapse after the Müller maneuver.

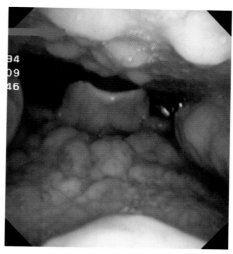

Figure 13.17 Nasendoscopic view of the oropharynx, retrolingual region: anteroposterior and lateral narrowing of retrolingual airway with enlarged right and left palatine tonsils and lingual tonsils against the epiglottis.

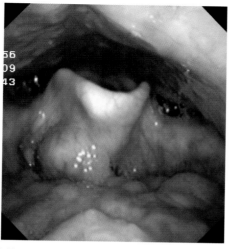

Figure 13.19 Nasendoscopic view of the hypopharynx: large mucocele pressing on right anterior epiglottis.

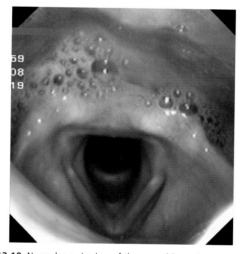

Figure 13.18 Nasendoscopic view of the normal hypopharynx.

posteriorly against the retropharyngeal wall. The hypopharynx is checked for any constrictions secondary to tumors growths, laryngeal or vocal chord abnormalities (Barkdull et al., 2008; Kim et al., 2010).

Orthodontic management

Given the complexity and multiple etiologies, interdisciplinary team management of the patient with OSA involving different specialists and coordination of treatments is essential. The sleep team comprises some or all of the following members depending on the needs of the patient: endocrinologist, general dentist, neurologist, nutritionist, oral and maxillofacial surgeon, orthodontist, otolaryngologist, prosthodontist, psychiatrist, and respiratory physician.

Treatment entails both general and specific measures to manage the varied causes and sequelae of OSA. Treatment is important in managing the patient's general health indicators: weight, cardiovascular health, respiratory and metabolic functions. Specific treatment decisions are based on the appropriate treatment modality for the probable cause or causes of airway obstruction while sleep-breathing.

Orthodontic treatment planning must take into consideration the tongue size, and location of any narrowings of the pharyngeal airway and the posterior airway space. Where appropriate, the treatment plan should enlarge the dental arches to within orthodontically acceptable limits rather than to extract teeth to relieve crowding in narrow maxillary and mandibular arches. Over-retraction of the upper incisors to compensate for a Class II Division 1 malocclusion with a retrusive mandible may position the tongue posteroinferiorly, posing a risk of obstructing an existing narrow oropharyngeal airway.

A combination of clinical, craniofacial, and polysomnographic variables are used to design effective prescriptions for oral appliance treatment. Positive predictors of successful outcomes with the use of oral appliances in OSA in patients with mild to moderate OSA are: AHI ≥5 to ≤30 events per hour (Schmidt-Nowara et al., 1995; Yow, 2009), posture-dependent or supine-related OSA (Marklund et al., 1998), retrognathic mandible, single-site obstruction at the retroglossal region, and an oropharyngeal lumen that is narrowed anteroposteriorly but not laterally. Negative predictors are: severe OSA with AHI >30 events/hour; BMI >30 kg/m^2; multiple level obstructions; nonpositional dependent OSA; inability to protrude the mandible >5 mm;

and Class III malocclusion with a large mandible (Johnston et al., 2002).

In adult patients with mild to moderate OSA, AHI ≥5 to ≤30, intra-oral appliances for mandibular advancement, similar in design to functional appliances for dentofacial growth in children, have been shown to be effective in managing OSA. However, mandibular advancement splints are not recommended as first-line treatment as they are not as efficacious as continuous positive air pressure therapy (CPAP), the latter being the gold standard in treating OSA (Barnes et al., 2004; Hoekema et al., 2004; Lim et al., 2006).

Oral appliance treatment in adult OSA increases the posterior airway space by enlarging the lumen of the pharyngeal airway, and increasing the muscular activity of the pharynx and tongue. Three-dimensional imaging and endoscopic studies of users of mandibular advancement splints have shown increased cross-sectional dimensions at the multiple levels of the pharynx (Liu et al., 2000). Anterior positioning of the mandible displaces the mandibular attachments away from the oropharynx, most importantly, the genioglossus. The upper airway muscle activity is increased through stretching the palatoglossus and palatopharyngeus (Lowe et al., 1990).

Different studies use different indicators to denote success in OSA management: some refer to AHI reduced by 50% as a success criterion while others maintain the polysomnographic yardstick of the norm as AHI ≤5 events/hour. Even though there is computerised tomographic evidence of enlarged airway measurements due to mandibular advancement appliances (Gale et al., 2000), follow-up polysomnography studies of the patient sleeping of the mandibular advancement splint are necessary to confirm the effectiveness in in OSA reduction (Kushida et al., 2005).

There are many types and designs of appliances used in OSA. The two main ones are the mandibular advancement and the tongue-retainer devices. The mandibular advancement device is the OSA appliance that is most widely used. Efficacy and outcomes of treatment with oral appliances with an anterior tongue-retention bulb, with or without mandibular advancement, are not well reported in the literature. The magnitude of mandibular advancement is an important factor in the reduction of AHI. A monobloc or a one-piece intra-oral appliance works well in patients who can manage good mandible protrusion of at least 5 mm. For the purposes of comfort and titratability, the initial mandibular advancement can be 75% of maximum protrusion. The desired mandibular position is achieved by using two-piece mandibular advancement splints with telescoping connectors, similar to the Herbst appliance or the twin-block appliance with anteroposterior screws for gradual titration of mandibular advancement. Oligodontia, with fewer than 10 teeth per jaw, is usually a contraindication to prescribing the use of an oral appliance. There are exceptions, however, and mandibular advancement appliances can sometimes be successfully worn by edentulous patients with good dentoalveolar ridges.

Tongue-retaining devices are monobloc appliances, with or without built-in mandibular advancement. The splint incorporates an anterior bulb, in front of the upper and lower incisors, for accommodating the tongue in a forward position. The tongue-retaining bulb is made from a soft polyvinyl material, which when squeezed, produces a negative pressure that draws the tongue forward into the retaining bulb. The best predictor of success of the tongue-retaining appliance is the presence of a single-site airway obstruction in supine-dependent OSA (Cartwright, 1985). Studies have shown no greater efficacy of the tongue-retaining device with regard to reduction of AHI as compared with the mandibular advancement splint. In a randomized controlled trial, more than 90% of patients preferred to use the mandibular advancement appliance without the tongue-retaining bulb (Deane et al., 2009). Patients also preferred mandibular advancement splints to CPAP, machines even though the oral appliance is less effective in relieving OSA. The reasons include effectiveness of the mandibular advancement appliance in managing mild to moderate OSA, fewer side effects and greater patient comfort (Ferguson et al., 1996). Furthermore, the oral appliance is small which makes it easy to carry while traveling, and it does not need to be powered by electricity like the CPAP machine. The lack of visibility of using an intraoral appliance is another incentive to wear it to bed; it does not come with the noise or cumbersome and unesthetic burden of the straps and tubes that accompany the use of a CPAP machine.

Oral appliance treatment does have its drawbacks too. Soreness of the teeth, occlusion changes, facial muscles and temporomandibular joint pain are commonly reported in the first few hours of waking. Long-term side effects occur after two or more years of oral appliance wear, and these include dental and skeletal changes. They present as: reduction of overbite and overjet, proclination and retroclination of the lower incisors and upper incisors, respectively, and about 26% of patients experience irreversible changes in their occlusion. Oral appliances with greater advancements of the mandible have greater impact on the skeletal system; there is downward and forward positioning of the mandible with increased anterior lower face height (Clark et al., 2000). In a report on the practice parameters of snoring and OSA, the American Academy of Sleep Medicine recommends fitting and follow-up of oral appliances by trained dental practitioners in dental sleep medicine. Follow-up overnight polysomnography is necessary to establish efficacy of the oral appliance with long-term monitoring of OSA signs and symptoms, dental and periodontal health as well as the occlusion (Kushida et al., 2006).

Orthognathic surgery management

Surgical treatment is considered when nonsurgical therapies have failed. The aims of surgical procedures are to improve the overall sleep pattern and decrease the amount of airway collapse, obstruction, and oxygen desaturations during sleep. The most common definition of a surgical cure for OSA is stated as a postoperative AHI of less than 20, together with a reduction of at least 50% of the preoperative value, infrequent oxygen desaturations of <90% and improvement of subjective symptoms.

Surgical treatment is divided into soft and hard tissue procedures. Multiple soft tissue procedures have been developed to treat OSA, from the external nasal valve to the larynx. Oral and maxillofacial surgery for OSA includes genioglossus advancement and maxillomandibular advancement (MMA), which involves the advancement of both the maxilla and mandible using traditional orthognathic surgical techniques. The first use of orthognathic surgery for the treatment of OSA was reported in 1979. Mandibular setback has been found to decrease the caliber of the posterior airway, while bimaxillary advancement significantly increases the posterior airway space. The estimated decrease in the anteroposterior dimension of the airway is 30–40% of the skeletal setback. This leads to the conclusion that the preoperative posterior airway space should be one of the variables checked during treatment planning for orthognathic surgery; large setbacks should be avoided and bimaxillary surgery used in place of any extreme setbacks that may have been indicated (Lye, 2008).

The positive effects of MMA arise from the advancement of the skeletal attachments of the associated muscles and tendons of the soft palate, tongue and pharynx, which results in the enlargement of the posterior airway and a decrease in laxity of the pharyngeal tissues. Overall, this procedure had a published short-term success rate of 97% (Hochban et al., 1997), and 100% (Prinsell, 1999), while a long-term success rate of 90% after a mean follow-up period of 4 years has also been reported (Li et al., 2000).

There are two principles underlying OSA therapy (Moore, 2000). The first states that in moderate and severe OSA, the entire upper airway is affected. The second states that the more severe the disorder, the more aggressive the surgical therapy has to be in order to achieve success. Based on these concepts, the indications for MMA are:

- AHI or RDI more than 15 events per hour with the lowest desaturation <90% and EDS;
- Conservative treatment and CPAP must have been unsuccessful or rejected;
- Extensive obstruction of the airway.

In addition, if there are coexisting dentofacial or skeletal deformities, MMA should be considered as the primary surgical procedure as it has multiple benefits. The contraindications to orthognathic management of OSA are the possibility of nonfulfillment of the indications, and patients are either medically unfit for the procedure or are unwilling to undergo an invasive surgical procedure.

MMA is usually carried out after a phase of presurgical orthodontics. However, the objectives are different from the treatment of routine dentofacial deformity cases. Presurgical orthodontic treatment is used to aid in maximizing the advancement of the maxillomandibular complex and for achieving proper occlusion postoperatively. A protrusive dentition is often retracted maximally in order to allow larger advancements of the jaws with minimal negative effect on the dentofacial esthetic outcome (Goh and Lim, 2003).

MMA involves a Le Fort I maxillary osteotomy and mandibular bilateral sagittal split osteotomy. The accepted magnitude of advancement is usually 10 mm, but this is not supported by research. It would be logical to customize the amount of movement based on the airway caliber and the severity of the OSA, but that information is currently unavailable. As the larger advancements may be susceptible to significant relapse, stabilization of the segments is important. Research has shown that with miniplate fixation and bone grafting, the relapse can be reduced to 10%, and hence, the risk of OSA recurrence (Waite et al., 1996). Details of the MMA technique can be found in the published literature (Lye and Deatherage, 2009).

Adjunctive procedures can also aid in the overall improvement of the airway. For example, nasal septal deviation and enlarged turbinates can be dealt with during the Le Fort advancement osteotomy. Another supplementary procedure is genioglossal advancement, which is a chin osteotomy to advance the genial tubercles and the attached muscles (Nagler and Laufer, 2002). Simultaneous pharyngeal soft issue procedures can also be executed, but with caution, as airway compromise secondary to bleeding and swelling may occur. These procedures include surgery to the soft palate, palatine tonsils, and the tongue.

Complications associated with MMA include permanent hypoesthesia of the lower lip and chin, malocclusion (if no orthodontic treatment was carried out in conjunction with MMA), temporary velopharyngeal insufficiency, minor speech difficulties, unesthetic facial changes, temporomandibular disorders, decreased range of motion, mild sinus dysfunction, and decreased bite force. Many of the complications are a result of the large magnitude of jaw advancements, or they occur in the older patient with medical comorbidities, or are due to adjunctive procedures performed. However, most complications are easily managed and do not result in serious, permanent problems for the patient.

An important consideration in planning orthognathic management of malocclusions in patients with pre-existing OSA is potential upper airway embarrassment. With the mandibular setback procedures, the degree of posterocaudal or clockwise rotation of the mandible correlates with airway narrowing (Liukkonen et al., 2002). Setback procedures are also associated with reduced posterior airway

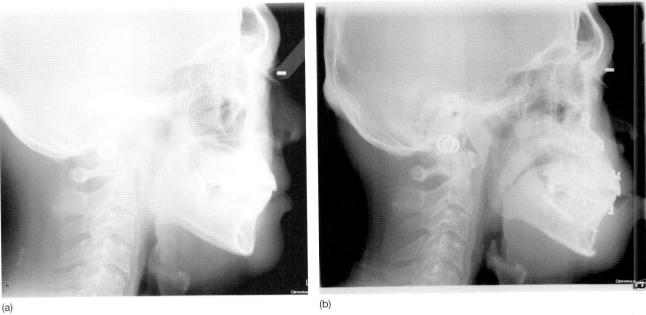

(a)   (b)

Figure 13.20 Pre (a) and post (b) maxillomandibular advancement (MMA) lateral cephalograms of a patient with severe obstructive sleep apnea and multi-level narrowing of airway. (b) Post-surgery with 100% increases in width in the oropharynx and hypopharynx.

space. The inferior repositioning of the hyoid bone and posterior displacement of the tongue and soft palate causes lateral as well as anteroposterior narrowing of the posterior airway space, and the effects are permanent. It is recommended that all patients planned for orthognathic surgery should be screened and examined to rule out pre-existing OSA. If OSA is confirmed, the orthognathic plan should be modified to improve the airway (Figure 13.20).

Conclusions

The causes of obstructive sleep-disordered breathing are multifactorial; the etiology and pathogenesis are neither well defined nor completely understood. Although the likely anatomical areas and obstructing structures in the nose and at different sites of the pharynx have been identified, their role in OSA may not always be one of direct cause and effect (Rivlin et al., 1984; Riley et al., 1985; Shepard et al., 1991).

In children, the important consideration in OSA management is to rule out the common causes of nasal and/or nasopharyngeal obstructions. Although surgical management by tonsillectomy and adenoidectomy is the mainstay in treatment of childhood OSA (Suen et al., 1995), treatment with dentofacial orthopedic appliances can alleviate compromised upper airways in growing patients where the adenotonsillar size is incompatible with upper airway function. The rationale behind the approach to treatment is to either increase the size of the hard tissue 'container' to accommodate the enlarged soft tissue contents, or to remove the contents that have become too large for the container. For some, especially in those with neuromuscular conditions, OSA can be a lifelong condition that requires comprehensive management of all possible causes, structural as well as nonstructural.

Currently, the first-line management strategy for OSA without nasal obstructions, in all patients of all ages, is the use of CPAP to pneumatically splint the airway open or to bypass the obstructed airway by using a nasopharyngeal breathing tube or by tracheotomy. The role of orthodontics in OSA management is emerging and constantly developing. Orthodontic treatment protocols include management of morphometric risk factors to alleviate OSA in the short term; long-term studies are needed to provide an evidence-based cure for OSA through widening the maxilla and protraction the retruded maxilla and mandible.

Caution should be exercised in certain surgical procedures that are known to cause OSA, such as pharyngoplasty to improve speech in cleft lip and palate patients, and orthognathic setback procedures of the mandible to manage dentofacial esthetics. There is evidence to substantiate that these surgeries can permanently reduce upper airway caliber. It is recommended to screen all patients for OSA before subjecting them to procedures that will reduce airway patency.

OSA is associated with a long list of medical comorbidities that adversely affects the cardiovascular and cerebrovascular systems as well as metabolic and neurocognitive functions. Evaluation with an interdisciplinary team trained in sleep medicine is vital for orthodontic or orthognathic patients presenting with sleep-disordered breathing for treatment. Identification of patients at risk of OSA preempts embarrassment of a narrow and/or collapsible upper airway. Communication with multiple specialists adds to the decision-making process in orthodontic or orthognathic treatment planning. Treatment aims to manage dentofacial esthetics and occlusion as well as to establish or maintain the patency of the upper airway.

The patient with OSA requires multiple treatment recommendations from the cardiologist, endocrinologist, neurologist, orthodontist, oral and maxillofacial surgeon, otorhinolaryngologist, pediatrician (for a child), psychiatrist, and respiratory physician. Dentists, orthodontists, and oral and maxillofacial surgeons, who have a good knowl-edge of sleep-disordered breathing, in close consultation with a sleep medicine team, can make informed decisions in managing OSA patients with dentofacial deformities and malocclusions.

An interactive, interdisciplinary approach is essential for optimal care of the OSA patient. The challenge for the orthodontist or dentist is in recognizing patients at risk of OSA for early investigation and intervention. Orthodontic patients can be easily screened using a combination of the sleep history, clinical and cephalometric findings (Boxes 13.1, 13.2 and Figure 13.21).

Box 13.1 Practice points in the work-up for the child with OSA and malocclusion

Questions for the patient's parent/caregiver
- Does the child have breathing difficulties when asleep?
- Does the child sleep in unusual positions or sleep sitting up?
- Is the child hyperactive and does the child have problems in school?

Screen for nonstructural causes
- Obesity BMI ≥95 percentile in age and gender cohorts
- Allergies and nasal congestion

Screen for structural causes
- Complex syndromes, craniofacial abnormalities, macroglossia
- Micrognathia or retrusion of the maxilla and/or mandible
- Hyotonia, muscular dystrophy or neurological disorders
- Look for oropharyngeal congestion – large tongue, enlarged tonsils and adenoids
- On the lateral cephalogram – check for adenoid hypertrophy, narrow upper airway in nasopharynx, oropharynx
- Nasendoscopic examination for nasal abnormalities, locations of upper airway narrowing, adenotonsillar size relative to upper airway size, airway collapsibility with Müller maneuver, airway caliber changes with mandibular advancement

Confirmation of OSA, other causes and comorbidities
- Refer to pediatric respiratory physician, otolaryngologist, endocrinologist and/or pediatrician

Orthodontic treatment recommendations
- Establish orthodontic diagnosis
- Define sites of dentofacial deformities
- Where appropriate, expand narrow maxilla, protract retruded/hypoplastic maxilla and use functional appliances to improve the position/size of a retrognathic/micrognathic mandible to orthodontically acceptable limits of occlusion and psychosocial function

Concomitant treatment recommendations
- Consultation with the patient's pediatric otolaryngologist, respiratory physician, endocrinologist, and/or the pediatrician for medical or surgical management of adenotonsillar hypertrophy, obesity, and other medical comorbidities related to OSA

Source: National Dental Centre, Singapore.

Box 13.2 Practice points in the work-up for an adult with OSA and malocclusion

Questions for the patient's bed-partner
- Does the patient snore habitually?
- Does the patient stop breathing while asleep?

Screen for systemic signs and symptoms
- Epworth Sleepiness Scale (ESS) ≥9
- Blood pressure >120/80 mmHg

Screen for nonstructural causes
- Neck circumference ≥37 cm (females); ≥43 cm (males)
- Obesity: BMI ≥28 for Asians; ≥30 for Caucasians
- Allergies and nasal congestion

Screen for structural causes of OSA
- Craniofacial abnormalities, syndromes or conditions with macroglossia
- Micrognathia or retrusion of the maxilla and/or mandible
- Myotonia, muscular dystrophy or neurological disorders
- Look for oropharyngeal congestion – large tongue, enlarged lingual tonsils and soft palate
- On the lateral cephalogram – check for narrow upper airway width and increased distance of hyoid to mandibular plane
- Nasendoscopic examination for nasal abnormalities, locations of upper airway narrowing, airway collapsibility with Müller maneuver, airway caliber changes with mandibular advancement

Confirmation of OSA, other causes, and comorbidities
- Refer to respiratory physician, otolaryngologist, endocrinologist and/or sleep medicine physician

Orthodontic treatment recommendations
- Establish orthodontic diagnosis
- Define sites of dentofacial deformities
- Expand transversely and anteroposteriorly rather than constrict maxillary and mandibular arches; treat to orthodontically acceptable limits of occlusion and psychosocial function
- Plan orthognathic surgery for bimaxillary correction of mandibular prognathism to reduce magnitude of mandibular setback
- Where appropriate, plan orthognathic procedures to advance rather than to set back the maxilla and mandible
- Screen for OSA in all patients planned for a mandibular setback procedure

Concomitant treatment recommendations
- Consultation with the patient's otolaryngologist, respiratory physician, endocrinologist, cardiologist and/or the sleep medicine physician for medical or surgical management of comorbidities related to OSA

Source: National Dental Centre, Singapore.

OSA EXAMINATION CHART PAGE 1

┌─────────────────────────────────┐
│   │   Weight: _____ kg
│   │
│   **Patient's Particulars**   │   Height: _____kg
│   │
│   │   BMI: _____ (at risk Asian ≥28 Caucasian ≥30)
│   │
└─────────────────────────────────┘   Neck circumference: __ cm (at risk ♀≥37 ♂ ≥43)

BP: Systolic/Diastolic_____ (at risk >120/80)

ESS: ____ (Excessive daytime sleepiness ≥ 9)

Referred by: _____

Complaint: _____

Previous OSA treatment, doctor and date: _____

Sleep history: _____

Child: Difficulty breathing during sleep: ☐Yes ☐No Unusual sleep posture: ☐Yes ☐No

Adult: Habitual snorer: ☐Yes ☐No   Witnessed apnea: ☐Yes ☐No

Medical history: _____

Medication: _____

Relevant dental history: _____

CPAP usage: ☐Yes ☐No From:_____ (year)   Current CPAP pressure: _____cmH$_2$O

Polysomnograph (PSG) results/date: _____
AHI: _____   AI: _____   Lowest SaO$_2$: _____%

Facial examination:

Deviation of nose	☐ Straight	☐ Right	☐ Left
Facial form	☐ Square	☐ Ovoid	☐ Tapering
Facial profile	☐ Convex	☐ Straight	☐ Concave
Maxilla	☐ Protrusive	☐ Normal	☐ Retrusive
Mandible	☐ Protrusive	☐ Normal	☐ Retrusive

Oropharyngeal examination:

Respiration	☐ Nasal	☐ Mouth	☐ Mixed
Nasal obstruction	☐ Right	☐ Left	
Swallowing	☐ Normal	☐ Abnormal	
Palatal vault	☐ Low	☐ Normal	☐ High

Tonsil size (Please circle the appropriate number) grade 0, 1, 2, 3, 4 (see Figure 13.5)
0: Tonsils fit within tonsillar fossa
1: Tonsils <25% of space between pillars
2: Tonsils <50% of space between pillars
3: Tonsils <75% of space between pillars
4: Tonsils >75% of space between pillars

Friedman palate/tongue position grade I, II, III, IV (please circle the appropriate number; see Figure 13.6)

Figure 13.21 Sample examination chart for obstructive sleep apnea. (Source: National Dental Centre, Singapore.)

In growing children with OSA, management involves a combined medical-surgical and orthodontic approach. Hyperplastic lymphoid tissues are the main structural causes of upper airway obstruction in children, and enlarged adenoids and tonsils are indications for inhalational corticosteroid treatment or they are removed surgically if deemed necessary by the pediatric otolaryngologists. Other pediatric OSA management modalities include weight loss and positive airway breathing using the CPAP machine. Orthodontic intervention is prescribed if there are concomitant maxillomandibular deficiencies: retrognathic maxilla and/or mandible. In protocols of adult (≥18 years) OSA management, CPAP is the gold standard. An oral appliance to advance the mandible during sleep is recom-

OSA EXAMINATION CHART PAGE 2

TMJ function: _____
(deviation, joint sounds, joint or muscle pain)

Range of motion:

Maximum mouth opening: _____mm

Lateral excursion: (right) _____mm   (Left) _____mm

Protrusion (max): _____mm   Deviation in protrusion: □ R   □ L

Intraoral exam:

Hygiene: □ Good   □ Adequate   □ Poor

Periodontal Status: _____

Dentition:

8	7	6	5	4	3	2	1	1	2	3	4	5	6	7	8

Occlusion:

Class   I   II/1   II/2   III   Overjet: ____ mm Overbite: ____ mm

Nasopharyngoscopic examination:

External nasal valve	□ Normal	□ Collapsed	
Deviated septum	□ None	□ Present	□ R / □ L
Turbinate hypertrophy	□ None	□ Present	□ R / □ L
Nasal polyps	□ None	□ Present	□ R / □ L
Sinusitis	□ None	□ Present	□ R / □ L
Adenoid hypertrophy	□ None	□ Present	
Retropalatal narrowing	□ None	□ Present	□ AP □ Lateral

Müller's maneuver   0   1   2   3   4

(0= no collapse, 1= 25% collapse, 2 = 50% collapse, 3= 75% collapse and 4=100% collapse)

Retrolingual narrowing	□ None	□ Present	□ AP □ Lateral
Lingual tonsils	□ Normal	□ Hypertrophy	
Hypopharynx	□ Normal	□ Anomaly:_____	

Radiographic examination:

OPG: _____

Lat ceph: Retropalatal airway space _____ mm Retrolingual airway space _____ mm (at risk <10mm)

Maxilla	□ Normal	□ Hypoplastic	□ Hyperplastic
Soft palate	□ Normal	□ Long	□ Thick
Mandible	□ Normal	□ Hypoplastic	□ Hyperplastic
Chin	□ Normal	□ Retrogenia	□ Progenia
Hyoid	□ Normal	□ Low _____ mm (At risk ≥24mm)	

Examiner's name and signature:_____   Date: _____

Figure 13.21 (*Continued*)

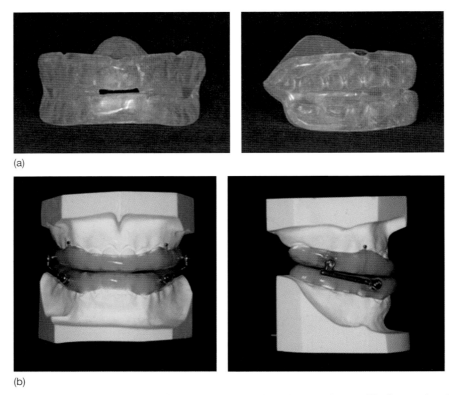

(a)

(b)

Figure 13.22 (a) Single-piece mandibular advancement splint for sleep-breathing, similar in design to the monobloc functional appliance. (b) Two-piece mandibular advancement splint for sleep-breathing, similar in design to the Herbst functional appliance.

mended for patients with mild to moderate OSA, who cannot use CPAP, and also in severe OSA patients who have failed CPAP treatment and who are poor surgical risks. The OSA mandibular advancement appliance is similar in design to functional appliances used in dentofacial orthopedic treatment of children (Figure 13.22). Follow-up efficacy check visits with polysomnography are necessary in OSA patients managed with mandibular advancement appliances. Patients must be followed up at regular intervals (6-monthly) for assessments of compliance with appliance wear, appliance deterioration or maladjustment, and to evaluate the general dental conditions: occlusion, dental, periodontal and temporomandibular joint health. Polysomnography will be be repeated whenever clinical signs and symptoms of OSA worsen or recur. The orthodontist should consider pre-existing narrow airway space and/or OSA during orthodontic and orthognathic planning. Orthodontic treatment in OSA cases may necessitate decompensation for maxillary and/or mandibular advancements rather than dentoalveolar compensation to treat maxillomandibular discrepancies. As mandibular setbacks can compromise posterior airway space, bimaxillary advancements are advocated. However, not all patients may desire surgery or they may not be surgically-fit. In these instances, CPAP or mandibular advancement splints will be the necessary aids in the management of sleep-breathing.

Improper care results from inadequate diagnosis or diagnostic errors, the prescription of inappropriate procedures and/or failure to treat the full spectrum of the condition. Obesity management, treatment of medical comorbidities of OSA and long-term follow-up of the patient are essential in the protocol for multidisciplinary care of OSA (Figure 13.23). It is advisable for the dental member of the sleep medicine team to stay current and conversant with practice and continuing education together with the team, so as to maintain clinical expertise in OSA diagnosis and provision of optimal treatment.

Acknowledgments

Special thanks are due to several people for their support, invaluable advice, and assistance in the preparation of illustrations, photographs, and the manuscript: Ms Kuah Ah San, Dr Kwa Chong Teck, Ms Jenny Lam, Ms Maple Lim, Ms Lio May Fern, Dr Eva Loh, Ms Roslinda bte Sabani, and Dr Lena Berglund-Stevenberg.

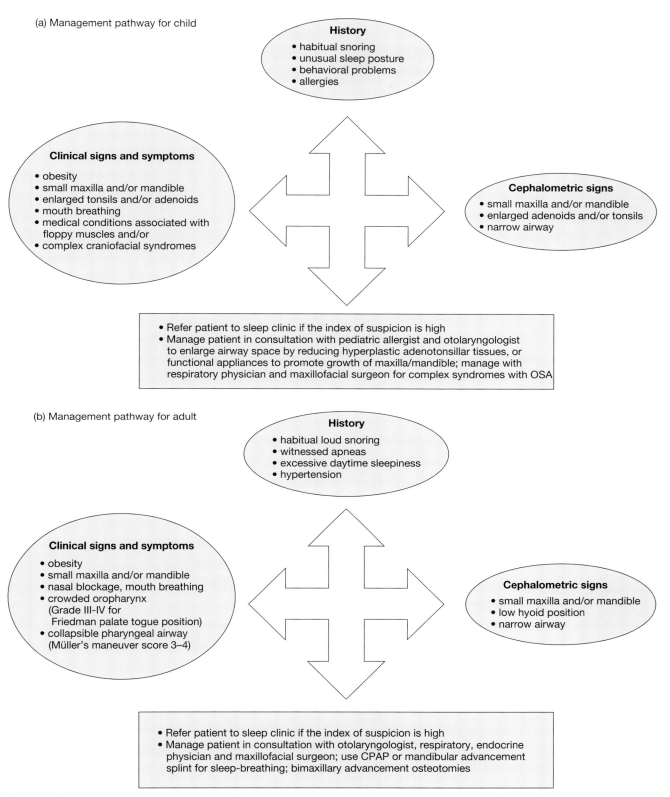

Figure 13.23 (a) Management pathway for a child with dentofacial deformity and malocclusion suspected of having OSA. (b) Clinical management pathway for an adult with dentofacial deformity and malocclusion, suspected of having OSA. (Source: National Dental Centre, Singapore.)

References

Ali NJ, Pitson DJ, Stradling JR (1993) Snoring, sleep disturbance and behaviour in 4–5 years-olds. *Archives of Disease in Childhood* 68: 360–6.

American Academy of Pediatrics, Section on Pediatric Pulmonology, Subcommittee on Obstructive Sleep Apnea Syndrome (2002) Clinical practice guideline: diagnosis and management of childhood obstructive sleep apnea syndrome. *Pediatrics* 109: 704–12.

American Academy of Sleep Medicine (2005) *The International Classification of Sleep Disorders*, 2nd edn. Diagnostic and Coding Manual. Westchester, IL: American Academy of Sleep Medicine.

American Academy of Sleep Medicine Task Force (1999) Sleep-related breathing disorders in adults: recommendations for syndrome definition and measurement techniques in clinical research. A report by the American Academy of Sleep Medicine Task Force. *Sleep* 22: 667–89.

American Thoracic Society (1999) Cardiorespiratory sleep studies in children. Establishment of normative data and polysomnographic predictors of morbidity. *American Journal of Respiratory and Critical Care Medicine* 160: 1381–7.

Anuntaseree W, Kuasirikul S, Suntornlohanakul S (2005) Natural history of snoring and obstructive sleep apnea in Thai school-age children. *Pediatric Pulmonology* 39(5): 415–20.

Arens R, McDonough JM, Corbin AM, et al. (2003) Upper airway size analysis by magnetic resonance imaging of children with obstructive sleep apnea syndrome. *American Journal of Respiratory and Critical Care Medicine* 167: 65–70.

Avrahami E, Englender M (1995) Relation between CT axial cross-sectional area of the oropharynx and obstructive sleep apnea syndrome in adults. *American Journal of Neuroradiology* 16(1): 135–40.

Baccetti T, Franchi L, Mucedero M, et al. (2010) Treatment and post-treatment effects of facemask therapy on the sagittal pharyngeal dimensions in Class III subjects. *European Journal of Orthodontics* 32: 346–50.

Bacon WH, Turlot JC, Kriegor J, et al (1990) Cephalometric evaluation of pharyngeal obstructive factors in patients with sleep apnea syndrome. *Angle Orthodontist* 60: 115–22.

Barkdull GC, Kohl CA, Patel M, et al. (2008) Computed tomography imaging of patients with obstructive sleep apnea. *Laryngoscope* 118(8): 1486–92.

Barnes M, McEvoy RD, Banks S, et al. (2004) Efficacy of positive airway pressure and oral appliance in mild to moderate obstructive sleep apnea. *American Journal of Respiratory and Critical Care Medicine* 170(6): 656–64.

Bannink N, Mathijssen IMJ, Joosten KFM (2010) Can parents predict obstructive sleep apnea in children with syndromic or complex craniosynostosis? *International Journal of Oral and Maxillofacial Surgery* 39: 421–3.

Berretin-Felix G, Yamashita R, Filho HN, et al. (2006) Short and long-term effect of surgically-assisted maxillary expansion on nasal airway size. *Journal of Craniofacial Surgery* 17(6): 1045–9.

Bixler EO, Vgontzas AN, Lin HM, et al. (2009) Sleep-disordered breathing in children in a general population sample: prevalence and risk factors. *Sleep* 32: 731–6.

Bradford A, McGuire M, O'Halloran KD (2005) Does episodic hypoxia affect upper airway dilator muscle function? Implications for the pathophysiology of obstructive sleep apnoea. *Respiratory Physiology and Neurobiology* 147(2–3): 223–34.

Brooks LJ, Stephens MB, Bacevice AM (1998) Adenoid size is related to severity but not the number of episodes of obstructive sleep apnea in children. *Journal of Pediatrics* 132: 682–6.

Brouillette RC, Fernbach SK, Hunt CE (1982) Obstructive sleep apnea in infants and children. *Journal of Pediatrics* 100: 31–40.

Brunetti L, Rana S, Lospalluti ML, et al. (2001)Prevalence of obstructive sleep apnea syndrome in a cohort of 1,207 children of southern Italy. *Chest* 120: 1930–5.

Burwell CS, Robin ED, Whaley RD, et al. (1994) Extreme obesity associated with alveolar hypoventilation – a Pickwickian syndrome. 1956. *Obesity Research* 2(4): 390–7.

Carroll JL (1996) Sleep-related upper airway obstruction in children and adolescents. *Child and Adolescent Psychiatric Clinics of North America* 5: 617–47.

Carroll JL, McColley SA, Marcus CL, et al. (1995) Inability of clinical history to distinguish primary snoring from obstructive sleep apnea syndrome in children. *Chest* 108: 610–18.

Cartwright RD (1985) Predicting response to the tongue retaining device for sleep apnea syndrome. *Archives of Otolaryngology* 111(6): 385–8.

Carvalho FR, Lentini-Oliveira D, Machado MA, et al. (2007) Oral appliances and functional orthopaedic appliances for obstructive sleep apnoea in children. *Cochrane Database System Review* 18(2): CD005520.

Castronovo V, Zucconi M, Nosetti L, et al. (2003) Prevalence of habitual snoring and sleep-disordered breathing in pre-school-aged children in an Italian community. *Journal of Pediatrics* 142(4): 377–82.

Ceroni CG, Tasca I, Alessandri-Bonetti G, et al. (2006) Acoustic rhinometric measurements in children undergoing rapid maxillary expansion. *International Journal of Pediatric Otorhinolaryngology* 70(1): 27–34.

Chan J, Edman JC, Koltai PJ (2004) Obstructive sleep apnea in children. *American Family Physician* 69: 1147–54.

Chay OM, Goh A, Abisheganaden J, et al. (2000) obstructive sleep apnea syndrome in obese Singapore children. *Pediatric Pulmonology* 29: 284–90.

Chervin RD, Archbold KH, Dillon JE, et al. (2002) Inattention, hyperactivity and symptoms of sleep-disordered breathing. *Pediatrics* 109: 449–56.

Chervin RD, Ruzicka DL, Giordani BJ, et al. (2006) Sleep-disordered breathing, behaviour and cognition in children before and after adenotonsillectomy. *Pediatrics* 117: e769–78.

Chng SY, Goh DY, Wang XS, et al. (2004) Snoring and atopic disease: a strong association. *Pediatric Pulmonology* 38: 210–16.

Ciscar MA, Jaun G, Martinez V, et al. (2001) Magnetic resonance imaging of the pharynx in OSA patients and healthy subjects. *European Respiratory Journal* 17: 79–86.

Clark GT, Sohn JW, Hong CN (2000) Treating obstructive sleep apnea and snoring: assessment of an anterior mandibular positioning device. *Journal of the American Dental Association* 131: 765–71.

Constantin E, Tewfik TL, Brouillette RT (2010) Can the OSA-18 Quality-of-Life Questionnaire detect obstructive sleep apnea in children? *Pediatrics* 125: e162–8.

Cozza P, Ballanti F, Prete L (2004) A modified monobloc for treatment of young children with obstructive sleep apnea. *Journal of Clinical Orthodontics* 38: 241–7.

Davila DG (1995) Medical considerations in surgery for sleep apnea. In: PD Waite (ed.) Oral and maxillofacial treatment of obstructive sleep apnea. *Oral Maxillofacial Surgery Clinics of North America* 7: 205–19.

Deane SA, Cistulli PA, Ng AT (2009) Comparison of mandibular advancement splint and tongue stabilizing device in obstructive sleep apnea: a randomized controlled trial. *Sleep* 32(5): 648–53.

deBerry-Borowiecki B, Kukwa A, Blanks RH (1988) Cephalometric analysis for diagnosis and treatment of obstructive sleep apnea. *Laryngoscope* 98: 226–34.

Defabjanis P (2003) Impact of nasal airway obstruction on dentofacial development and sleep disturbances in children: preliminary notes. *Journal of Clinical Pediatric Dentistry* 27(2): 95–100.

Dempsey JA, Veasey SC, Morgan BJ, et al. (2010) Pathophysiology of sleep. *Physiological Reviews* 90: 47–112.

Dickens C (1837) *The Posthumous Papers of the Pickwick Club*, 1st edn. London: Chapman and Hall.

Dyken ME, Lin-Dyken DC, Poulton S, et al. (2003) Prospective polysomnographic analysis of obstructive sleep apnea in Down syndrome. *Archives of Pediatric and Adolescent Medicine* 157(7): 655–60.

Enoki C, Valera FC, Lessa FC, et al. (2006) Effect of rapid maxillary expansion on the dimension of the nasal cavity and on nasal air resistance. *International Journal of Pediatric Otorhinolaryngology* 70(7): 1225–30.

Ferguson KA, Ono T, Lowe AA, et al. (1996) A randomized crossover study of an oral appliance vs nasal-continuous positive airway pressure in the treatment of mild-moderate obstructive sleep apnea. *Chest* 109(5): 1269–75.

Ferreira AM, Clemente V, Gozal D, et al. (2000) Snoring in Portuguese primary school children. *Pediatrics* 106(5): e64.

Ferris B, Mead J, Opie L (1964) Partitioning of respiratory flow resistance in man. *Journal of Applied Physiology* 19: 653–8.

Fregosi RF, Quan SF, Kaemingk KL, et al. (2003) Sleep disordered breathing, pharyngeal size and soft tissue anatomy in children. *Journal of Applied Physiology* 95: 2030–8.

Friedman M, Tanyeri H, La Rosa M, et al. (1999) Clinical predictors of obstructive sleep apnea. *Laryngoscope* 109(12): 1901–7.

Gale DJ, Sawyer RH, Woodcock A, et al. (2000) Do oral appliances enlarge the airway in patients with obstructive sleep apnoea? A prospective computerized tomographic study. *European Journal of Orthodontics* 22: 159–68.

Goh YH, Lim KA (2003) Modified maxillomandibular advancement for the treatment of obstructive sleep apnea: a preliminary report. *Laryngoscope* 113(9): 1577–82.

Goldhart AD, Krishna J, Li RC, et al. (2006) Inflammatory mediators in exhaled breath condensate of children with obstructive sleep apnea syndrome. *Chest* 130(1): 143–8.

Gottlieb DJ, Young TB (2009) Natural history of sleep-disordered breathing: shedding light on the early years. *Sleep* 32(6): 715–16.

Gottlieb DJ, Chase C, Vezina RM, et al. (2004) Sleep disordered breathing symptoms are associated with poorer cognitive function in 5 year old children. *Journal of Pediatrics* 145: 458–64.

Gozal D, O'Brien LM (2004) Snoring and obstructive sleep apnoea in children: why should we treat? *Paediatric Respiratory Review* 5(Suppl A): S371–6.

Gozal D, Pope DW (2001) Snoring during early childhood and academic performance at ages thirteen to fourteen. *Pediatrics* 107: 1394–9.

Griffith JL, Ramadan HH, Wetmore SJ (1993) Laryngocele: a cause of stridor and airway obstruction. *Otolaryngology Head and Neck Surgery* 108: 760–2.

Guilleminault C, van den Hoed J, Mitler M (1978) Clinical overview of the sleep apnea syndrome. In: C Guilleminault, WC Dement (eds) *Sleep Apnea Syndromes*. New York, NY: Alan R Liss, pp. 1–12.

Guilleminault C, Korobkin R, Winkle R (1981) A review of 50 children with obstructive sleep apnea syndrome. *Lung* 159: 275–87.

Guye AA (1889) On aprosexia, being the inability to fix attention and other allied troubles in the cerebral functions caused by nasal disorders. *British Medical Journal* 28: 2(1500): 709–11.

Hall GL, Hantos Z, Petak F, et al. (2000) Airway and respiratory tissue mechanics in normal infants. *American Journal of Respiratory and Critical Care Medicine* 162: 1397–402.

Handelman CS, Osborne G (1976) Growth of the nasopharynx and adenoid development from one to eighteen years. *Angle Orthodontist* 46(3): 243–59.

Hartgerink DV, Vig PS, Abbott DW (1987) The effect of rapid maxillary expansion on nasal airway resistance. *American Journal of Orthodontics and Dentofacial Orthopedics* 92: 381–9.

Hill W (1889) On some causes of backwardness and stupidity in children: and the relief of these symptoms in some instances by naso-pharyngeal scarifications. *British Medical Journal* 2(1500): 711–12.

Hochban W, Conradt R, Brandenburg U, et al. (1997) Surgical maxillofacial treatment of obstructive sleep apnea. *Plastic and Reconstructive Surgery* 99: 619–26.

Hoekema A, Stegenga B, de Bont LG (2004) Efficacy and co-morbidity of oral appliances in the treatment of obstructive sleep apnoea-hypopnoea: a systematic review. *Critical Reviews of Oral Biology Medicine* 15(3): 137–55.

Hoffstein V, Szalai JP (1993) Predictive value of clinical features in diagnosing obstructive sleep apnea. *Sleep* 16(2): 118–22.

Horner RL, Shea SA, McIvor J, et al. (1989) Pharyngeal size and shape during wakefulness and sleep in patients with obstructive sleep apnoea. *Quarterly Journal of Medicine* 72: 719–35.

Hsu PP, Tan AK, Chan YH, et al. (2005) Clinical predictors in obstructive sleep apnoea patients with calibrated cephalometric analysis – a new approach. *Clinical Otolaryngology* 30: 234–41.

Hudgel DW (1988) Palate and hypopharyx – sites of inspiratory narrowing of the upper airway during sleep. *American Review of Repiratory Diseases* 138: 1542–7.

Hui DS, Ko FW, Chu AS, et al. (2003) Cephalometric assessment of craniofacial morphology in Chinese patients with obstructive sleep apnoea. *Respiratory Medicine* 97: 640–6.

Ingman T, Nieminen T, Hurmerinta K (2004) Cephalometric comparison of pharyngeal changes in subjects with upper airway resistance syndrome or obstructive sleep apnoea in upright and supine positions. *European Journal of Orthodontics* 26: 321–6.

Isono S, Shimada A, Utsugi M, et al. (1998) Comparison of static mechanical properties of the passive pharynx between normal children and children with sleep-disordered breathing. *American Journal of Respiratory and Critical Care Medicine* 157(4): 1204–12.

Isono S, Tanaka A, Tagaito Y, et al. (2004) Influences of head positions and bite opening on collapsibility of the passive pharynx. *Journal of Applied Physiology* 97: 339–46.

Issa FG, Sullivan CE (1984) Upper airway closing pressures in snorers. *Journal of Applied Physiology* 57: 528–35.

Johns MW (1991) A new method for measuring daytime sleepiness: the Epworth Sleepiness Scale. *Sleep* 14(6): 540–5.

Johns MW (1992) Reliability and factor analysis of the Epworth Sleepiness Scale. *Sleep* 15(4): 376–81.

Johnston CD, Gleadhill IC, Cinnamond MJ, et al. (2002) Mandibular advancement appliances and obstructive sleep apnea: a randomized clinical trial. *European Journal of Orthodontics* 24(3): 251–62.

Jordan AS, White DP (2008) Pharyngeal motor control and the pathogenesis of obstructive sleep apnea. *Respiratory Physiology and Neurobiology* 160(1): 1–7.

Katz I, Stradling J, Slutsky AS, et al. (1990) Do patients with obstructive sleep apnea have thick necks? *American Review of Respiratory Disease* 141(5 Pt 1): 1228–31.

Kaygisiz E, Tuncer BB, Yüksel S, et al. (2009) Effects of maxillary protraction and fixed appliance therapy on the pharyngeal airway. *Angle Orthodontist* 79(4): 660–7.

Kennedy JD, Blunden S, Hirte C, et al. (2004) Reduced neurocognition in children who snore. *Pediatric Pulmonology* 37(4): 330–7.

Kim YJ, Hong JS, Hwang YI, et al. (2010) Three-dimensional analysis of pharyngeal airway in preadolescent children with different anteroposterior skeletal patterns. *American Journal of Orthodontics and Dentofacial Orthopedics* 137(3): 306, e1–11.

Kushida CA, Efron B, Guilleminault C (1997) A predictive morphometric model for the obstructive sleep apnea syndrome. *Annals of Internal Medicine* 127(8 Pt 1): 581–7.

Kushida CA, Littner MR, Morgenthaler T, et al. (2005) Practice parameters for the indications for polysomnography and related procedures: an update for 2005. *Sleep* 28(4): 499–521.

Kushida CA, Morgenthaler TI, Littner M, et al. (2006) Practice parameters for the treatment of snoring and obstructive sleep apnea with oral appliances: an update for 2005. *Sleep* 29(2): 240–3.

Kyzer S, Charuzi I (1998) Obstructive sleep apnea in the obese. *World Journal of Surgery* 22(9): 998–1001.

Lamm C, Mandeli J, Kattan M (1999) Evaluation of home audiotapes as an abbreviated test for obstructive sleep apnea syndrome in children. *Pediatric Pulmonology* 27: 267–72.

Larkin EK, Rosen CL, Kirchner HL et al (2005) Variation of C-reactive protein levels in adolescents: association with sleep-disordered breathing and sleep duration. *Circulation* 111: 1978–84.

Launois SH, Feroah TR, Campbell WN, et al. (1993) Site of pharyngeal narrowing predicts outcome of surgery for obstructive sleep apnea. *American Review of Respiratory Diseases* 147: 182–9.

Lavie P, Fischel N, Zomer J, et al. (1983) The effects of partial and complete mechanical occlusion of the nasal passages on sleep structure and breathing in sleep. *Acta Otolaryngology* 95: 161–6.

Leach J, Olson J, Hermann J, et al. (1992) Polysomnographic and clinical findings in children with obstructive sleep apnea. *Archives of Otolaryngology Head and Neck Surgery* 118: 741–4.

Lechner DE (1990) *The New Lexicon Webster's Dictionary of the English Language, Encyclopedic Edition*. New York, NY: Lexicon Publications, Inc.

Li AM, Chan MH, Yin J, et al. (2008) C-reactive protein in children with obstructive sleep apnea and the effects of treatment. *Pediatric Pulmonology* 43(1): 34–40.

Li KK, Powell NB, Riley RW, et al. (2000) Long-term results of maxillomandibular advancement surgery. *Sleep and Breathing* 4(3): 137–40.

Lim J, Lasserson T, Fleetham J, et al. (2006) Oral appliances for obstructive sleep apnoea. *Cochrane Database Systematic Review* 1: CD004435.

Linder-Aronson S (1970) Adenoids: their effect on mode of breathing and nasal airflow and their relationship to characteristics of the facial skeleton and the dentition. A biometric, rhinomanometric and cephalometro-radiographic study on children with and without adenoids. *Acta Otolaryngology Supplement* 265: 1–132.

Linder-Aronson S, Leighton BC (1983) A longitudinal study of the development of the posterior nasopharyngeal wall between 3 and 16 years of age. *European Journal of Orthodontics* 5(1): 47–58.

Liu Y, Zeng X, Fu M, et al. (2000) Effects of a mandibular repositioner on obstructive sleep apnea. *American Journal of Orthodontics and Dentofacial Orthopedics* 118(3): 248–56.

Liukkonen M, Vähätalo K, Peltomäki T, et al. (2002) Effect of mandibular setback surgery on the posterior airway size. *International Journal of Adult Orthodontics and Orthognathic Surgery* 17: 41–6.

Lowe AA, Gionhaku N, Takeuchi K, et al. (1986) Three-dimensional CT reconstructions of tongue and airway in adult subjects with obstructive sleep apnea. *American Journal of Orthodontics and Dentofacial Orthopedics* 90(5): 364–74.

Lowe AA, Fleetham JA, Ryan F, et al. (1990) Effects of a mandibular repositioning appliance used in the treatment of obstructive sleep apnea on tongue muscle activity. *Progress in Clinical and Biology Research* 345: 395–405.

Lowe AA, Fleetham JA, Adachi S, et al. (1995) Cephalometric and computed tomographic predictors of obstructive sleep apnea severity. *American Journal of Orthodontics and Dentofacial Orthopedics* 107: 589–95.

Lye KW (2008) Effect of orthognathic surgery on the posterior airway space (PAS). *Annals of the Academy of Medicine Singapore* 37(8): 677–82.

Lye KW, Deatherage JR (2009) Surgical Maxillomandibular Advancement Technique. *Seminars in Orthodontics* 15(2): 99–104.

Malhotra A, Trinder J, Fogel R, et al. (2004) Postural effects on pharyngeal protective reflex mechanisms. *Sleep* 27(6): 1105–12.

Mallory GB, Fiser DH, Jackson R (1989) Sleep associated breathing disorders in morbidly obese children and adolescents. *Journal of Pediatrics* 115: 892–7.

Marcus CL, Keens TG, Baustista DB, et al. (1991) Obstructive sleep apnea in children with Down syndrome. *Pediatrics* 88: 132–9.

Marcus CL, Omlin KJ, Basinski DJ, et al. (1992) Normal polysomnographic values for children and adolescents. *American Review of Respiratory Diseases* 146: 1235–9.

Marklund M, Persson M, Franklin KA (1998) Treatment success with mandibular advancement device is related to supine-dependent sleep apnea. *Chest* 114(6): 1630–5.

Mathur R, Douglas NJ (1995) Family studies in patients with the sleep apnea-hypopnea syndrome. *Annals of Internal Medicine* 122(3): 174–8.

McNicholas WT (2002) Impact of sleep on respiratory muscle function. *Monaldi Archives for Chest Disease* 57(5–6): 277–80.

Mei Z, Grummer-Strawn LM, Pietrobelli A, et al. (2002) Validity of body mass index compared with other body-composition screening indexes for the assessment of body fatness in children and adolescents. *American Journal of Clinical Nutrition* 75: 978–85.

Miles PG, Vig PS, Weyant RJ, et al. (1996) Craniofacial structure and obstructive sleep apnea syndrome – a qualitative analysis and meta-analysis of the literature. *American Journal of Orthodontics and Dentofacial Orthopedics* 109: 163–72.

Montgomery-Downs HE, Gozal D (2006) Snores associated sleep fragmentation in infancy: mental development effects and contribution of secondhand cigarette smoke exposure. *Pediatrics* 117: 496–502.

Moore K (2000) Site-specific versus diffuse treatment/presenting severity of obstructive sleep apnea. *Sleep and Breathing* 4(4): 145–6.

Morgenthaler TI, Kagramanov V, Hanak V, et al. (2006) Complex sleep apnea syndrome: is it a unique clinical syndrome? *Sleep* 29(9): 1203–9.

Morrison DL, Launois SH, Isono S, et al. (1993) Pharyngeal narrowing and closing pressures in patients with obstructive sleep apnea. *American Review of Respiratory Diseases* 148: 606–11.

Nagler RM, Laufer D (2002) Genioglossal advancement – a simple surgical procedure for sleep apnea. *European Surgical Research* 34: 373–7.

Neeley WW, Edgin WA, Gonzales DA (2007) A review of the effects of expansion of the nasal base on nasal airflow and resistance. *Journal of Oral and Maxillofacial Surgery* 65(6): 1174–9.

Ng DK, Hui HN, Chan CH, et al. (2006) Obstructive sleep apnea in children with Down syndrome. *Singapore Medical Journal* 47(9): 774–9.

Ogawa T, Enciso R, Shintaku WH, et al. (2007) Evaluation of cross-section airway configuration of obstructive sleep apnea. *Oral Surgery, Oral Medicine, Oral Pathology, Oral Radiology and Endodontics* 103(1): 102–8.

Oktay H, Ulukaya E (2008) Maxillary protraction appliance effect on the size of the upper airway passage. *Angle Orthodontist* 78(2): 209–14.

Oosterkamp BC, Remmelink HJ, Pruim GJ, et al. (2007) Craniofacial, craniocervical, and pharyngeal morphology in bilateral cleft lip and palate and obstructive sleep apnea patients. *Cleft Palate Craniofacial Journal* 44(1): 1–7.

Partinen M, Guilleminault C, Quera-Salva MA, et al. (1988) Obstructive sleep apnea and cephalometric roentgenograms. The role of anatomic upper airway abnormalities in the definition of abnormal breathing during sleep. *Chest* 93: 1199–205.

Pracharktam N, Hans MG, Strohl KP, et al. (1994) Upright and supine cephalometric evaluation of obstructive sleep apnea syndrome and snoring subjects. *Angle Orthodontist* 64: 63–73.

Prinsell JR (1999) Maxillomandibular advancement surgery in a site-specific treatment approach for obstructive sleep apnea in 50 consecutive patients. *Chest* 116: 1519–29.

Remmers JE, DeGrott WT, Sauerland EK, et al. (1978) Pathogenesis of upper airway occlusion during sleep. *Journal of Applied Physiology* 44(6): 931–8.

Resta O, Foschino-Barbaro MP, Legari G, et al. (2001) Sleep-related breathing disorders, loud snoring and excessive daytime sleepiness in obese subjects. *International Journal of Obesity and Related Metabolic Disorders* 25(5): 669–75.

Ricketts RM (1954) The cranial base and soft structures in cleft palate speech and breathing; *Plastic and Reconstructive Surgery* 14: 47–61.

Riley R, Guilleminault C, Herran J, et al. (1983) Cephalometric analyses and flow-volume loops in obstructive sleep apnea patients. *Sleep* 6: 303–11.

Riley R, Guilleminault C, Powell NB, et al. (1985) Palatopharyngoplasty failure, cephalometric roentgenograms, and obstructive sleep apnea. *Otolaryngology – Head and Neck Surgery* 93: 240–4.

Rivlin J, Hoffstein V, Kalbfleisch J, et al. (1984) Upper airway morphology in patients with idiopathic obstructive sleep apnea. *American Review of Respiratory Disease* 129: 355–60.

Roberts JL, Reed WR, Mathew OP, et al. (1985) Assessment of pharyngeal airway stability in normal and micrognathic infants. *Journal of Applied Physiology* 58: 290–9.

Roberts JL, Reed WR, Mathew OP, et al. (1986) Control of respiratory activity of the genioglossus muscle in micrognathic infants. *Journal of Applied Physiology* 61(4): 1523–33.

Robin P (1934) Glossoptosis due to atresia and hypotrophy of the mandible. *American Journal of Diseases of Children* 48: 541–7.

Rosen CL, Storfer-Isser A, Taylor HG, et al. (2004) Increased behavioural morbidity in school-aged children with sleep-disordered breathing. *Pediatrics* 114(6): 1640–8.

Scammon R (1930) The measurement of the body in childhood. In: JA Harris, CM Jackson, DG Paterson, et al. (eds) *The Measurement of Man.* Minneapolis, MN: University of Minnesota Press.

Schmidt-Nowara W, Lowe AA, Wiegand L, et al. (1995) Oral appliances for the treatment of snoring and obstructive sleep apnea: a review. *Sleep* 18(6): 501–10.

Schulof RJ (1978) Consideration of airway in orthodontics. *Journal of Clinical Orthodontics* 12: 440–4.

Schwab RJ (2003) Pro: Sleep apnea is an anatomic disorder. *American Journal of Respiratory and Critical Care Medicine* 168(3): 270–1.

Schwab RJ, Gefter WB, Hoffman EA, et al. (1993) Dynamic upper airway imaging during awake respiration in normal subjects and patients with sleep disordered breathing. *American Review of Respiratory Disease* 148: 1385–400.

Schwab RJ, Pasirstein M, Pierson R, et al. (2003) Identification of upper airway anatomic risk factors for obstructive sleep apnea with volumetric magnetic resonance imaging. *American Journal of Respiratory and Critical Care Medicine* 168: 522–30.

Schwab RJ, Kuna ST, Remmers JE (2005) Anatomy and physiology of upper airway obstruction. In: MH Kryger, T Roth, WC Dement (eds) *Principles and Practice of Sleep Medicine*, 4th edn. Philadelphia, PA: Elsevier/WB Saunders, pp. 983–1000.

Sériès F (2002) Upper airway muscles awake and asleep. *Sleep Medicine Reviews* 6(3): 229–42.

Shakespeare W (circa 1611) (1987) Act II Scene 1. In: S Orgel (ed.) *The Tempest*. Oxford: Oxford University Press.

Shepard JW Jr, Thawley SE (1989) Evaluation of the upper airway by computerized tomography in patients undergoing uvulopalatopharyngoplasty for obstructive sleep apnea. *American Review of Respiratory Diseases* 140: 711–16.

Shepard JW Jr, Gefter W, Guilleminault C, et al. (1991) Evaluation of the upper airway in patients with obstructive sleep apnea. *Sleep* 14: 361–71.

Shintani T, Asakura K, Kataura A (1998) The effect of adenotonsillectomy in children with OSA. *International Journal of Pediatric Otorhinolaryngology* 44(1): 51–8.

Silvestri JM, Weese-Mayer DE, Bass MT, et al. (1993) Polysomnography in obese children with a history of sleep-associated breathing disorders. *Pediatric Pulmonology* 16: 124–9.

Strauss RA, Burgoyne CC (2008) Diagnostic imaging and sleep medicine. *Dental Clinics of North America* 52(4): 891–915, viii.

Suen JS, Arnold JE, Brooks LJ (1995) Adenotonsillectomy for treatment of obstructive sleep apnea in children. *Archives of Otolaryngology – Head and Neck Surgery* 121: 525–30.

Suto Y, Matsuo T, Kato T, et al. (1993) Evaluation of the pharyngeal airway in patients with sleep apnea: Value of ultrafast MR imaging. *American Journal of Roentgenology* 160: 311–14.

Suzuki M, Kirchner JA (1969) The posterior cricoarytenoid as an inspiratory muscle. *Annals of Otology, Rhinology and Laryngology* 78: 849–64.

Terris DJ, Hanasono MM, Liu YC (2000) Reliability of the Müller maneuver and its association with sleep-disordered breathing. *Laryngoscope* 110(11): 1819–23.

Tishler PV, Larkin EK, Schluchter MD, et al. (2003) Incidence of sleep-disordered breathing in an urban adult population: the relative importance of risk factors in the development of sleep-disordered breathing. *Journal of the American Medical Academy* 289(17): 2230–7.

Trudo FJ, Gefter WB, Welch KC, et al. (1998) State-related changes in upper airway caliber and surrounding soft tissue structures in normal subjects. *American Journal of Respiratory and Critical Care Medicine* 158: 1259–70.

Verhulst SL, van Gaal L, de Backer W, et al. (2008) The prevalence, anatomical correlates and treatment of sleep-disordered breathing in obese children and adolescents. *Sleep Medicine Reviews* 12: 339–46.

Vig KW (1998) Nasal obstruction and facial growth: the strength of evidence for clinical assumptions. *American Journal of Orthodontics and Dentofacial Orthopedics* 113(6), 603–11.

Villa MP, Bernkopf E, Pagani J, et al. (2002) Randomized controlled study of an oral jaw-positioning appliance for the treatment of obstructive sleep apnea in children with malocclusion. *American Journal of Respiratory and Critical Care Medicine* 165(1): 123–7.

Villa MP, Malagola C, Pagani J, et al. (2007) Rapid maxillary expansion in children with obstructive sleep apnea syndrome: 12-month follow-up. *Sleep Medicine* 8: 128–34.

Viva E, Stefini S, Annibale G, et al. (1992) Aspects of prevention of obstructive sleep apnea syndrome in developing children. *Advances in Otorhinolaryngology* 47: 284–9.

Waite PD, Tejera TJ, Anucul B (1996) The stability of maxillary advancement using Le Fort I osteotomy with and without genial bone grafting. *International Journal of Oral and Maxillofacial Surgery* 25(4): 264–7.

Weitzman ED, Pollak CP, Borowiecki B, et al. (1978) The hypersomnia-sleep apnea syndrome: Site and mechanism of upper airway obstruction. In: C Guilleminault, WD Dement (eds) *Sleep Apnea Syndromes*. New York, NY: Alan R Liss, pp. 235–48.

White DP, Lombard RM, Cadieux RJ, et al. (1985) Pharyngeal resistance in normal humans: influence of gender, age, and obesity. *Journal of Applied Physiology* 58: 365–71.

White SC, Pharoah MJ (2008) The evolution and application of dental maxillofacial imaging modalities. *Dental Clinics of North America* 52(4): 689–705, v.

WHO Expert Consultation (2004) Appropriate body-mass index for Asian populations and its implications for policy and intervention strategies. *Lancet* 363(9403): 157–63.

Wyke B (1974) Respiratory activity of intrinsic laryngeal muscles. An experimental study. In: BD Wyke (ed.) *Ventilatory and Phonatory Control Systems*. London: Oxford University Press, pp. 408–21.

Young T, Plata M, Dempsey J, et al. (1993) The occurrence of sleep-disordered breathing among middle-aged adults. *New England Journal of Medicine* 328: 1230–5.

Yow M (2009) An overview of oral appliances and management of the airway in obstructive sleep apnea. *Seminars in Orthodontics* 15(2): 88–93.

14

Acute and Chronic Infections Affecting the Oral Cavity: Orthodontic Implications

Vinod Krishnan, Gunnar Dahlén, Ze'ev Davidovitch

Summary

Infectious diseases occur worldwide, posing multilevel challenges to orthodontists everywhere. Each new patient must be examined thoroughly to uncover the possible presence of infections that could be potentially dangerous for others. Recognition of pathological conditions in a patient's orofacial region before or during treatment requires a precise diagnostic technique to eliminate all potential health risks to other patients and staff in the orthodontic clinic. In those cases where patients have such infections, it is advisable to promptly interact with pertinent medical specialists to obtain confirmation of the disease identity, its treatment, and any bearing of the disease and medications on the orthodontic treatment plan and projected outcome. Both infectious diseases and the medications taken for their treatment may affect the tissue remodeling response to orthodontic forces. This chapter discusses the features of infectious diseases, both acute and chronic, that may profoundly affect the diagnosis, course, and outcome of orthodontic treatment. These infectious diseases are caused by bacteria, viruses, fungi, and parasites and some may be potentially lethal. The goal of this chapter is to stress the importance of identifying these diseases during the diagnostic phase of orthodontic therapy and of seeking advice from medical specialists to prevent the spread of the diseases and achieving optimal orthodontic outcomes.

Introduction

Orthodontics, a specialty based on solid scientific foundations, is being practiced predominantly as a mechanical art, due, at least in part, to its close association with dentofacial esthetic dogmas. Orthodontists are keen to correct facial and dental disfigurements, but often little attention is paid to the general health status of patients, as if the dentofacial region exists in isolation from the rest of the body. This approach can be termed as 'regional diagnosis', where an emphasis is placed on the face and oral cavity while ignoring the overwhelming evidence on an intimate association between dentofacial events and a multitude of pathophysiological developments throughout the rest of the body (Moore, 1939). Such a narrow approach to orthodontic diagnosis and treatment planning, which overlooks basic biological principles, may not only jeopardize treatment outcomes but also the wellbeing of the patients. Thus it is essential to shift the paradigm of orthodontic patient evaluation to encompassing all aspects, both medical and dental, in the diagnostic datasheet, with due consideration of all health-related issues.

Orthodontic tooth movement results from profound remodeling activities of all dental and paradental tissues in response to the application of mechanical forces to the crowns of the teeth. These remodeling activities are performed by various cells, including cells of the nervous, immune, endocrine, and skeletal systems, providing tooth movement with a noticeable systemic involvement. Therefore, orthodontics should be considered as an integral part of medicine, and aiming to treat and correct malocclusions while weighing the possible effects of each patient's systemic condition on his/her orthodontic diagnosis and treatment plan. This definition introduces biological factors into orthodontic practice, and increases the probability of attaining pleasing and durable results (Childs, 1933).

Orthodontists often see patients with acute or chronic infectious diseases or with adverse reactions to the mechanotherapeutics they practice. It is helpful to refer these patients to competent physicians for advice that will enable the orthodontist to expand the boundaries of the diagnostic process, and craft detailed individual treatment plans. Creation of such a communication bridge will augment the union between orthodontics and medicine to the benefit of all individuals in need of orthodontic care (Dunning, 1941).

The close relationship that an orthodontist should maintain with other medical and dental specialists depends on the extent of his or her knowledge base, on which depends the ability to identify conditions requiring and/or justifying patient referral to appropriate medical professionals (Weinberger, 1938). An orthodontic practice might encounter patients with oral manifestations of a variety of diseases. Recognizing these signs and symptoms should prompt the practitioner to perform specific laboratory tests to facilitate making the correct diagnosis, identifying the course of the disease process, and assessing its effects on the treatment plan and the course of treatment. Such a routine could include differentiation between infectious and noninfectious diseases, and aid in deciding whether orthodontic treatment can be provided without further delay, or if a referral to a medical specialist for consultation is deemed necessary prior to formulating a comprehensive diagnosis. Lack of adequate knowledge of infectious diseases can cause unnecessary delays in instituting appropriate therapy, and at the same time lead to failure in implementing proper safety measures for prevention of disease transmission to the orthodontic office personnel. This chapter will concentrate on non-odontogenic infections and their possible orthodontic implications (odontogenic infections are discussed in subsequent chapters of this book). Systemic infectious diseases with oral manifestations and with a high degree of microbiological specificity are discussed, providing a clear guide to distinguish between bacterial, viral, fungal and parasitic infections.

In many systemic infectious diseases, the salient causative organisms have been identified and characterized as bacteria, viruses, fungi, or parasites. The infectious nature of these diseases requires the implementation of strict hygienic procedures and disinfection, to avoid any chance of contamination and transmission of the disease in the orthodontic office. To achieve this goal, it is imperative to identify at the first appointment itself, patients who may be carriers of such diseases, prior to proceeding with any clinical activities. However, in addition to the efforts to eliminate the risk of spreading an infectious disease to other people in the orthodontic office, orthodontists should realize that infectious diseases, with no exception, modify the immune system of each infected person. Such modifications may have profound effects on the paradental cellular and tissue response to orthodontic forces. Inflammation is a major part of this response, intimately involved in every step of the tissue remodeling process that facilitates tooth movement. Signaling molecules produced by migratory primed inflammatory cells reaching the mechanically stressed periodontal ligament (PDL) are capable of both accelerating and inhibiting the rate of tooth movement, depending on the nature of the specific molecules involved. Moreover, patients who have been diagnosed as having acute or chronic infectious diseases are usually being treated with medications that may markedly alter the course and outcome of orthodontic therapy, primarily by affecting the patient's immune system and the paradental inflammatory process. All these facets of infectious diseases dictate that a consultation with a physician specializing in treating patients with these diseases is imperative prior to the onset of any orthodontic treatment. This communication between the orthodontist and the physician must continue throughout the course of treatment in the event of any change in the health status of the infected patient during this period.

Bacterial infections

The resident and transient microflora of the oral cavity consists of more than 700 bacterial species or phylotypes, providing a useful defense mechanism against the establishment of more pathogenic species (Aas et al., 2005). The resident oral flora can be divided into the indigenous flora, that is, those are found in almost all humans irrespective of environmental conditions (e.g. species of *Streptococcus*, *Actinomyces*, *Haemophilus*, *Neisseria*, *Fusobacterium*, and *Prevotella*), and the supplemental flora, which have specific requirements for adhesion, nutrition, redox potential, and pH levels (Dahlèn, 2009). The species of transient flora do not permanently colonize the oral cavity, have low virulence and live in harmony with the hosts. This might include some opportunistic pathogens, such as *Staphylococcus aureus*, pneumococci, enterococci, enteric rods, and yeasts. If the host's immunity becomes impaired, these bacteria might initiate an infectious process (Kononen, 2000). Moreover, impairment of the host immune response destroys the microbial homeostasis, which allows some pathogens to grow in greater numbers and cause an infection characterized by increased pathogen load and inflammation.

Mucosal lesions of uncertain microbiological basis

Mucositis

Mucositis is a form of mucosal barrier injury, characterized clinically by oral erythema, ulceration, and pain (Figure 14.1). It is a common complication of therapeutic procedures involving chemotherapy, radiotherapy, or both, and in patients receiving bone marrow transplants, which are damaging to the epithelial cells (Scully et al., 2003). The role of microorganisms in mucositis is uncertain as regards whether they have a role in the initiation of the lesion, or whether they secondarily infect the damaged area or the

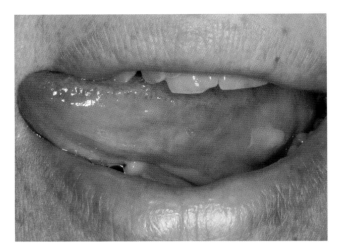

Figure 14.1 Oral mucositis. (Courtesy of Dr Nathaniel S Treister.)

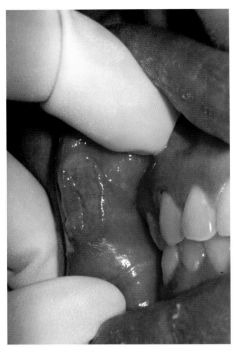

Figure 14.2 Major aphthous ulceration.

ulcer. Commonly, the oral manifestation of cancer therapy is a generalized stomatitis whose association with the primary underlying infection is more obvious (For further details, see 'Oral mucosal bacterial infections', p. 243). Secondary bacterial infections may also arise in bite wounds, and in viral stomatitis and aphthous ulcerations, and lead to streptococcal bacteraemia in any area of the mouth, such as the tongue, buccal mucosa, floor of the mouth, palate, and gingiva.

In addition, there is increased occurrence of opportunistic pathogens such as aerobic Gram-negative bacilli (AGNB) including enterics (*Escherichia coli, Enterobacter* spp.) and pseudomonads, as well as yeasts (*Candida* spp), in mucositic lesions. If xerostomia prevails, oral health can be seriously compromised (Sonis, 2007). Xerostomia can lead to decreased clearance of oral microorganisms, along with decreased pH, resulting in increased colonization by lactobacilli, *Candida albicans*, and other opportunistic microorganisms, such as *Staphylococcus aureus*, enterococci, and enteric rods (Pajukoski et al., 2001).

Recurrent aphthous stomatitis

Otherwise known as canker sore, this is the most common nontraumatic type of oral ulcer (Figure 14.2). The sore is often mistaken for a virus infection (herpes simplex), and is differentiated by appearance only in the nonkeratinized mucosa, such as the labial mucosa, buccal mucosa, ventral tongue, and vestibule (Ship et al., 2000). Based on their clinical appearance, aphthous ulcers can be classified as minor (<1 cm in diameter), major (>1 cm diameter), and herpetiform, in which multiple minute ulcers and which might coalesce to form plaques (Woo and Sonis, 1996). Most aphthae are of the minor variety, and heal within 10 days. Factors predisposing to this condition include stress,

poor nutrition, infection, hormonal fluctuation, and trauma (McCullough et al., 2007). The disease is usually self–limiting, and nutritional supplementation, alleviation of stress, and warm saline rinses have been found to help in its management. Orthodontic attachments are considered to be one among the main reasons for triggering their appearance. If the ulcers appear following orthodontic bonding, the irritating attachment can be either covered with orthodontic wax or removed to prevent further irritation aggravating the process.

Burning mouth syndrome

Scala et al. (2003) defined the burning mouth syndrome as a chronic pain syndrome that mainly affects middle-aged/ older women with hormonal changes or psychological disorders. This disorder reduces the quality of life, especially with large psychological implications. Although the etiology of this syndrome remains unclear, the presence of salivary gland dysfunction or systemic diseases, such as diabetes, makes a patient prone to it. In addition, patients with chronic pulmonary diseases, asthma, and rheumatic arthritis can develop epithelial atrophia, glossitis, xerostomia, and the burning mouth syndrome. All these symptoms are due to superimposing fungal and bacterial infections that follow adverse reactions to immunosuppressive medications and reduced salivary flow. Chemotherapeutic agents also have the potential to induce changes in the oral epithelium, leading to superinfection (Lopez-Jornet et al., 2010).

Oral mucosal bacterial infections

Acute mucosal infections of the oral cavity may appear locally, or as generalized stomatitis, and can be asymptomatic or accompanied by mild discomfort or severe pain (Dahlèn, 2009). Patients often neglect these conditions, unless they become bothersome. The most common symptoms are burning sensations, followed by clinical signs of redness and epithelial atrophy or desquamation. Helovuo et al. (1993) observed an increased prevalence of *E. coli*, *Enterobacter* spp, and *Staph. aureus* after treatment with penicillin and erythromycin. Patients with conditions causing immunocompromise, such as leukemia and other malignancies, are at high risk of developing oral mucosal ulcerations due to drug consumption and development of granulocytopenia. Similar conditions have been found in patients with organ transplants and rheumatic arthritis (Dahlèn, 2009). As a result of decreasing general health and increased medication intake, older people are more prone to develop oral mucosal lesions (Sweeney et al., 1994). Dahlèn et al. (2009) recently confirmed that bacterial mucosal infections are more prevalent than fungal infections in the oral cavity. They also observed a marked decline in the levels of normal mucosal bacteria, such as viridians streptococci (α-streptococci), *Neisseria*, and *Haemophilus* spp.

Dentists, more specifically orthodontists, frequently ignore such conditions, and/or leave them underdiagnosed. Infections associated with the oral cavity have a unique microbiological base, often a mixed one, making it difficult to identify a specific, salient microorganism. The best diagnostic approach starts with comprehensive history taking, which should be followed by a thorough physical examination. Microbiological laboratory investigations and antibiotic susceptibility tests should be conducted routinely on orthodontic patients with oral lesions, so that the conditions can be effectively and properly managed. An orthodontist accepting patients in this category should emphasize the importance of maintaining impeccable oral hygiene to postpone or minimize the development of oral mucosal ulcerations. It is also highly recommended to refer any patient with an oral microbiological infection that might be contagious, for a consultation to a physician. The infections arising in the oral cavity are listed in Table 14.1.

Aerobic infections of the oral cavity

Microorganisms causing oral mucosal infection have a predominantly aerobic character, and in the majority comprise staphylococci, enterococci, AGNB, and yeasts. They are all categorized as classical opportunists, and are commonly associated with immunocompromise (Dahlèn et al., 2009), although they have been noted in healthy individuals. These aerobic infections are difficult to treat due to a pronounced resistance against common antibiotics by these microorganisms and a low response as long as the compromised condition prevails. A microbiological diagnosis is strongly recommended since the treatment strategy may be quite different, depending on the identity of the involved microorganisms. Treatment of these infections is also sometimes challenging due to a combination of infections caused by two or more of these opportunists. A brief description of bacteria commonly producing oral mucosal infections is provided below. Yeasts involved in the process are discussed on page 256–259.

Staphylococcus aureus

Staph. aureus is considered to be a relevant pathogen in symptomatic oral mucosal lesions. Until then, if isolated, it was considered to be a part of a transient microbial flora that seems to increase with advanced age. This bacterium is frequently isolated from infections of the facial skin and lips (Faergemann and Dahlèn, 2009). Angular cheilitis is commonly secondarily infected by *Staph. aureus* (Figure 14.3), with a particular predilection in young individuals and those with dry skin. If a healthy individual harbors high numbers of salivary *Staph. aureus* (>100 000 colony-forming units/mL) over an extended period of time, they are considered to be healthy carriers (Dahlèn, 2009). Infected medical and dental professionals pose a risk of transmitting it to other individuals visiting them. A serious concern in this regard is the infection caused by methicillin-resistant *Staph. aureus*. Treatment of infection with *Staph. aureus* typically included penicillinase-stable penicillins, such as cloxacillin, dicloxacillin, or flucloxacillin, because of the risk of developing resistant strains (Dahlèn, 2009).

Enterococci

Enterococci, particularly *Enterococcus faecalis*, are commonly involved in oral mucosal infections. These infections occur sporadically in the oral mucosa and around the teeth in healthy individuals but enterococci are a typical opportunist in immunocompromised patients, often in combination with other opportunists such as enterics and yeasts (Dahlèn, 2009). Enterococci are of particular interest to dentists due to their persistence even after treatment of endodontically involved teeth.

Enterococci were known as streptococci for a long time, and were classified as Lancefield group D. However, owing to their survival in harsh environments (temperature, dryness, salts, dyes, antiseptics, and antibiotics), they were classified as a new genus, which normally resides in a significant part of the upper intestine and is resistant to bile salts. It is spread to the oral cavity by vomiting and faecal contamination. Enterococci are commonly used in the food processing, e. g. cheese, and spread through food cannot be excluded (Templer et al., 2008). It is resistant to penicillin V and clindamycin, and broad-spectrum penicillins such as ampicillin and amoxicillin remain the drugs of choice (Dahlén et al., 2009).

Table 14.1 Bacterial infections of the oral cavity

Type of infection Bacterial infections of the oral cavity and its environment	Main causative agent	Prevalence in the disease[a]	Prevalence in the resident flora of the oral cavity[b]	Treatment
Oral mucosal infections (including bacterial associated lesions)	Staph. aureus	++	+	Cloxacillin, clindamycin, vancomycin
	Strep. pyogenes[c]	+	(+)	Penicillin V
	Enterococcus faecalis	++	+	Amoxicillin/ampicillin
	Aerobic Gram-negative bacilli	+++	+	Multi-resistance drugs (ciprofloxacin)
	Yeasts[d]	+++	++	Mucostatins, amphotericin, azoles
Acute necrotizing ulcerative gingivitis	Treponema spp.	+++	+	Penicillin V
	Anaerobes (Fusobacterium spp., Prevotella spp.)	++	+++	
Peritonsillar abscess	Strep. pyogenes[c]	+++	(+)	Penicillin V
Lemierre disease	Anaerobes (Fusobacterium spp., Prevotella spp.)	+	+++	Metronidazole
	F. necrophorum	+++	(+)	Metronidazole, surgery
Suppurative parotitis	Staph. aureus	+	+	Cloxacillin, clindamycin
	Anaerobes	+	+++	Penicillin V
Non-infectious rhinitis	Allergy	+++	?	–
Rhinitis and sinusitis	Primary infection – viral	++	+	Penicillin V, amoxicillin
	Secondary infection –Facultative bacteria (Strep. pneumoniae, H. influenzae) and less commonly facultative bacteria (Staph. aureus, Strep. pyogenes)	+	+++	Penicillin V, macrolides
	Third phase infection – anaerobes	+++	+++ (nostrils)	Cloxacillin, clindamycin
Chronic rhinitis	Staph. aureus			
Epiglottitis	H. influenzae	+++	+	Amoxicillin, ceftriaxone, penicillin V, ampicillin, chloramphenicol
Chronic infections with oral manifestations				
Actinomycosis	Actinomycosis israelii	+++	+	Penicillin V (long time, high doses)
Gonorrhea	Neisseria gonorrhea	+++	–	Penicillin V
Mycobacterial infections	Mycobacterium tuberculosis	+++	–	Rifampicin
	Mycobacterium leprae	+	–	
Syphilis	Treponema pallidum	+	–	Penicillin V

[a]Prevalence: + <10%, ++ <30%, +++ >30%.
[b]Not isolated, (+) sporadically present in low numbers, + present in <10% and in low numbers, ++ commonly present <30% sparsely or in moderately heavy growth, +++ usually present and in the predominant flora.
[c]Group A hemolytic streptococci.
[d]Candida spp.

AGNB, including E. coli, Enterobacter spp., Klebsiella spp., Proteus spp. and more, are typically involved in human opportunistic infections, including oral mucosal infections. AGNB are part of the normal resident intestinal flora, frequent participants in nosocomial infections, and cause the classic opportunistic infections affecting the oral cavity. Transmission of these bacteria to the oral cavity can occur through poor personal hygiene, or through food and drinking water. They are frequently associated with periodontitis and peri-implantitis. They rapidly become drug-resistant, and the drug to be used should be selected only after a susceptibility test, although the choices are more or less exhausted. Quinolones (ciprofloxacin, norfloxacin) are the drugs of choice for the infections with AGNB, but should be prescribed only under proper medical supervision. Empirically, it has been observed that it is difficult to harm the bacteria and for the infection to heal as long as the patient is in a compromised state (Dahlèn et al., 2009).

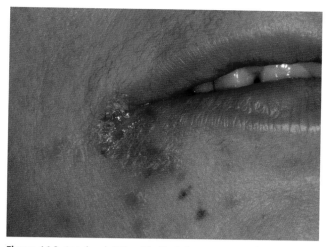

Figure 14.3 Angular cheilitis with *Staphylococcus aureus*. (Courtesy of Dr Maria Westin.)

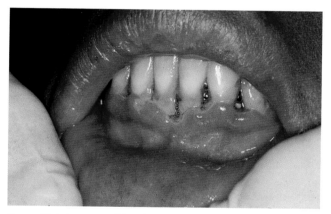

Figure 14.4 Acute necrotizing ulcerative gingivitis (ANUG). (Courtesy of Dr. Martin S Spiller.)

Acute necrotizing ulcerative gingivitis

Acute necrotizing ulcerative gingivitis (ANUG) is an infectious disease of the gingiva (Figure 14.4), caused by a mixed flora consisting of spirochetes, fusobacteria, *Prevotella intermedia*, *Veillonella* species, and streptococci (Rivera-Hidalgo and Stanford, 1999). This disease often results in gingival bleeding, ulceration, and episodes of severe pain. Factors predisposing to this condition include stress, smoking, malnutrition, and poor oral hygiene (Horning and Cohen, 1995). ANUG is common in patients with human immunodeficiency virus (HIV) infection. If it is associated with rapid alveolar bone loss, it is categorized as necrotizing ulcerative periodontitis, in which severe deep aching pain is a characteristic feature (Murayama et al.,

1994). The treatment of this condition is directed towards debridement of affected soft tissues and teeth, along with antibiotic therapy (Rivera-Hidalgo and Stanford, 1999). A referral to a competent periodontist, if an orthodontist encounters such a condition, can be of great value in its management.

Acute pharyngitis

Acute pharyngitis, otherwise known as a sore throat, can have either viral or bacterial etiology. The most common bacterium involved is *Streptococcus pyogenes* (β-hemolytic streptococci or group A streptococci [GAS]) (Peterson and Thomson, 1999). During the acute phase of the disease, these microorganisms can be detected in the saliva. This disease is among the 20 most common diseases that occur without any age, sex, or racial predilection. The exotoxins produced in this infection by the β-hemolytic streptococci act as superantigens that up-regulate the T lymphocytes, prompting the release of proinflammatory cytotoxins, and have synergistic effects along with the lipopolysaccharides of the extracellular matrix. The superantigens then evade the pharyngeal immune response, resulting in proliferation of *Strep. pyogenes*. The most common symptoms of acute pharyngitis are sore throat, odynophagia, headache, nausea, vomiting, and abdominal pain. On physical examination, the patient may have fever, tonsillopharyngeal erythema, exudates, beefy red swollen uvula, anterior cervical tender lymph nodes, petechiae on the palate, and scarlatiniform rash. The gold standard diagnostic test for acute pharyngitis is throat culture, but unfortunately this test takes 24–48 hours to be completed (Halsey, 2009). Instead, rapid antigen detection tests (RADTs) with commercial kits are available but these are relatively expensive. Samples for throat culture or RADTs should be obtained from the posterior pharynx or the tonsils. Imaging studies have no role in the diagnosis of this disease.

Oral penicillin V is the drug of choice for this disease. Amoxicillin remains a better alternative, but tetracyclines or sulfamethoxazole should not be used due to the high resistance rate. In the case of penicillin allergy, cephalosporins, which contain a β-lactam ring, can be used with caution. In rare cases, the pharyngitis spreads to adjacent areas, forming abscesses requiring surgical drainage. Surgery is an option, especially if the history reveals recurrent tonsillitis (Brook, 2009). The patient should be allowed to eat a normal diet and drink warm liquids that provide symptomatic relief (Halsey, 2009). An otorhinolaryngologist should be consulted for local suppurative complications such as peritonsillar abscess and mastoiditis. An infectious disease expert should be consulted for patients with immunocompromising conditions, or when HIV infection is suspected.

A rare but often underdiagnosed form of an oropharyngeal infection is the Lemierre syndrome, an infection caused by *Fusobacterium necrophorum* (Karkos et al., 2009), which

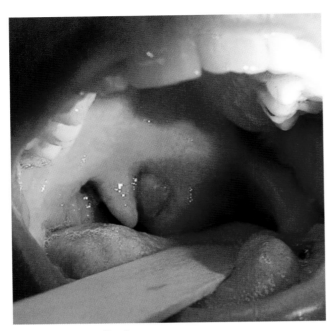

Figure 14.5 Peritonsillar abscess.

occurs in adolescents and young adults as a complication of tonsillitis ('sore throat'), especially in recurrent forms (Klug et al., 2009). It is life-threatening if neglected, and should be treated aggressively with antibiotics (metronidazole) and/or surgery (Ridgway et al., 2010).

Peritonsillar abscess

Peritonsillar abscess (PTA) is a localized accumulation of pus in the peritonsillar tissues, which forms as a result of suppurative tonsillitis (Figure 14.5). The peritonsillar space is bounded by the tonsillar pillars anteroposteriorly, piriform fossa inferiorly, and the hard palate superiorly. The area can be infected with both aerobic (*S. pyogenes*) and anaerobic (*Prevotella* and *Peptostreptococcus* spp.) bacteria. The infection begins superficially, progresses into deep tissues and has no age, sex, or racial predilection. The symptoms include sore throat, dysphagia, and change in the voice, headache, malaise, fever, neck pain, otalgia, and odynophagia. Physical examination reveals mild to moderate discomfort, fever, tachycardia, dehydration, drooling of saliva, trismus, cervical lymphadenitis, asymmetric tonsillar hypertrophy, inferior and medial displacement of a tonsil, contralateral deviation of the uvula, and erythema and exudates from the tonsils. No investigations are required to diagnose PTA but if a need is assumed, needle aspiration followed by culture of the fluid obtained can be performed (Peterson and Thomson, 1999; Mehta et al., 2009). Patients are often managed in the outpatient department, unless they show signs of airway obstruction, sepsis, toxicity, or other complications. Along with incision and drainage, analgesics, and throat wash, antibiotics are often prescribed for complete resolution of PTA. A combination therapy of penicillin and metronidazole is often preferred. Clindamycin is a good choice in people with penicillin allergy. Consultation with an otorhinolaryngologist should be sought whenever a PTA is recognized, before, during, or after the onset of orthodontic treatment, for proper management of these patients. Help from an anesthetist might sometimes be required if the patient develops difficulty in maintaining airway patency.

Suppurative parotitis/sialadenitis

Acute suppurative parotitis (ASP) is an infectious process of the parotid gland, usually seen in elderly people who are dehydrated, malnourished, or recovering from surgery (Raad et al., 1990). Although the infection is usually confined to the parotid capsule, it can occasionally spread to cervical fascial planes. Immunosuppression states such as diabetes, alcoholism, HIV infection, autoimmune disorders (e.g. Sjögren's syndrome), poor oral hygiene, decreased salivary flow, postsurgical dehydration, sialolithiasis, tumors or foreign bodies in the duct, can increase the risk for ASP. The most common clinical manifestation of ASP is an indurated, erythematous, warm swelling of the cheek. The patient will also have mild fever along with pain. Intraorally, the orifice of Stensen's duct will be red, and pus may be expelled while palpating it (Brook, 2009). In rare instances, facial nerve dysfunction may be the end result (Noorizan et al., 2009). Diagnosis can be established by a thorough clinical examination, along with a complete blood count and chemistry, and culture and sensitivity. Radiological evaluation should include CT scanning with an intravenous contrast medium, ultrasound scanning for detection of abscesses and also sialography.

Traditionally, the main causative agent of ASP is thought to be *Staph. aureus*. However, Brook et al. (1991) have isolated strict anaerobes such as *Peptostreptococcus* spp. and Gram-negative anaerobic rods from ASP lesions. The key treatment for ASP is rehydration and supportive treatment, which should include intravenous fluids, nutritional support, a warm compress, sialogogs, good oral hygiene, and antibiotic therapy. The drugs of choice in ASP are penicillin, first-generation cephalosporins or clindamycin, however, more important is the selection of the drug in relation to the causative agent. Intraductal injections of antibiotics usually lead to improvement in the condition. If there is lack of improvement after 3–5 days of antibiotic treatment, and if there is facial nerve involvement or involvement of adjacent vital structures, surgical opinion must be sought; usually incision and drainage via a standard parotidectomy incision will be the preferred treatment. Proper follow-up, repeated clinical examinations, fine needle biopsy, and imaging should be performed on a regular basis to ensure the absence of any neoplastic changes in the gland (Brook, 2009).

Rhinitis and sinusitis

Rhinitis implies a heterogeneous group of nasal disorders, characterized by sneezing, nasal itching, rhinorrhea, and nasal congestion, which can be allergic, nonallergic, infectious, occupational, or hormonal in nature. Recently Dykewicz and Hamilos (2010) suggested that in approximately 44–87% of patients with rhinitis, the condition is either allergic or non-allergic in nature. Common allergens causing the problem include proteins and glycoproteins in airborne dust, mite fecal particles, cockroach residues, animal dander, moulds, and pollens. Within minutes of inhalation, these allergens are recognized by IgE antibody bound to mast cells and basophils, causing degranulation and release of preformed mediators, such as histamine and tryptase, and inflammatory mediators, such as leukotrienes and prostaglandin D2. These mediators cause plasma extravasation from blood vessels, with consequent edema, pooling of blood in cavernous sinusoids, and occlusion of nasal passages. These developments are accompanied by active secretion of mucus from glandular and goblet cells, and release of histamine, which manifests as itching, rhinorrhea, and sneezing. In late stages, a prominent nasal congestion develops, as these early phase reactions set off by around 4–8 hours (Rosenwasser, 2007). Rhinitis is often accompanied by non-nasal symptoms, such as allergic conjunctivitis, and it is frequently associated with allergic asthma, pathophysiologically and epidemiologically.

Diagnosis should include evaluation of all specific symptoms and the pattern of occurrence of the symptoms (infrequent/intermittent, seasonal and perennial) along with identification of predisposing factors, previous responses to medication, and coexisting diseases. A hand-held otoscope or head lamp with nasal speculum permits viewing of the anterior third of the nasal airway, including the anterior tip of the inferior turbinates. Determination of specific antibody involvement can be made through skin testing, which has high sensitivity, and at the same time is simple, easy, and can be rapidly performed (Wallace et al., 2008). The main treatment for rhinitis is directed towards avoidance of the inciting factors, such as allergens and irritants. A multitude of drugs are available for the management of this disease, including antihistamines, corticosteroids, oral and nasal decongestants, leukotriene receptor antagonists, etc. For the orthodontist, making a referral to an otorhinolaryngologist is an important step in managing the condition. The specialist will determine an individualized treatment approach for each patient, based on their responses, preferences, and cost–effectiveness of the treatment options (Dykewicz and Hamilos, 2010).

Sinusitis or rhinosinusitis is defined as inflammation of the nose and the paranasal sinuses, and is usually infectious in nature (Meltzer et al., 2004). Typically, sinusitis follows, from a microbiological point of view, a characteristic pattern, starting as a viral infection, followed by superinfection with facultative bacteria after a couple of days and, after 1 week, showing anaerobes as the predominant organisms (Brook, 2009). Acute rhinosinusitis is diagnosed when there is purulent nasal drainage of with up to 4 weeks, accompanied by nasal obstruction, facial pain, pressure, fullness, or both. The pain is usually described as being dull, or felt as pressure in the upper cheeks, between the eyes, or in the forehead. The most common bacteria isolated from sites of acute rhinosinusitis are *H. influenzae, Strept. pneumoniae, Moraxella catarrhalis* and sometimes *Staph. aureus.* Disturbances in the sense of smell, which occur in sinusitis, can be either partial (hyposmia) or complete (anosmia), and are usually associated with mucosal thickening or opacification in the anterior ethmoid sinuses, which can be seen a hyperdense areas in an orthopantomograph and computed tomography (CT) images (Dykewicz and Hamilos, 2010) (Figure 14.6). An initial period of watchful

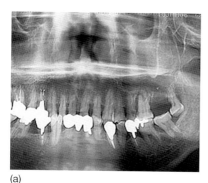 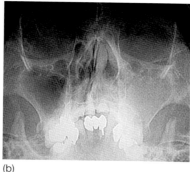 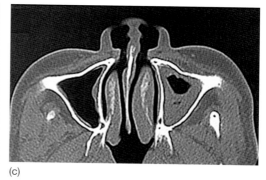

(a)   (b)   (c)

Figure 14.6 (a–c) Radiological appearances of sinusitis in various radiographs. (Courtesy of Akitoshi Kawamata, Asahi University School of Dentistry, Gifu, Japan.)

waiting without initiation of antibiotics is the best treatment for acute rhinosinusitis.

An important aspect of the diagnosis of sinusitis is to differentiate between bacterial and viral causes, as only bacterial infections respond to antibiotic therapy. Clinical signs suggestive of bacterial infection include symptoms that last for more than 7 days. Patients with more severe forms of the disease can be treated with antibiotics, and if this approach is decided on, amoxicillin is the drug of choice. If the patient is allergic to penicillin, a combination of trimethoprim and – sulfamethoxazole (not used in Scandinavian countries) or macrolide antibiotics can be considered. Intranasal decongestants can be prescribed, but for no more than 3 days, to avoid rebound decongestions (Brook, 2010).In contrast to acute rhinosinusitis, chronic rhinosinusitis (CRS) is defined as an inflammatory condition involving the paranasal sinuses and nasal passages over a minimum duration of 8–12 weeks, despite attempts at medical management (Meltzer et al., 2004). Superimposed bacterial infections further complicate the process. The four major symptoms of CRS are: anterior, posterior, or mucopurulent drainage; nasal obstruction or blockage; facial pain, pressure, or fullness; and decreased sense of smell (Meltzer et al., 2004). The bacteria can also form a biofilm over the sinus epithelium. Sequestration of bacteria within biofilms allows the bacteria to resist antibiotic treatment and persist as a low-grade infection within the sinus mucosa. Topical corticosteroid nasal sprays are preferred for all forms of CRS, along with antihistamines for underlying allergic causes, and antibiotics (penicillin V, amoxicillin, or cloxacillin) are prescribed when nasal purulence is present (Dykewicz and Hamilos, 2010). Functional endoscopic sinus surgery (FESS) is the management of choice of chronic refractory rhinosinusitis.

Epiglottitis

Epiglottitis, or inflammation of the epiglottis, is considered to be a medical emergency, as it can lead to airway obstruction and death. It follows oral infection with *H. influenzae* (Peterson and Thomson, 1999). This microorganism is abundant in the oral mucosal surfaces and in dental plaque. However, certain capsulated strains are considerably more virulent and are thought to be a major pathogen in the respiratory tract, causing otitis, sinusitis, and pharyngitis. The major symptoms are fever, difficulty swallowing, drooling, hoarseness of voice, and stridor. The diagnosis is often confirmed by examination with a laryngoscope, which will show cherry-red and swollen epiglottis and arytenoids (Jenkins and Saunders, 2009). This condition requires immediate medical attention, with urgent endotracheal intubation, to protect the airway. This procedure should be performed by a competent anesthetist, with the help of a respiratory therapist and otorhinolaryngologist (D'Agostino, 2010). In addition, the patient should be given antibiotics,

such as ceftriaxone or chloramphenicol, either alone or in combination with penicillin or ampicillin, for streptococcal coverage.

Chronic infections with oral manifestations

Actinomycosis

Actinomycosis is a chronic disease characterized by formation of abscesses, fibrosis, and draining sinuses (Figure 14.7). The causative agent is the nonspore-forming anaerobic or microaerophilic bacterial species of the genus *Actinomyces* (most commonly *Actinomyces israelii*), which are normal inhabitants of cervicofacial, thoracic, and abdominal areas (Rivera-Hidalgo and Stanford, 1999). A similar infection, nocardiosis, is caused by the related facultative *Nocardia* spp. Cervicofacial actinomycosis is the most common form of the disease (Laskaris, 1996). Actinomyces get access to the host tissues when there is an interruption in the mucosal barrier, caused by procedures such as tooth extraction and endodontic infection and treatment. Following this initial superficial invasion, the infection spreads deep into the tissues and a hard, slow growing, relatively tender swelling may form with multiple drainage areas or sinus tracts. The discharge from these tracts typically contains the visible yellowish colonies of the microorganisms and are termed 'sulfur granules'. If left untreated osteomyelitis with extensive bone destruction will result (Feder, 1990; Brook, 2008). Diagnosis can be confirmed by isolation of *Actinomyces* species from clinical specimens. Indirect immunofluorescence can also be utilized for this purpose (Gohean et al., 1990). The demonstration of actinomycotic granules, which consist of tangled filaments of organisms, in the exudates or histological sec-

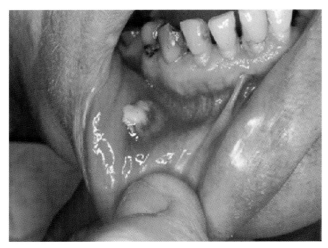

Figure 14.7 Oral actinomycosis. (Image reprinted with permission from Medscape.com, 2011.)

tions, confirms the diagnosis. *Actinomyces* species are susceptible to several antibiotics such as penicillins, tetracyclines, erythromycin, clindamycin, and ciprofloxacin. Antibiotics need to be given at high doses for longer periods (2–6 weeks) for a complete cure. Surgery might be required in some cases to aspirate or surgically drain the abscesses (Brook, 2008). Consultation with an oral medicine specialist and with an otorhinolaryngologist will be of great help in managing these patients.

Gonorrhea

Gonorrhea is the most frequently encountered sexually transmitted disease, caused by *Neisseria gonorrhea*, a non-motile spherical oval coccus. The organism is aerobic, Gram-negative and cannot penetrate an intact stratified squamous epithelium, such as that of the skin and oral mucous membrane (Rivera-Hidalgo and Stanford, 1999). However, it can directly invade the urethra, cervix, pharynx, and conjunctiva, because of the presence of columnar and transitional epithelium in these areas. From these sites, infection may spread readily along mucosal surfaces, or systemically, resulting in disseminated disease (Guinta and Fiumara, 1986). Humans are the only known hosts for *N. gonorrhea*, and the organism has been cultured from saliva of infected individuals. Twenty percent of patients with gonorrhea have oral, pharyngeal, and tonsillar involvement. The tonsils are red and swollen, with grayish exudates. Lesions in the oral mucosa may appear as fiery red and edematous, and occasionally there may be painful ulcerations. Diagnosis is established by culture and identification of *N. gonorrhoeae* (Laskaris, 1996; Bruce and Rogers, 2004). Sugar fermentation tests aid in species differentiation, and fluorescent antibody techniques have been used for rapid identification of gonococci. Penicillin is the drug of choice for this infection, and in drug-resistant patients ceftriaxone and ciprofloxacin have been used successfully (Chue, 1975).

Mycobacterial infections

The most common mycobacterial infections are tuberculosis, caused by the tubercle bacilli, *Mycobacterium tuberculosis*, and leprosy, caused by *Mycobacterium leprae*. There are also numerous nontuberculous mycobacteria, such as *M. kansasii*, *M. chelonei*, and *M. avium* – intercellular complex (Weg, 1976; Rivera-Hidalgo and Stanford, 1999), which cause most of the medical infections. These infections are noncommunicable from person to person, and do not require long-term systemic medication as in the case of tuberculosis (Rivera-Hidalgo and Stanford, 1999).

Tuberculosis

Tuberculosis is a chronic infectious disease caused by the airborne mycobacterium tubercle bacilli, and spreads almost exclusively via droplets from a person with active disease. Tuberculosis is still among the most life-threatening infectious diseases in humans and one-third of the world's population comes in contact with the disease at some stage in their life (Kakisi et al., 2010). It commonly affects the lungs, but can occur in any part of the body, and is characterized by formation of granulomas with caseation necrosis caused by cell-mediated response. Primary tuberculosis is seen in patients who have had no previous exposure to the disease and initially is predominantly subclinical. Secondary tuberculosis is seen in previously sensitized patients (Phalen et al., 1996). Oral lesions are rare (0.1–5%, Kakisi et al., 2010), but if they occur, they appear as chronic, painless, irregular ulcers, with a vegetative surface covered by grayish or yellow exudates. The dorsal surface of the tongue is a common site of secondary tuberculous infection, followed by the palate, gingiva, buccal mucosa, and lips (Hale and Tucker, 2008). Diagnosis is reached based on the medical history, identification of acid-fast mycobacteria in clinical specimens, a positive delayed hypersensitivity skin reaction to purified protein derivative, and chest radiograph findings, which includes infiltrates or consolidations and/or cavities in the upper lungs with or without mediastinal or hilar lymphadenopathy. Recent developments in rapid detection and identification of tuberculous bacteria are reducing the laboratory time in the diagnostic process (Ellner et al., 1988). If a patient has tuberculosis, all orthodontic procedures should be carried out under strict medical or a pulmonologist's supervision, in order to prevent the spread of the disease, as well as its aggravation.

Leprosy

Leprosy is a chronic disease caused by *M. leprae*, and is characterized by damage to the nerves and skin, resulting in deformities and disability. *M. leprae* is a Gram-positive, acid-fast, nonspore-forming, nonmotile, pleomorphic bacillus, which causes four types of leprosy: indeterminate, tuberculoid, borderline, and lepromatous (Rivera-Hidalgo and Stanford, 1999). Oral lesions have been demonstrated in tuberculoid, borderline, and lepromatous leprosy. The lesions present as nodules/lepromas that progress to necrosis and ulcerations. The ulcers may heal with scarring or progress to produce further tissue destruction. Lepromas are filled with *M. leprae*, and might occur in the palate, dorsum of the tongue, uvula, and the lips. When left untreated, these lesions can cause extensive destruction of the oral tissues (Ghosh et al., 2009). The diagnosis is based on clinical signs such as anesthetic skin lesions, enlarged peripheral nerves, and the presence of acid-fast bacilli in smears taken from skin lesions.

Syphilis

Syphilis caused by the spirochete *Treponema pallidum* is a venereal disease, with a decreasing prevalence rate.

Syphilis can be either congenital (when the fetus becomes infected *in utero*), or acquired (contracted by sexual contact, direct inoculation, or by transfusion with fresh human blood). Early congenital syphilis may manifest itself as papulosquamous lesions of the skin and the oral mucous membranes. The lesions at the commissures of the lips, angle of the nose, and eyes heal with radiating scars called 'rhagades' (Rivera-Hidalgo and Stanford, 1999). Oral manifestations of late congenital syphilis include Hutchinson's triad of deafness, interstitial keratitis, and malformed incisors, along with other dental anomalies such as hypoplastic molars with poorly developed cusps, called mulberry molars.

Acquired syphilis has three classic phases. Primary syphilis is characterized by chancre, a centrally ulcerated granulomatous lesion with a raised, indurated border; the lesion is painless and resolves within 2–8 weeks. Secondary syphilis is the systemic or disseminated phase, and may occur 2–12 weeks after contact. Signs and symptoms consist of fever, headache, malaise, a symmetrical rash, and mucous patches in the oral cavity. The oral lesions appear as grayish-white, glistening patches on the soft palate, tongue, and buccal mucosa, but rarely on the gingiva. After this stage, the patient enters a latent stage and 30–40% of untreated patients develop tertiary syphilis, which includes multiorgan involvement. Gumma is the characteristic lesion in this phase and is seen in the hard palate. This phase is not infectious (Little, 2005). Clinical examination and serological tests aid in the diagnosis of syphilis. Dark field microscopy can sometimes be useful when serological test results are negative but there is a high index of suspicion (Seigel, 1996). Penicillin is the pharmaceutical agent of choice in this disease.

The three mycobacterial infections, tuberculosis, leprosy, and syphilis, are highly contagious, posing a serious danger to all the people in the orthodontic office, including the orthodontist, the patients, and the staff. It is, therefore, essential to identify suspected carriers of these diseases, and refer them promptly to a physician for a definitive diagnosis. Failure to recognize and appropriately refer potential carriers and proceeding to address only their malocclusion may endanger all personnel and patients visiting an orthodontic office.

Viral infections

Oral diseases and infections of viral etiology are common in dental, as well as orthodontic practices, and awareness of these can effectively prevent their spread. Viruses contain one type of nucleic acid alone, either DNA or RNA. They often require a host, who provides them with ribosomes, which they need to multiply to produce disease conditions. Nearly all viruses are icosahedral, and possess a protein shell or nucleocapsid; protein spikes project from the surface of the viral nucleocapsids. The proteins are usually glycoproteins, participating in viral attachment and infection of the host. Viral infections have two stages: attachment and penetration. Viruses attach to their host cells by the way of cellular receptors, and after getting enveloped, they fuse with the host cell membrane. Receptor-mediated endocytosis is the process through which enveloped and naked viruses gain entry into host cells. The outcome of viral infection depends on the viral state. If the virus is in a lytic stage, the host cell is destroyed. In lysogeny, the virus enters and integrates with the host cell, and is reactivated at a later date to become lytic in nature. In latent stage, a form of lysogeny, the viral genome stays in the host cell, but is not necessarily incorporated. Once the viral gene is released, early gene transcription begins, the products of which are proteins that regulate the transcription of further genes and viral DNA replication (McCullough and Savage, 2005b). Viral diseases may be the direct result of cell destruction by a virus, or a consequence of host immune reactions against viral proteins. Viruses may encode homologs of host cytokines and decoy receptors capable of binding and neutralizing host-derived cytokines. The rapid rate of mutation in critical viral genes can help viruses to overcome adaptive host defenses (Slots, 2009). The most common viral infections that are relevant to dentists and orthodontists are listed in Table 14.2.

Herpesvirus

This virus belongs to the family Herpetoviridae, and consists of a double-stranded DNA molecule surrounded by an icosahedral capsid, a proteinaceous tegument, and a lipid-containing envelope with embedded viral glycoproteins (Greenberg, 1996). Around 300 different types of herpesvirus have been identified, of which eight human herpesvirus species with distinct biological and clinical implications have been classified in three groups (Slots, 2009):

- Alpha group: includes herpes simplex virus 1 (HSV-1), the herpes simplex virus 2 (HSV-2) and varicella zoster (VZ) virus
- Beta group: human cytomegalovirus, human herpesvirus 6 and human herpesvirus 7
- Gamma group: Epstein–Barr virus (EBV) and human herpesvirus 8.

Primary herpetic gingivostomatitis

The primary infection with herpes simplex virus, which usually occurs in infants and children, often goes unnoticed, being subclinical in nature (Scott et al., 1997). There may be a prodrome of fever, malaise, and nausea. The infection might also present as vesicles on the mucosa of the mouth and pharynx. The vesicles break down to form clusters of small, round or irregular superficial ulcers with yellowish base and red margins. There is a characteristic widespread inflammation of the gingivae, which appear

Table 14.2 Viral infections of relevance for the dentist and orthodontist

Virus family	Virus name	Viral disease	General clinical or oral appearance	Treatment
Herpes viruses				
Alfa group	Herpes simplex (HSV – 1 and 2)	Primary infection gingivostomatitis	Swollen and red gingiva, sometimes with ulcers, multiple vesicles in mucosa	Aciclovir
	Varicella zoster (VZ or herpes virus 3)	Recurrent infection: herpes labialis and intraoral herpes	Lesions on lips (usually unilateral), perioral skin, intraoral ulcer lesions, trigeminal neuralgia	Aciclovir
		Shingles	'Belt of roses', rash and neuralgia with pain commonly from the trigeminal nerve (15%), on one or sometimes both sides of the face	Palliative
Beta group	Cytomegalovirus (CMV or herpesvirus 5)	CMV infection	May infect fetus during pregnancy	Ganciclovir
Gamma group	Epstein–Barr virus (EBV or herpesvirus 4)	Infectious mononucleosis	Tonsillitis	Palliative
Morbilli virus	Morbilli virus	Measles	Cough, conjunctivitis, fever, photophobia, rhinitis, Koplik spots, skin rash	Vaccine
Paramyxoma	Mumps virus	Mumps (parotitis)	Glandular infection especially of salivary glands, which become swollen and painful – unilaterally or bilaterally	Vaccine
Papovavirus	Human papillomavirus (HPV)	Papilloma	Squamous cell papilloma – cauliflower-like lesions, narrow base, pink, exophytic growth	Surgery
			Verruca vulgaris – wartlike and broader base	
Retroviruses	HIV-1, HIV-2	Acquired immune deficiency syndrome (AIDS)	Hairy leukoplakia	Retarding medicine – highly active antiretroviral therapy (HAART)
		Acute and chronic (years)	Candidiasis and other fungal infections	
			Aggressive periodontitis	
			Kaposi sarcoma	
			Frequently mucosal infections	
Picorna virus	Coxsackie virus	Herpangina	Clustered petechiae in the soft palate that becomes ulcerated in a few days	Palliative
Picorna virus	Enterovirus	Hand, foot and mouth disease	Ulcerations on the buccal mucosa and soft palate often in conjunction with ulcers on the hands and feet	Benign and heals within 7–10 days
Hepatitis virus	Hepatitis B virus (HBV)	Liver infection	Jaundice (yellow skin and eye)	Aciclovir HBV – vaccine
	Hepatitis C virus (HCV)		HBV – acute infections and 5% develop the chronic, benign carrier state	HBC – no vaccine, aciclovir
			HCV – 60% develop chronic liver disease and 80% of these develops cirrhosis	

Adapted from Sällberg (2009) and Slots (2009).

pinkish red and swollen (Figure 14.8). The patient will experience difficulty eating and swallowing, and the condition, which is self-limiting, heals without scars in about 10 days. The lesion is always accompanied by cervical lymphadenopathy, and may be more severe if it occurs in adults (Tovaru et al., 2009).

After primary infection, the virus remains dormant in the sensory and autonomic trigeminal or sacral ganglia, and is reactivated at a later stage, when host immunity is compromised. Recurrent infections are observed in 20–40% of individuals after a primary infection. The reappearance of the infection shows regional predilection with the type 1 virus (mostly activated from trigeminal ganglia) producing oral infections, and type 2 (activated from sacral ganglia) producing genital lesions. The typical picture of the intraoral recurrent lesions is a cluster of small ulcers in the attached gingivae, which are initially discrete and painful and then coalesce at a later stage to form

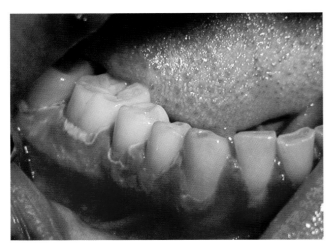

Figure 14.8 Acute herpetic gingivostomatitis. (Courtesy of Professor Mats Jontell.)

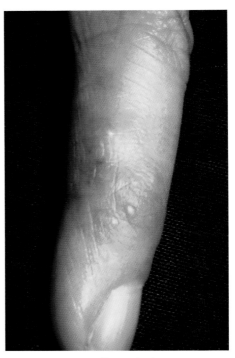

Figure 14.10 Herpetic whitlow affecting the fingers.

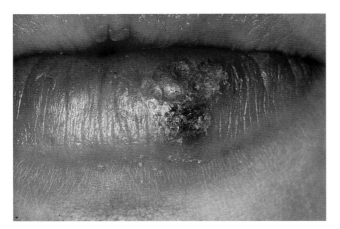

Figure 14.9 Herpes labialis.

larger lesions that heal in 10–12 days (Arduino and Porter, 2008).

Herpes labialis/cold sores (Figure 14.9) is a common recurrent herpes infection. A prickling sensation precedes blister formation. These blisters enlarge, coalesce, rupture, and become crusted before healing within 7–10 days. The lesions usually appear on the lips and perioral skin, often triggered by ultraviolet radiation. In some cases, trigeminal neuralgia has been described in conjunction with episodes of herpes labialis, suggesting induction of neurosensory abnormalities (Treister and Woo, 2010). Herpetic whitlow (Figure 14.10), a herpetic infection of the fingers, is an occupational hazard as far as dental professionals are concerned, consisting of severely painful localized lesions, but which can spread following surgical intervention (Wu and Schwartz, 2007).

Clinical features are usually sufficient for diagnosis of herpes infection, the major differential diagnosis of which is recurrent aphthous ulceration (p. 242). The diagnosis can be confirmed with the help of cultures and enzyme-linked immunosorbent assay (ELISA), polymerase chain reaction (PCR), or direct immunofluorescence (Rivera-Hidalgo and Stanford, 1999).

Aciclovir has been recommended for treatment of this condition, but should be prescribed only under strict medical guidance. It should be supplemented with bed rest, fluids, and soft diet, along with antipyretics for fever reduction (Wilson et al., 2009). Patients should be discouraged from touching the lesions, in order to reduce the risk of spreading the infection.

Varicella zoster infection

The primary infection from varicella virus is chicken pox, which occurs mainly in children. The virus remains in a latent state in dorsal root ganglia, and is reactivated, when host immunity is compromised at a later stage to produce herpes zoster or shingles. Varicella is a highly infectious disease, transmitted by inhalation of infective droplets and by direct contact with the lesions. The pruritic skin rash progresses through macules, papules, vesicles, drying vesicles and scabs, with healing occurring over 2–3 weeks. Intraoral vesicles are commonly seen on the tongue, buccal mucosa, gingiva, palate (Figure 14.11), and oropharynx, and are generally not painful (Birek, 2000). A number of predisposing factors can lead to recurrence of the infection

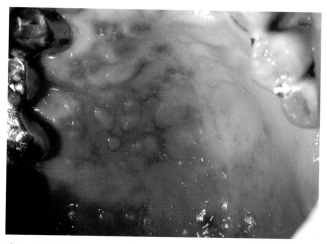

Figure 14.11 Herpes zoster. (Courtesy of Professor Mats Jontell.)

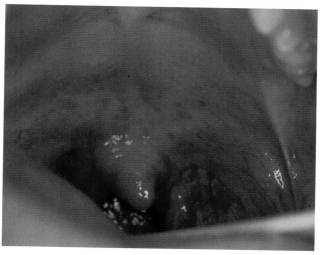

Figure 14.12 Infectious mononucleosis.

in tissues supplied by sensory nerves, such as immunosuppression with cytotoxic drugs, radiation, internal malignancies, malnutrition, old age, alcohol, and substance abuse. In immunocompromised patients, including those infected with HIV, the recurrence rate of herpes infection is increased (Civen et al., 2009). Occasionally, dental manipulation can also lead to recurrence. The first signs are pain and tenderness in the dermatome corresponding to the sensory ganglion, following which vesicles appear on one side of the face or along the distribution area of one branch of the trigeminal nerve. The unilateral vesicles form clusters with areas of surrounding erythema, ending abruptly in the midline. The lesions often heal with scarring, and areas of hypo/hyperpigmentation may be seen. When the facial and auditory nerves are affected, there is facial paralysis, vesicles in external ear, tinnitus, deafness, and vertigo, the combination of which is called 'Ramsay–Hunt syndrome' (Persson et al., 2009). A residual complication of herpes zoster infection is postherpetic neuralgia, which occurs in 10% of patients, and manifests as unilateral persistent pain in the affected area (Gilden et al., 2010). Treatment of this infection is supportive and symptomatic, with topical, as well as systemic antipruritics and analgesics that do not contain aspirin. A high dose of aciclovir (800 mg five times daily for 7 days) is recommended.

Epstein–Barr virus

EBV is the causative agent in infectious mononucleosis or 'kissing disease' in young adults and children, transmitted mainly through blood and saliva (Rivera-Hidalgo and Stanford, 1999). The disease manifestations include fever, lymphadenopathy, malaise, and sore throat. Oral ulcers, multiple palatal petechiae, gingival ulcerations, and enlarged

tonsils (Figure 14.12), are the reported oral manifestations (Mendoza et al., 2008). This virus is also implicated in oral hairy leukoplakia, which is seen in HIV-infected patients, and in malignancies (nasopharyngeal carcinoma, Burkitt lymphoma, and oral squamous cell carcinoma) and periodontal disease (Mendoza et al., 2008; Hoelzer, 2009). EBV and cytomegalovirus have been associated with multiple autoimmune disorders, such as systemic lupus erythematosus, rheumatoid arthritis, multiple sclerosis, pemphigus vulgaris, Sjögren syndrome, Wegener granulomatosis, and polyarteritis nodosa (Barzilai et al., 2007). Diagnosis is established with a monospot test, and the disease is usually self-limiting with bed rest and analgesics. Aciclovir has no role in its treatment.

Cytomegalovirus infection

This is the least common of the herpes viral infections, as is herpes 6, 7 and 8 viral infections. Human cytomegalovirus infection presents as mainly three syndromes: perinatal and human cytomegalovirus inclusion disease, acute acquired human cytomegalovirus infection, and human cytomegalovirus disease in immunocompromised hosts (Rivera-Hidalgo and Stanford, 1999). Oral manifestations are observed in the latter two syndromes, which are together called heterophil-negative infectious mononucleosis. Infection often arises after blood transfusion or sexual contact (Miller, 1996). Sahin et al. (2009) recently identified the saliva of patients with chronic periodontitis as the source for human cytomegalovirus and EBV, from where the reactivation process can start. These viruses become very active in immunocompromised patients and are often associated with malignancies such as oral squamous cell carcinoma and cervical carcinoma (Miller, 1996).

Palliative treatment is the management choice in these conditions.

Measles

An enveloped virus belonging to the family Morbillivirus causes measles. This is a highly communicable disease, transmitted by inhalation of infective droplets with an incubation period of 10–14 days. It is an acute systemic condition, the prodrome of which consists of cough, conjunctivitis, fever, malaise, photophobia, rhinitis, and Koplik spots, which appear on the mucosa next to the molars as bluish-gray specks on a red base. The spots start to appear 48 hours before the development of the irregular red-brick maculopapular rash characteristic of measles, and may last 4 days (Steichen and Dautheville, 2009). Shedding of measles virus starts in the prodromal stage, and continues through the acute stage. Measles remains a major cause of childhood mortality in developing countries (Rivera-Hidalgo and Stanford, 1999). However, vaccination can prevent its occurrence.

Mumps

Mumps, or epidemic parotiditis, is caused by the mumps virus, which belongs to the Paramyxoma virus genus. The parotid salivary gland infection may appear either unilaterally or bilaterally, and viremia can lead to complications such as orchitis in males, oophoritis in females, pancreatitis, deafness, and aseptic meningitis and encephalitis. Affected salivary glands will appear swollen, and will be accompanied by swelling of Stensen's duct, erythema, and pain. It is a highly communicable disease, transmitted by inhalation of infective droplets, with an incubation period of 14–21 days. Clinical diagnosis is based on the classic parotid swelling, while laboratory diagnosis is based on the isolation of the virus, detection of viral nucleic acid, or serological confirmation with the presence of IgM mumps antibodies. Vaccination can prevent mumps; one dose of vaccine is about 80% effective against the disease (Hviid et al., 2008).

Orthodontic treatment should not be carried out during the infectious stages of these diseases, as inter-personnel transfer occurs rapidly. If the orthodontist is unaware of the disease process, its clinical signs and symptoms, especially the initial oral manifestations, he or she might contract the infection and become a carrier. Thus for ethical reasons, an orthodontist, as part of the healthcare system, should be aware of the signs and symptoms of all these diseases along with the methods of identification and management/referral strategies, not only to protect him or herself but also their office staff and patients from contacting it.

Human papillomavirus infections

Human papillomavirus is composed of more than 60 serological types, and produces lesions in many areas of the body, such as the trachea, esophagus, genitalia, nasal cavity, larynx, and the mouth (Dhariwal et al., 1995). The classical oral lesions associated with papillomavirus infection are squamous cell papilloma, condyloma acuminatum, verruca vulgaris, and focal epithelial hyperplasia (Chaudhary et al., 2009). Squamous cell papilloma is a slow growing, solitary, painless, exophytic, cauliflower-like, small, pink mucosal lesion with a narrow base. It can occur at any age, but is most commonly seen between 30 and 50 years of age, with predilection for the tongue, lip, and soft palate (Carneiro et al., 2009). Verruca vulgaris or the common wart is a narrow exophytic growth with a wider base, that is sessile, and firm. Oral lesions arise through autoinoculation, with the labial mucosa, tongue, and gingiva as the preferred sites. The most common site is the buccal mucosa, and the infection is strongly associated with oral habits such as areca quid chewing and cigarette smoking (Wang et al., 2009). Condyloma acuminatum is usually found in the genitalia, with occasional occurrence in the oral cavity. Oral infections are predominantly transmitted through oral–genital sexual contact, and consist of multiple cauliflower-like lesions; the labial mucosa, lingual frenulum, and the soft palate are the sites of preferred invasion. Kui et al. (2003) traced the occurrence of condyloma acuminatum to infection by human papillomavirus, and suggested sexual abuse as the most common route of transmission. Focal epithelial hyperplasia, or Heck disease, usually presents as multiple plaque-like lesions, which are the same color as the mucosa and have a smooth surface. Individual lesions tend to be small (0.3–1 cm), but they coalesce and cluster, giving the mucosa a cobblestone or fissured surface. Lesions occur exclusively in the oral mucosa, and often present as asymptomatic papules (Bennett and Hinshaw, 2009). Other lesions such as erythroplakia, proliferative verrucous leukoplakia, candidal leukoplakia, squamous cell carcinoma, and lichen planus have also been associated with papillomavirus infection (Rivera-Hidalgo and Stanford, 1999). Most often, the treatment objective is to surgically excise the lesion if it causes esthetic problems, or is chronically injured.

Retroviral infections

Retroviral species, which inhabit almost all vertebrates, have seven established genera. HIV and T-lymphocytic viruses are considered to be the human pathogens in this group. The name retrovirus has its origin in its unique mode of replication. After entering a cell, the viral RNA is transcribed by viral reverse transcriptase into a DNA molecule, which is integrated as a provirus into the host chromosomal DNA. The provirus DNA serves as a template for the formation of viral RNA and the proteins used in the assembly of new virions. The ability of a provirus to remain transcriptionally inactive enables retroviruses to maintain persistent infection despite a functional host immune system (Slots, 2009). HIV belongs to the Lentivirus genus, and HIV-1 and HIV-2 are its two subspecies. HIV-1 is the most virulent type, and is responsible for the majority of HIV infections globally. The most common mode of spread is through the sexual route, followed by blood or blood products infusion, and mother-to-child transmission *in utero*. HIV uses the CD4 receptor and chemokine co-receptor (CCR5) for entry into susceptible cells, and results in selective depletion of CD4+ T lymphocytes by apoptosis or necrosis. This process leads to progressive loss of cell-mediated immunity (Sallberg, 2009). The course of infection can be primary or acute, or chronic, finally culminating in acquired immune deficiency syndrome (AIDS). In the early stages, there is development of oral and vaginal candidiasis along with pneumococcal infections, tuberculosis, and reactivation of herpes simplex and vari- cella infections. Later stages involve infections caused by *Candida, Pneumocystis jiroveci, Histoplasma, Toxoplasma,* and *Cryptococcus* species (Reichart, 2003; Slots, 2009). Malignancies in HIV patients are often viral related, and EBV lymphomas, human herpesvirus, Kaposi sarcoma, and papillomavirus sarcomas predominate (Slots, 2009).

Oral hairy leukoplakia presents as a white, vertically cor- rugated, nonremovable lesion on the lateral or ventral margin of the tongue. The lesion is caused by EBV and has no premalignant potential (McCullough and Savage, 2005b; Gonzalez et al., 2010). Kaposi sarcoma is characterized by erythematous or violaceous plaque-like lesions that develop into tumorous growths over time. Large lesions may get ulcerated and become painful, and interfere with function. Hairy leukoplakia is predominantly seen in the palate or in the attached gingiva (Van Heerden, 2006). Other HIV- related oral lesions include pseudomembranous candidia- sis, non-Hodgkin lymphoma, linear gingival erythema, necrotizing ulcerative periodontitis, and necrotizing ulcera- tive gingivitis (Leao et al., 2009). Current therapy for HIV infection is termed as HAART, or highly active antiretrovi- ral therapy, and it includes at least two classes of antiretro- viral agents. These may be a combination of two nucleoside analog inhibitors of reverse transcriptase, together with a protease inhibitor or a non-nucleoside reverse transcriptase inhibitor. If immune reconstitution had not happened, there may be a rebound of symptoms, such as oral candi- diasis and parotid gland enlargement (Ortega et al., 2008). If the patient is resistant to antiretroviral agents, the newer classes of drugs such as CCR5 antagonists can be prescribed (Slots, 2009).

If an orthodontist fails to identify this highly contagious, globally prevalent viral infection, for which no effective treatment has yet been developed, this will be considered highly negligent and dangerous. There is every chance that infected individuals will request correction of their maloc- clusion, but treating them without taking proper precau- tionary measures may lead to transmission of the infection. It is, therefore, imperative to obtain a detailed medical history, and to perform a thorough orofacial examination, in both young and adult candidates for orthodontic treat-

ment, in order to detect those who may have symptoms suggestive of these viral infections. Provision of orthodon- tic care for patients with these viral diseases requires close and continuous interaction with the physicians treating these individuals.

Herpangina

Herpangina is an acute febrile illness of sudden onset, char- acterized by the presence of ulcerations, vesicles, and diffuse erythema of the soft palate (Figure 14.13), fauces, and ton- sillar areas. It commonly occurs in children, mainly during the summer, with a sudden onset of malaise, fever, and sore throat. The absence of oral lesions on the hard palate, and the acute onset and short period of morbidity, help to dif- ferentiate herpangina from other infectious processes. It is more frequently caused by the Coxsackie group A serotypes (Figure 14.14), and less frequently by group B serotypes,

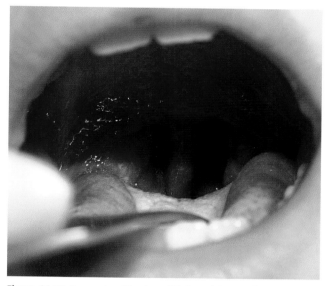

Figure 14.13 Herpangina. (Courtesy of Dr Peter Johansson.)

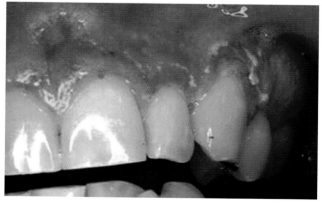

Figure 14.14 Coxsackievirus infection of the gingiva. (Courtesy of Professor Mats Jontell.)

echovirus, and enterovirus. Usually the disease is self-limiting (Rivera-Hidalgo and Stanford, 1999; McCullough and Savage, 2005b; Van Heerden, 2006; Slots, 2009).

Hand, foot, and mouth disease

Hand, foot, and mouth disease is a mild exanthematous lesion, most commonly seen in children aged 1–5 years, but older children and young adults are not spared. Several enteroviruses are thought to be causative, and the most important ones are human enterovirus-71 and Coxsackievirus serotype (Kushner and Caldwell, 1996). The typical feature is exanthematous illness with vesicular lesions, 2–10 mm in diameter, of the hands, feet, and mouth. The cutaneous vesicles can resemble chicken pox (Slots, 2009). Oral lesions appear as ulcerations in the buccal mucosa (square blisters) and soft palate. Aciclovir has been found to be useful in the treatment of hand, foot, and mouth disease (Shelley et al., 1996). Sometimes the disease is self-limiting, with only symptomatic treatment indicated, to alleviate pain and associated fever. Non-aspirin antipyretics and topical anesthetics are of great help in these patients (Rivera-Hidalgo and Stanford, 1999; McCullough and Savage, 2005b; Van Heerden, 2006; Slots, 2009).

Viral hepatitis

Viral hepatitis does not have any oral manifestations, but is important because it can spread through the oral route. Dentists and orthodontists treating patients with this disease should be aware of its signs and symptoms, so that they can prevent the spread of the infection to themselves and to their patients and clinical staff.

Infection with hepatitis B virus has three distinct phases: the first phase is acute, and is either subclinical or shows the classic signs of liver disease. This phase is seen mainly in adults. Children show the other two stages: chronic infection, in which there is a high rate of viral replication, and later on a latent phase, where the virus maintains a lower replication rate. During the infectious phase, the child is highly contagious and the risk for severe liver disease is increased (Broderick and Jonas, 2003). The disease can be easily transmitted via an accidental needle stick injury, or a bite, through just 1 mL of blood, which contains 10^5–10^7 viral genomes. Dental staff should be vaccinated against hepatitis B, as once infected they can become lifelong carriers. Treatment for hepatitis B infection requires a combinatorial approach, as in HIV-infected patients, and it requires drugs that attack the various stages of viral replication (Sallberg, 2009).

Hepatitis C is quite rare in childhood, but can be seen owing to vertical transmission (from mother to child) or through a nosocomial route. This virus can also lead to a serious liver disorder, and children are often treated with interferon gamma and riboflavin combination regimen. No vaccine is presently available for hepatitis C (Fischler, 2007; Sallberg, 2009).

Fungal infections

The most common fungal infections affecting the oral cavity and of interest to dental surgeons and especially orthodontists are listed in Table 14.3.

Table 14.3 Fungal infections of relevance to the dentist and orthodontist

Type of fungi	Type of fungal infection	Common species	Clinical manifestations	Treatment
Oral yeast infections	Candidiasis	C. albicans C. glabrata	Acute pseudomembranous	Mucostatin Amphotericin
	Candida-associated lesions	C. tropicalis C. krusei	Chronic hyperplastic or erythematous (atrophic)	Azoles
		C. dublinensis	Hyperkeratinized (white) or atrophic (red) mucosal lesions from which Candida can be isolated	
Systemic mycoses by molds	Aspergillosis	A. fumigates	Pulmonary	Amphotericin B Azoles
	Cryptococcosis	C. neoformans	Pulmonary	Amphotericin B Flucytosine
	Blastomycosis	B. dermatitidis	Pulmonary, cutaneous	Amphotericin B Azoles
	Mucormycosis	Mucorales spp.	Pulmonary	Amphotericin Surgery
	Histoplasmosis	H. capsulatum	Pulmonary, cutaneous	Amphotericin B Azoles
	Paracoccidioidomycosis	P. brasilisensis	Pulmonary	Amphotericin B Azoles
	Sporotrichosis	S. schenckii	Cutaneous	Amphotericin B

Adapted from Samaranayake et al., 2009.

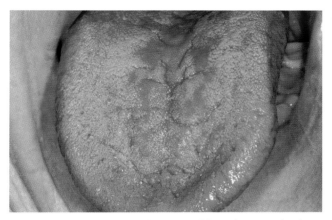

Figure 14.15 Acute pseudomembranous candidiasis. (Courtesy of Professor Mats Jontell.)

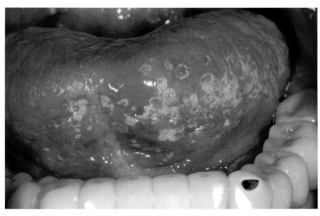

Figure 14.16 Acute erythematous candidiasis. (Courtesy of Dr Bengt Hasseus.)

Candidiasis is the most common oral mycotic infection, and *Candida albicans* is the organism most commonly associated with it. Other species observed in oral fungal infections are *Candida tropicalis, Candida glabrata, Candida krusei*, and *Candida dublinensis*. Clinically, candidiasis can be the cause of oral discomfort or pain, dysgeusia, and aversion to food (Samaranayake et al., 2009). Oral candidal infections are categorized as primary and secondary; primary candidiasis is confined to the oral and peri-oral tissues. If oral candidiasis is a manifestation of systemic disease, it is categorized as secondary candidiasis (Axell et al., 1997). Primary oral candidiasis is further subdivided into pseudomembranous, erythematous, and hyperplastic types. Pseudomembranous candidiasis (Figure 14.15), otherwise known as thrush, is characterized by white patches on the labial and buccal mucosa, tongue, and soft palate. The lesions often resemble milk curd, and can be wiped off very easily with the help of a tongue blade, to reveal an erythematous, erosive base. The white mass consists of a tangled mass of fungal hyphae, bacteria, inflammatory cells, fibrin, and desquamated epithelial cells. Erythematous candidiasis (Figure 14.16) occurs as a consequence of persistent acute pseudomembranous candidiasis and it is the most common form seen in HIV-infected patients. It consists of red patches, often in the mid-dorsum of the tongue, palate, and buccal mucosa. Palatal erythematous lesions, otherwise known as 'kissing' lesions, are a common finding in HIV infection. Motta-Silva et al. (2010) recently concluded that oral erythematous candidiasis is more prevalent in patients with controlled diabetes mellitus type 2. Hyperplastic candidiasis, or candidal leukoplakia (Figures 14.17, 14.18), is the least common form, appearing as chronic, discrete, slightly raised lesions that vary from small palpable, translucent, whitish areas, to large, dense, opaque plaques, with hard and rough areas evident on palpation (Sitheeque and Samaranayake, 2003). Fifteen percent of candidal leukopla-

kia tends to have a tendency towards malignant conversion (McCullough and Savage, 2005a; Samaranayake et al., 2009).

Other conditions caused by *Candida* species are chronic atrophic candidiasis or denture sore mouth, linear gingival erythema, secondary oral candidiasis, and chronic mucocutaneous candidiasis syndromes. In denture sore mouth (Figure 14.19), which can be seen in patients wearing removable orthodontic appliances, there is overgrowth of *C. albicans* on the fitting surface of a denture or a removable orthodontic appliance. The patient may complain of angular cheilitis (Figure 14.20a,b), or occasional burning or tingling sensation beneath the acrylic baseplate. This can be prevented by educating the patient about the importance of oral hygiene measures, and cleaning and proper follow-up of inserted dentures and removable orthodontic appliances (Coelho et al., 2004).

Linear gingival erythema is defined as nonplaque-induced gingivitis, presenting as a distinct erythematous band of at least 2 mm along the margin of the gingiva, with either diffuse or punctate erythema of the attached gingiva. The lesions may be localized to one or two teeth, or can be generalized, and may or may not be accompanied by occasional bleeding and discomfort. *C. dubliniensis* has been implicated in linear gingival erythema, and is one of the common oral manifestations of HIV infection (Zhang et al., 2009). Treatment of this condition does not require antifungal medications, but rather professional periodontal scaling and debridement, along with effective plaque control at home, and twice daily mouth rinses with 0.12% chlorhexidine gluconate for 2 weeks.

Secondary candidiasis occurs consequent to HIV infection, hematological malignancies, and aggressive treatment with cytotoxic agents. Chronic mucocutaneous candidiasis syndrome is a persistent candidiasis that

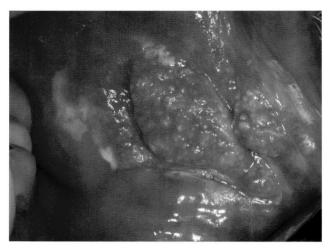

Figure 14.17 Chronic nodular candidiasis in the buccal mucosa. (Courtesy of Professor Mats Jontell.)

responds poorly to topical antifungal agents (Samaranayake et al., 2009).

Treatment of candidal infections ranges from topical delivery of polyene agents up to four times a day, to systemic delivery of azole agents ranging from a weekly single dose, to a single dose per day for a week (Greenspan, 1994; Laudenbach and Epstein, 2009). Two polyenes are commonly used for antifungal treatment: nystatin and amphotericin B, of which nystatin is more commonly used. It has fungicidal and static activity, and is available as creams, tablets, suspensions, oral gels, rinses, and pastilles. Nystatin is not absorbed when given orally, and is too toxic for parenteral use. In such cases, amphotericin B is preferred, but it has a serious systemic adverse effect, that is, nephrotoxicity. Hypokalemia and anemia are

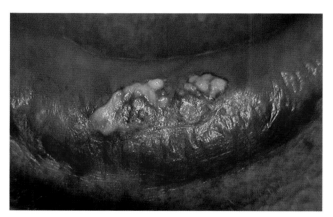

Figure 14.18 Chronic nodular candidiasis of the lip. (Courtesy of Dr Per-Olov Rödström.)

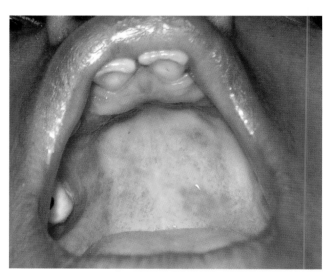

Figure 14.19 Denture sore mouth with secondary *Candida* infection. (Courtesy of Dr Ranimol Sreekumar.)

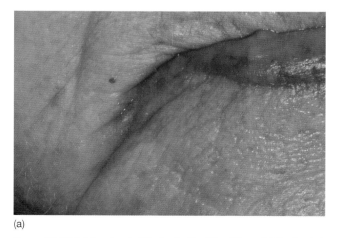

(a)

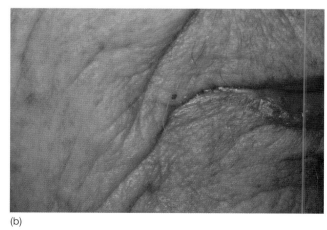

(b)

Figure 14.20 (a) Angular cheilitis due to *Candida albicans*. (b) Healing lesions in the same patient as in Figure 14.20a. (Courtesy of Professor Mats Jontell.)

also common, along with anaphylaxis, fever, headache, vomiting, and anorexia. Amphotericin B is available as lozenges, ointment, suspensions, and cream. Azole antifungal agents are imidazoles (clotrimazole, econazole, isoconazole, miconazole), and triazoles (fluconazole and itraconazole). Clotrimazole has a broad spectrum of activity, and is mainly fungistatic. It is available in the form of 1% cream, lozenges, vaginal creams, and tablets. Miconazole, which also has a broad spectrum of activity, is also effective against some Gram-positive bacteria, such as staphylococci (Isham and Ghannoum, 2010). Fluconazole is the drug of choice in oropharyngeal candidiasis in HIV-infected patients, due to its high systemic absorption rate. It is available as capsular and intravenous formulations, with a dosage of 100 mg daily for 7–14 days (Samaranayake et al., 2009; Martinez-Beneyto et al., 2010).

Orthodontic appliances, removable, fixed, or functional ones, by virtue of preventing proper performance of oral hygiene measures can promote candidal overgrowth. Orthodontists should be equipped for management of these lesions after appropriate identification, as well as differential diagnosis to eliminate serious underlying disorders. They should be aware of the available antifungal preparations and their dosages, so that minor problems can be tackled in the orthodontic office. Major problems should be identified, followed by referral to an oral medicine specialist or to a physician, so that the patient's wellbeing and quality of life are not compromised.

Some uncommon systemic mycoses with oral lesions

An increasing number of immunocompromised patients are attending dental as well as orthodontic offices; thus a number of uncommon mycotic lesions are now being first detected by dental surgeons and orthodontists. Aspergillosis is the second most common opportunistic mycotic infection and affects the paranasal sinuses, the nasal cavity and oral mucosa, as well as the facial skin. It is caused by several *Aspergillus* species, of which *Aspergillus fumigates* is the most common. It is generally contracted through inhalation of spores, leading to both upper and lower respiratory tract infection, and to bronchopulmonary aspergillosis. Oral aspergillosis lesions are yellow or black in color, with a necrotic ulcerated base, typically seen in the posterior palate or posterior tongue (Iatta et al., 2009). The hyphae may penetrate the walls of small-to-medium sized arteries and veins and cause infarction, thrombosis, and necrosis, leading to systemic spread (Sales Mda, 2009). Systemic amphotericin B is the treatment of choice, along with topical clotrimazole or ketoconazole (Samaranayake et al., 2009).

Cryptococcosis is a chronic fungal disease involving the lungs, the central nervous system, and occasionally the skin and the mouth. The causative agent is *Cryptococcus neofor-*mans (Swe Han et al., 2009). The disease is usually a pulmonary infection, but oral lesions occur in the disseminated form. Oral lesions range from violaceous nodules of granulation tissue, swelling, to ulcers, and are usually seen in the gingiva, hard and soft palate, pharynx, oral mucosa, and in tooth sockets after extraction (Iatta et al., 2009). Diagnosis is confirmed by microscopy, and systemic amphotericin B, supplemented with flucytosine, is the drug of choice for treatment (Samaranayake et al., 2009).

Blastomycosis, caused by *Blastomycosis dermatitidis*, is a relatively uncommon male-predominant disease, presenting as pulmonary, disseminated or localized cutaneous lesions. The disease is initiated upon inhalation of the spores, and the clinical and histopathological findings are similar to those of squamous cell carcinoma. Oral blastomycosis is uncommon, but when present, it is seen as single or multiple ulcerations, sessile projections, and granulomatous or verrucous lesions (Kruse et al., 2010). Diagnosis is based on biopsy, smear, and culture. Amphotericin, ketoconazole, miconazole, and itraconazole are all effective in treating this disease (Samaranayake et al., 2009).

Mucormycosis, caused by the saprophytic fungus *Mucorales*, is often found in the nasal cavity of healthy individuals. Infection arises through inhalation of spores that are deposited in the pulmonary alveoli and spreads to different locations, such as the paranasal, rhino-orbital, rhinocerebral, cerebral, pulmonary, and gastrointestinal areas. The fungi erode the arteries, resulting in thrombosis and subsequent necrosis of surrounding tissues. Auluck (2007) described maxillary erosion (which is rare due to high vascularity) by mucormycosis in a patient with uncontrolled diabetes, outlining its severity. Six cases with mucormycosis affecting the periodontal ligament have been described in the literature (McDermott et al., 2010). Oral ulcerations, sinusitis, and facial cellulitis are common with mucormycosis, along with blood-tinged nasal discharge, and unilateral facial pain or numbness (Tabachnick and Levine, 1975). Diagnosis is confirmed by smear and histological demonstration of tissue invasion by hyphae. Treatment involves correction of acidosis, antifungal therapy with amphotericin B, and surgical debridement (Samaranayake et al., 2009).

Histoplasmosis, a localized or systemic fungal infection, caused by *Histoplasma capsulatum*, appears when microconidiae or hyphae are inhaled into the lungs. Clinical presentation of this infection includes acute or chronic pulmonary cutaneous histoplasmosis, with or without disseminated disease. Oral lesions are mostly chronic, with nodular, indurated or granular masses and ulceration affecting the oral mucosa, tongue, palate, gingiva, and the periapical region of the teeth (Epifanio et al., 2007; Narayana et al., 2009). Diagnosis is confirmed by microscopy, culture, and serology. Amphotericin B is the drug of choice, with fluconazole and itraconazole as alternatives (Samaranayake et al., 2009).

Paracoccidioidomycosis is caused by *Paracoccidioides brasiliensis*, which produces a granulomatous disease, primarily affecting the lungs and then disseminating to the nasal mucosa and other organ systems. The disease is restricted to south and central America, especially Brazil, hence the name South American blastomycosis. The source of the organism is the soil, and infection occurs through inhalation or by direct contact (Ramos-E-Silva and Saraiva, 2008). Oral manifestations are common, and the lesions usually appear as small papules and vesicles, which then ulcerate to form shallow ulcers with a rolled edge and a white exudative base studded with small hemorrhagic dots (Jham et al., 2008). In severe cases, infection may penetrate deep into the bone with perforation of the hard palate. Lesions can occur anywhere in the oral cavity, including the hard and soft palate, tongue, gingiva, and tonsils, and may lead to mobility of teeth due to periodontal infection. The face becomes readily swollen (Godoy and Reichart, 2003; Silva et al., 2007). Diagnosis is usually confirmed by histology and culture. Sulphonamide or amphotericin B alone, or in combination, is the treatment of choice. Ketoconazole can also be used (Samaranayake et al., 2009).

Sporotrichosis is a chronic nodular mycotic disease, the causative agent of which is *Sporotrichium schenckii*, a fungus found in soil and rotting wood. The fungi gain access through traumatic ulcerations, and usually affect the skin (Mahlberg et al., 2009). Proliferation of the organism leads to formation of a nodule or small ulcer. The nodules turn into 'bumps' on the skin and after several weeks the initial lesions heal with scarring, as new nodules and new bumps develop in other areas. Oral lesions are initially erythematous, ulcerative, and suppurative, but eventually become granulomatous, vegetative, and papillomatous. These lesions are painful, with enlarged and hard regional lymph nodes, and may resemble aphthous ulcerations, lichen planus, or cutaneous leishmaniasis (Aarestrup et al., 2001). Diagnosis is confirmed by histology and culture. Oral potassium iodide is the treatment of choice, followed by Amphotericin B, itraconazole and terbinafine (Kusuhara, 2009).

Parasitic infections

The common parasitic infections of particular interest to dentists and orthodontists are listed in Table 14.4.

Local protozoan infections, caused by *Trichomonas tenax* and *Entamoeba gingivalis*, which may occur as harmless commensals of the oral cavity, are observed in conditions of poor oral hygiene and in people with a low standard of living. The etiological role of these organisms in oral infections is unclear, but they have been isolated from periodontal tissues of immunocompromised patients with necrotic gingivitis. This finding has led to an assumption that parasitic infections are uncommon in healthy individuals and are more frequently observed in immunocompromised individuals. Diagnosis is based on microscopic examination of tissue scrapings after Giemsa staining, or after preculture in specific media, such as Kupferberg Trichomonas broth. In addition, polymerase chain reaction (PCR) amplification techniques can also be employed. Metronidazole is the drug of choice in both *Trichomonas* and *Entamoeba* infections, with a dosage of 400 mg three times daily for 1 week. There are no vaccines for these diseases (Bergquist, 2009).

Leishmaniasis, the systemic parasitic infection, is caused by *Leishmania*, a protozoan parasite that is found worldwide. Transmission relies on the sand fly, which constitutes a vector for the parasite and is part of the life cycle of *Leishmania*. Leishmaniasis has a spectrum of clinical symptoms ranging from superficial self-resolving skin patches, to systemic mutilating forms resembling leprosy (Motta et al., 2007). The clinical spectrum also includes cutaneous, mucocutaneous, and visceral leishmaniasis. Cutaneous leishmaniasis, often referred to as oriental sore, is a localized skin lesion that does not spread beyond the area of inoculation. This is the least serious form of the disease (Reithinger et al., 2007). When the organism invades

Table 14.4 Parasitic infections of interest to dentists and orthodontists

Type of infection	Microorganisms involved	Clinical manifestation	Treatment	Comment
Local oral parasitic infection	*Entamoeba gingivalis*	Associated with aggressive periodontitis in immunocompromised patients	Metronidazole	
	Trichomonas tenax	Associated with aggressive periodontitis in immunocompromised patients	Metronidazole	
Systemic parasitic infections (leishmaniasis)	*Leishmania brasiliensis*, *L. mexicana* (in the mucocutaneous form)	Cutaneous, mucocutaneous and visceral forms	No efficient drugs available	Transmitted by a vector (sand fly)
		The mucocutaneous forms may have oral manifestations	Amphotericin B and antimonite have some effect	

Adapted from Bergquist (2009).

mucosal tissues, it is called as mucocutaneous leishmaniasis, and has a predilection for oto-nasopharyngeal areas. The most common symptom is nasal irritation or stiffness due to infiltration of the parasite into the septum and inferior turbinates. Extension of this lesion can lead to granulomas in the oral, laryngeal and pharyngeal areas, and as the disease progresses, severe facial deformities develop, sometimes resulting in total loss of the nose and upper lip (Di Lella et al., 2006). The involvement of the palate, tongue, pharynx, and larynx can lead to dysphagia or dysphonia. Bacterial superinfections can occur over these areas, further complicating the problem (Bergquist, 2009). Visceral leishmaniasis is otherwise known as kala azar, in which there is hematogenous dissemination of *Leishmania* species, which then infect macrophages in the liver, spleen, bone marrow, and lymph nodes. This condition usually develops gradually, and the patient becomes progressively weak with abdominal distension, nausea, and vomiting, followed by lymphadenopathy, petechiae, ecchymoses, and edema. The skin becomes dry and scaly, and can acquire a grayish tone, especially on the hands and face (Gupta et al., 2010).

Aspirates and biopsy specimens from the raised edges of skin lesions can be used to make a direct diagnosis. Giemsa staining will reveal amastigotes, which tend to be found in the periphery of infected host cells (Bergquist, 2009). Aspirates can be cultured in specialized media such as Novy-McNeal-Nicolle medium (Limoncu et al., 2004). Several rapid and reliable tests are available, such as Montenegro skin test, immunochromatographic test, and molecular diagnostic tests using PCR (Bergquist, 2009). Pentavalent antimonials, such as sodium stibogluconate (Pentostam) and methylglucamine antimonite (Glucantime), are the drugs used in treatment of leishmaniasis of all forms. A dose of 20 mg/kg/day is recommended, and should be administered only under medical supervision. The second line of drugs such as pentamidine, amphotericin B, and macrolide polyenes can also be used, from which amphotericin B has the highest cure rate (Bergquist, 2009; van Griensven et al., 2010). There is no vaccine available for this disease, and prevention is the only option. Use of insecticide-treated nets is a good method and is recommended as a preventive measure (Bergquist, 2009).

The oral cavity as a source for focal infections

Focal oral infections can be defined as infections occurring in different locations in the human body which are caused by microorganisms normally inhabiting the oral cavity or their products. Dental procedures such as tooth extraction, endodontic treatment, periodontal surgery, orthodontic separator placement, banding and debonding procedures, can introduce oral microorganisms into the blood stream and the lymphatic system. The number of bacteria in the blood stream required to cause transient bacteremia is around 1–10 per mL of blood; this usually lasts for no more than 15–30 minutes. The bacterial spread is mainly by three routes (Gendron et al., 2000):

- Metastatic infection – caused by translocation of bacteria
- Metastatic injury – through microbial toxins
- Metastatic inflammation – due to immune injury.

Recent studies have confirmed the role of oral microorganisms in focal infections that can lead to coronary heart disease, pre-term low birthweight babies, and aspiration pneumonia (Destefano et al., 1993; Offenbacher et al., 1996; Scannapieco et al., 1998). The susceptibility of certain groups of individuals, such as older patients and the immunocompromised (HIV infected, organ transplanted), to this process is well established (Gendron et al., 2000).

Infective endocarditis

Infective endocarditis is the most common heart disease caused by oral bacterial metastasis. Congenital heart diseases, presence of valvular defects and a previous history of congestive cardiac diseases, all predispose patients to infective endocarditis when exposed to surgical dental procedures (Bascones-Martinez et al., 2009). The outcome of the disease varies from debilitation to death due to valvular malfunction, congestive cardiac failure, or renal complication. About 50% of the cases are due to viridans streptococci (alpha streptococci), more particularly the polysaccharide-producing *Strep. sanguinis*, *Strep. mutans*, *Strep. oralis*, *Strep. mitis*, and *Strep. salivarius* (Douglas et al., 1993). Production of extracellular polysaccharide glucan by these bacteria favors their attachment to heart surfaces or fibrin-platelet clots. Fiehn et al. (1995) reported that bacteria colonizing in the oral cavity may invade through the blood stream and cause infective endocarditis. It has been reported that cardiovascular complications are more frequent in patients with periodontitis, and studies have provided evidence of a close association between periodontitis and myocardial infarction, atherosclerosis or stroke, and fatal coronary artery diseases (Scannapieco et al., 2010). For a more detailed discussion of the subject and the management strategies see Chapter 8 in *Biological Mechanisms of Tooth Movement* (Krishnan and Davidovitch (eds), Oxford, Wiley Blackwell, 2009).

Brain abscess

A focal suppurative process in the brain parenchyma can result from transient bacteremia from oral infections or dental treatment. Around 0.09–0.84 cases of brain abscess reported per million population per year can be attributed to oral infectious causes. In most cases of brain abscess from oral infections, the lesions are located in the frontal or temporal lobes, and reach the brain via direct extension or cavernous sinus thrombosis through the hematogenous or anatomical routes (Gendron et al., 2000). Syrjanen et al. (1989) found an increased prevalence of periodontitis, periapical abscess, poor oral hygiene, and carious lesions in patients with ischemic cerebral infarction. All types of microorganisms, Gram-positive cocci, Gram-negative cocci and rods, and anaerobic bacteria have been isolated from brain abscess lesions (Schuman and Turner, 1994).

Chronic meningitis

Various oral infections, such as dental abscesses and dental caries, have been implicated in chronic meningitis. Bacteria found at these sites can contaminate the cerebrospinal fluid, and reach the central nervous system. Moreover, the spread of oral infections into the tissues surrounding the oral cavity may give rise to chronic maxillary sinusitis and facial plane infections. The extreme form of infection in this regard is Ludwig angina, which involves life-threatening swelling of the posterior floor of the mouth as it can cause obstruction of the airway (Gilon et al., 2002; Jimenez et al., 2004). Oral infections have also been implicated in eye infections such as uveitis, endophthalmitis, and chronic conjunctivitis (Gendron et al., 2000).

Pneumonia

Pneumonia is infection of the pulmonary parenchyma caused by anaerobic bacteria and a dental source of the infection has been demonstrated in the form of dental plaque, associated with periodontitis (Sharma and Shamsuddin, 2011). Lung abscesses caused by *Streptococcus intermedius*, *Actinomyces* species, and *Campylobacter rectus* have been reported to originate from oral infectious sources and dental treatment-induced bacteremia (Scannapieco and Mylotte, 1996). Dental plaque containing *Pseudomonas aeruginosa* has been implicated in the development of chronic infection of the respiratory tract in patients with cystic fibrosis. The mechanisms by which these bacteria produce respiratory infections have been described by Scannapieco (1999), who suggests that the host-derived enzymes in the saliva uncover receptors on the mucosal surface allowing colonization by respiratory pathogens. From this site, periodontal pathogens such as *Porphyromonas gingivalis* and *A. actinomycetemcomitans*, are aspirated into the lung where they initiate infections. At the same time, cytokines derived from periodontal tissues may alter the respiratory epithelium, promoting infection by respiratory pathogens.

Helicobacter pylori infection

H. pylori, which persist in dental plaque even after its eradication with triple drug therapy, may get reactivated in some instances to produce reinfection. Zaric et al. (2009) reported that 77.3% of their patients treated with combined periodontal therapy and triple therapy with antibiotics, antimicrobials, and proton pump inhibitors, showed successful eradication of gastric *H. pylori* infection in comparison with 47.6%, who received only triple therapy. Oral microorganisms such as *A. actinomycetemcomitans*, *Fusobacterium nucleatum*, *Prevotella intermedia* and *Peptostreptococcus micros* (now *Parvimonas micra*) can also cause skin infections following direct inoculation (Gendron et al., 2000). In the same way, chronic urticaria can be triggered by pathogenic oral microorganisms that favor release of histamine from mast cells, or formation of circulating immune complexes (Thyagarajan and Kamalam, 1982).

Osteomyelitis

Osteomyelitis has been reported in association with *A. actinomycetemcomitans*, *P. micros*, and *E. corrdens*. In addition, fusobacteria and *C. albicans* have been implicated in some cases of osteomyelitis following dental treatment (Hudson, 1993; Navazesh and Mulligan, 1995; Gendron et al., 2000).

Pre-term birth

Approximately 7% of all infants weigh less than 2500 g at birth, and these infants account for two-thirds of neonatal deaths. There are many risk factors involved in pre-term birth, such as maternal smoking, alcohol abuse, drug use, and infection. Periodontal disease has also been recently implicated as a risk factor in this phenomenon. It had been suggested that periodontal disease provides a chronic systemic source of lipopolysaccharides, which stimulate the production of interleukin-1β and prostaglandin E2, which are closely associated with pre-term delivery (Heimonen et al., 2009; Kumar and Samelson, 2009). Katz et al. (2009) isolated *P. gingivalis* colonies from the placental tissue of women delivering pre-term babies. Han et al. (2004) proposed *F. nucleatum* as a cause of pre-term delivery. However, further evidence is required to clarify the precise role of this microorganism.

Conclusions

Orthodontic care is available to people regardless of age, sex, and geographical location. Most orthodontic patients are healthy, or have health problems that are of minor sinificance as far as mechanotherapeutics is concerned. However, some individuals have pre-existing conditions that may endanger their wellbeing, and sometimes their life. Some of these diseases may be contagious and spread to other people, who are otherwise healthy. The individuals at risk are the orthodontist, the orthodontic office staff, and all other patients who are being treated in the same clinic.

Therefore, it is of prime importance for the orthodontist to identify patients who carry these diseases, in the initial diagnosis. The most important duty of orthodontists is to protect themselves, their assistants, and all their patients from being infected by contagious diseases carried by some persons who are receiving orthodontic care in the same office.

The orthodontist may be the first to diagnose a contagious disease in a patient before or during orthodontic treatment. In addition to looking for physical evidence of specific pathological conditions, many laboratory tests are available, which can confirm or alter the initial diagnosis. The orthodontist may prescribe medications for the diagnosed diseases, based on his or her knowledge, but frequently they would benefit from seeking the advice of the infected patient's physician, or a specialist in contagious diseases.

In addition to the external dangers associated with contagious diseases, these pathological conditions and the medications used to treat them may affect adversely the biological response to orthodontic forces. Tooth movement is facilitated by the remodeling of mineralized and non-mineralized tissues, under the control of the nervous, immune, and endocrine systems. Changes in any or all of these systems, caused by either the disease or its medications, may affect processes such as inflammation, which is a core part of the cellular and tissue response to mechanotherapy. Little is known about these associations and their effects on the course and outcome of orthodontic treatment, but our knowledge about the nature of these diseases and the development of means to cure them effectively continues to grow, enabling the orthodontist to provide the best care, alongside protection from undesirable diseases.

References

Aarestrup FM, Guerra RO, Vieira BJ, et al. (2001) Oral manifestation of sporotrichosis in AIDS patients. *Oral Diseases* 7: 134–6.

Aas JA, Paster BJ, Strokes LN, et al. (2005) Defining the normal bacterial flora of the oral cavity. *Journal of Clinical Microbiology* 43: 5721–32.

Arduino PG, Porter SR (2008) Herpes simplex virus type 1 infection: overview of relevant clinic-pathologic features. *Journal of Oral Pathology and Medicine* 37: 107–21.

Auluck A (2007) Maxillary necrosis by mucormycosis: a case report and literature review. *Medicina Oral Pathologia Oral y Cirugia Bucal* 12: E360–4.

Axell T, Samaranayake LP, Reichart PA, et al. (1997) A proposal for reclassification of oral candidosis. *Oral Surgery Oral Medicine Oral Pathology Oral Radiology and Endodontics* 84: 111–12.

Barzilai O, Sherer Y, Ram M, et al. (2007) Epstein-Barr virus and cytomegalovirus in autoimmune diseases: are they truly notorious? A preliminary report. *Annals of the New York Academy of Sciences* 1108: 567–77.

Bascones-Martinez A, Munoz-Corcuera M, Meurman JH (2009) Odontogenic infections in the etiology of infective endocarditis. *Cardiovascular and Hematologic Disorders Drug Targets* 9: 231–5.

Bennett LK, Hinshaw M (2009) Heck's disease: diagnosis and susceptibility. *Pediatric Dermatology* 26: 87–9.

Bergquist R (2009) Parasitic infections affecting the oral cavity. *Periodontology 2000* 49: 96–105.

Birek C (2000) Herpes virus induced diseases: oral manifestations and current treatment options. *Journal of California Dental Association* 28: 911–21.

Broderick AL, Jonas MM (2003) Hepatitis B in children. *Seminars in Liver Diseases* 23: 59–68.

Brook I (2008) Actinomycosis: diagnosis and management. *Southern Medical Journal* 101: 1019–23.

Brook I (2009) Current management of upper respiratory tract and head and neck infections. *European Archives of Otorhinolaryngology* 266: 315–23.

Brook I (2010) Treatment modalities for bacterial rhinosinusitis. *Expert Opinion on Pharmacotherapy* 5: 755–69.

Brook I, Frazier EH, Thompson DH (1991) Aerobic and anaerobic microbiology of acute suppurative parotitis. *Laryngoscope* 101: 170–2.

Bruce AJ, Rogers RS 3rd (2004) Oral manifestations of sexually transmitted diseases. *Clinics in Dermatology* 22: 520–7.

Carneiro TE, Marinho SA, Verli FD, et al. (2009) Oral squamous papilloma: clinical, histologic and immunohistochemical analysis. *Journal of Oral Science* 51: 367–72.

Chaudhary AK, Singh M, Sundaram S, et al. (2009) Role of human papilloma virus and its detection in potentially malignant and malignant head and neck lesions: an updated review. *Head and Neck Oncology* 1: 22.

Childs WB (1933) The value of orthodontia as a health service. *International Journal of Orthodontia and Dentistry for Children* 19: 184–90.

Chue PW (1975) Gonorrhea – its natural history, oral manifestations, diagnosis, treatment and prevention. *Journal of American Dental Association* 90: 1297–301.

Civen R, Chaves SS, Jumaan A, et al. (2009) The incidence and clinical characteristics of herpes zoster among children and adolescents after implementation of varicella vaccination. *Pediatric Infectious Disease Journal* 28: 954–9.

Coelho CM, Sousa YT, Dare AM (2004) Denture-related oral mucosal lesions in a Brazilian school of dentistry. *Journal of Oral Rehabilitation* 31: 135–9.

D'Agostino J (2010) Pediatric airway nightmares. *Emergency Medicine Clinics of North America* 28: 119–26.

Dahlén G (2009) Bacterial infections of the oral mucosa. *Periodontology 2000* 49: 13–38.

Dahlén G, Blomquist S, Carlen A (2009) A retrospective study on the microbiology in patients with oral complaints and oral mucosal lesions. *Oral Diseases* 15: 265–72.

Destefano F, Anda RF, Kahn S, et al. (1993) Dental disease and risk of coronary heart disease and mortality. *British Medical Journal* 306: 688–91.

Dhariwal SK, Cubie HA, Southam JC (1995) Detection of human papilloma virus in oral lesions using commercially developed typing kits. *Oral Microbiology and Immunology* 10: 60–3.

Di Lella F, Vincenti V, Zennaro D, et al (2006) Mucocutaneous leishmaniasis: report of a case with massive involvement of nasal, pharyngeal and laryngeal mucosa. *International Journal of Oral and Maxillofacial Surgery* 35: 870–2.

Douglas CWI, Hearth J, Hampton KK, et al. (1993) Identity of viridians streptococci isolated from cases of infective endocarditis. *Journal of Medical Microbiology* 39: 179–82.

Dunning SH (1941) Medico-dental cooperation in the field of oral and physical diagnosis. *American Journal of Orthodontics and Oral Surgery* 27: A347–9.

Dykewicz MS, Hamilos DL (2010) Rhinitis and sinusitis. *Journal of Allergy and Clinical Immunology* 125: S103–115.

Ellner PD, Kiehn TE, Cammarata R, et al. (1988) Rapid detection and identification of pathogenic mycobacteria by combining radiometric and nucleic acid probe methods. *Journal of Clinical Microbiology* 26: 1349–52.

Epifanio RN, Brannon RB, Muzyka BC (2007) Disseminated histoplasmosis with oral manifestation. *Special Care in Dentistry* 27: 236–9.

Faergemann I, Dahlèn G (2009) Facial skin infections. *Periodontology 2000* 49: 194–209.

Feder HM (1990) Actinomycosis manifesting as an acute painless lump of the jaw. *Paediatrics* 85: 858–63.

Fiehn NE, Gutschik E, Larsen T, et al. (1995) identity of streptococcal blood isolates and oral isolates from tow patients with infective endocarditis. *Journal of Clinical Microbiology* 33: 1399–401.

Fischler B (2007) Hepatitis C virus infection. *Seminars in Fetal Neonatology and Medicine* 12: 168–73.

Gendron R, Grenier D, Maheu-Robert LF (2000) The oral cavity as a reservoir of bacterial pathogens for focal infections. *Microbes and Infection* 2: 897–906.

Ghosh S, Gadda RB, Vengal M, et al. (2009) Orofacial aspects of leprosy: report of two cases with literature review. *Medicina Oral Patologia Oral Y Cirugia Bucal* 15: e459–62.

Gilden D, Cohrs RJ, Mahalingam R, et al. (2010) Neurological disease produced by varicella zoster virus reactivation without rash. *Current Topics in Microbiology and Immunology* 342: 243–53.

Gilon Y, Brandt L, Lahaye T, et al. (2002) Systemic infections of dental origin. *Reveue de Stomatologie et de Chirurgie Maxilla-Faciale* 103: 26–9.

Godoy H, Reichart PA (2003) Oral manifestations of paracoccidiodomycosis: report of 21 cases from argentina. *Mycoses* 46: 412–17.

Gohean RJ, Pantera EA, Schuster SG (1990) Indirect immunofluorescence microscopy for the identification of Actinomyces sp. in endodontic disease. *Journal of Endodontics* 16: 318–22.

Gonzalez X, Correnti M, Rivera H, et al. (2010) Epstein Barr virus detection and latent membrane protein 1 in oral hairy leukoplakia in HIV+ Venezuelan patients. *Medicina Oral Pathologia Oral Ycirugia Bucal* 15: e297–e302.

Greenberg MS (1996) Herpesvirus infections. *Dental Clinics of North America* 40: 359–68.

Greenspan D (1994) Treatment of oropharyngeal candidiasis in HIV positive patients. *Journal of American Academy of Dermatology* 31: S51–5.

Guinta JL, Fiumara NJ (1986) Facts about gonorrhoea and dentistry. *Oral Surgery Oral Medicine Oral Pathology Oral Radiology and Endodontics* 62: 529–31.

Gupta S, Pal A, Vyas SP (2010) Drug delivery strategies for therapy of visceral leishmaniasis. *Expert Opinion on Drug Delivery* 7: 371–402.

Hale RG, Tucker DI (2008) Head and neck manifestations of tuberculosis. *Oral and Maxillofacial Surgery Clinics of North America* 20: 635–42.

Halsey ES (2009) *Pahryngitis, Bacterial*. Available at: http://emedicine.medscape.com/article/225243-overview (accessed 10 June 2010).

Han YW, Redline RW, Li M, et al. (2004) Fusobacterium nucleatum induces premature and term stillbirths in pregnant mice: implication of oral bacteria in preterm birth. *Infection and Immunity* 72: 2272–9.

Heimonen A, Janket SJ, Kaaja R, et al. (2009) Oral inflammatory burden and preterm birth. *Journal of Periodontology* 80: 884–91.

Helovuo H, Hakkarainen K, Paunio K (1993) Changes in the prevalence of subgingival enteric rods, staphylococci and yeasts after treatment with penicillin and erythromycin. *Oral Microbiology and Immunology* 8: 75–9.

Hoelzer D (2009) Update on Burkitt lymphoma and leukemia. *Clinical Advances in Hematology and Neurology* 7: 728–9.

Horning GM, Cohen ME (1995) Necrotizing ulcerative gingivitis, periodontitis and stomatitis: clinical staging and predisposing factors. *Journal of Periodontology* 66: 990–8.

Hudson JW (1993) Osteomyelitis of jaws: a 50 year perspective. *Journal of Oral and Maxillofacial Surgery* 51: 1294–301.

Hviid A, Rubin S, Muhlemann K (2008) Mumps. *Lancet* 371: 932–44.

Iatta R, Napoli C, Borghi E, et al. (2009) Rare mycoses of the oral cavity: a literature epidemiologic review. *Oral Surgery Oral Medicine Oral Pathology Oral Radiology and Endodontics* 108: 647–55.

Isham N, Ghannoum MA (2010) Antifungal activity of miconazole against recent candida strains. *Mycoses* 53: 434–7.

Jenkins IA, Saunders M (2009) Infections of the airway. *Paediatric Anesthesia* 19: 118–30.

Jham BC, Fernandes AM, Duraes GV, et al. (2008) The importance of intraoral examination in the differential diagnosis of paracoccidioidomycosis. *Brazilian Journal of Otorhinolaryngology* 74: 946.

Jimenez Y, Bagan JV, Murillo J, et al. (2004) Odontogenic infections, complications, systemic manifestations, *Medicina Oral Patologia Oral Ycirugia Bucal* 9: 139–47.

Kakisi OK, Kechagia AS, Kakisis IK, et al. (2010) Tuberculosis of the oral cavity: a systematic review. *European Journal of Oral Sciences* 118: 103–9.

Karkos PD, Asrani S, Karkos CD, et al (2009) Lemierre's syndrome. A systematic review. *Laryngoscope* 119: 1552–9.

Katz J, Chengini N, Shiverick KT, et al. (2009) Localization of P. gingivalis in preterm delivery placenta. *Journal of Dental Research* 88: 575–8.

Klug TE, Rusan M, Fuursted K, et al (2009) Fusobacterium necrophorum: most prevalent pathogen in peritonsillar abscess in Denmark. *Clinical Infectious Diseases* 49: 1467–72.

Kononen E (2000) Development of oral bacterial flora in young children. *Annals of Medicine* 32: 107–12.

Kruse AL, Zwahlen RA, Bredell MG, et al. (2010) Primary blastomycosis of oral cavity. *Journal of Craniofacial Surgery* 21: 121–3.

Kui LL, Xiu HZ, Ning LY (2003) Condyloma acuminatum and human papilloma virus infection in the oral mucosa of children. *Pediatric Dentistry* 25: 149–53.

Kumar J, Samelson R (2009) Oral health care during pregnancy – recommendations for oral health professionals. *The New York State Dental Journal* 75: 29–33.

Kushner D, Caldwell BD (1996) Hand-foot and mouth disease. *Journal of American Pediatric Medical Association* 86: 257–9.

Kusuhara M (2009) Sporotrichosis and dematiaceous fungal skin infections. *Japanese Journal of Medical Mycology* 50: 213–17.

Laskaris G (1996) Oral manifestations of infectious diseases. *Dental Clinics of North America* 40: 395–423.

Laudenbach JM, Epstein JB (2009) Treatment strategies for oropharyngeal candidiasis. *Expert Opinion on Pharmacotherapy* 10: 1413–21.

Leao JC, Ribeiro CM, Carvalho AA, et al. (2009) Oral complications of HIV disease. *Clinics (Sao Paulo)* 64: 459–70.

Limoncu ME, Ozbilgin A, Balcioglu IC, et al. (2004) Evaluation of three new culture media for cultivation and isolation of Leishmania parasites. *Journal of Basic Microbiology* 44: 197–202.

Little JW (2005) Syphilis: an update. *Oral Surgery Oral Medicine Oral Pathology Oral Radiology and Endodontics* 100: 3–9.

Lopez-Jornet P, Camacho-Alonso F, Andujar-Mateos P, et al. (2010) Burning mouth syndrome: An update. *Medicina Oral Patologia Oral Ycirugia Bucal* 15: e562–8.

Mahlberg MJ, Patel R, Rosenman K, et al. (2009) Fixed cutaneous sporotrichosis. *Dermatology Online Journal* 15: 8.

Martinez-Beneyto Y, Lopez-Jornet P, Velandrino-Nicolas A, et al. (2010) Use of antifungal agents for oral candidiasis: results of a national survey. *International Journal of Dental Hygiene* 8: 47–52.

McCullough MJ, Savage NW (2005a) Oral candidosis and therapeutic use of antifungal agents in dentistry. *Australian Dental Journal* 50: S36–9.

McCullough MJ, Savage NW (2005b) Oral viral infections and the therapeutic use of antiviral agents in dentistry. *Australian Dental Journal* 50: s31–5.

McCullough MJ, Abdel-Hafeth S, Scully C (2007) Recurrent aphthous stomatitis revisited: clinical features, associations and new association with infant feeding practices? *Journal of Oral Pathology and Medicine* 36: 615–20.

McDermott NE, Barrett J, Hipp J, et al. (2010) Successful treatment of periodontal mucormycosis: report of a case and literature review. *Oral Surgery Oral Medicine Oral Pathology Oral Radiology and Endodontics* 109: e64–9.

Mehta N, Silverberg MA, Kazzi AA, et al. (2009) *Peritonsillar Abscess*. Available at: http://emedicine.medscape.com/article/764188-overview (accessed 10 June 2010).

Meltzer EO, Hamilos DL, Hadley JA, et al. (2004) Rhinosinusitis: establishing definitions for clinical research and patient care. *Journal of Allergy and Clinical Immunology* 114: 155–212.

Mendoza N, Diamantis M, Arora A, et al. (2008) Mucocutaneous manifestations of Epstein-barr virus infection. *American Journal of Clinical Dermatology* 9: 295–305.

Miller CS (1996) Viral infections in the immunocompromised patient. *Dermatologic Clinics* 14: 225–41.

Moore HN (1939) Changing concepts in diagnosis. *American Journal of Orthodontics and Oral Surgery* 25: 875–82.

Motta ACF, Lopes MA, Ito FA, et al. (2007) Oral leishmaniasis: a clinicopathological study of 11 diseases. *Oral Diseases* 13: 335–40.

Motta-Silva AC, Aleva NA, Chavasco JK, et al. (2010) Erythematous oral candidiasis in patients with controlled type II diabetes mellitus and complete dentures. *Mycopathologia* 169: 215–23.

Murayama Y, Kurihara H, Nagai A, et al. (1994) Acute necrotizing ulcerative gingivitis: risk factors involving host defence mechanisms. *Periodontology 2000* 6: 116–24.

Narayana N, Gifford R, Giannini P, et al. (2009) Oral histoplasmosis: an unusual presentation. *Head and Neck* 31: 274–7.

Navazesh M, Mulligan R (1995) Systemic dissemination as a result of oral infection in individuals 50 years of age and older. *Special Care Dentist* 15: 11–19.

Noorizan Y, Chew YK, Khir A, et al. (2009) parotid abscess: an unusual case of facial nerve palsy. *Medical Journal of Malaysia* 64: 172–3.

Offenbacher S, Katz V, Fertik G, et al. (1996) Periodontal disease as a possible risk factor for preterm low birth weight. *Journal of Periodontology* 67: 1103–13.

Ortega KL, Ceballos-Salobrena A, Gaitan-Cepeda LA, et al. (2008) Oral manifestations after immune reconstitution in HIV patients on HAART. *International Journal of STD and AIDS* 19: 305–8.

Pajukoski M, Meurman JH, Halonen P, et al. (2001) Prevalence of subjective dry mouth and burning mouth in hospitalized elderly patients and outpatients in relation to saliva, medication and systemic diseases. *Oral Surgery Oral Medicine Oral Pathology Oral Radiology and Endodontics* 92: 641–9.

Persson A, Bergstrom T, Lindh M, et al. (2009) Varicella Zoster virus CNS disease- viral load, clinical manifestations and sequels. *Journal of Clinical Virology* 46: 249–53.

Peterson LR, Thomson RB (1999) Use of clinical microbiology laboratory for the diagnosis of infectious diseases related to the oral cavity. *Infectious Disease Clinics of North America* 13: 775–95.

Phalen JA, Jimenez V, Tompkins DC (1996) Tuberculosis. *Dental Clinics of North America* 40: 327–41.

Raad IL, Sabbagh MF, Caranasos GJ (1990) Acute bacterial sialadenitis: A study of 29 cases and review. *Reviews of Infectious Diseases* 12: 591–602.

Ramos-E-Silva M, Saraiva Ldo E (2008) Paracoccidioidomycosis. *Dermatologic Clinics* 26: 257–69.

Reichart PA (2003) Oral manifestation in HIV infection: fungal and bacterial infections, Kaposi's sarcoma. *Medical Microbiology and Immunology* 192: 165–9.

Reithinger R, Dujardin JC, Louzir H, et al. (2007) Cutaneous leishmaniasis. *Lancet Infectious Diseases* 7: 581–96.

Ridgeway JM, Parikh DA, Wright R et al (2010) Lemierre syndrome: a pediatric case series and review of literature. *American Journal of Otolaryngology* 31: 38–45.

Rivera-Hidalgo F, Stanford TW (1999) Oral mucosal lesions caused by infective microorganisms I. Viruses and bacteria. *Periodontology 2000* 21: 106–24.

Rosenwasser L (2007) New insights into the pathophysiology of allergic rhinitis. *Allergy and Asthma Proceedings* 28: 10–15.

Sahin S, Saygun I, Kubar A, et al. (2009) Periodontitis lesions are the main source of salivary cytomegalovirus. *Oral Microbiology and Immunology* 24: 340–2.

Sales Mda P (2009) Chapter 5-Aspergillosis: from diagnosis to treatment. *Journal Brasiliero De Pnemologia* 35: 1238–44.

Sällberg M (2009) Oral viral infections of children. *Periodontology 2000* 49: 87–95.

Samaranayake LP, Keung Leung W, Jin L (2009) Oral mucosal fungal infections. *Periodontology 2000* 49: 39–49.

Scala A, Checchi L, Montevecchi M, et al. (2003) Update on burning mouth syndrome: overview and patient management. *Critical Reviews in Oral Biology and Medicine* 14: 275–91.

Scannapieco FA (1999) Role of oral bacteria in respiratory infection. *Journal of Periodontology* 70: 793–802.

Scannapieco FA, Mylotte JM (1996) Relationships between periodontal disease and bacterial pneumonia. *Journal of Periodontology* 67: 1114–22.

Scannapieco FA, Papandonatos GD, Dunford RG (1998) Associations between oral conditions and respiratory disease in a national sample survey population. *Annals of Periodontology* 3: 251–6.

Scannapieco FA, Dasanayake AP, Chhun N (2010) Does periodontal therapy reduce the risk of systemic diseases? *Dental Clinics of North America* 54: 163–81.

Schuman NJ, Turner JE (1994) Brain abscess and dentistry: a review of literature. *Quintessence International* 25: 411–13.

Scott DA, Coulter WA, Biagioni PA, et al. (1997) Detection of herpes simplex virus type I shedding in the oral cavity by polymerase chain reaction and enzyme linked immunosorbant assay at the prodromal stage of recrudescent herpes labialis. *Journal of Oral Pathology and Medicine* 26: 305–9.

Scully C, Epstein J, Sonis S (2003) Oral mucositis: A challenging complication of radiotherapy, chemotherapy and radiochemotherapy: Part I pathogenesis and prophylaxis of mucositis. *Head and Neck* 25: 1057–70.

Seigel MA (1996) Syphilis and gonorrhoea. *Dental Clinics of North America* 40: 369–83.

Sharma N, Shamsuddin H (2011) Association between respiratory disease in hospitalized patients and periodontal disease: A cross-sectional study. *Journal of Periodontology* 10 January [Epub ahead of print].

Shelley WB, Hashim M, Shelley ED (1996) Acyclovir in the treatment of hand-foot and mouth disease. *Cutis* 57: 232–4.

Ship JA, Chavez EM, Doerr PA, et al. (2000) Recurrent aphthous stomatitis. *Quintessence International* 31: 95–112.

Silva CO, Almeida AS, Pereira AA, et al. (2007) Gingival involvement in oral paracoccidiodomycosis. *Journal of Periodontology* 78: 1229–34.

Sitheeque MA, Samaranayake LP (2003) Chronic hyperplastic candidosis/candidiasis (candidal leukoplakia). *Critical Reviews in Oral Biology and Medicine* 14: 253–67.

Slots J (2009) Oral viral infections of adults. *Periodontology 2000* 49: 60–86.

Sonis ST (2007) Pathobiology of oral mucositis: Novel insights and opportunities. *Journal of Supportive Oncology* 5: 3–11.

Steichen O, Dautheville S (2009) Koplik spots in early measles. *Canadian Medical Association Journal* 180: 583.

Swe Han KS, Bekker A, Greeff S, et al. (2009) Cryptococcus meningitis and skin lesions in an HIV negative child. *Journal of Clinical Pathology* 61: 1138–9.

Sweeney MP, Bagg J, Fell GS, et al. (1994) The relationship between micro-nutrient depletion and oral health in geriatrics. *Journal of Oral Pathology and Medicine* 23: 168–71.

Syrjanen J, Peltola J, Vatonen V, et al. (1989) Dental infections in association with cerebral infection in young and middle aged men. *Journal of Internal Medicine* 225: 179–84.

Tabachnick TT, Levine B (1975) Mucormycosis of the craniofacial structures. *Journal of Oral Surgery* 33: 464–9.

Templer SP. Rohner P, Baumgartner A (2008) Relation of *Enterococcus faecalis* and *Enterococcus faecium* isolates from foods and clinical specimens. *Journal of Food Protection* 71: 2100–4.

Thyagarajan K, Kamalam A (1982) Chronic urticaria due to abscessed teeth roots. *International Journal of Dermatology* 21: 606.

Tovaru S, Parlatescu I, Tovaru M, et al. (2009) Primary herpetic gingivostomatitis in children and adults. *Quintessence International* 40: 119–24.

Treister NS, Woo SB (2010) Topical n-docosanol for management of recurrent herpes labialis. *Expert Opinion on Pharmacotherapy* 11: 853–60.

van Griensven J, Balasegaram M, Meheus F, et al. (2010) Combination therapy for visceral leishmaniasis. *Lancet Infectious Diseases* 10: 184–94.

Van Heerden WFP (2006) Oral manifestations of viral infections. *SA Family Practice* 48: 20–4.

Wallace DV, Dykewicz MS, Bernstein DI, et al. (2008) Joint task force on practice: American academy of allergy, asthma and immunology. The diagnosis and management of rhinitis: an updated practice parameter. *Journal of Allergy and Clinical Immunology* 122: S1–84.

Wang YP, Chen HM, Kuo RC, et al. (2009) Oral verrucous hyperplasia: histologic classification, prognosis and clinical implications. *Journal of Oral Pathology and Medicine* 38: 651–6.

Weg JG (1976) Diagnostic standards of tuberculosis – revised. *Journal of the American Medical Association* 235: 1329–30.

Weinberger BW (1938) Medical problems relating to orthodontia. *American Journal of Orthodontics and Oral Surgery* 24: 213–34.

Wilson SS, Fakioglu E, Herold BC (2009) Novel approaches in fighting herpes simplex virus infections. *Expert Review of Anti-Infective Therapy* 7: 559–68.

Woo SB, Sonis ST (1996) Recurrent aphthous ulcers; a review of diagnosis and treatment. *Journal of American Dental Association* 127: 1202–13.

Wu IB, Schwartz RA (2007) Herpetic whitlow. *Cutis* 79: 193–6.

Zaric S, Bojic B, Jankovic LJ, et al. (2009) Periodontal therapy improves gastric helicobacter pylori eradication. *Journal of Dental Research* 88: 946–50.

Zhang X, Reichart PA, Song Y (2009) Oral manifestations of HIV/AIDS in china: a review. *Oral and Maxillofacial Surgery* 13: 63–8.

15

Orthodontics and Pediatric Dentistry: Two Specialties, One Goal

Elliott M Moskowitz, George J Cisneros, Mark S Hochberg

Summary

The pediatric dentist and orthodontist share many professional interests by virtue of the fact that they both are treating the same patient often on a regular and sustained basis. Furthermore, the treatment delivered by both specialties often has profound overall effects upon the function and esthetics of these young patients as they approach adulthood. Each clinician has the opportunity to support the other's therapeutic efforts; however, there appears to be a significant 'disconnect' in treatment focus and inter-specialty communication and overall interactivity. Individual patient care suffers as the potential synergistic collaboration of the pediatric dentist and orthodontist is never fully realized. The ongoing sharing of new information between both specialties is critical, as is coordination of pediatric dental and orthodontic treatment. This chapter explores some of the existing problems of communication and inter-specialty interactivity. Several commonly encountered clinical scenarios are presented to illustrate these problems as well as to suggest changes in future pediatric dental and orthodontic education, clinical practice, and ongoing assessments of respective specialty guidelines.

Introduction

The pediatric dentist is a unique dental clinician as he or she is both a primary care dental health provider and specialist. As such, the pediatric dentist has an extraordinary responsibility in treating, triaging, and coordinating dental healthcare for infants, children, and adolescents. The pediatric dentist will most likely interface with the orthodontist on a daily basis far more than any other dental clinician for the obvious reason that many pediatric dental patients will be under the care of both clinicians during the same and often extended time period. Both the orthodontist and pediatric dentist will be applying therapies to their mutual patient and in many instances, these therapeutic decisions will impact on the immediate and long-term esthetic and functional status of their patient. It is the authors' belief that new and more profoundly effective avenues of communication and interaction between the orthodontist and pediatric dentist need to be established and maintained if individual patients and the public at large are to benefit from modern orthodontic and pediatric dental care. Additionally, achieving meaningful and consequential interactivity and communication between both specialties will require a re-examination of orthodontic and pediatric dental postgraduate curricula as well as existing guidelines that have been established by each respective specialty.

Both specialties need to inculcate core information that crosses traditionally defined borders of academic and clinical interest. Some of these areas might include caries management, enamel decalcification, fluoride use, ectopic and impacted teeth, timing of orthodontic treatment, overall benefit of extraction strategies in orthodontic treatment, management of third molars, dental trauma, patient management, root resorption, and treatment options in cases of missing permanent teeth. Additionally, the pediatric dentist needs more core information on both evidence-based and evidence-'bolstered' information about a number of initial orthodontic strategies and midcourse orthodontic treatment changes that might become necessary as a result of adverse dentofacial growth and development and/or poor patient compliance. Similarly, the orthodontist should appreciate the incontrovertible value of faithful routine pediatric dental recall visits of patients undergoing active

Integrated Clinical Orthodontics, First Edition. Edited by Vinod Krishnan, Ze'ev Davidovitch.
© 2012 Blackwell Publishing Ltd. Published 2012 by Blackwell Publishing Ltd.

orthodontic treatment. Both clinicians require a new thinking of integrating 'best evidence' with clinical experience and individual patient or parental values. Finally, the orthodontist and pediatric dentist must establish mutually acceptable and practical communication protocols to ensure that any or all of these clinical insights will ultimately result in a consistently higher level of patient care for each individual patient. While it would be impossible for the authors to cover all of the aforementioned clinical situations that the orthodontist and pediatric dentist will encounter in the mixed dentition stage of dental development in one chapter, several commonly encountered clinical entities will be included in an effort to emphasize the importance of clinician interactivity between these two specialties.

Coordinating orthodontic and pediatric dental appointments in a group or solo practitioner setting

In order for the pediatric dentist and orthodontist to be optimally supportive of each other's efforts, several conditions need to be met. An understanding of the overall emphasis of comprehensive care for the pediatric dental and orthodontic patient must be appreciated by both clinicians. Most important is the development and maintenance of ongoing communication paths, so that each clinician is maximally apprised of the treatment that might already be in progress and/or will be contemplated for the immediate or long-term future. There is a growing trend all over the world for the formation of consequential ethical professional partnerships or group types of practice that include the participation of pediatric dentists and orthodontists. One would think that such a consortium or association would facilitate streamlining communication efforts between the orthodontist and pediatric dentist. However, unless such group practices develop new and unprecedented communication avenues, the net result would be no better than what is observed in other types of traditional treatment settings in which the orthodontist and pediatric dentist frequently are virtually working independently in their own milieu, unaware of each other's treatment plan and its progress.

A glaring, but rather basic example of this point is the pediatric dental recall visit schedule for patients undergoing orthodontic treatment. It is a frequent complaint of the pediatric dentist that some patients undergoing orthodontic treatment do not faithfully keep their regular pediatric dental recall appointments during the often-extended period of orthodontic treatment. The reason for this occurrence might be a misunderstanding of parents who mistakenly confuse monthly visits to the orthodontist as substitutes for semi-annual or annual visits to the pediatric dentist while their child is undergoing orthodontic treatment. The pediatric dentist might therefore be denied an opportunity

to observe important developmental changes in the dentition and beyond during orthodontic treatment. It is the authors' belief that the orthodontist should bear responsibility in assisting the pediatric dentist in ensuring that all patients are receiving regularly scheduled pediatric dental appointments during orthodontic treatment.

Figure 15.1 shows a typical orthodontic appointment schedule in a group orthodontic/pediatric dental practice. At the bottom of the page there are several columns that were derived from scheduling information supplied to the orthodontist from the pediatric dental section of the practice. The first column at the bottom of the page has a list of patients who will be seen by the orthodontist and already have pediatric dental appointments scheduled. This section is helpful in coordinating orthodontic treatment and pediatric dental treatment in the near future. For example, timely prescriptions (removal of primary or permanent teeth, oral hygiene recommendations and/or concerns, etc.) can be prepared in advance of the individual patient's pediatric dental appointment. The second column has a list of patients who will also be seen by the pediatric dentist that particular day. This information may help overall pediatric dental concerns as posterior orthodontic bands can be removed, a thorough caries check can be performed, and the bands can be replaced that very same day. Additionally, oral hygiene concerns or any unusual in-treatment findings can be discussed directly with the pediatric dentist and dental hygienist. The third column shows patients who the orthodontist will be seeing, but are overdue for their pediatric dental appointments. It is perhaps, this particular column that is most important, for it identifies patients undergoing orthodontic treatment and who are not being seen by the pediatric dentist during the course of orthodontic treatment. Identifying these potentially 'high risk patients' gives the orthodontist an opportunity to have frank conversations with the parents of these patients about the importance of regular pediatric dental appointments during the course of orthodontic treatment, and encourage them to make pediatric dental appointments while they are being seen that day for their child's orthodontic appointment. This protocol has greatly improved oral hygiene efforts and decreased the incidence of white spot lesions and any associated liability in our practice during orthodontic treatment, as the orthodontist, pediatric dentist, patient, and parent are optimally apprised of any adverse conditions during orthodontic treatment, and appropriate strategies (bolstered oral hygiene instruction, use of fluoride varnishes, etc.) can be administered on a regular and thoroughly coordinated basis.

For those solo orthodontic practitioners who might be interested in a more proactive method of encouraging their patients to keep routine pediatric dental appointments during orthodontic treatment, a similar strategy can be employed. Figure 15.2 is a chart that the orthodontist sends to the pediatric dentist along with a note that the listed

APPOINTMENT BOOK VIEW (6/10/2010)
East Side Orthodontic Dental Group

| Date: | 6/10/2010 | | | | Page: | 1 |

Wednesday, June 10, 2010

	OP 1	OP 2	OP 3	OP 4
9:00 am				
:15				
:30				
:45				
10:00 am	Clinton, Chelsea	Fields, Mrs.	Shepard, Sam	Do Not Book
:15	Marley, Bob	Fields, Sarah	Jones, Allan	Do Not Book
:30	Thomas, Dylan	VanGogh, Vincent	Marley, Marie	Do Not Book
:45	Tutu, Desmond	Monet, Claude	Lady Gaga	Whelan, Jenny
11:00 am	Jones, Sarah	Dylan, Robert	Ferguson, Sarah	Smith, Jada P.
:15	Bennett, Anthony	Tutu, Desmond	Griffin, Merv	Smith, Johnny
:30	Whelan, Cathy	Jones, Sarah	Povich, Maurie	Presley, Elvis
:45	Jones, Spike	Bennett, Anthony	Cooper, Peter	Jackson, Michael
12:00 pm	Smith, Johnny	Kahn, Genghis	Bernhardt, Sarah	Cardinale, Claudia
:15	Sing, Li	Jones, Catherine Z.	Lama, Dahli	King, Peggy
:30	Cary, Harry	Zimmerman, Bob	Buffett, Warren	Welsch, Racquel
:45	Leno, J.	Pearl, Minnie	Trump, Don	Smith, Adam
1:00 pm				
:15				
:30				
:45				
2:00 pm	Noth, Christopher	Woods, Tiger	Jennings, Whelan	Do Not Book
:15	Parker, S. J.	Smits, Jimmy	Orbach, Jerry	Do Not Book
:30	Monk, Thelonius	Smith, Johnny	Winfrey, Oprah	Martin, Dean
:45	Mariner, Silas	Foster, P.	McGhee, Bobby	Lewis, Jerry
3:00 pm	Paige, Pattie	Simmons, Jean	Jones, Tom	Crosby, Bing
:15	Rose, S.	Garbo, Greta	Jones, Star	Sirrus, Miley
:30	Combs, Sean	May, Pearlie	Latifah, Queen	Lauren, Sophia
:45	Thomas, Danny	Kadiddlehoffer, C.	Kimmel, James	Lauder, Estee
4:00 pm	Heinz, B.	Bond, James	Cooper James F.	Ono, Yoko
:15	Wall, Jon	Veneer, Fred	Zuckerberg, Mark	Yip, John
:30	Black, Jack	Diver, Pearl	Gates, Bill	Donovan, James
:45	Hanks, Thomas	Upton, Sinclair	Gates, Melinda	Crow, Russ
5:00 pm	Stein, Sally	Bundy, George	Bloomberg, Mike	Armstrong, Louis
:15	Shaw, Dinah	Whitiger, Forrest	Sandler, Adam	Phelps, Mike
:30	Streisand, B.	Harden, Marcia G.	Turner, Ted	Letterman, Dave
:45	Brecht, Berthold	Lewis, Sinclair	Seinfeld, Jerry	Christopherson, C.
6:00 pm				
:15				
:30				
:45				

Scheduled Pedo Appt
Chris Noth 6/9
J. Leno 5/5
Tom Dylan 5/28
Minnie Pearl 6/8
Bob Marley 6/10

Scheduled for Pedo Today
George Bundy 6/9
Spike Jones @ 11:45 am
Sarah Jones @ 11 am

Overdue for Pedo
Sammy Kahn 4/18
John Leeds 3/9
Ilya Kazan 5/1
Jason Bateman 4/30
Sidney Ceasar 3/30
Chris Lee 5/9

Figure 15.1 Appointment schedule of an orthodontic/pediatric dental group, which faithfully tracks the individual orthodontic patient's pediatric dental appointments during orthodontic treatment.

Dr. John Doe – Pediatric Dentist	
Mary Smith	- August 2009
Jim Cohen	- June 2009
William Burk	- Sept. 2008
Andrea Wilks	- Feb. 2008
Simon Grove	May 2009

Figure 15.2 A list of orthodontic patients (and their commencement date of active orthodontic treatment) who are also being treated by the pediatric dentist, Dr John Doe.

Dr. John Doe – Pediatric Dentist	
Mary Smith	- August 2009
Jim Cohen	- June 2009 overdue 4mos.
William Burk	- Sept. 2008
Andrea Wilks	- Feb. 2008 overdue 8mos.
Simon Grove	May 2009

Figure 15.3 The returned list indicating which patients are overdue for their pediatric dental appointments.

patients are under the care of the orthodontist, and Figure 15.3 is the returned chart with any of the patients listed who are overdue for their pediatric dental appointments. The orthodontist can now speak to the parents at their child's next orthodontic appointment and inform them that one of the requirements of quality orthodontic treatment is to ensure that patient's overall pediatric oral health needs are met during the course of orthodontic treatment. This single measure is well appreciated by the referring pediatric dentist and represents the orthodontist's 'team' participation in the overall care of the orthodontic/pediatric dental patient.

Identifying orthodontic and pediatric dental problems earlier than later

The pediatric dentist is often the first clinician to recognize malocclusions in the mixed dentition. Figure 15.4 is a chart that should assist the pediatric dentist and dental hygienist in quickly assessing any deviations from the ideal or norm and serve as a useful adjunct to the routine overall pediatric dental examination as well as an important vehicle of communication to the referred orthodontist. The orthodontist, similarly, can utilize this check-off assessment chart to further augment his or her traditional orthodontic examination and study of current orthodontic diagnostic records. The pediatric dentist should obtain a panoramic radiograph as an integral part of any initial orthodontic examination in the mixed dentition. Without the use of such a

screening image, missing, supernumerary or ectopic teeth and a number of other salient underlying deviations and/ or frank pathology will go unnoticed. Radiographs obtained by the pediatric dentist or orthodontist need to be shared so that each clinician is maximally informed at each juncture of patient assessment efforts. Routine yearly panoramic images obtained by the treating orthodontist should also be sent to the pediatric dentist. The modern age of digital or electronic capabilities make this a seamless routine for both clinicians and should be faithfully included in each other's basic communication protocols.

Figure 15.5 is a panoramic radiograph of a patient undergoing orthodontic treatment in the mixed dentition. Despite the less than average quality of this panoramic radiograph, the pediatric dentist viewing this radiograph noticed possible developmental caries in the mandibular second molars. Further specific periapical radiographs were then taken, the parents were apprised of this finding early on, and the matter was reassessed and managed after the eruption of the mandibular second molars. After confirmation of caries, the teeth were appropriately and conservatively restored (Figure 15.6). Figure 15.7 is an intraoral view of a patient, HW, in the mixed dentition, who, after examination by the pediatric dentist, was considered to have seemingly unremarkable orthodontic issues that would require later rather than earlier (i.e. orthodontic treatment in the permanent rather than mixed dentition stage) orthodontic treatment. The screening panoramic radiograph, however (Figure 15.8), suggested otherwise. The path of eruption of the canines and several other teeth was notably altered. There is considerable evidence, not only from the authors' clinical observations, but from other investigators as well, to support the supposition that the majority of observed ectopically developing maxillary canines that are predisposed to becoming frank impactions can be conservatively managed by appropriate orthodontic intervention if such treatment is commenced earlier rather than later (Leonardi et al., 2004; Baccetti et al., 2009). HW was comprehensively treated utilizing maxillary expansion, removal of the maxillary primary canines, and fixed edgewise orthodontic appliances. Figure 15.9 is an in-treatment panoramic radiographic view and Figure 15.10 is an intraoral view of the maxillary canines mid-treatment and already well positioned into the dental arch. The overall pediatric dental and orthodontic management of this patient was considerably helped by the recognition of the benefits of panoramic 'screening' radiographs obtained in the mixed dentition for pediatric dental patients.

It is the authors' belief that the pediatric dentist should serve as the most important screening clinician for orthodontic problems for children in his or her practice. The clinical examination (utilizing the aforementioned orthodontic examination checklist) during a routine pediatric dental appointment and a panoramic radiograph should be sufficient for identifying many early developing

OCCLUSAL AND FUNCTIONAL ASSESSMENT

EXTRAORAL EVALUATION

Frontal: [ ] dolichofacial [ ] mesofacial [ ] brachyfacial

[ ] symmetrical [ ] asymmetrical
[ ] skeletal [ ] functional

Profile: [ ] convex [ ] Mx prognathic [ ] Md retrognathic [ ] BiMax prognathic
[ ] straight
[ ] concave [ ] Mx retrognathic [ ] Md prognathic [ ] BiMax retrognath

Anterior display: Dental: [ ] excessive @ rest [ ] wnl [ ] minimal @ rest
Gingival: [ ] excessive @ rest [ ] wnl [ ] minimal @ rest

INTRAORAL EVALUATION

Dental Development: [ ] ahead for age [ ] WNL [ ] behind for age
[ ] aplasias [ ] ectopias [ ] supernumeraries

Occlusion: Left Molar: [ ] Class II [ ] End on [ ] Class I [ ] Class III
Right Molar: [ ] Class II [ ] End on [ ] Class I [ ] Class III
Left Canine: [ ] Class II [ ] End on [ ] Class I [ ] Class III
Right Canine: [ ] Class II [ ] End on [ ] Class I [ ] Class III

Overbite: [ ] Deep [ ] WNL [ ] Open

Overjet: [ ] Excessive [ ] WNL [ ] Negative

Transverse: [ ] Anterior X-bite [ ] Posterior X-bite
[ ] w/ shift [ ] w/o shift [ ] w/shift [ ] w/o shift
[ ] bilateral [ ] unilateral

Midlines: [ ] Mx & Md Coincident w/ face
[ ] Mx off
[ ] Md off If yes: [ ] skeletal asymm [ ] funct asymm [ ] dental asymm

Crowding: Mx: [ ] none [ ] mild [ ] moderate [ ] severe
Md: [ ] none [ ] mild [ ] moderate [ ] severe

Spacing: Mx: [ ] none [ ] mild [ ] moderate [ ] severe
Md: [ ] none [ ] mild [ ] moderate [ ] severe

Frenal concern: [ ] no [ ] yes
[ ] max [ ] mand [ ] lingual

FUNCTIONAL EVALUATION

TMJ / MPD [ ] yes [ ] no

Habits [ ] yes [ ] no

Figure 15.4 Orthodontic status assessment chart that can be incorporated into the examination protocol of a pediatric dental practice.

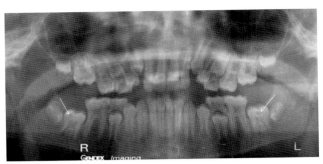

Figure 15.5 Panoramic radiograph obtained during the course of orthodontic treatment suggests developmental caries in the unerupted mandibular second molars.

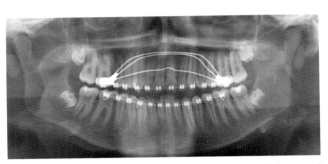

Figure 15.6 Removal of caries and restoration of the mandibular second molars.

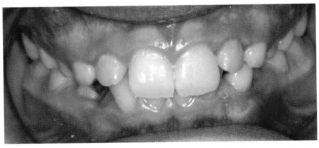

Figure 15.7 Intraoral view of a young patient (HW) undergoing a clinical examination, with what appears to be minor deviations from the expected 'norms'.

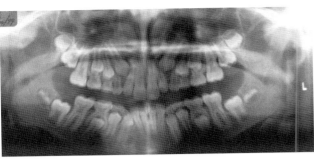

Figure 15.8 Panoramic radiograph of HW revealed altered path of eruption of canine and other teeth.

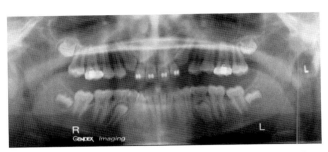

Figure 15.9 In-treatment radiograph of HW with initial orthodontic objectives of redirecting the ectopic path of eruption of the maxillary permanent canines.

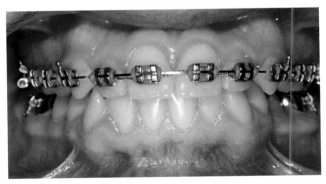

Figure 15.10 In-treatment intraoral view of the maxillary permanent canines successfully and conservatively redirected into the dental arch.

orthodontic problems. The panoramic radiograph should be considered indispensable to any clinical examination and should be obtained by the age of 7–8 years. Prompt treatment (when appropriate) and/or referral to an orthodontic colleague for an assessment of the need and timing of earlier (mixed dentition) rather than later orthodontic intervention (in the adult permanent dentition) can be more proactively managed in many instances prior to the onset of more serious and sometimes irreversible adverse developmental problems. While it is generally accepted that many malocclusions can benefit from earlier rather than later orthodontic treatment, some other clinicians think that this might not result in an overall benefit to individual patients. And while controversy in some instances might

exist with respect to both timing and specific treatment strategy, suffice to say that the early recognition of any developing orthodontic deviation can and should serve as the beginning of an important dialog between the pediatric dentist and orthodontic clinician.

Restoring form and function – revisiting the unilateral posterior crossbite with a functional mandibular shift

The unilateral posterior crossbite is a commonly observed clinical finding in the mixed dentition. Posterior crossbites in the mixed or permanent dentition represent deviations from the normal buccolingual occlusal relationships.

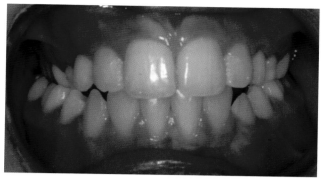

Figure 15.11 Lingual crossbite of several teeth in a patient in the mixed dentition.

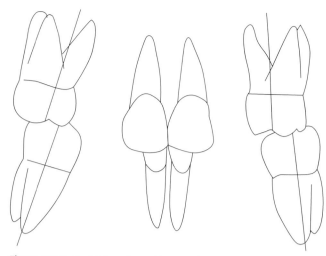

Figure 15.12 Dental lingual crossbite caused by malpositions of individual teeth. The maxillary and mandibular dental midlines are coincident.

Posterior crossbites can be caused by malpositions of individual or groups of posterior teeth (dental crossbites), malpositions of posterior teeth accompanied by a functional shift of the mandible (functional crossbites), or transverse disharmonies of the maxilla and mandible (skeletal crossbites) (Moskowitz, 2005). Posterior crossbites are frequently observed as palatal crossbites (Figure 15.11), but may occur in buccal crossbite relationship as well. There is a wide range of reported prevalence of unilateral posterior crossbites in the primary and mixed dentition – from 7% to 23% (Kutin and Hawes, 1969; Day and Foster, 1971; Infante, 1976; Kurol and Bergland, 1982; De Vis et al., 1984; Thilander et al., 1984; Heikinheimo and Salmi, 1987; Hannuksela et al., 1988). They have been reported to develop between 19 months and 5 years of age, with approximately 80% being accompanied by functional shifts of the mandible (Gottlieb et al., 2004).

Unilateral posterior crossbites with functional shifts of the mandible should be differentiated from unilateral posterior crossbites without shifts of the mandible. Figure 15.12 is a posterior dental crossbite caused by an individual tooth malposition of the maxillary left molar. Note that the maxillary and mandibular dental midlines coincide. This type of crossbite can be treated by moving the tooth (or teeth) in crossbite into normal position. However, the situation in Figure 15.13 is quite different. The observed crossbite relationship in the maximum intercuspation position appears to be identical to the dental crossbite anomaly. A closer look, however, reveals a notable disparity between the maxillary and mandibular dental midlines. The mandible has shifted (to the side of the observed crossbite) as it encountered prematurities upon closure. If we were to place the mandible in its normal transverse position (lining up the true maxillary and mandibular dental midlines), we would observe the actual transverse relationship between the maxillary and mandibular posterior teeth (Figure 15.14). It becomes apparent that both the right and left sides of the maxillary posterior segments are lingually displaced. Consequently, the functional crossbite (even though it resembles the dental posterior crossbite in the maximum

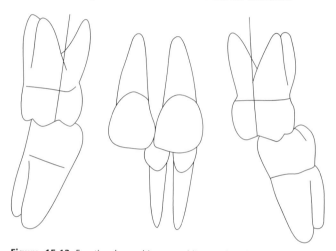

Figure 15.13 Functional crossbite resembling a dental lingual crossbite, however, the maxillary and mandibular dental midlines are not coincident. This situation represents a functional shift of the mandible on closure to the patient's left side.

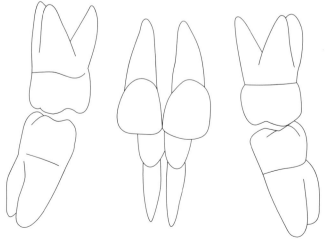

Figure 15.14 As a diagnostic aid, placing the midlines in their correct coincident positions will reveal the bilateral constriction of the maxilla and suggest the need for bilateral expansion of the maxillary dental arch.

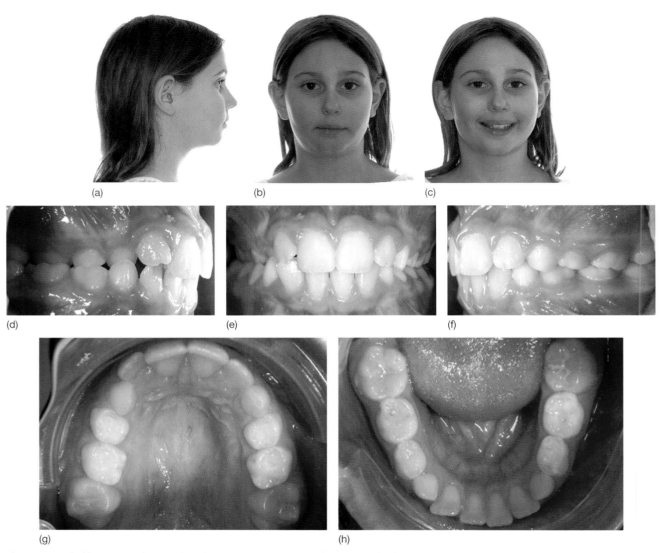

Figure 15.15 (a–h) Patient EH has a unilateral posterior crossbite with a functional shift of the mandible to the right side on closure and dental midline disharmony.

intercuspation position) is a result of a bilateral constriction or narrowness of the maxillary dental arch and, therefore, requires bilateral expansion.

The patient EH is a young female in the mixed dentition with a unilateral posterior crossbite (Figure 15.15). Note the disparity between the maxillary and mandibular dental midlines which is reflective of the mandibular shift to the right side upon closure and resultant facial asymmetry (Figure 15.16). Maxillary expansion (Hyrax palatal expander) as part of a 'Phase I' type of treatment in the mixed dentition was used to accomplish the goal of bilateral maxillary posterior expansion (Figure 15.17). Phase I treatment resulted in the normal transverse relationship of the mandible in relation to the maxilla and improvement in facial symmetry and extended approximately 12 months (Figure 15.18).

Undoubtedly, orthodontic treatment can often significantly improve both dental and facial esthetics. Quantifying functional benefits of orthodontic treatment outcomes has been a difficult task for the orthodontic specialty for specific types of orthodontic problems. The unilateral posterior crossbite with a functional shift is one opportunity, however, for the orthodontist and pediatric dentist to restore function and balance within the dentofacial complex. There is evidence that untreated unilateral posterior crossbite accompanied by transverse functional shifts of the mandible in still growing patients may result in morphological asymmetries in addition to translational disharmonies (Pinto et al., 2001). Such transverse translational and morphological disparities may further result in notable facial asymmetries as well as predispositions to temporomandibular joint-related pathology (Sonnesen et al., 2001;

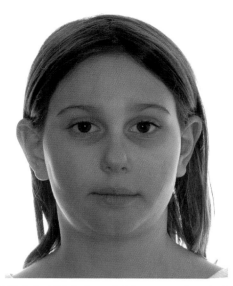

Figure 15.16 Patient EH displays a facial asymmetry from the frontal view as a result of the imposed improper position of the mandible in centric occlusion.

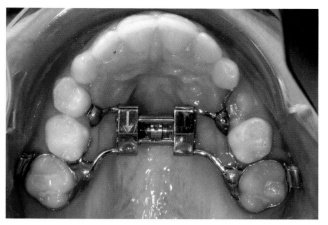

Figure 15.17 Maxillary bilateral posterior expansion achieved with a fixed palatal expanding appliance.

Moskowitz, 2003). Figure 15.19 shows an adult patient, GL, with an obvious facial asymmetry as a result of a longstanding and untreated unilateral crossbite. Figure 15.20 shows the crossbites on the left side and mandibular shift on closure to the patient's left side. Note that the maxillary and mandibular dental midlines do not coincide. This longstanding inter-dental arch occlusal condition has contributed to profound morphological differences on the left and right sides as evidenced in both the frontal facial photograph and the anteroposterior cephalometric radiograph (Figure 15.21). The distance from the condylar to antegonial areas (ramal length) is remarkably different on the two sides. Although orthodontic treatment at this juncture for this patient could improve some of the translation or positional issues associated with a deviated mandible as a result of prematurities of the occlusion, it is obvious that establishing a fully symmetrical mandible with equal ramal length would involve a coordinated orthodontic and orthognathic surgical procedure.

The earlier dentofacial orthopedic possibilities rather than those employed in later stages for patients exhibiting unilateral posterior crossbites with functional shifts might be analogous to our orthopedic medical colleagues who choose to treat scoliosis (Figure 15.22) in a growing child quite differently from patients who have already completed their growth. In the former situation, patients are treated with an orthopedic brace for the spine and in the latter situation, surgery is often performed. Pinto et al. (2001) have demonstrated that orthodontic patients exhibiting morphological differences in cases of unilateral posterior crossbite with functional shifts have a remarkable capacity to rebound to normal as a result of treatment during the active

growth years. It would be interesting and beneficial for future investigations to determine if there is an identifiable timeline threshold beyond which individual patients are incapable of such a dramatic reversal in condylar and ramal asymmetry corrections via conventional orthodontic/dentofacial treatment.

Congenitally missing maxillary lateral incisors – who does what, when, and how?

The congenitally missing lateral incisor either unilaterally or bilaterally presents a unique challenge to the orthodontic clinician in many respects. First, a decision needs to be made as to whether or not the maxillary permanent canines will be used as a substitute for the missing lateral incisors or whether the treatment plan will dictate creating adequate space for an implant and subsequent implant-supported restoration. It should be appreciated that decisions made with respect to the appropriate treatment plan for individual patients with missing maxillary lateral incisors will indeed impact on the esthetics and function of the young patient as he or she matures into and beyond the adult permanent dentition. Second, utilizing the modern implant modality requires exquisite coordination between several clinicians other than the pediatric dentist.

Figure 15.23 is representative of a typical young patient who may be referred to the orthodontist by the pediatric or general dentist. The patient has a malocclusion caused in great measure by a congenitally missing maxillary left lateral incisor, undersized maxillary right lateral incisor, and resulting shifting of the maxillary central incisors. This seemingly routine and frequently encountered type of malocclusion requires a considerable degree of treatment planning prior to orthodontic treatment, during orthodontic treatment, and following orthodontic treatment in order to provide comprehensive care consistent with modern

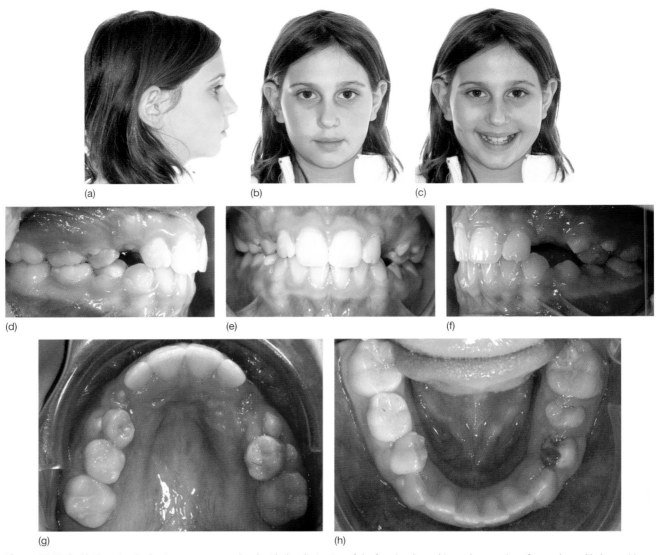

Figure 15.18 (a–h) Phase I orthodontic treatment completed with the elimination of the functional crossbite and restoration of normal mandibular position.

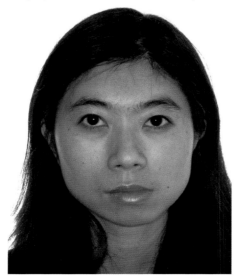

Figure 15.19 Patient GL has a significant facial asymmetry due to a long-standing and untreated unilateral crossbite with a functional shift.

orthodontic, pediatric dental, periodontal, prosthodontic and restorative requirements. The specific needs of this young patient at each juncture of their chronological and developmental age should dictate which clinician makes the appropriate decision impacting on the immediate and long-term needs of the patient. The orthodontist will need to coordinate orthodontic treatment, as some of the salient considerations beyond the usual orthodontic requirements include the precise amount of space to be left between the maxillary permanent left central incisor and permanent maxillary canine at the coronal, gingival, and apical levels, the amount of space to be created in the area of the existing undersized maxillary right lateral incisor, the selection of the most effective type of esthetic and functional retentive device, the timing of the implant placement in the area of the missing maxillary left lateral incisor, and the choice of implant and implant-supported restoration, which are all

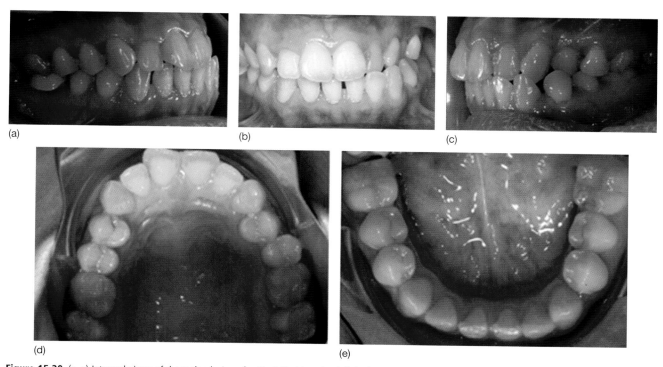

(a)

(b)

(c)

(d)

(e)

Figure 15.20 (a–e) Intraoral views of the malocclusion of patient GL. Note the definite lingual crossbite of the maxillary left canine and first premolar as well as the dental midline discrepancy.

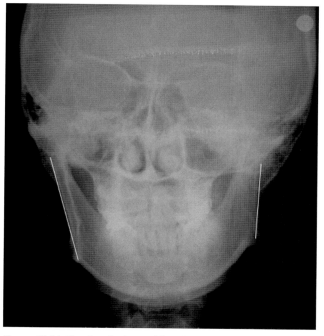

Figure 15.21 The disparity in ramal lengths in patient GL as a result of a longstanding imposed mandibular malposition during the many growth cycles of development.

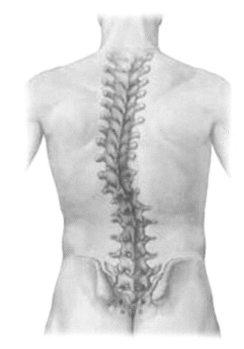

Figure 15.22 Scoliosis of the spine, representing an orthopedic developmental anomaly.

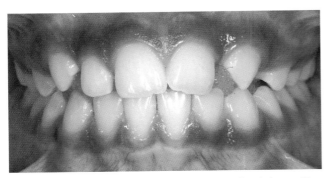

Figure 15.23 Pediatric dental patient with a congenitally missing maxillary left lateral incisor and undersized maxillary right lateral incisor, who will be undergoing orthodontic treatment.

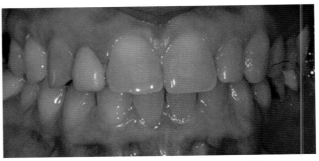

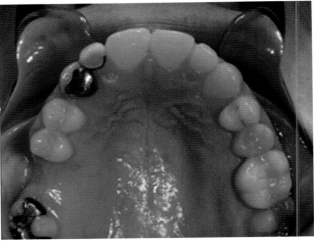

Figure 15.26 The missing maxillary right lateral incisor was replaced by a cantilever bridge due to the lack of space for a conventional implant.

Figure 15.24 Interaction between different specialties is needed when long-term treatment plans are formulated for pediatric dental patients.

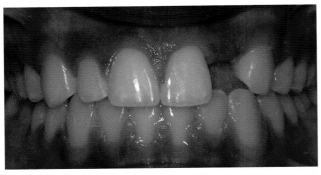

Figure 15.25 Orthodontics completed in the patient in Figure 15.23, with appropriate space created for the future implant-supported restoration.

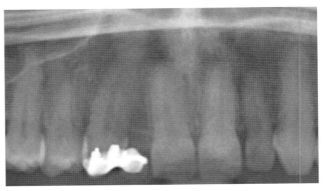

Figure 15.27 Radiograph showing the inadequate space for an appropriate implant due to the convergence of the roots of the adjacent teeth.

important details to satisfying modern caveats of esthetics, function, and stability.

Figure 15.24 depicts the interaction sequence that might follow an initial referral of a young patient with a congenital missing maxillary lateral incisor to an orthodontist and several other clinicians who might be consulted during the orthodontic treatment period. Figure 15.25 shows the same patient discussed above immediately following fixed appliance removal, and Figures 15.26 and 15.27 illustrate the consequences of the lack of such coordination. The patient

had received orthodontic treatment in which little to no consideration was given to the size of the resulting space requiring future replacement, as well as the lack of divergence of the roots of teeth adjacent to the missing maxillary right lateral incisor. A cantilever bridge intended to replace the missing maxillary right lateral incisor was deemed the only long-term solution to this clinical dilemma. As an alternative to the existing situation, further orthodontic treatment was planned to re-create the appropriate space needed, respecting the caveats of modern implant place-

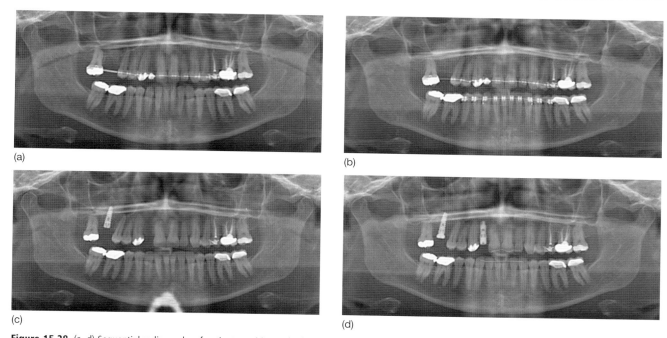

Figure 15.28 (a–d) Sequential radiographs of patient requiring orthodontic treatment to accommodate future implants.

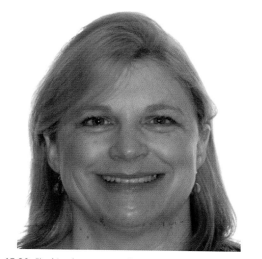

Figure 15.29 Final implant-supported restorations and veneers placed after orthodontic treatment.

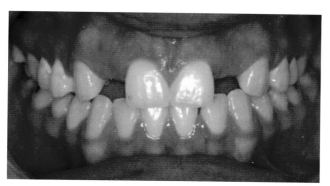

Figure 15.30 Post-orthodontic patient requiring implants to replace congenitally missing maxillary lateral incisors.

ment and implant supported restorations (Figure 15.28). The orthodontic objectives included diverging the roots of the maxillary right central incisor and maxillary right canine to accommodate an appropriate implant and implant supported restoration. The implant placement (Figure 15.28d) and final restorations (Figure 15. 29) were coordinated with the orthodontic treatment to assure that implant and prosthodontic needs were properly met. This type of coordination, once again, should have taken place during the earlier pediatric/orthodontic treatment experience of this patient, thereby avoiding orthodontic re-treatment in adulthood.

Retention considerations and beyond

The retention of the corrected malocclusions of individual patients who will be receiving implants for missing anterior teeth needs to be coordinated as well. Patients receiving implants immediately following orthodontic treatment, such as the patient depicted in Figure 15.30 might fare well with either a conventional Hawley type of retainer (Figure 15.31) or a typical 'flipper' type of removable appliance which provides for the maintenance of beneficial tooth movements achieved during orthodontic treatment, pontic replacement of the missing maxillary lateral incisors, and some function. However, removable appliances with traditional labial bows are not esthetic and present long-term issues such as interference with settling of the occlusion and tissue irritation (Figure 15.32), hygienic issues, and, when used, simple 'flipper' types cannot prevent the reconvergence of the adjacent roots in the implant site. Short-term esthetic retention alternatives include the use of thermoplastic (Essix-type) removable devices with a pontic replacement in the area of the missing teeth (Figure 15.33). Long-term retention in post-orthodontic patients who will not be receiving implants until clinicians are reasonably assured of the cessation of any significant dentofacial growth, however, requires a more sophisticated type of retentive device.

The patient ID (Figure 15.34) underwent orthodontic treatment for a malocclusion complicated by the absence of the maxillary right lateral incisor and peg-shaped maxillary left lateral incisor. Figure 15.35 shows the completed treatment with appropriate space left for the implant and subsequent implant-supported restoration as well as needed space for the peg-shaped maxillary left lateral incisor restoration. However, this patient will not be receiving an implant for approximately 2–3 years. Once again, the orthodontist and pediatric dentist need to interact on behalf of this patient so that the most appropriate retentive device can be planned. Such interaction might very well ultimately direct this patient to a general dentist or prosthodontist who is capable of fabricating a bonded resin type of bridge. A bonded resin bridge was used to replace the maxillary right lateral incisor with some esthetic bonding with composite of the maxillary left peg shaped lateral incisor (Figure 15.36). This type of more sophisticated prosthesis/retainer will serve this patient well until an implanted supported restoration can be placed for the missing maxillary right lateral incisor and a veneer is placed on the maxillary left lateral incisor. As can be appreciated, these seemingly 'routine' types of cases indeed require a considerable degree of coordination and interactivity among the orthodontist, referring pediatric dentist, and several other specialists.

Enamel demineralization during orthodontic treatment – who takes responsibility for prevention?

Orthodontic treatment with fixed appliances offers many distinct advantages to the patient and orthodontic clinician.

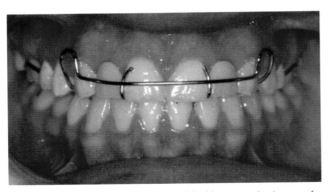

Figure 15.31 Removable retainer with a labial bow to maintain space for future implants in the maxillary lateral incisor area.

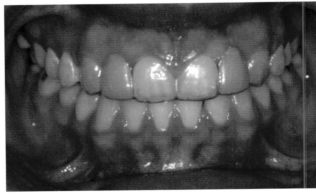

Figure 15.33 Essix-type thermoplastic retainers are excellent short-term retentive devices for patients missing maxillary lateral incisors.

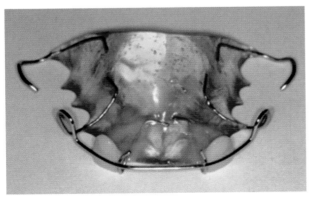

Figure 15.32 Long-term removable appliance wear for post-orthodontic/preimplant patients pose hygienic issues as well potential areas of palatal tissue irritations.

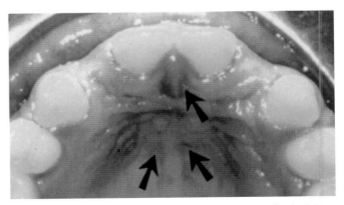

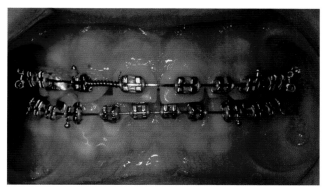

Figure 15.34 Patient ID: appropriate space being created for an implant-supported restoration of the maxillary right lateral incisor and a veneer for the peg-shaped maxillary left lateral incisor.

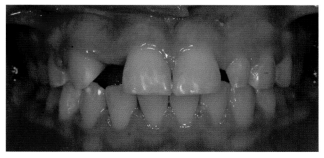

Figure 15.35 Patient ID, post-orthodontic treatment, requiring planning for an appropriate retainer prior to implant placement.

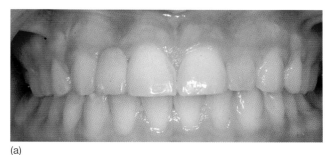

(a)

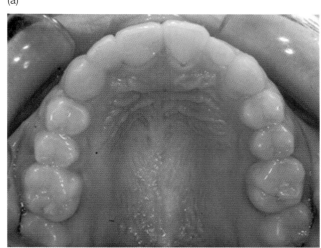

(b)

Figure 15.36 (a,b) The bonded resin bridge replacing the maxillary right lateral incisor and bonded composite resin restoration on the maxillary left lateral incisor will serve as excellent long-term (2–3 years) transitional retentive devices until the patient is ready for an implant and veneer.

These advantages include a broad capability in the management of inter- and intra-arch tooth movements during orthodontic treatment. Regrettably, however, one disadvantage is that fixed orthodontic appliances can present significant oral hygiene challenges to the young orthodontic patient. Consequently, increased plaque retention around orthodontic brackets can contribute to enamel demineralization, resulting in unsightly white spot lesions with or without cavitation. Figure 15.37 depicts a teenage patient with notably poor oral hygiene during orthodontic treatment and resulting enamel demineralization with both noncavitated and cavitated white spot lesions. The patient had missed his monthly orthodontic visits for 6 months and failed to keep his regular pediatric dental examination appointments. Such adverse occurrences seriously question any perceived benefit (esthetic or otherwise) of the orthodontic service itself. Clinician-prescribed fluoride rinses and gels, although remarkably effective for orthodontic patients with scrupulous oral hygiene, are predictably ineffective for patients who demonstrate poor oral hygiene compliance.

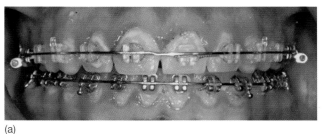

(a)

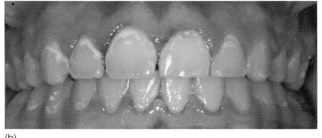

(b)

Figures 15.37 (a,b) A teenage patient with notably poor oral hygiene during orthodontic treatment and resulting enamel demineralization with both non-cavitated and cavitated white spot lesions.

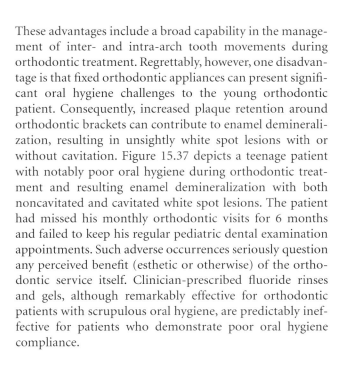

Geiger et al. (1988, 1992) found poor compliance with a preventive fluoride rinse program occurred in 50% of the patients. Along with other orthodontic and pediatric dental colleagues, the authors have utilized fluoride varnishes for patients undergoing active orthodontic treatment with fixed orthodontic appliances in an effort to either completely prevent or at least minimize the occurrence of white spot lesions during orthodontic treatment. Duraflor (Pharmascience Inc., Montreal, Canada) is a fluoride varnish that contains 5% sodium fluoride by weight in a natural colophony base. An *ex vivo* study by Todd et al. (1999) as well as a recent *in vivo* investigation by Farhadian et al. (2008) have reported a measureable benefit of fluoride varnish to significantly minimize white spot lesions in the orthodontic population with fixed orthodontic appliances. Coordinating the use of these new varnishes between the pediatric dentist and orthodontist remains a notable challenge to attain the maximum benefit and avoid any possible overdosing of fluoride. This is yet another example of the need for a smooth and continual interaction between the pediatric dentist and orthodontist so that therapeutic compounds can be judiciously prescribed at optimal efficacy levels. Our orthodontic group has been using such varnishes at 3-monthly intervals and this protocol needs to be transmitted to the pediatric dentist to avoid unnecessary overlapping and duplication of effort.

While the pediatric dentistry specialty has vast experience with fluoride compounds and their uses, this area is relatively new to the orthodontic specialty. In the absence of acceptable bond strength associated with fluoride-releasing orthodontic bonding resins, orthodontists should consider routinely incorporating fluoride varnishes in their clinical protocols. Finally, both the orthodontist and pediatric dentist need to take responsibility for recognizing orthodontic patients at risk for developing white spot lesions and take appropriate and coordinated proactive measures to minimize such occurrences.

Conclusions

We conclude this chapter by revisiting our original intention – that is, to emphasize the profound need for a greater interactivity and communication between the orthodontist and pediatric dentist in order to optimize the treatment of individual patients. Each specialist must be educated to appreciate the goals and objectives of each other, and when necessary, be prepared to call on the expertise of other medical and dental specialists, as required for the specific needs of each individual patient. We recommend a reassessment of respective postgraduate curricula, re-examination of each specialty's clinical 'guidelines', and increased effort of each specialty association to encourage ongoing interdisciplinary forums, so that orthodontists and pediatric dentists will continue to travel along parallel and intersecting paths together in harmony with the singular purpose of providing the most modern, evidence-based, and practically high-quality oral healthcare to our mutual patients.

References

Baccetti T, Mucedero M, Leonardi M, et al. (2009) Interceptive treatment of palatal impaction of maxillary canines with rapid palatal expansion: a randomized clinical trial. *American Journal of Orthodontics and Dentofacial Orthopedics* 136: 657–61.

Day AJ, Foster TD (1971) An investigation into the prevalence of molar crossbite and some associated etiological conditions. *Dental Practice* 21: 402–10.

De Vis H, de Boever JA, van Cauwenberge P (1984) Epidemiologic survey of functional conditions of the masticatory system in Belgium children aged 3–6 years. *Community Dentistry Oral Epidemiology* 12: 203–7.

Farhadian N, Miresmaeili A, Eslami B, et al. (2008) Effect of fluoride varnish on enamel demineralization around brackets: An in-vivo study. *American Journal of Orthodontics and Dentofacial Orthopedics* 133: S95–8.

Geiger AM, Gorelick L, Gwinnett AJ, et al. (1988) The effect of a fluoride program on white spot formation during orthodontic treatment. *American Journal of Orthodontics and Dentofacial Orthopedics* 93: 929–38.

Geiger AM, Gorelick L, Gwinnett AJ, et al. (1992) Reducing white spot lesions in orthodontic populations with fluoride rinsing. *American Journal of Orthodontics and Dentofacial Orthopedics* 101: 403–7.

Gottlieb E, Cozzani M, de Harfin JF, et al. (2006) JCO roundtable, stability of orthodontic treatment, Part 2. *Journal of Clinical Orthodontics* 40(2): 83–94.

Hannuksela A, Laurin A, Lehmus V, et al. (1988) Treatment of crossbite in early mixed dentition. *Proceedings of Finnish Dental Society* 84: 175–82.

Heikinheimo K, Salmi K (1987) Need for orthodontic intervention in five-year-old Finnish children. *Proceedings of Finnish Dental Society* 83: 165–9.

Infante PF (1976) An epidemiologic study of finger habits in preschool children as related to malocclusion, socioeconomic status, race, sex, and size of community. *Journal of Dentistry for Children* 1: 33–8.

Kurol J, Bergland L (1982) Longitudinal study and cost-benefit analysis of the effect of early treatment of posterior crossbites in the primary dentition. *European Journal of Orthodontics* 14: 173–9.

Kutin G, Hawes RR (1969) Posterior crossbites in the deciduous and mixed dentition. *American Journal of Orthodontics* 56: 491–504.

Leonardi M, Armi P, Franchi L, et al. (2004) Two interceptive approaches to palatally displaced canine: a prospective longitudinal study. *Angle Orthodontist* 74: 581–6.

Moskowitz E (2003) Orthodontics in the progressive dental practice. In: R Edwab (ed.) *Essential Dental Handbook.* Tulsa, OK: PennWell Corp, pp. 387–430.

Moskowitz E (2005) The unilateral posterior functional crossbite, an opportunity to restore form and function. *New York State Dental Journal* Aug/Sept: 36–9.

Pinto AS, Buschang PH, Throckmorton GS, et al. (2001) Morphological and positional asymmetries of young children with functional unilateral posterior crossbite. *American Journal of Orthodontics and Dentofacial Orthopedics* 20: 513–20.

Sonnesen L, Bakke M, Solow B (2001) Bite force in pre-orthodontic children and unilateral crossbite. *European Journal of Orthodontics* 23: 741–9.

Thilander B, Wahlund S, Lennartsson B (1984) The effect of early interceptive treatment in children with posterior posterior crossbite. *European Journal of Orthodontics* 6: 25–34.

Todd M, Staley R, Kanellis M, et al. (1999) Effect of a fluoride varnish on demineralization adjacent to orthodontic brackets. *American Journal of Orthodontics and Dentofacial Orthopedics* 116: 159–67.

16

Dental Caries, Tooth Fracture and Exposed Dental Pulp: The Role of Endodontics in Orthodontic Treatment Planning and Mechanotherapy

Neslihan Arhun, Ayca Arman-Ozcirpici, Mete Ungor, Omur Polat Ozsoy

Primum non nocere

> Hipoccrates (c.460 to c.377 BC)

Summary

For the past 15–20 years, social scientists and observers of contemporary life have been commenting on the dramatic change in the way business is done in both the public and private sectors. The change that has attracted so much attention and commentary is a significant increase in teamwork and collaborative efforts: *people with different views and perspectives are coming together, putting aside their narrow self-interests, and discussing issues openly and supportively in an attempt to solve a larger problem or achieve a broader goal.* Teams come together for a number of different reasons, but their goals are the same – to achieve peak performance and experience success. We as dental specialists share the same goal. We want to have happy and satisfied patients with acceptable, even better, facial and dental esthetics with healthy, functional, and stable occlusions. In a beauty-addicted society where a good smile is a powerful weapon, the demand for orthodontic treatment is increasingly rising, and in challenging situations, input from a number of dental disciplines is required to construct detailed treatment plans.

This chapter comprises a comprehensive review of topics requiring interactive cooperation or teamwork between the orthodontist, endodontist, and/or conservative dentistry specialist. Topics such as enamel demineralization around orthodontic attachments, pulpal reactions, root resorption or invasive cervical resorption due to orthodontic treatment, and special considerations about dental trauma will be discussed in detail.

Introduction

An increased desire towards improved facial esthetics and dental appearance is the key motivating factor for orthodontic treatment in every population. These appearance-conscious patients and/or their families request esthetic treatment plans that usually require a comprehensive interactive approach. Coordinated orthodontic, endodontic, and restorative treatments, with careful consideration of patients' and their families' expectations and requests are critical for successful outcomes and patient satisfaction (Vitale et al., 2004). Clearly, it is the orthodontist's responsibility to take a proactive role in forming close cooperation between the disciplines to reach the ultimate goal of achieving healthy esthetics and function, while at the same time limiting undesirable consequences and risks of mechanotherapeutics.

Optimized treatment outcomes necessitate close collaboration between the disciplines to evaluate, diagnose and resolve problems at the following stages of the treatment life cycle:

- Pretreatment evaluation and the early stages of the orthodontic treatment
- Orthodontic treatment
- Emergency orthodontic treatment in trauma cases
- Immediate post-orthodontic period and during orthodontic retention.

Integrated Clinical Orthodontics, First Edition. Edited by Vinod Krishnan, Ze'ev Davidovitch.
© 2012 Blackwell Publishing Ltd. Published 2012 by Blackwell Publishing Ltd.

This chapter reviews and summarizes the need and benefit of interactions between orthodontists, endodontists, and/or conservative dentistry specialists according to the stages of orthodontic treatment mentioned above.

Pretreatment evaluation and early orthodontic treatment

Successful orthodontic therapy relies on the accurate assessment of the pretreatment dental and gingival health status with the aid of other dental disciplines. The assessment should include a determination of systemic and/or local factors, and obtaining a detailed history of previous trauma to the oral tissues. The initial clinical examination should precede basic radiographic evaluation, which will help the clinician to decide on precautions to minimize the undesirable effects of orthodontic mechanics. It should not be forgotten that every patient is unique, and demands and merits a unique treatment plan customized for his/her specific needs.

Endodontically treated teeth

The decision of whether or not to extract tooth/teeth is an important step in designing concrete orthodontic treatment procedures. If the orthodontist judges a case as one requiring extraction, the next step will be the decision regarding which tooth/teeth to extract (Yagi et al., 2009). There may be multiple options and choosing one of the potential teeth requires consideration of parameters that might require a consultation with specialists from other disciplines. For example, a history of root canal treatment or the presence of periapical lesions, restorations, and carious teeth complicates the decision about the site of extraction. In such cases, the decision should be the one that optimizes the orthodontic treatment prognosis with less invasive operative intervention.

Successful root canal treatment relies on adequate removal of microorganisms and prevention of re-colonization or re-infection through the placement of a root canal filling that obliterates the canal space and a restoration with good coronal seal (Briggs and Scott, 1997). The benefits of root canal treatment are: retention of the natural tooth in the dental arch and facilitation of the restoration to conserve the remaining crown and root structures, preservation of the alveolar bone and accompanying papillae, and maintenance of pressure and tension perception by paradental mechanoreceptors. However, such a retained tooth may be at risk of a future root fracture and development of caries or periodontal disease after orthodontic treatment (Torabinejad et al., 2007). Epidemiological radiographic surveys have revealed a relatively low frequency of high-quality root canal fillings, ranging from 14% to 65% (Eriksen et al., 2002).

Endodontic outcomes are difficult to predict since non-endodontic factors such as the quality of the subsequent restoration and the remaining tooth structure contribute to the true prognosis. Whenever the decision has to be made about whether to perform endodontic treatment or to extract a tooth, orthodontists should consult with endodontists taking into account pre-, intra-, and postoperative factors, such as the patient's age, socioeconomic class, vital or necrotic pulp, and presence of periapical infections (Travassos et al., 2003). It is important to realize that the presence of periapical lesions, increased age, and the presence of irregular canal anatomies especially in molars may compromise the endodontic outcome. Moreover, procedural errors during canal instrumentation, rinsing with irrigation solutions, and medicaments and fillings may play a crucial role in long-term prognosis. These factors should be evaluated based on good clinical judgment along with input from endodontists, so that the patient is provided with an optimized treatment plan, which is at the same time cost-effective.

Endodontically treated teeth can be moved orthodontically as readily as teeth with vital pulps. If teeth require root canal treatment during orthodontic movement, it is recommended that the root canals be cleaned, shaped, and an interim dressing of calcium hydroxide be placed. Canal obturation is accomplished after orthodontic treatment (Hamilton and Gutmann, 1999). If orthodontic treatment might take too long to finish, a gutta-percha filling should be placed in-treatment, because the calcium hydroxide filling may make the tooth prone to fracture during this period.

Cariogenic potential and white spot lesions

After the decision about the final treatment plan, before the full bond-up appointment, the clinician should take measures against cariogenic challenge. Dental caries in the enamel is unique among other infective diseases in the human body, as enamel is both acellular and avascular; thus enamel cannot heal itself by a cellular repair mechanism (Zero, 1999). In orthodontic patients, caries starts as decalcification areas adjacent to fixed orthodontic appliances. Earlier studies demonstrated increased cariogenic risk associated with a rapid increase in the volume of dental plaque, which has a lower pH and significantly elevated levels of acidogenic bacteria such as *Streptococcus mutans* around orthodontic attachments than in nonorthodontic patients (Chatterjee and Kleinberg, 1979; Gwinnett and Ceen, 1979). These acidogenic bacteria produce byproducts of organic acids in the presence of fermentable carbohydrates, further lowering the pH of the plaque. As the pH drops below the threshold for remineralization (pH = 4.5), enamel demineralization/decalcification occurs. The first clinical evidence of this demineralization is visualized as a white spot lesion (WSL), which has been defined as 'sub-surface enamel porosity from carious demineralization' that represents itself as 'a milky white opacity' caused by the changes in enamel translucency and light scattering (Bishara and Ostby, 2008).

WSLs are clinically induced in less than 4 weeks (Ogaard et al., 1988), and their prevalence is reported to vary from 4.9% (Gorelick et al., 1982) to 84% (Mizrahi, 1982) of tooth surfaces. More than 50% of subjects may experience an increase in the number of WSLs with fixed orthodontic appliance therapy (Artun and Brobakken, 1986). Boersma et al. (2005) observed that 97% of all their subjects and on average 30% of the buccal surfaces in a person were affected. Again, on average, 40% of the surfaces in males and 22% in females showed white spot lesions. Briefly, any tooth in the mouth can be affected, with the common ones being the maxillary lateral incisors, maxillary canines, and mandibular premolars. Diagnosis, prevention, and treatment of WSLs are all crucial to prevent tooth decay as well as to minimize the tooth discoloration that could compromise the smile esthetics.

The acquired biofilm (the pellicle) in the intact enamel surface participates in dynamic physico-chemical equilibrium with the oral fluids (Zero, 1999; Ten Cate and van Loveren, 1999). When the pH of the oral fluids goes below the physiological norm, calcium and phosphate ions diffuse from the hydroxyapatite mineral in the enamel to the pellicle and into the oral cavity (demineralization). When the pH of the oral fluids rises to the norm, the calcium and phosphate ions in the supersaturated saliva are transmitted through the pellicle into the enamel following the laws of chemical equilibrium (remineralization). Within this cycle, destructive demineralization and restorative remineralization occur either simultaneously or alternately. If this cycle is not prevented and demineralization predominates, WSLs will be the result and once established, it is extremely difficult, or sometimes impossible, to achieve complete remineralization.

The most important prophylactic measure against WSLs is implementation of a good dietary and oral hygiene regimen along with proper tooth brushing with a fluoridated dentifrice. The remineralization process is greatly enhanced by the low levels of fluoride in the saliva and plaque (Ten Cate and van Loveren, 1999). According to Lima et al. (2008), by controlling biofilm accumulation with a fluoride-containing dentifrice, the lesions can not only be arrested but also be partially repaired. Dentifrices typically contain sodium fluoride, monofluorophosphate, stannous fluoride, amine fluoride, or a combination of these compounds, but the maximum concentration allowed in the European community is 0.15%. Ogaard et al. (2004) demonstrated a dose–response effect and a fluoride concentration above 0.1% in dentifrices is recommended for orthodontic patients, because of their increased risk of WSLs.

Stannous fluoride, which interferes with the adsorption of plaque bacteria to the enamel surface, offers beneficial effects not only against caries but also against plaque-induced gingival diseases during orthodontic treatment (Ogaard et al., 1980; Boyd and Chun, 1994). Tin atoms in stannous products block the passage of sucrose into bacterial cells, inhibiting acid production. Ogaard et al. (2006) demonstrated an inhibiting effect of a combined stannous fluoride/amine fluoride toothpaste/mouth rinse against both decalcification and gingival bleeding in a prospective, randomized clinical study. Titanium tetrafluoride solutions through formation of the retentive, titanium-rich, glaze-like surface coating on treated enamel surfaces inhibit caries lesion development in patients wearing fixed appliances. At a low pH, titanium binds with an oxygen atom of a phosphate group to form Ti-O-Ti-O-chains on the tooth surface and this covalently bound titanium covers the tooth surface by formation of a strong complex. This surface coating resists cariogenic challenges even under extreme alkaline and acidic conditions (Büyükyılmaz et al., 1994).

The effect of fluoride is limited when the pH level drops to lower than the solubility product of pure fluoroapatite (pH = 4.5). When this pH is exceeded, the liquid phase of the plaque will be undersaturated with hydroxyapatite and fluoroapatite making remineralization no longer possible (Larsen, 1990). A dose response to fluoride may not be apparent in this stage and more fluoride may not produce a better clinical effect (Ogaard, 2001). Briefly, if the patient is noncompliant with the implemented hygiene and dietary precautions, the use of a fluoridated dentifrice alone may not be effective in preventing the development of WSLs (O'Reilly and Featherstone, 1987). Supplemental professional sources of fluoride and other antimicrobial agents in the forms of varnishes, solutions or gels are often recommended. Fluoridated mouth rinses containing 0.05% sodium fluoride used daily have been shown to significantly reduce lesion formation beneath bands. These mouth rinses may be combined with antimicrobial agents such as chlorhexidine (CHX), octenidine dihydrochloride, benzydamine, triclosan, or zinc to improve their cariostatic effect (Kocak et al., 2009). CHX varnishes for long-term use have been introduced (Ogaard et al., 2001) but are not recommended because of the metallic taste and frequent discoloration it causes to the teeth and tongue.

An in-office application of a high concentration of fluoride in the form of a varnish or sealant may be beneficial in noncompliant patients. This exposure to fluoride is limited to office-only application, because of the temporary discoloration of the teeth and the gingival tissues, and, at the same time, increasing expense to the patient and/or chair-time to the clinician (Bishara and Ostby, 2008). With topical fluoride application, a calcium-fluoride like material (CaF_2) builds up in plaque, on the tooth surface (enamel/dentin), or in incipient carious lesions, which acts as a reservoir for fluoride release when the pH is lowered (Ogaard, 1990). Vivaldi-Rodrigues et al. (2006) found that the application of the fluoride varnish resulted in a 44.3% reduction in enamel demineralization in orthodontic patients. The Cochrane systematic reviews have not been able to reach a consensus on any topical preparation or schedule that would provide the greatest benefit for preventing enamel demineralization (Benson et al., 2004; Derks et al., 2004; Chadwick et al., 2005). In fact, Benson and co-workers recommended daily fluoride mouth rinsing (0.05% NaF) similar to Zachrisson more than 30 years ago (Benson et al., 2004).

Glass ionomer cements (GICs) and resin-modified glass ionomer (RMGI) cements were introduced as orthodontic bonding adhesives to take advantage of some of their sustained fluoride release capabilities (Swift, 1989; McCourt et al., 1990) but their bond strength was found to be equivocal while the concentration of fluoride released decreased with time (Miguel et al., 1995; Miller et al., 1996; Bishara et al., 2007). Nowadays, bioactive adhesive systems with antibacterial effects or intensive remineralization ability are considered to be beneficial. Recently, a fluoride-releasing antibacterial adhesive system has been developed that combines the physical advantages of dental adhesive technology with antibacterial effects. MDPB (12-methacryloyloxydodecyl-pyridinium bromide) is potentially applicable with various restorative materials since it allows immobilization of the antibacterial component by polymerization, halts the deterioration in the mechanical properties of cured resins, and improves inhibitory effects against bacterial growth on their surfaces (Imazato, 2009). The use of argon laser for curing composite resins used for orthodontic attachments has been tried as it saves time and alters the enamel structure, rendering it less susceptible to demineralization. Combining laser irradiation with fluoride treatment can have a synergistic effect on acid resistance, thus preventing formation of WSLs (Hicks et al., 1995).

Interactive collaboration during orthodontic treatment

Orthodontic treatment will succeed when its advantages outweigh any adverse sequelae. To prevent, minimize, and manage iatrogenic effects of orthodontic mechanics, the clinician should examine both the hard and soft oral tissues that may be affected by the orthodontic treatment (Shaw et al., 1991).

Cariogenic challenge

WSL development is a very rapid process and may be apparent within 4 weeks after orthodontic bond-up appointment (Ogaard et al., 1988). Excess of bonding material around the attachment base may exacerbate the problem by creating retentive areas where the acidogenic bacteria can adhere and cause demineralization. Complicated appliance designs with loops, auxiliary archwires, springs, coils, and some Class II correctors create non-cleanable areas even in highly motivated patients. In most cases, the lesions are small and restricted to forming narrow white bands around the bracket bases or in the areas between the brackets and the gingival margin (Ogaard, 2008). The demineralized enamel is porous and absorbs stain from daily diet, representing esthetic challenges on the labial surfaces of the affected tooth. In some patients, who are noncompliant with oral hygiene and fluoride regimens, lesion development may be extensive and require premature debonding.

Tooth-conserving and time-saving adhesive methods of retaining orthodontic attachments are replacing traditional methods and procedures. However, despite these advances, caries risk under and in the vicinity of the multibonded appliances is of concern (Ogaard, 1989). Microleakage, an important post-restorative complication, is defined as the seeping and leaking of fluids and bacteria in the tooth–restoration interface (Gladwin and Bagby, 2004). The concept of microleakage has been underestimated by the orthodontists. Formation of WSL at and under the adhesive–enamel interface is often due to microleakage that may be of clinical importance (Arhun et al., 2006b; Arıkan et al., 2006). Expansion and contraction occur when the teeth are subjected to temperature changes by the ingestion of hot or cold foods. The linear thermal coefficients of expansion of enamel and ceramic or metal brackets and the adhesive systems do not match closely. Metal brackets repeatedly contract and expand more than ceramic brackets, enamel, or the adhesive systems, producing microgaps between the bracket and the adhesive system, resulting in leakage of oral fluids and bacteria beneath the brackets. However, if microleakage cannot be prevented, inactivation of bacteria will be a direct strategy to prevent development of WSLs. Antimicrobial adhesive systems may be beneficial in such situations, ensuring antimicrobial effect at the site of therapeutic importance, which is the enamel surface under the bracket in this circumstance (Arhun et al., 2006b).

Pulpal reactions to orthodontic forces

The dental pulp is a specialized type of loose connective tissue, rich in cells such as odontoblasts, fibroblasts, and cells of the immune, nervous, and vascular systems (Leone et al., 2009). While performing complex functions such as having a nervous and vascular supply for vitality, carrying sensory impulses and formation of protective secondary dentin, it is responsive to peripheral impacts, such as orthodontic forces. Morphological and structural changes occur in dental pulps subjected to such forces (Anstendig and Kronman, 1972; Delivanis and Gauer, 1980; Popp et al., 1992; Kayhan et al., 2000). Although reports on these changes present conflicting data, most show degenerative changes that may have harmful effects on tooth vitality.

Circulatory disturbances, vascular compression, and formation of secondary dentin after orthodontic force application have been reported (Stenvik and Mjör, 1970; Anstendig and Kronman, 1972). Radiorespirometric techniques, which measure the tissue respiration rate, indicated depression of the oxygen utilization system within the pulp cells after the application of orthodontic forces (Hamersky et al., 1980; Unsterseher et al., 1987). An average of 27% reduction in pulpal respiration has been seen after 3 days of orthodontic force application (Unsterseher et al., 1987) and this might compromise the long-term vitality of the tooth (Popp et al., 1992). Hypoxia in pulp cells due to reduced blood flow may negatively enhance mitochondrial function and proliferative activity (Amemiya et al., 2003). Significant elevation of aspartate aminotransferase (AST) activity, an enzyme that is released into the extracellular environment following cell death, has been demonstrated after 1 week of intrusive force application (Veberiene et al., 2009). Likewise, Perinetti et al. (2004) observed elevated AST activity in orthodontically treated teeth and found these levels comparable to reversible pulpitis. It has been hypothesized that increased AST levels could be the result of circular disruption, reduction in oxygen levels, and pulp tissue apoptosis. Furthermore, an increased response to electrical pulp testing was seen, which is positively correlated to anatomical features such as pulpal weight and root surface area (Veberiene et al., 2009).

Several authors have detected formation of calcified deposits in the dental pulps of teeth undergoing orthodontic treatment (Stenvik and Mjör, 1970; Delivanis and Gauer, 1980; Popp et al., 1992). However, Stenvik and Mjör (1970) concluded that these changes were not different from those in untreated teeth. Loss of tooth vitality during orthodontic treatment has also been reported, especially in previously traumatized teeth. Histologically, cell death can be seen as either cellular necrosis and/or apoptosis. Even though previous studies named the changes in teeth undergoing orthodontic treatment as necrosis, the term apoptosis is more suitable for nontraumatized teeth. Rana et al. (2001) investigated apoptotic changes with orthodontic mechanics in detail and could observe maximum rate after 3 days of force application.

Several other factors are also involved in pulpal reactions to orthodontic force, the main one being the type of tooth movement. Intrusion, the movement that has the greatest impact on the root apex, is capable of occluding the pulpal blood supply (Vandevska-Radunovic et al., 1994; Sano et al., 2002). Moreover, Kvinnsland et al. (1989) and Nixon et al. (1993) reported a substantial increase in pulpal blood flow and in the number of capillaries after application of extrusive orthodontic forces. Mostafa et al. (1991) observed vacuolization and severe odontoblastic degeneration in dental pulps undergoing orthodontic extrusion for 7 days. McDonald and Pitt Ford (1994) found decreased human blood flow after continuous light tipping forces, using laser Doppler flowmetry. Since orthodontic treatment involves complex three-dimensional tooth movements, it is not always possible to avoid movements that are relatively more detrimental.

Since the first rule of orthodontic mechanics is to avoid poorly controlled and jiggling forces (Krishnan and Davidovitch, 2009), the magnitude of the applied force is another important factor. Controlled intraoral orthodontic mechanics do not require heavy forces for tooth movement, but orthopedic treatment requiring forces over 500 g may have deleterious effects on the dental pulp. In a histological study, Küçükkeleş and Okar (1994) reported degeneration of vessel walls in teeth undergoing rapid palatal expansion treatment. However, contrary to the results of previous studies, a histomorphometric evaluation by Kayhan et al. (2000) has shown no pulpal differences between control teeth and teeth undergoing RPE.

The degree of pulpal reaction to orthodontic forces also depends on individual factors such as the age of the patient and the size of the apical foramen (Butcher and Taylor, 1951; Stenvik and Mjör, 1970). Hamersky et al. (1980) reported positive correlations between age and the rate of tissue respiratory depression. Therefore, the maturity of a tooth is an important aspect in preserving tooth vitality during orthodontic treatment and clinicians should be cautious while moving teeth with closed apices.

As pulpal tissue is susceptible to thermal stress, temperature generating orthodontic procedures such as stripping, thermal debonding, and residual adhesive removal after debonding requires extra attention. The heat generated during rotary instrumentation may result in irreversible trauma to the pulp. Among the different modalities used for instrumentation, such as handheld stripper, rotary disks and air-rotor stripping that utilizes diamond burs, the handheld stripper, which does not need any rotary instrument, has been found to be the safest method (Baysal et al., 2007). Thermal debonding using carbon dioxide laser (Ma et al., 1997) is considered safest for debonding orthodontic brackets. Clean-up of residual resin using high-speed handpieces may cause vascular injuries and pulp necrosis. Zach and Cohen (1965) stated that a temperature rise of more than 5.5°C will result in pulpal inflammation and an increase of 11°C resulted in necrosis. Uysal et al. (2005) reported that clean-up of residual resin should be performed with adequate water-cooling to avoid temperature changes exceeding the critical value. Eminkahyagil et al. (2006) concluded that tungsten carbide burs used at low speed may be the method of choice for adhesive clean-up.

Technological advancements in laser dentistry may be useful in the future for avoiding severe pulpal reactions. In a recent study performed on rats, it has been shown that the use of low level laser therapy (LLLT) during tooth movement results in increase in vascularization and faster repair of pulpal tissue. The therapeutic effects of LLLT, such as pain relief, acceleration of tissue healing, repair and neo-vascularization, increased fibroblast and collagen fiber proliferation, and decrease in the immune response, may provide an insight for optimization of orthodontic treatment (Abi-Ramia et al., 2010).

Despite all these efforts to minimize adverse pulp reactions, it seems almost impossible to avoid hyperemia or reversible pulpitis during the early stages of orthodontic tooth movement. As shown by Popp et al. (1992), the signs of hyperemia diminish as blood flow returns to normal in 72 hours. These mild pulpitis reactions can be detected 2 hours after bonding/banding. Moderate pain caused by pulp hyperemia can last up to at least 7 days (Polat and Karaman, 2005). Mild pain can be noted after each appointment due to the change in archwires, but pulp vitality is unaffected in most of these cases.

Differential diagnosis between symptoms of tooth movement and an inflamed tooth is very difficult, especially if there is a history of a trauma. A patient with severe pain or pain that lasts for more than 10 days or who has darkening of the crown should consult a restorative specialist, preferably an endodontist. Radiographic evidence of an apical radiolucency may necessitate endodontic therapy (Hamilton and Gutmann, 1999), although orthodontic movement can be continued afterward.

Orthodontically induced root resorption

Both external and internal root resorption are challenging for the clinician since the exact nature of irreversible loss of tooth substance is not known and treatment of aggressive forms is difficult. Several predisposing factors have been suggested and the application of faulty mechanics has been proposed as the main cause of iatrogenic external root resorption. This section provides an overview of two types

of external root resorption: external apical root resorption and invasive cervical root resorption.

Alveolar bone resorption is the basis of orthodontic tooth movement. Bone resorption occurs in a usual healthy periodontal environment, while the highly mineralized cementum is more resistant to the resorption process, because of its fluoride content and vascular nature. Moreover, the cemental surface is covered by a pre-cemental layer that is resistant to resorption (Reitan, 1974). The inflammatory process, incident and essential for tooth movement, is also a reason for orthodontically induced root resorption. Orthodontically induced inflammatory root resorption (OIRR) frequently determines the success of orthodontic treatment (Mohandesan et al., 2007). If the duration of orthodontic treatment or the magnitude of the force is increased, the risk of root resorption increases and results in exposure of the dentin layer under the resorbing cementum, which heightens the osteoclastic attack and leads to progressive root resorption until all orthodontic forces are stopped. When the forces are relieved, repair commences from the periphery with fibroblast and cementoblast-like cells synthesizing collagenous fibrillar material and a new periodontal ligament (PDL). Most of the resorbed lacunae are frequently repaired with secondary cementum (Reitan, 1985). According to Owman-Moll and Kurol (1998), 6–7 weeks after the termination of force, the amount of repair rises to 82%.

Root resorption caused by orthodontic therapy occurs in two locations: superficial surface resorption or in the apical third of the root (Figure 16.1). The increased incidence can be explained in two ways (Huang et al., 2005).

- First, the fulcrum of the tooth is more coronal to the apical third of the root and due to the differences in the direction of the PDL fibers, forces are more traumatic to the apical region than to the coronal.
- Second, the middle and gingival thirds of the root are covered with acellular cementum, whereas the apical

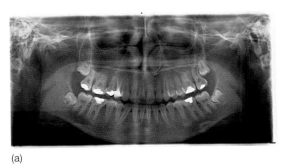 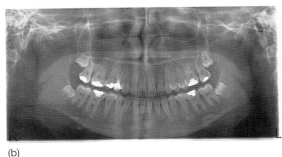 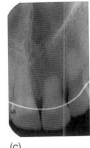

(a)   (b)   (c)

Figure 16.1 Orthodontically induced apical root resorption in the apical third of the root. (a) At the end of fixed appliance treatment. (b) At 1-year follow up. (c) Periapical radiograph at 14-month follow-up. Resorption has not progressed: however the tooth has been splinted with a flexible wire retainer due to slight mobility.

third is covered with cellular cementum, containing cells and blood vessels that have been damaged by heavy forces (Rygh, 1977).

Predisposing factors for root resorption can be divided into biological factors and factors related to orthodontic mechanics. Among the biological factors, chronological age, dental age, gender, tooth structure, root morphology, presence of previous resorption, trauma and endodontic therapy, autotransplantation, alveolar bone density, malocclusion type, periodontal disease, occlusal forces, habits, absence of teeth, impacted canines, and systemic conditions, have been listed. Treatment and appliance type, amount of tooth displacement, type of tooth movement, duration, degree and amount of orthodontic force, intermaxillary elastic usage and application of orthopedic forces are among the mechanical factors related to root resorption. However, a major factor for the occurrence of root resorption is individual susceptibility (Rygh, 1977). The susceptibility to root resorption differs among individuals, as well as within the same individual at different periods of time. Hormones, body type and the metabolic rate trigger signals that initiate fluctuations in osteoclastic and osteoblastic activities. In certain systemic diseases such as allergy and asthma there is increased susceptibility to resorption (Davidovitch, 1996; McNab et al., 1999; Davidovitch et al., 2000). The maxillary and mandibular incisors, maxillary first molars, maxillary first and second premolars, and the maxillary canines are the teeth that are more prone to root resorption. One reason for the high prevalence of root resorption among incisors may be their thin root morphology, but it is more likely due to the excessive movement during orthodontic treatment, that is, round tripping, and contact with the cortical plates of alveolar bone, particularly during the use of intra-slot torque, which generates very heavy forces (De Angelis and Davidovitch, 2009).

The presence of root resorption can be established using conventional radiographic methods such as periapical radiography, orthopantomograms, or lateral cephalograms. However, these routinely used methods are not helpful in the detection of lateral and early lesions, since resorption cannot be radiographically seen before some amount of apical root shortening occurs (Brezniak and Wasserstein, 2002). The periapical method seems to be the best conventional method, with minimal distortion and superimposition of anatomic structures. Computed tomography (CT), either computed medical or dental cone beam, is far superior to conventional dental radiography for locating early resorptive areas (Ericson and Kurol, 2000). However, the routine clinical use of CT is limited by its high radiation dose and expense (Sameshima and Asgarifar, 2001). Cone-beam dental CT offers lower radiation dose, fewer artifacts, and faster image projection than a conventional CT (Dudic et al., 2009).

Resorption is observed in teeth subjected to faulty mechanics in the early stages of treatment, such as in uncontrolled tipping of maxillary incisors in order to reduce excessive overjet (De Angelis and Davidovitch, 2009). Root resorption can be diagnosed with the help of dentinal proteins such as dentin matrix protein 1 and dentin phosphophoryn, which are released into the gingival crevicular fluid during active root resorption (Mah and Prasad, 2004). If there was pretreatment root resorption, the rate might increase from 4% to 77% during treatment (Goldson and Henrikson, 1975). Previously traumatized teeth present an important risk for OIRR (Linge and Linge, 1991), but Malmgren et al. (1982) concluded that resorption rates do not increase in the presence of trauma if a normal PDL environment is maintained (as a result of applying appropriate mechanics). Although Wickwire et al. (1974) found a greater incidence of resorption during orthodontic treatment in 53 endodontically treated teeth, Spurrier et al. (1990) and Remington et al. (1989) found lower resorption rates in such teeth due to their increased dentin hardness and density after the orthodontic treatment (Figure 16.2).

Treatment plans for patients with predisposing factors should ensure that teeth will not be moved unnecessarily and into contact with cortical plates of alveolar bone, in order to avoid any additional resorption. During treatment, evaluation should be done 6 months after the onset of treatment (Levander and Malmgren, 1988). If any sign of resorption is seen in the radiographs (which implies that faulty mechanics had been used), the application of orthodontic force can be interrupted for 2–4 months to allow for repair (Reitan, 1964; Levander and Malmgren, 1988), but more importantly, the appliances should be adjusted to deliver the appropriate mechanical forces. Severe resorption should never occur when biomechanical principles are followed correctly, with close attention to the unique anatomical features of each patient. Iatrogenic root resorption usually does not progress once orthodontic force is discontinued.

A tooth with severe resorption and increased mobility can be splinted to the neighboring teeth. The patient should be informed about the situation and advised to be careful during the use of these teeth. Root canal treatment is usually not needed but can be performed if excessive loss of root length has occurred (Malmgren and Levander, 2004). In rare cases, resorption continues despite termination of orthodontic treatment and does not stop until splinting and endodontic therapy is performed (Gholston and Mattison, 1983). For severe, active lesions, endodontic treatment should be performed with a calcium hydroxide paste, but if the resorption has ceased, the canal can be filled with gutta-percha. During the retention period, the clinician should prevent occlusal trauma to the resorbed teeth through modification in the retainers (Dougherty, 1968). A crown/root ratio of 1 : 1 is sufficient for maintaining the

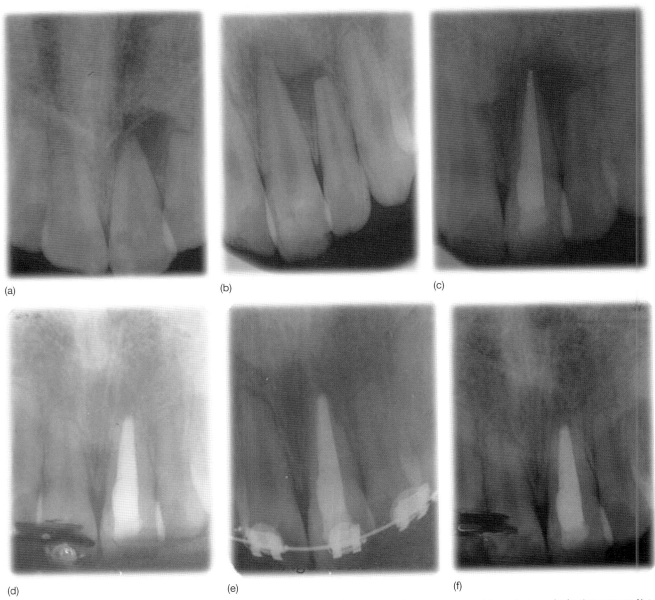

Figure 16.2 Root resorption due to orthodontic treatment. (a,b) The talon cusp of the left central incisor was ground down during orthodontic treatment. Note that only this tooth did not demonstrate apical resorption, as it was nonvital due to pulp/dentin exposure, which was not diagnosed during the grinding procedure. (c,d) Treatment of chronic apical periodontitis with root canal treatment and apical resection. (e) Patient was re-treated orthodontically. (f) After the second orthodontic treatment, the left central incisor showed no resorption and was also asymptomatic without any mobility.

tooth. If the root length is shorter than this, the tooth is likely to be unable to bear the functional loads of mastication. Although vitality is rarely affected, endodontic treatment should be performed if the crown/root ratio is less than 1 : 1 . A search for pharmacological agents capable of repairing root resorption revealed that bisphosphonates (Liu et al., 2004), echistatin (Talic et al., 2006) and low doses of corticosteroids (Ashcraft et al., 1992) (1 mg/kg) have positive effects, whereas high doses (15 mg/kg) have a reverse effect.

Invasive cervical resorption is an aggressive type of external root resorption that leads to progressive destruction of tooth structure. It usually affects single teeth, but in rare cases multiple teeth are affected (Coyle et al., 2006). Cervical location is the characteristic feature, and resorption of coronal dentin and enamel creates a pinkish color as the vascular tissues become visible (Heithersay, 2004) (Figure 16.3). The lesions are characterized by highly vascular fibrous tissue with osteoclasts arising from the PDL (Smidt et al., 2007). Since microorganisms are rarely found,

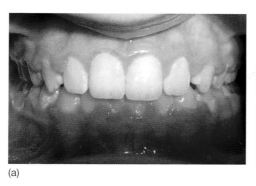
(a)

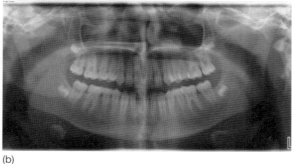
(b)

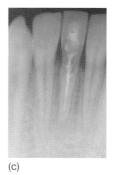
(c)

Figure 16.3 (a,b) Invasive cervical resorption after orthodontic treatment, demonstrating a pinkish color. (c) Patient was referred to an experienced endodontic specialist for treatment of invasive cervical resorption by elimination of the actively resorbing tissue and restoration of the defect with a suitable filling material (mineral trioxide aggregate [MTA]). However, conventional root canal treatment was carried out by a general practitioner and the prognosis remained poor.

microbial involvement in these lesions is doubtful (Heithersay, 1999; Trope, 2002). A study of 222 patients who displayed invasive cervical resorption showed that orthodontic treatment, trauma, intracoronal bleaching, and surgery involving the cementoenamel junction were the major predisposing factors. In that study, 21.2% of patients were reported to have a history of orthodontic treatment. Again, this type of root resorption implies that inappropriate mechanics had been applied in these patients.

Invasive cervical resorption is painless and rarely symptomatic. The resorption process starts below the gingival margin and extends apically and coronally along the root dentin (Smidt et al., 2007). The lesion is often separated from the pulp by the predentin layer, which is the last to resorb (Heithersay, 2004). A clinical feature is a pink coronal discoloration close to the gingival margin. It can go unnoticed for months to years and only become evident on routine radiography. Conventional radiographs taken from different angles can identify the involved surfaces but a three-dimensional visualization of the exact size and location of the lesion requires a CT scan (Kim et al., 2003; Gulsahi et al., 2007). Two important features of invasive cervical resorption differentiate it from internal root resorption. One is the absence of pulpal signs and the other is the radiographic appearance of the pulp canal size (Gulabivala and Searson, 1995; Smidt et al., 2007). In invasive cervical resorption the canal space is unchanged and the radiolucency extends coronally and apically in the dentin.

Invasive cervical resorption is quite aggressive, therefore the orthodontist should refer the patient as soon as the lesion is diagnosed. The treatment should be performed by experienced specialists to prevent tooth loss. The rationale for treatment of invasive cervical resorption is the elimination of the actively resorbing tissue and restoration of the defect with a suitable filling material (Figure 16.4). Both nonsurgical and surgical treatment approaches can be used. Nonsurgical regimens involve topical application

of a 90% aqueous solution of trichloroacetic acid for the induction of coagulation necrosis to the lesion area, curettage, endodontic treatment if pulpal perforation is present, and glass ionomer cement restoration. The use of calcium hydroxide for neutralization of the lesion, elimination of microorganisms and inactivation of toxic products is also recommended (Frank, 1981). If the margin of the lesion is below the cervical line, orthodontic extrusion can be performed. Extrusive orthodontic forces can be applied for 4–6 weeks and during the extrusion, crown shortening can be performed if premature contact occurs. Fiberotomy can be performed for the maintenance of the extruded tooth (Smidt et al., 2007). However, the clinician should keep in mind the possibility of ankylosis, which is not seen in cases of cervical resorption (Figure 16.5).

Surgical treatment involves periodontal flap surgery, curettage, and restoration of the defect. Restorative materials that have been used previously include amalgam, composite resin, and glass ionomer cement (Lustmann and Ehrlich, 1974; Frank, 1981; Frank and Blakland, 1987). Currently, mineral trioxide aggregate (MTA) is recommended to restore the resorptive cementum in cervical resorption cases (Frank and Torabinejad, 1998; White and Bryant, 2002; Yilmaz et al., 2010). Baek et al. (2005) have shown that the type of cementum coverage achieved using MTA had not been achieved with any other material. White and Bryant (2002) reported an increase in radiodense crestal bone when MTA was used with guided tissue regeneration to fill an external root resorption site with a bone defect. A platelet-enriched fibrin sealant (Tisseel) has been in use for a long time for sinus floor augmentation, treatment of peri-implantitis, intrabony periodontal defects, and alveolar ridge reconstruction. Ren et al. (2000) have demonstrated that Tisseel enhances the healing of exposed pulp tissue in dogs. Though dentinal bridge formation was not present in a majority of cases, the authors concluded that fibrin sealant was a promising material as a bioactive pulp capping agent.

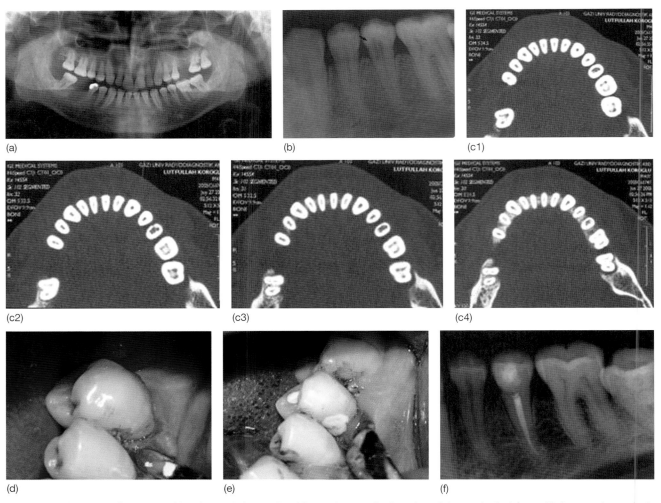

Figure 16.4 Diagnosis and treatment of invasive cervical resorption. (a) Note the extensive irregular radiolucency in the left mandibular second premolar in the panoramic radiograph. (b) The periapical radiograph of the left mandibular second premolar tooth shows an irregular radiolucent area in the tooth crown (arrow). (c) Axial computed tomography (CT) scans taken from coronal to apical and obtained with a bone window setting showing extensive resorption in the mesial cervical area of the left mandibular second premolar. (d) Intraoral appearance of the resorption area. (e) Intraoral appearance after the root canal treatment and restoration of the resorbed area. (f) Periapical radiograph at 6-month follow-up. (From Gulsahi A, Gulsahi K, Ungor M (2007) Invasive cervical resorption: clinical and radiological diagnosis and treatment of 3 cases. *Oral Surgery Oral Medicine Oral Pathology Oral Radiology and Endodontics* 103(3): e65–72.)

Emergency orthodontic treatment in trauma cases

There are instances where other dental disciplines may require orthodontic collaboration such as in trauma patients referred from emergency clinics. Trauma to the orofacial region occurs frequently and comprises 5% of all injuries that require treatment (Glendor et al., 2007). Dental injuries, which are the most common among all facial injuries, are experienced by more than 20% of children, mostly between the ages of 8 and 12 (Glendor et al., 2007; Moule and Moule, 2009). Boys sustain dental injuries about twice as often as girls do. Most dental injuries involving the maxillary incisors occur in cases of Class II Division 1 malocclusion with increased overjet and inadequate lip closure (Forsberg and Tedestam, 1993; Burden, 1995).

Emergency management of traumatized teeth is usually performed by a pediatric dentist, or an endodontic/conservative dentistry specialist, but an interactive approach involving the orthodontist in the trauma management team is advised. Orthodontic treatment planning for patients with previously traumatized teeth often requires decisions regarding the long-term viability of the traumatized teeth and effects of trauma on the developing dentoalveolar complex.

Treatment of an uncomplicated crown fracture can be accomplished quite successfully by either a build-up with acid-etch composite resin, or by reattaching the fractured segment, if available, using an adhesive bonding system (Figure 16.6). The expected outcome for either approach is excellent with nearly 100% pulp survival regardless of root developmental status (Robertson et al., 2000). The

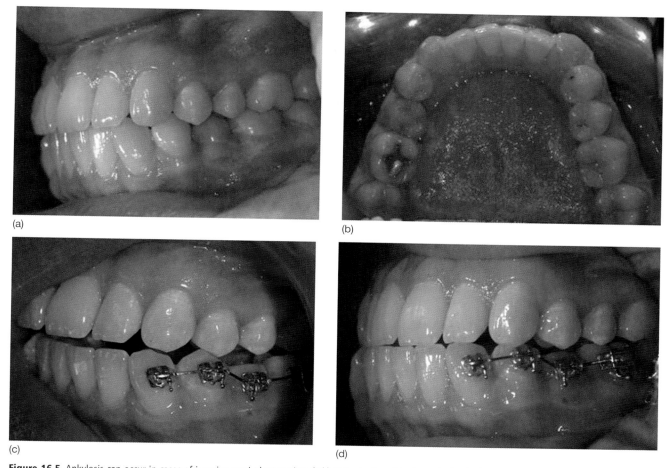

Figure 16.5 Ankylosis can occur in cases of invasive cervical resorption. (a,b) Patient referred to the orthodontic clinic for treatment of cervical resorption via orthodontic extrusion after periodontal curettage. (c) Orthodontic force was applied after occlusal grinding. (d) No movement occurred following 3 months of force application as the tooth was ankylosed, it was then extracted.

appropriate time for evaluating the vitality of the tooth is 8 weeks after the trauma.

A fracture involving dentin exposes dentinal tubules in direct communication with the pulp. Therefore, timely protection of the exposed dentin is advisable to prevent the pulp from undergoing infection-related necrosis. Complicated fractures of the primary teeth require decisions based on life expectancy of the primary tooth and vitality of the pulpal tissue (Flores, 2002). If the fracture occurs in an adult with fully formed roots it will be more practical to perform root canal treatment prior to the prosthetic restoration and/or orthodontic treatment. On the other hand, it is very important to make every effort to preserve pulp vitality in young patients with developing permanent teeth as continued pulp vitality facilitates root development (Fuks et al., 1987). The exposed pulp will develop granulation tissue to protect the exposed wound and bacteria will invade the pulp tissue gradually. However, it may take many days for bacteria to penetrate even a few millimeters so the pulp can be preserved even if it has

been exposed for more than 24–48 hours (Heide, 1991). Therefore, complicated fractures should not be viewed as hopeless situations for pulp survival in young patients. Miomir Cvek (1978) introduced a procedure known as the *Cvek pulpotomy technique,* which employs calcium hydroxide for pulp capping. This vital pulpotomy technique should be performed as soon as possible after the trauma. As long as the pulp is alive and is properly protected, continued root development can be expected.

If pulpal necrosis accompanies the fracture, the general treatment protocol involves root canal treatment followed by protective permanent restorations. The open and sometimes divergent apical morphology and weak root dentinal walls make endodontic procedures challenging and present restorative problems. More definitive treatment options such as implant supported crowns or fixed prostheses may not be feasible until craniofacial growth is complete, which can be up to the age of 25 years (Op Heij et al., 2006).

Apexification is a method of inducing a calcified apical barrier in an incompletely formed root of a pulpless tooth,

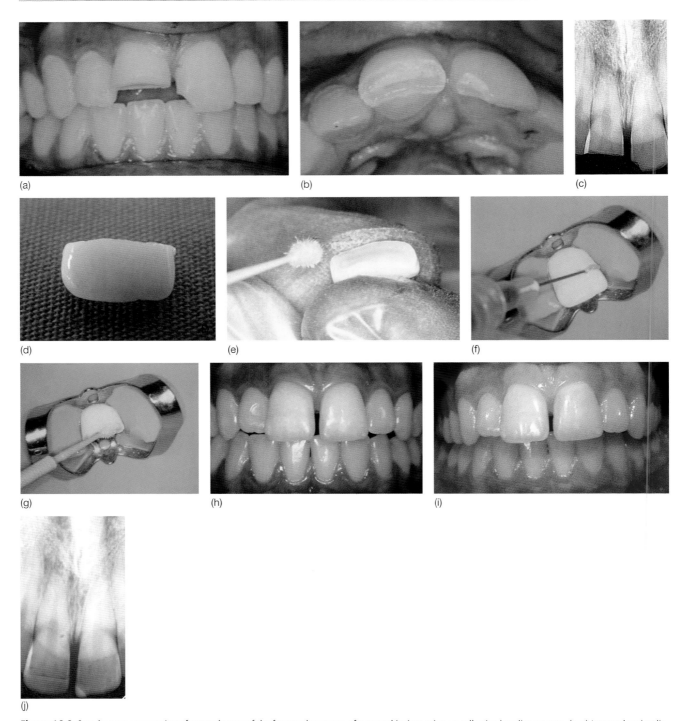

Figure 16.6 Step-by-step progression of reattachment of the fractured segment of a central incisor using an adhesive bonding system. (a–c) Intraoral and radiographic views before treatment. (d) Broken fragment of tooth. (e–g) Re-attachment procedure. (h) After re-attachment and polishing. (i,j) 1-year follow-up. The tooth was vital. (From Arhun N, Ungor M [2007] Re-attachment of a fractured tooth: a case report. *Dental Traumatology* 23(5): 322–6. Courtesy of John Wiley and Sons.)

which has now become a routine endodontic procedure. The treatment involves the use of calcium hydroxide to fill a debrided, biomechanically prepared immature root canal. The calcium hydroxide leaches from the canal over time and needs to be replenished every 3–6 months. Apexification

may take between 6 and 24 months to promote formation of a hard apical barrier to allow condensation of a gutta-percha root filling (Rafter, 2005). Recent studies suggest using MTA as an apical plug as it reduces the duration of time required for the calcium hydroxide dressing and

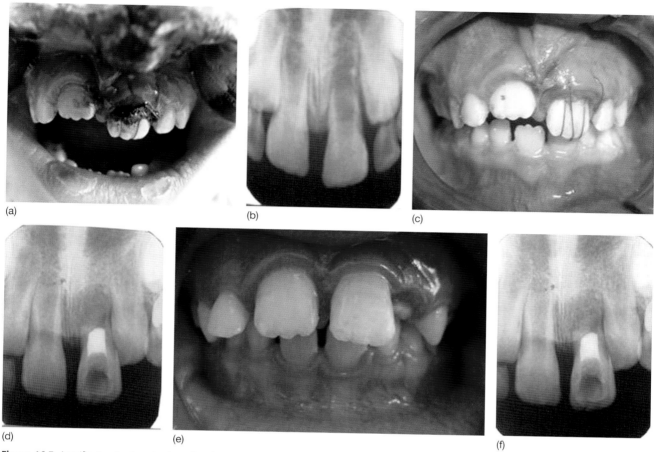

Figure 16.7 Apexification treatment using mineral trioxide aggregate (MTA) as an apical plug. (a) Replantation of avulsed left central incisor 1 hour after trauma. (b,c) 3 days after replantation. (d) Apexification treatment using mineral trioxide aggregate (MTA) as an apical plug. (e,f) At the 3-month follow-up. (Courtesy of Dr Sevi Burçak Çehreli, Associate Professor and Head, Department of Pediatric Dentistry, Faculty of Dentistry, Baskent University, Ankara, Turkey.)

overall treatment (Felippe et al., 2006; Simon et al., 2007) (Figure 16.7).

Some patients requiring apexification might be under orthodontic treatment or are at an age when orthodontic treatment should be initiated. Delaying orthodontic treatment in these patients will prevent achieving optimal treatment results, which are usually obtained in the growing stages. Steiner and West (1997) showed successful formation of the apical barrier in two incisors of an 11-year-old patient with apexification performed simultaneously with orthodontic treatment. Fully formed apical barriers were evident after 2 years of endodontic treatment and orthodontic treatment was completed 6 months later. Anthony (1986) also reported a successful apexification procedure during active orthodontic movement. These reports demonstrate that a calcified barrier develops even with ongoing resorption and apposition during orthodontic movement.

Another common problem in teeth with open and divergent apical root areas is the high risk of cervical fracture during or after the root canal treatment. Most fractures are observed within 3 years of commencing long-term calcium

hydroxide treatment. The frequency ranges from 77% in teeth with the least root development to 28% in teeth with the fully developed roots (Cvek, 1992). The adverse effects of long-term calcium hydroxide administration on the physical properties of the root dentin were studied (Andreasen et al., 2002; Rosenberg et al., 2007). Andreasen et al. (2006) recommend placing calcium hydroxide for a maximum of 4 weeks followed by filling the canal with MTA. Other methods proposed to reduce the fracture risk include use of composite resin in the root canal and metallic posts embedded in MTA. Current evidence suggests that placement of composite resin materials deep into the coronal aspect of the root canal imparts superior fracture resistance (Desai and Chandler, 2009). Reducing the amount of coronal root canal filling and replacing it with composite resin should have the secondary benefit of reducing coronal leakage and contributing to endodontic success.

Even with the increased risk of fracture, these teeth should not be arbitrarily extracted because they help to maintain the developing alveolar ridge, act as a space

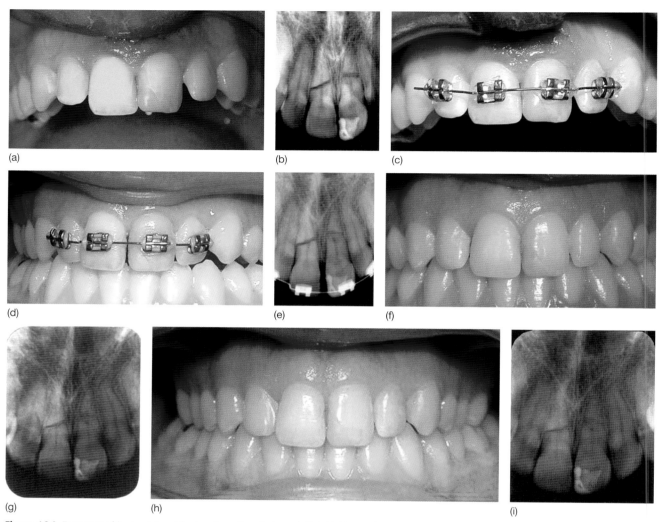

Figure 16.8 Treatment of horizontal root-fractured maxillary incisors. (a,b) Initial intraoral and radiographic views. (c) Orthodontic brackets and an .016 inch stainless steel archwire for splinting. First and second order bends were made in the archwire to retain forward positioning of the incisors during splinting in order to prevent the traumatized incisors from contacting the lower teeth. (d,e) Day 20: note the color change in the tooth. (f,g) Intraoral and periapical views after removal of brackets at week 14. (h,i) Clinical and radiographic appearance after 9-month follow-up. (From Polat-Ozsoy O, Gülsahi K, Veziroğlu F [2008] Treatment of horizontal root-fractured maxillary incisors – a case report. *Dental Traumatology* 24(6): e91–5. Courtesy of John Wiley and Sons.)

maintainer, and preserve the natural appearance of the site. If the tooth eventually fractures after the completion of dentofacial growth, a permanent replacement can be more favorably placed. Root fractures, which comprise 0.5–7% of all trauma cases, are more likely to be observed in the maxillary anterior region of males in the 11–20-year age group (Andreasen et al., 2007). Radiographs may reveal one or more radiolucent lines separating the tooth fragments and multiple angled radiographs can confirm these findings (American Academy of Pediatric Dentistry, 2004).

Main factors influencing the healing process of root fractures include the amount of displacement of the coronal segment, the stage of root development, and the severity of the trauma. Ideally root fractures are repaired with hard tissue, but sometimes there is also redundant healing with

connective or granulation tissue (Skaare and Jacobsen, 2003). In permanent teeth, the location of the root fracture has not been shown to affect pulp survival after injury (Andreasen and Andreasen, 2000). Therefore, root fractures occurring in either the tooth's cervical third or apical third can be treated successfully by stabilization of the repositioned fragment (Figure 16.8).

According to the guidelines of the International Association of Dental Traumatology, for treatment of root fractures, the coronal segment should be repositioned as soon as possible and then stabilized in its anatomically correct position with a flexible splint for 4 weeks (Flores et al., 2007). Avoidance of any occlusal contact is of prime importance (Hovland, 1992; Yates, 1992). Various types of splint have been introduced over the years for stabilization of fractured segments, including splinting via orthodontic brackets (Mackie and Warren, 1988; Cengiz et al., 2006). Orthodontic splints are often advantageous in multiple tooth injuries as any tooth included in the splint can be removed from the splint or aligned into the desired position if needed.

Many authors have reported successful healing of crown/ root or root fractures without any endodontic treatment (Poi et al., 2002; Erdemir et al., 2005). The communication of the fracture line with the oral environment, which may promote bacterial contamination, determines the healing process (Hovland, 1992). If the apical root fragment is long enough to support a coronal restoration, the definitive treatment alternatives are to remove the coronal fragment and perform endodontic treatment, followed by a supragingival restoration or necessary gingivectomy, osteotomy, and surgical or orthodontic extrusion to prepare for restoration (Andreasen and Andreasen, 2000).

Orthodontic treatment of the teeth with repaired root fractures is possible, even if the fracture at the time of the accident is extensive, with marked fragment dislocation. In cases where the repair occurs without separation of the fragments, the apical fragment may remain attached to the coronal portion throughout and following orthodontic treatment. On the other hand, separation of the segment may be enhanced by orthodontic tooth movement (Hamilton and Gutmann, 1999). It is recommended that teeth with these types of fractures be observed for at least 2 years before initiating orthodontic treatment. Hovland et al. (1983) presented a successful case followed up for 8 years, in which a maxillary central incisor with a transverse fracture at the junction of the apical and middle third of the root was moved palatally and intruded during orthodontic treatment. Erdemir et al. (2005) also demonstrated satisfactory healing of a horizontal root fractured maxillary incisor without treatment, which was moved orthodontically a long time after the trauma (Figure 16.9).

Orthodontic extrusion of teeth, or so-called 'forced eruption', was first described by Ingber (1974), for treatment of one-wall and two-wall bony pockets that were difficult to manage with conventional therapy alone. The criteria to help determine whether the tooth should be forcibly erupted or extracted are: root length, root form, level of the fracture, relative importance of the tooth, esthetics, and endo/perio prognosis (Kokich, 2002). Orthodontic extrusion can be achieved with various kinds of fixed or removable orthodontic appliances (Cengiz et al., 2005; Yüzügüllü et al., 2008). Bonding an attachment to the remaining root fragment might be difficult sometimes because of lack of available tooth tissue and difficulties in isolating the bonding interface from the gingival crevicular fluid and blood. Metal endodontic posts may be useful for extrusion of the root without buccal tipping (Arhun et al., 2006a) (Figure 16.10). A more esthetic approach for bonding is building a composite core using a tooth-colored glass-fiber post (Yüzügüllü et al., 2008) (Figure 16.11). It is possible to use a T-loop or a spring, as well as an elastic module, to apply vertical extrusive force. In order to achieve controlled root movement in the vertical and anteroposterior direction, first and second order bends on the main archwire can be used as well (Proffit, 2000; Arhun et al., 2006a). A force of only 20–30 g is sufficient for extrusion, however, some clinicians prefer higher forces of 50–60 g for rapid extrusion of traumatized teeth (Malmgren et al., 1994). After adequate extrusion is achieved by forced eruption, a fiberotomy of the stretched periodontal fibers is usually performed to prevent relapse (Heithersay and Moule, 1982; Malmgren et al., 1994).

A special type of dental trauma for which an interactive strategy is required is intrusive luxation, common in the deciduous dentition. This might result in unexpectedly severe complications, such as pulp necrosis, inflammatory root resorption, ankylosis, replacement resorption, and loss of marginal bone support. Different approaches have been suggested for tooth repositioning, such as observation for spontaneous re-eruption, surgical crown exposure, orthodontic extrusion (with or without previous luxation of the intruded tooth), and surgical repositioning (Turley et al., 1987; Oulis et al., 1996). Immediate application of orthodontic force on traumatically intruded teeth facilitates extrusion, allowing early endodontic access. It can prevent ankylosis, however, it may increase the risk of external root resorption and marginal bone loss (Oulis et al., 1996; Chaushu et al., 2004a; de Alencar et al., 2007). The most appropriate time of initiating orthodontic extrusion after an injury is still controversial. It is customary to delay orthodontic tooth movement until the teeth are symptomless for at least a few months. However, although the risk of root resorption is reduced, this observation period may result in the development of ankylosis and delay endodontic access (Turley et al., 1987). A high rate of success (95.4%) was observed in orthodontically extruded teeth, both immediately (within 10 weeks posttrauma) and later (after 3 months) (Medeiros and Mucha, 2009) (Figures 16.12, 16.13). Using the adjacent teeth as anchorage for extrusion should be avoided, as they may also be affected by the trauma, and unwanted tipping or intrusion may result. In order to prevent side effects, adjacent teeth can be splinted or palatal arches soldered to molar bands, and self-supporting labial arches can be used. Fixed retainers should be used for retention (Chaushu et al., 2004a).

Tooth avulsion is defined as complete displacement of a tooth from its socket, severing the pulpal blood supply and exposing the cells of the PDL to the external environment (Andersson, 2007). The reported incidence of tooth avulsions ranges from 1% to 16% of all traumatic injuries of the permanent dentition. The most common age of occurrence is around 8–12 years, a time when the loosely structured PDL surrounding the erupting teeth provides only

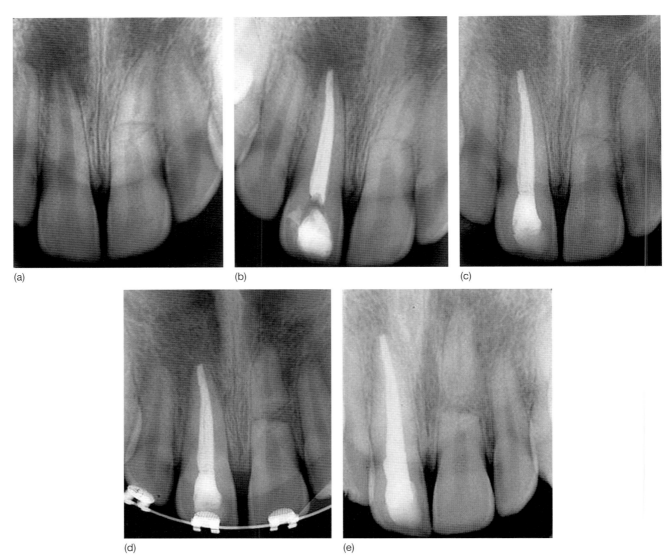

(a)　　　　　　　　(b)　　　　　　　　(c)

(d)　　　　　　　　(e)

Figure 16.9 Orthodontic movement of a horizontally fractured tooth. (a) Periapical radiograph showing a radiolucency in maxillary right central incisor and a horizontal root fracture in the left central incisor. (b) Postoperative radiograph. No treatment performed in the maxillary right incisor as there was no evidence of pathology and pulp tests were positive. (c) 6 months following endodontic treatment. The right central incisor has healed without treatment. (d) Radiograph 1 year after the endodontic treatment. Note the orthodontic brackets on the teeth. The orthodontic treatment was started 3 months previously. The coronal fragment of the right central incisor had moved relative to the apical. The orthodontic treatment was stopped as the orthodontic problem was mild. Pulp tests remained positive, but mobility increased slightly. (e) 12 years post-trauma and 6 years after orthodontic treatment. Tooth was asymptomatic and showed a good appearance clinically and radiographically. (From Erdemir A, Ungor M, Erdemir EO [2005] Orthodontic movement of a horizontally fractured tooth: a case report. *Dental Traumatology* 21: 160–4. Courtesy of John Wiley and Sons.)

minimal resistance to an extrusive force (Andreasen and Andreasen, 2007). Treatment of avulsions is directed towards avoiding or minimizing the effects of the two main complications, namely: attachment damage and pulpal infection. While it is not possible for the original blood supply to be re-established after avulsion, under special circumstances it is possible for the replanted tooth to become revascularized. If the tooth is immature with an open apex, efforts should be made to promote revascularization of the pulp. In the tooth with a closed or open apex in which the revascularization is unsuccessful, treatment

efforts should be aimed at elimination of potential bacterial toxins from the root canal space (Lee et al., 2001). Replantation of teeth has been considered a temporary measure because many replanted teeth ultimately succumb to root resorption. However, many cases have been reported in which teeth have survived successfully for 20–40 years, with a normal PDL. The success rate of replanted teeth has been reported to be as low as 4% and as high as 50% (Andreasen et al., 1995b).

The success of replantation is dependent on many factors, such as the time period the tooth was out of the mouth

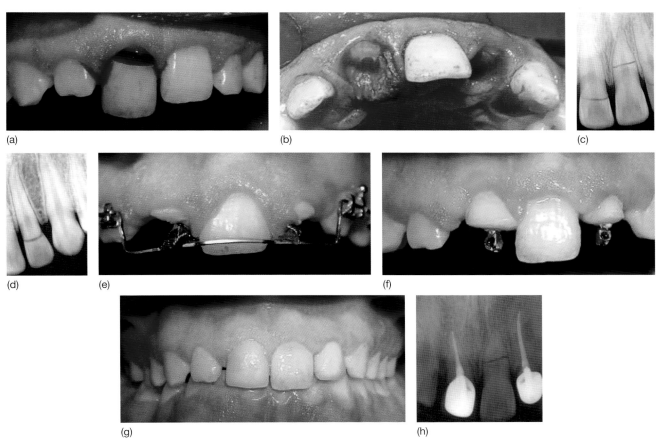

Figure 16.10 Orthodontic extrusion or forced eruption of roots via metal endodontic posts. (a–d) Fractured anterior teeth in a 19-year-old male patient as a result of a road traffic accident. Right central incisor and lateral incisor was treated endodontically while, left central incisor was untouched and observed. (e) Metal endodontic post with a drilled hole for orthodontic force application. (f) Orthodontic extrusion with posts. (g) The roots after extrusion. (h) Final restoration after gingival recontouring and fiberotomy. (i) At 19 months follow-up (From Arhun N, Arman A, Ungor M, et al. [2006a] A conservative multidisciplinary approach for improved aesthetic results with traumatised anterior teeth. *British Dental Journal* 201: 509–12.)

(Kenny and Barrett, 2001), the type of splinting, and the duration of splinting. Adhesive-bonded composite resin splints such as wire-composite splints and titanium trauma splints are recommended because semi rigid or flexible splinting allows physiological tooth movement, and such functional stimuli promote healing (Ram and Cohenca, 2004). In view of long-term splinting causing ankylosis, it is recommended that teeth should be splinted for up to 2 weeks rather than 6 weeks as previously practiced; splinting for 1 week may be adequate for periodontal healing (Andreasen et al., 1995b; Andreasen and Andreasen, 2007).

The timing of endodontic treatment of a replanted avulsed tooth depends on the maturity of the tooth and, if it is immature, the amount of time it was outside the mouth. Clinical guidelines recommend avoiding endodontic treatment of immature teeth, unless obvious signs of non-revascularization are present or the period outside the mouth has been prolonged (Gregg and Boyd, 1998). Extirpation may be delayed in immature teeth if there is a

chance that the pulp is vital; root growth may then continue. The frequency of revascularization of a replanted immature incisor has been reported as 18% (Kling et al., 1986) and 34% (Andreasen et al., 1995a), being influenced by the extraoral time. The timing of pulpal extirpation is crucial and it should be performed within the first 3 weeks to prevent the development of inflammatory resorption in mature teeth (Gregg and Boyd, 1998; Hinckfuss and Messer, 2009). Calcium hydroxide is recommended generally as the intracanal medicament for 6–12 months or until the entire lamina dura is apparent radiographically prior to gutta-percha obturation. Systemic antibiotic therapy (doxycycline or penicillin V) is recommended to prevent bacterial infection (Gregg and Boyd, 1998).

In 7–8% of injuries, the avulsed tooth cannot be replanted or the replanted tooth develops progressive root resorption or there are crown/root or root fractures, all of which lead to tooth loss (Borum and Andreasen, 2001). In such situations, the treatment modalities including no treatment, orthodontic space closure, conventional bridges, adhesive

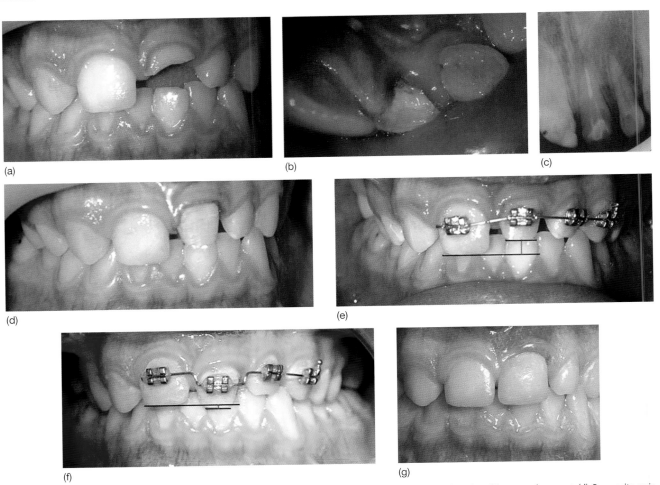

Figure 16.11 Orthodontic extrusion with a glass-fiber post and composite core. (a,b) Before treatment. (c) After glass-fiber post placement. (d) Composite resin crown for bracket attachment. (e) Initiation of orthodontic treatment with horizontal lines showing the incisal edges before extrusion. (f) At the end of orthodontic treatment. (g) Final restoration with porcelain fused to metal crown. (From Yüzügüllü B, Polat O, Ungör M [2008] Multidisciplinary approach to traumatized teeth: a case report. *Dental Traumatology* 24: e27–30. Courtesy of John Wiley and Sons.)

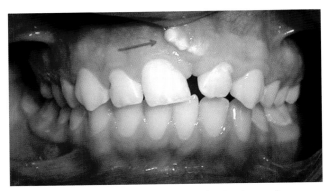

Figure 16.12 Traumatic intrusion of left central incisor (arrowed).

bridges, removable prosthetic appliances, or single tooth implants, and autotransplantation should also be considered (Andreasen et al., 2009) (Figure 16.14). Apart from orthodontic space closure, autotransplantation of teeth appears to be the most biologically oriented approach due

to its bone-generating capacity and because it allows orthodontic treatment to be performed at an early age (10–12 years). Progressive root resorption, necrosis of the pulp, ankylosis, and infraocclusion are commonly reported problems related to autotransplantation (Schwartz et al., 1985). Successful autotransplantation depends on several factors, such as the age at transplantation, the developmental stage of the tooth, donor type, the duration of extraoral exposure of the donor tooth during surgery, damage to the root cementum and the PDL, and the experience of the oral surgeon (Ahlberg et al., 1983; Schwartz et al., 1985). Zachrisson et al. (2004) stated that the optimal time for autotransplantation of premolars to the maxillary anterior region is when root development has reached two-thirds or two-fourths of the final length, enhancing the prognosis.

Various techniques have been described for stabilization including splinting with orthodontic brackets, ligatures, sutures, and composite resins. Long-term success rates vary between 74% and 100% (Lundberg and Isaksson, 1996;

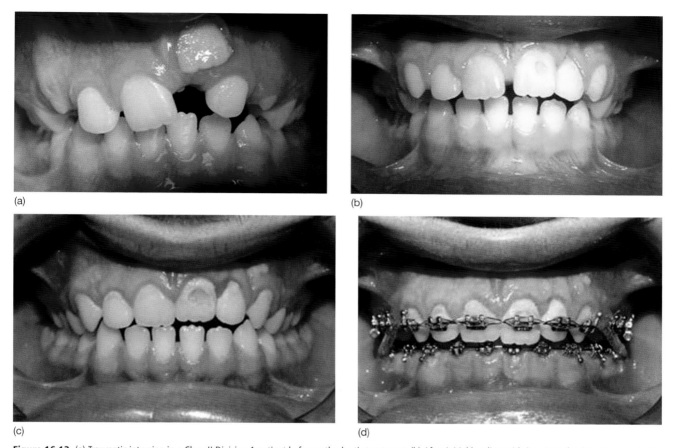

Figure 16.13 (a) Traumatic intrusion in a Class II Division 1 patient before orthodontic treatment. (b) After initial leveling with 2 × 4 mechanics prior to activator treatment. (c) At the end of functional treatment. Note the relapse in the vertical position of the traumatized tooth. (d) Intraoral view of the second stage of fixed appliance treatment.

Gault and Warocquier-Clerout, 2002). More recently, Kvint et al. (2010) reported an 81% success rate in 215 consecutively transplanted teeth with the highest success rate (100%) in transplantation of premolars to the maxillary incisor region. Autotransplantation of cryopreserved teeth has also been reported (Schwartz and Rank, 1986; Temmerman et al., 2006). This procedure requires a special facility and expertise to avoid damage to the PDL and dental pulp. The main advantage is that the transplanted teeth can be moved orthodontically (Fujita et al., 2008; Andreasen et al., 2009).

Special attention should be given to the pulpal response of orthodontically moved autotransplanted teeth as transplantation of teeth leads to interruption of the pulpal vascular and neural supply. As Skoglund et al. (1981) stated, pulpal necrosis occurs in most transplanted teeth. Repair includes revascularization, but pulpal obliteration mostly cannot be avoided. Although revascularization can be observed at the end of the first month (Skoglund et al., 1978), pulpal reinnervation may not be apparent even after 3 months (Robinson, 1983). Since sensory pulpal nerves are essential for regulating blood flow via release of

vasoactive neuropeptides, reduced pulpal innervations may compromise vasodilatation and angiogenesis and, as a result, pulp survival (Kerezoudis et al., 1995; Berggreen and Heyeraas, 1999). Paulsen et al. (1995) reported occurrence of late pulpal necrosis 5 years after orthodontic derotation of premolars. Bauss et al. (2004) evaluated the influence of derotation and extrusion on pulps of autotransplanted third molars and found that these movements were not associated with any additional risks to the long-term survival of transplanted single-rooted third molars. However, the authors concluded that special care should be taken while derotating autotransplanted multirooted molars.

Root resorption occurs when a donor tooth with partial or total lack of vital PDL is transplanted. It is categorized as replacement resorption, inflammatory resorption, and surface resorption (Andreasen, 1992) (Figure 16.15). Metabolic byproducts produced by bacteria present in necrotic pulp initiate periodontal inflammation, leading to inflammatory resorption of the transplanted tooth. Therefore, root canal treatment is often necessary for satisfactory clinical results in transplanted or replanted teeth

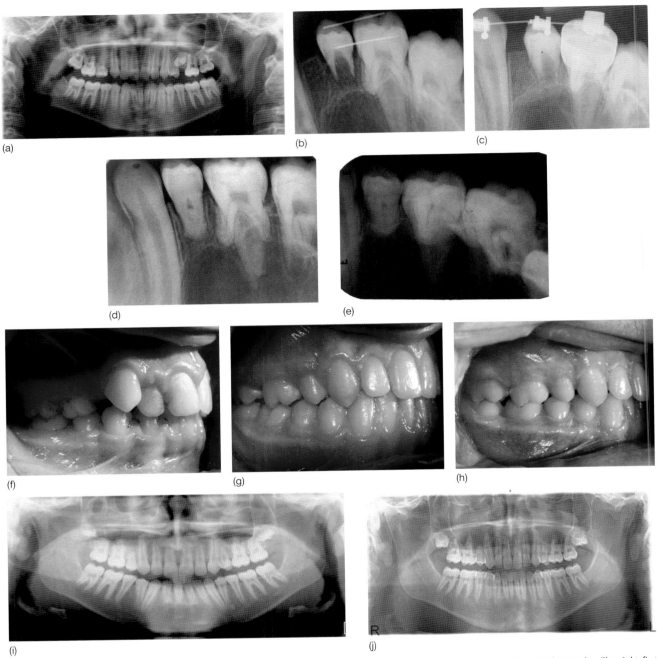

Figure 16.14 Autotransplantation. A boy aged 11 years, 3 months presented with a congenitally missing maxillary right second premolar. The right first premolar was also missing due to intentional extraction in order to correct the position of the buccally positioned canine. The treatment plan was to transplant the left second premolar germ in the place of the missing premolars on the right side. (a) Pretreatment panoramic radiograph. (b–e) The donor tooth after splinting (b), after placement of brackets (c), after orthodontic treatment (d), and after 7 years' follow-up (e). (f–h) Intraoral right views at the beginning, end of treatment and at the 7-year follow up. (i) Panoramic radiograph at the end of the fixed appliance treatment. (j) Panoramic radiograph 7 years after finishing of active treatment.

with complete root formation (Schwartz et al., 1985; Eliasson et al., 1988). Unlike replacement resorption, inflammatory resorption can be arrested by root canal therapy if it is performed early. According to Andreasen and Hjorting-Hansen (1966) endodontic treatment should be started only when a tooth becomes symptomatic or when bone lesions develop. Inflammatory resorption usually occurs 3–4 weeks after transplantation, whereas replacement resorption (ankylosis) takes 3–4 months to 1 year to become evident (Thomas et al., 1998). Most authors recommend endodontic treatment 7–14 days after transplantation as this time period is considered sufficient for the

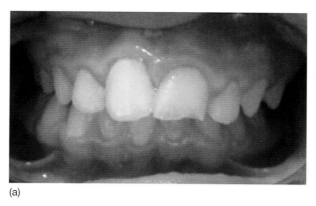 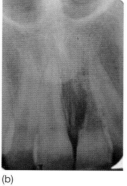

(a)   (b)

Figure 16.15 (a,b) The maxillary left central incisor was replanted 2 years ago, however no endodontic treatment was carried out. Both inflammatory and replacement resorption is evident radiographically. (Courtesy of Dr Sevi Burçak Çehreli, Associate Professor and Head, Department of Pediatric Dentistry, Faculty of Dentistry, Baskent University, Ankara, Turkey.)

start of possible pulp necrosis and inflammatory resorption (Andreasen, 1992; Thong et al., 2001; Pohl et al., 2005).

Autotransplantation of teeth offers an effective treatment option, particularly when combined with an appropriate orthodontic treatment plan. Subsequent to autotransplantation, a delay of at least 3 months, but preferably 6 months, has been recommended before applying active orthodontic forces (Lagerström and Kristerson, 1986). On the other hand, Fujita et al. (2008) have recommended using stable light orthodontic forces (using superelastic nickel-titanium alloy archwires) after just a short period of splinting (4 weeks) in order to avoid ankylosis and inflammatory root resorption. Berglund et al. (1996) reported that the use of orthodontic force (jiggling force) on the tooth to be transplanted prior to autotransplantation decreased the risk of damage to the PDL. Nishimura et al. (2009) reported on successful 10-year follow-up of an orthodontic case with an autotransplanted mature tooth with prior application of jiggling forces. Fukui et al. (2009) recommended monitoring of transplanted teeth during and after orthodontic treatment because of their susceptibility to inflammatory root resorption.

Primary failure of eruption (PFE) is a non-syndromic failure of permanent teeth eruption in the absence of mechanical intrusion (Frazier-Bowers et al., 2010). Recent studies have suggested that this dental phenotype is inherited and that mutations in parathyroid hormone receptor 1 genes can explain several familial cases of PFE. In these cases, a posterior open bite malocclusion accompanies normal vertical facial growth and the infraoccluded teeth cannot be moved orthodontically (Figure 16.16).

Ankylosis of teeth can lead to serious clinical problems such as tilting or migration of adjacent teeth, supraeruption of the opposing teeth, impaction of the succeeding permanent teeth or eruption delay, midline deviation, alveolar bone loss, and lack of alveolar bone development of the involved area (Becker and Karnei-R'em, 1992a,b; Becker et al., 1992; Kurol, 2002, 2006). Early clinical diagnosis of

ankylosis is based on the typical metallic sound heard on percussion of the tooth, marked decrease in the normal physiological facial-lingual excursion, and the lack of tooth mobility. Ankylosis can be evidenced on a periapical radiograph as an interruption of the PDL in a small area. However, early detection of ankylosis on dental radiographs is often difficult because the areas of ankylosis are very small, often located on the labial or lingual surface of the root, and are not visible on the two-dimensional radiograph (Isaacson et al., 2001). A more acceptable and reliable sign of ankylosis is infraocclusion, as only a third of ankylosed teeth will have a metallic sound on percussion or show loss of PDL space in radiographs (Raghoebar et al., 1989). The diagnosis of ankylosis can be confirmed when the affected tooth does not move when subjected to orthodontic forces.

Ankylosis in deciduous teeth is about 10 times more likely than in the permanent dentition (Mullally et al., 1995) and twice as likely in the mandibular than in the maxillary arch, with higher incidence in the molar region. With a permanent successor in a normal position, a 6-month delay in shedding time can be expected for ankylosed deciduous molars compared with normal teeth. Thus, early extraction of the ankylosed deciduous molar is unnecessary (Kurol and Koch, 1985). If the permanent successor is missing, spontaneous exfoliation is not likely. However, root resorption might continue, and an impaired vertical position might occur due to ankylosis (Kurol and Thilander, 1984). If the loss of height is mild or moderate, this situation can be accepted or the occlusal height can be restored. In severe infraocclusion, extraction is recommended as early as possible to promote spontaneous mesial migration of the permanent molars (Nishimura et al., 2009).

Retention of a permanent ankylosed tooth in a young patient is complicated by the arrested development of the alveolar ridge, coupled with the continuing facial growth of the child. It has been proposed to remove the ankylosed

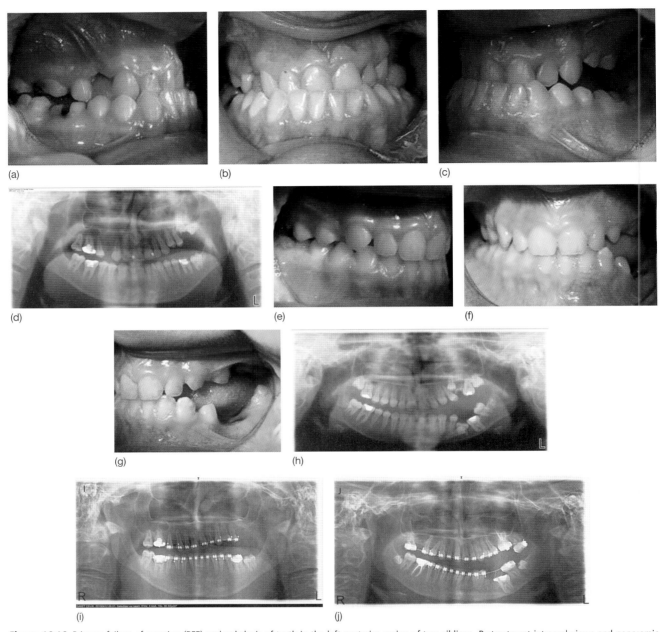

Figure 16.16 Primary failure of eruption (PFE) and ankylosis of teeth in the left posterior region of two siblings. Pretreatment intraoral views and panoramic radiographs of (a–d) the brother and (e–h) the sister. (i,j) In PFE, the affected teeth cannot be moved with conventional orthodontic mechanics.

tooth at the start of the rapid phase of adolescent growth (Steiner and West, 1997). Ankylosed teeth are excellent sources of rigid anchorage and a number of reports have been published on the use of the remaining ankylosed teeth as anchorage for orthodontic or orthopedic movement (Roberts, 2000).

Extraction is not the only treatment approach for an ankylosed tooth. Prosthetic build-up is also possible in mild cases, if the infraocclusion is less than 5 mm (Mullally et al., 1995; Chaushu et al., 2004b). If the ankylosed tooth is extracted and replaced with a prosthetic restoration, the results may not be esthetically acceptable due to the presence of an alveolar defect. Additional surgical procedures, such as ridge augmentation or onlay bone grafts may be required (Isaacson et al., 2001). Malmgren et al. (1984) described a method in which only the crown is removed and the ankylosed root is left in place. As the root is resorbed and replaced by bone (replacement resorption), the height and width of the ridge is maintained, allowing for placement of a more natural-looking restoration. Lee et al. (2009) suggested using miniscrew implants and cantilever uprighting springs to achieve root movement of the adjacent tooth into the extraction space of an ankylosed molar in order to restore the alveolar bone defect.

Orthodontic treatment combined with surgical luxation might be an acceptable approach in some cases, although there are associated risks, including fracture, recurrence of ankylosis, need for endodontic treatment, and intrusion of adjacent teeth (Razdolsky et al., 2004; Kofod et al., 2005; Lim et al., 2008). The ankylosed tooth can be extracted and reimplanted into the socket thus created, but this may result in external root resorption (Proffit, 1986). Another treatment alternative is mobilization of the anky- losed tooth along with surrounding bone by interdental osteotomy and repositioning of the tooth–bone segment in its proper position, followed by fixation with an archwire or acrylic splints (Medeiros and Bezerra, 1997). Surgical repositioning is one of the best treatment alternatives, but total mobilization of the segment and separation of the palatal mucosa may compromise the blood supply of the segment, and the gingival tissues may not follow the move- ment of the tooth–bone segment, resulting in areas of gin- gival recession and differences in the gingival margin level (Alcan, 2006). Distraction osteogenesis is a promising tech- nique for moving ankylosed teeth as it induces expansion and regeneration of soft tissues along with that of the bone. The most important advantage of distraction osteogenesis is bringing the clinical crown, incisal edge, and gingival margin into their appropriate position relative to the neigh- boring teeth (Razdolsky et al., 2004; Susami et al., 2006). Management of ankylosed teeth with distraction osteogen- esis can be performed with orthodontic tooth-borne dis- tractors or internal bone-supported screw distracters, followed by leveling with archwires (Isaacson et al., 2001; Kinzinger et al., 2003; Razdolsky et al., 2004; Kofod et al., 2005; Alcan, 2006) (Figure 16.17). Because of the bulky nature and cost factors along with the difficulty in place- ment of distraction devices, Dolanmaz et al. (2010) pro- posed conventional orthodontic treatment mechanics instead of additional devices.

More than 20% of children experience damage to their permanent dentition by 14 years of age and many trauma- tized permanent incisors are candidates for orthodontic therapy. Bauss et al. (2008) found that previously trauma- tized maxillary incisors with severe periodontal injuries were more susceptible to pulp necrosis during orthodontic intrusion than non-traumatized teeth. Impaired pulpal blood flow during orthodontic intrusion, with reduced capacity of the apical vessels, has been suggested as an explanation for the significantly increased rate of pulp necrosis in teeth with a history of trauma.

Immediate post-orthodontic period, and the long-term retention requirements for avoiding relapse

After the completion of orthodontic treatment, the ortho- dontist should evaluate in detail the oral hard and soft tissues for any iatrogenically induced pathologies. If any finding justifies seeking advice from medical or dental spe- cialists, a prompt referral should be made.

Debonding reduces or eliminates the cariogenic poten- tial and increases accessibility of mechanical cleaning. However, resin remnants may present a potential risk for plaque accumulation on the posterior and mandibular teeth where brackets are bonded close to the gingival margin (Fjeld and Ogaard, 2006). Any WSLs that have developed might reduce to some extent, depending on the severity of the lesions, due to the continuous wear caused by tooth brushing rather than due to remineralization after debonding (Artun and Thylstrup, 1986). Willmot (2004) reported a rapid reduction in size in most cases during the first 12 weeks after appliance removal, with little reduction observed after 26 weeks. A 'remineralizing therapy' should follow two fundamental principles:

- The presence of the dental biofilm should be removed with tooth brushing

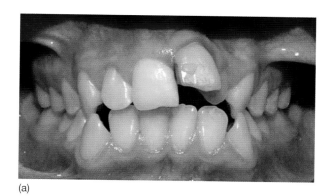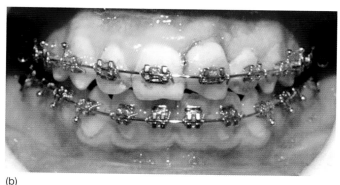

(a) (b)

Figure 16.17 Treatment of ankylosis with osteotomy and orthodontic mechanics. (a) Before treatment (ankylosed maxillary central incisor 4 years after reimplantation). (b) Alignment following osteotomy and orthodontic mechanics over a period of 4 weeks.

- Fluoride should be prescribed either to arrest existing lesions or to reduce the progression of new lesions (Kudiyirickal and Ivancakova, 2008).

Natural remineralization produces greater resistance to further dissolution as the mineral components are replaced with a less soluble substance that may have larger crystal size (Silverstone, 1983). Applying high concentrations of fluoride to WSLs may seem to be the best method for remineralization; however, a high fluoride concentration may immediately remineralize the most superficial layer of enamel, leaving the deeper enamel crystals relatively unaffected (Bishara and Ostby, 2008). To avoid this problem, low-dose fluoride applications have been recommended to enhance subsurface remineralization. A 50 ppm fluoride mouth rinse was shown to be more efficacious with regard to remineralization than a control solution or a regular mouth rinse containing 250 ppm fluoride (Linton, 1996). These arrested lesions may persist lifelong, keeping their white color or they may take up exogenous stains from foods, with a change in color to yellowish to dark brown. Acid etching of fluoride-treated lesions increases the surface porosity and facilitates remineralization of the lesion by oral fluids (Hicks et al., 1984).

Casein phosphopeptide or amorphous calcium phosphate (CPP-ACP) – a product derived from milk casein – is capable of being absorbed through the enamel surface (Reynolds, 1987). CPP-ACP is a delivering system that allows freely available calcium and phosphate ions to attach to enamel and re-form into calcium phosphate crystals. The free calcium and phosphate ions move out from CPP-ACP and into the enamel rods and free themselves to form apatite crystals (Reynolds, 1997). A number of different media have been developed to deliver CPP-ACP, including a water-based mousse, a topical cream, chewing gum, mouth rinses, and sugar-free lozenges. Studies of the effects of CPP-ACP have shown promising dose-related increases in enamel remineralization in demineralized lesions (Reynolds et al., 2003; Sudjalim et al., 2006). The addition of fluoride to this paste should further enhance the precipitation of this mineral into subsurface incipient lesions (Donly and Sasa, 2008). The use of sugar-free gums, such as xylitol, for their salivary stimulation effects has been recommended after the removal of fixed orthodontic appliances, although as yet there is a lack of quantitative data to help evaluate whether the effect is clinically beneficial (Willmot, 2008).

Caries infiltration is an alternative, and promising, therapeutic approach for preventing further progression of enamel lesions that are not expected to remineralize or arrest with noninvasive measures. This treatment aims to occlude the microporosities within the lesion by infiltration with low-viscosity light-curing resins that have been optimized for rapid penetration into the porous enamel (infiltrants). In contrast to fissure sealing, where the diffusion barrier is placed on the top of the lesion surface, the infiltration technique aims to create the diffusion barrier within the lesion, by replacing lost mineral with resin (Paris et al., 2007). After surface conditioning using hydrochloric acid (HCl) gel, a resin infiltrant is applied on top of the lesion (Meyer-Lueckel et al., 2007). The resin penetrates into the lesion body, driven by the capillary forces, and excess material is removed from the surface before the resin is light cured (Meyer-Lueckel and Paris, 2008). A positive 'side' effect of resin infiltration is that the WSLs lose their whitish appearance when their microporosities are filled with the resin, and look similar to sound enamel. Thus, this treatment may be used not only to arrest enamel lesions but also to improve the esthetic appearance of buccal white spots (Paris and Meyer-Lueckel, 2009). In orthodontic patients with WSLs, the best results are achieved if the infiltration treatment is started shortly after debonding, targeting the relatively active lesions. With regard to possible side effects, a short contact time with HCl does not cause any considerable alterations in the gingiva, although exposures of 30 seconds or more might evoke ulceration (Croll et al., 1990). It has been argued that irrespective of the seal, bacteria trapped in the apical end of the lesion could trigger the caries process. However, there is good evidence that entrapped bacteria are not harmful if the lesion has been properly sealed (Kidd, 2004).

Microabrasion, whose use has been advocated for the removal of post-orthodontic demineralized white lesions, is merely the application of an acidic and abrasive compound on the surface of the enamel for the removal of superficial, noncarious enamel defects (Croll and Bullock, 1994; Croll and Helpin, 2000). Research indicates that a 1-minute application of a commercially available microabrasion compound will remove 12 μm on the first application and 26 μm on subsequent applications, leaving a highly polished enamel surface (Waggoner et al., 1989). This phenomenon of less removal of enamel on the first application than on subsequent applications is due to the fluoride-rich surface enamel. Following microabrasion, a 4-minute, 2% sodium fluoride treatment is recommended. Only a few quantitative studies have assessed the success of the microabrasion technique in improving the cosmetic appearance of post-orthodontic, demineralized enamel lesions. If the outcome is found to be unsatisfactory, vital tooth bleaching can be considered as the next step, which is a treatment that camouflages mild and moderate fluorosis or WSLs by whitening the surrounding enamel surfaces.

The last step in meeting the esthetic objectives of the patient and the clinician involves the placement of composite restorations or ceramic veneers. The latter treatment requires the removal of sound tooth structure and is typically more costly. The patient and the family should be informed about the damages versus the benefits and the duration of the operative interventions, with an emphasis on the sacrifice of sound tooth structure. However, this option might be the most successful option in addressing the esthetic concerns of the patient in severely compromising situations (Bishara and Ostby, 2008).

The caries risk does not diminish after debonding. Precautions, including proper diet and oral hygiene maintenance, should continue because bonded retainers might also provoke a cariogenic challenge. After debonding, it is advisable to test the vitality of the teeth. Only a few studies have evaluated the long-term vitality of orthodontically treated teeth. Although pulpal changes such as root canal obliteration and loss of tooth vitality have been observed in some patients, Popp et al. (1992) found no differences in pulpal changes in patients 5 years out of retention and in untreated controls.

Conclusion

In a beauty-addicted society, where a pleasing smile serves as a powerful weapon, the demand for orthodontic treatment is increasing. Treating uncomplicated, caries-free adolescent patients with good oral hygiene is every clinician's dream, but this is not always the case for several reasons, such as a requirement for complex restorative procedures, trauma that occurred before the onset of orthodontic treatment, or complications evolving during or at the end of mechanotherapy. The management of these problems often requires interactive collaboration between orthodontic, endodontic and restorative dentistry specialists. In this situation, the orthodontist should assume the leading role as coordinator of the various treatment phases, thus optimizing the outcome by minimizing the risks. By forming close cooperative links between the different disciplines the ultimate goal of a healthy, esthetic and functional oral rehabilitation can be attained. Each of these specialties is constantly advancing and improving due to ongoing research in the biological and physical sciences. Therefore, having thorough knowledge about contemporary restorative and endodontic treatment approaches (which was the main thrust of this chapter) is a must for an orthodontist. By becoming familiar with these developments, and interacting with other experts, orthodontists can enhance the quality of orthodontic care, and preserve the favorable outcome of the interactive effort for a long time.

References

Abi-Ramia LBP, Stuani AS, Stuani AS, et al. (2010) Effects of low-level laser therapy and orthodontic tooth movement on dental pulps in rats. *Angle Orthodontist* 80: 116–22.

Ahlberg K, Bystedt H, Eliasson S, et al. (1983) Long-term evaluation of autotransplanted maxillary canines with completed root formation. *Acta Odontologica Scandinavia* 41: 23–31.

Alcan T (2006) A miniature tooth-borne distractor for the alignment of ankylosed teeth. *Angle Orthodontist* 76: 77–83.

Amemiya K, Kaneko Y, Muramatsu T, et al. (2003) Pulp cell responses during hypoxia and reoxygenation in vitro. *European Journal of Oral Sciences* 111: 332–8.

American Academy of Pediatric Dentistry (2004) Clinical guideline on management of acute dental trauma. *Pediatric Dentistry* 26: 120–7.

Andersson L (2007) Tooth avulsion and replantation. *Dental Traumatology* 23: 129.

Andreasen FM, Andreasen JO, Tsukiboshi M (2007) Examination and diagnosis of dental injuries. In: JO Andreasen, FM Andreasen, L Andersson (eds) *Textbook and Color Atlas of Traumatic Injuries to the Teeth*. Oxford: Blackwell/Munksgaard, pp. 255–74.

Andreasen JO (1992) *Atlas of Replantation and Transplantation of Teeth*. Philadelphia, PA: WB Saunders.

Andreasen JO, Andreasen FM (2000) *Essentials of Traumatic Injuries to the Teeth*, 2nd edn. Copenhagen: Munksgaard/Mosby, pp. 9–154.

Andreasen JO, Andreasen FM (2007) Avulsions. In: JO Andreasen, FM Andreasen, L Andersson (eds) *Textbook and Color Atlas of Traumatic Injuries to the Teeth*. Oxford: Blackwell/Munksgaard, pp. 444–80.

Andreasen JO, Hjorting-Hansen E (1966) Replantation of teeth. I. Radiographic and clinical study of 110 human teeth replanted after accidental loss. *Acta Odontologica Scandinavia* 24: 263–86.

Andreasen JO, Borum MK, Jacobsen HL, et al. (1995a) Replantation of 400 avulsed permanent incisors. 2. Factors related to pulpal healing. *Endodontics and Dental Traumatology* 11: 59–68.

Andreasen JO, Borum MK, Jacobsen HL, et al. (1995b) Replantation of 400 avulsed permanent incisors. 1. Diagnosis of healing complications. *Endodontics and Dental Traumatology* 11: 51–8.

Andreasen JO, Farik B, Munksgaard EC (2002) Long-term calcium hydroxide as a root canal dressing may increase risk of root fracture. *Dental Traumatology* 18: 134–7.

Andreasen JO, Munksgaard EC, Bakland LK (2006) Comparison of fracture resistance in root canals of immature sheep teeth after filling with calcium hydroxide or MTA. *Dental Traumatology* 22: 154–6.

Andreasen JO, Schwartz O, Kofoed T, et al. (2009) Transplantation of premolars as an approach for replacing avulsed teeth. *Pediatric Dentistry* 31: 129–32.

Anstendig H, Kronman J (1972) A histologic study of pulpal reaction to orthodontic tooth movement in dogs. *Angle Orthodontist* 42: 50–5.

Anthony DR (1986) Apexification during active orthodontic movement. *Journal of Endodontics* 12: 419–21.

Arhun N, Arman A, Ungor M, et al. (2006a) A conservative multidisciplinary approach for improved aesthetic results with traumatised anterior teeth. *British Dental Journal* 201: 509–12.

Arhun N, Arman N, Çehreli SB, et al. (2006b) Microleakage beneath metal and ceramic brackets bonded with a conventional and an antibacterial adhesive system. *Angle Orthodontist* 76: 1028–34.

Arıkan S, Arhun N, Arman A, et al. (2006) Microleakage beneath ceramic and metal brackets photopolymerized with LED or conventional light curing units. *Angle Orthodontist* 76: 1035–40.

Artun J, Brobakken BO (1986) Prevalence of carious white spots after orthodontic treatment with multibonded appliances. *European Journal of Orthodontics* 8: 229–34.

Artun J, Thylstrup A (1986) Clinical and scanning electron microscopic study of surface changes of incipient caries lesions after debonding. *Scandinavian Journal of Dental Research* 94: 193–201.

Ashcraft MB, Southard KA, Tolley EA (1992) The effect of corticosteroid-induced osteoporosis on orthodontic tooth movement. *American Journal of Orthodontics and Dentofacial Orthopedics* 102: 310–19.

Baek SH, Plenk H Jr, Kim S (2005) Periapical tissue responses and cementum regeneration with amalgam, superEBA and MTA as root-end filling materials. *Journal of Endodontics* 31: 444–9.

Bauss O, Schwestka-Polly R, Kiliaridis S (2004) Influence of orthodontic derotation and extrusion on pulpal and periodontal condition of autotransplanted immature third molars. *American Journal of Orthodontics and Dentofacial Orthopedics* 125: 488–96.

Bauss O, Röhling J, Sadat-Khonsari R, et al. (2008) Influence of orthodontic intrusion on pulpal vitality of previously traumatized maxillary permanent incisors. *American Journal of Orthodontics and Dentofacial Orthopedics* 134: 12–17.

Baysal A, Uysal T, Usumez S (2007) Temperature rise in the pulp chamber during different stripping procedures. *Angle Orthodontist* 3: 478–82.

Becker A, Karnei-R'em RM (1992a) The effects of infraocclusion: Part 2. The type of movement of the adjacent teeth and their vertical development. *American Journal of Orthodontics and Dentofacial Orthopedics* 102: 302–9.

Becker A, Karnei-R'em RM (1992b) The effects of infraocclusion: Part 1. Tilting of the adjacent teeth and local space loss. *American Journal of Orthodontics Dentofacial Orthopedics* 102: 256–64.

Becker A, Karnei-R'em RM, Steigman S (1992) The effects of infraocclusion: Part 3. Dental arch length and the midline. *American Journal of Orthodontics and Dentofacial Orthopedics* 102: 427–33.

Benson PE, Parkin N, Millett DT, et al. (2004) Fluorides for the prevention of white spots on teeth during fixed brace treatment. *Cochrane Database Systematic Reviews* 3: CD003809.

Berggreen E, Heyeraas KJ (1999) The role of sensory neuropeptides and nitric oxide on pulpal blood flow and tissue pressure in the ferret. *Journal of Dental Research* 78: 1535–43.

Berglund L, Kurol J, Kvint S (1996) Orthodontic pre-treatment prior to autotransplantation of palatally impacted maxillary canines: case reports on a new approach. *European Journal of Orthodontics* 18: 449–56.

Bishara SE, Ostby AW (2008) White spot lesions: formation, prevention and treatment. *Seminars in Orthodontics* 14: 174–82.

Bishara SE, Ostby AW, Laffoon J, et al. (2007) Shear bond strength comparison of two adhesive systems following thermocycling: a new self-etch primer and resin modified glass ionomer. *Angle Orthodontist* 77: 337–41.

Boersma JG, van der Veen MH, Lagerweij MD, et al. (2005) Caries prevalence measured with QLF after treatment with fixed orthodontic appliances: influencing factors. *Caries Research* 39: 41–7.

Borum MK, Andreasen JO (2001) Therapeutic and economic implications of traumatic dental injuries in Denmark: an estimate based on 7549 patients treated at a major trauma centre. *International Journal of Pediatric Dentistry* 11: 249–58.

Boyd RL, Chun YS (1994) Eighteen month evaluation of the effects of a 0.4% stannous fluoride gel on gingivitis in orthodontic patients. *American Journal of Orthodontics and Dentofacial Orthopedics* 105: 35–41.

Brezniak N, Wasserstein A (2002) Orthodontically induced inflammatory root resorption. Part II: The clinical aspects. *Angle Orthodontist* 72: 180–4.

Briggs PF, Scott BJ (1997) Evidence based dentistry; endodontic failure – now should it be managed? *British Dental Journal* 183: 159–64.

Burden DJ (1995) An investigation of the association between overjet size, lip coverage, and traumatic injury to maxillary incisors. *European Journal of Orthodontics* 17: 513–17.

Butcher EO, Taylor AC (1951) The effects of denervation and ischemia upon the teeth of the monkey. *Journal of Dental Research* 30: 265–75.

Büyükyılmaz T, Tangugsorn V, Ogaard B, et al. (1994) The effect of titanium tetrafluoride (TiF4) application around orthodontic brackets. *American Journal of orthodontics and Dentofacial Orthopedics* 105: 293–6.

Cengiz SB, Kocadereli I, Gungor HC, et al. (2005) Adhesive fragment reattachment after orthodontic extrusion: a case report. *Dental Traumatology* 21: 60–4.

Cengiz SB, Stephan Atac A, Cehreli ZC (2006) Biomechanical effects of splint types on traumatized tooth: a photoelastic stress analysis. *Dental Traumatology* 22: 133–8.

Chadwick BL, Roy J, Knox J, et al. (2005) The effect of topical fluorides on decalcification in patients with fixed orthodontic appliances: a systematic review. *American Journal of Orthodontics and Dentofacial Orthopedics* 128: 601–6.

Chatterjee R, Kleinberg I (1979) Effect of orthodontic band placement on the chemical composition of human incisor plaque. *Archives of Oral Biology* 24: 97–100.

Chaushu S, Shapira J, Heling I, et al. (2004a) Emergency orthodontic treatment after the traumatic intrusive luxation of maxillary incisors. *American Journal of Orthodontics and Dentofacial Orthopedics* 126: 162–72.

Chaushu S, Becker A, Chaushu G (2004b) Orthosurgical treatment with lingual orthodontics of an infraoccluded maxillary first molar in an adult. *American Journal of Orthodontics and Dentofacial Orthopedics* 125: 379–87.

Coyle M, Toner M, Barry H (2006) Multiple teeth showing invasive cervical resorption-an entitiy with little known histologic features. *Journal of Oral Pathology and Medicine* 35: 55–7.

Croll TP, Bullock GA (1994) Enamel microabrasion for removal of smooth surface decalcification lesions. *Journal of Clinical Orthodontics* 28: 365–70.

Croll TP, Helpin ML (2000) Enamel microabrasion: a new approach. *Journal of Esthetic Dentistry* 12: 64–71.

Croll TP, Killian CM, Miller AS (1990) Effect of enamel microabrasion compound on human gingiva: report of a case. *Quintessence International* 21: 959–63.

Cvek M (1978) A clinical report on partial pulpotomy and capping with calcium hydroxide in permanent incisors with complicated crown fracture. *Journal of Endodontics* 4: 232–7.

Cvek M (1992) Prognosis of luxated non-vital maxillary incisors treated with calcium hydroxide and filled with gutta-percha. A retrospective clinical study. *Endodontics and Dental Traumatology* 8: 45–55.

Davidovitch Z (1996) Etiologic factors in force-induced root resorption. In: Z Davidovitch, LA Norton (eds) *Biological Mechanisms of Tooth Movement and Craniofacial Adaptation*. Boston, MA: Harvard Society for the Advancement of Orthodontics, pp. 349–55.

Davidovitch Z, Lee YJ, Counts AL, et al. (2000) The immune system possibly modulates orthodontic root resorption. In: Z Davidovitch, J Mah (eds) *Biological Mechanisms of Tooth Movement and Craniofacial Adaptation*. Boston, MA: Harvard Society for the Advancement of Orthodontics, pp. 207–17.

de Alencar AH, Lustosa-Pereira A, de Sousa HA, et al. (2007) Intrusive luxation: a case report. *Dental Traumatology* 23: 307–12.

De Angelis V, Davidovitch Z (2009) Biologically and clinically, what are optimal orthodontic forces and how are they applied in selective common malocclusions? In: V Krishnan, Z Davidovitch (eds) *Biological Mechanisms of Tooth Movement*. Oxford: Wiley-Blackwell, pp. 180–200.

Delivanis HP, Gauer GJ (1980) Incidence of canal calcification in the orthodontic patient. *American Journal of Orthodontics* 82: 58–61.

Derks A, Katsaros C, Frencken JE, et al. (2004) Caries inhibiting effect of fluoride measures during orthodontic treatment with fixed appliances: a systematic review. *Caries Research* 38: 413–20.

Desai S, Chandler N (2009) The restoration of permanent immature anterior teeth, root filled using MTA: a review. *Journal of Dentistry* 37: 652–7.

Dolanmaz D, Karaman AI, Pampu AA, et al. (2010) Orthodontic treatment of an ankylosed maxillary central incisor through osteogenic distraction. *Angle Orthodontist* 80: 391–5.

Donly KJ, Sasa IS (2008) Potential remineralization of postorthodontic demineralized enamel and the use of enamel microabrasion and bleaching for esthetics. *Seminars in Orthodontics* 14: 220–5.

Dougherty HL (1968) The effect of mechanical forces upon the mandibular buccal segments during orthodontic treatment. Part II. *American Journal of Orthodontics* 54: 83–103.

Dudic A, Giannopoulou C, Leuzinger M, et al. (2009) Detection of apical root resorption after orthodontic treatment by using panoramic radiography and cone-beam computed tomography of super-high resolution. *American Journal of Orthodontics and Dentofacial Orthopedics* 135: 434–7.

Eliasson S, Laftman AC, Strindberg L (1988) Autotransplanted teeth with early-stage endodontic treatment: a radiographic evaluation. *Oral Surgery Oral Medicine Oral Pathology* 65: 598–603.

Eminkahyagil N, Arman A, Çetinşahin A, et al. (2006) Effect of resin-removal methods on enamel and shear bond strength of rebonded brackets. *Angle Orthodontist* 76: 314–21.

Erdemir A, Ungor M, Erdemir EO (2005) Orthodontic movement of a horizontally fractured tooth: a case report. *Dental Traumatology* 21: 160–4.

Ericson S, Kurol J (2000) Resorption of incisors after ectopic eruption of maxillary canines. A CT study. *Angle Orthodontist* 70: 415–23.

Eriksen HM, Kirkevang LL, Petersson K (2002) Endodontic epidemiology and treatment outcome: general considerations. *Endodontic Topics* 2: 1–9.

Felippe WT, Felippe MC, Rocha MJ (2006) The effect of mineral trioxide aggregate on the apexification and periapical healing of teeth with incomplete root formation. *International Endodontic Journal* 39: 2–9.

Fjeld M, Ogaard B (2006) Scanning electron microscopic evaluation of enamel surfaces exposed to 3 orthodontic bonding systems. *American Journal of Orthodontics and Dentofacial Orthopedics* 130: 575–81.

Flores MT (2002) Traumatic injuries in the primary dentition. *Dental Traumatology* 18: 287–98.

Flores MT, Andersson L, Andreasen JO, et al. (2007) Guidelines for the management of traumatic dental injuries. I. Fractures and luxations of permanent teeth. *Dental Traumatology* 23: 66–71.

Forsberg CM, Tedestam G (1993) Etiological and predisposing factors related to traumatic injuries to permanent teeth. *Swedish Dental Journal* 17: 183–90.

Frank AL (1981) External-internal progressive resorption and its non-surgical correction. *Journal of Endodontics* 7: 473–6.

Frank AL, Blakland LK (1987) Nonendodontic therapy for supra osseous extra-canal invasive resorption. *Journal of Endodontics* 13: 348–87.

Frank AL, Torabinejad M (1998) Diagnosis and treatment of extracanal invasive resorption. *Journal of Endodontics* 24: 500–4.

Frazier-Bowers SA, Simmons D, Wright JT, et al. (2010) Primary failure of eruption and PTH1R: the importance of a genetic diagnosis for orthodontic treatment planning. *American Journal of Orthodontics and Dentofacial Orthopedics* 137: 160, e1–7.

Fujita K, Kanno Z, Otsubo K, et al. (2008) Autotransplantation combined with orthodontic treatment in adult patients. *Orthodontic Waves* 67: 128–34.

Fuks AB, Cosack A, Klein H, et al. (1987) Partial pulpotomy as a treatment alternative for exposed pulps in crown-fractured permanent incisors. *Endodontics and Dental Traumatology* 3: 100–2.

Fukui T, Choi YB, Yamaguchi H, et al. (2009) Treatment of a horizontal open bite with an invisible multiloop appliance in a girl with tooth trauma. *American Journal of Orthodontics and Dentofacial Orthopedics* 136: 596–606.

Gault PC, Warocquier-Clerout R (2002) Tooth auto-transplantation with double periodontal ligament stimulation to replace periodontally compromised teeth. *Journal of Periodontology* 73: 575–83.

Gholston L, Mattison G (1983) An endodontic-orthodontic technique for esthetic stabilization of externally resorbed teeth. *American Journal of Orthodontics* 83: 435–40.

Gladwin M, Bagby M (2004) *Clinical Aspects of Dental Materials Theory, Practice and Cases*. Baltimore, MD: Lippincott Williams & Wilkins.

Glendor U, Marcenes W, Andreasen JO (2007) Classification, Epidemiology and Etiology. In: JO Andreasen, FM Andreasen (eds) *Textbook and Color Atlas of Traumatic Injuries to the teeth*. Oxford: Blackwell/Munksgaard, pp. 217–44.

Goldson L, Henrikson CO (1975) Root resorption during Begg treatment. A longitudinal roentgenologic study. *American Journal of Orthodontics* 68: 55–66.

Gorelick L, Geiger AM, Gwinnett AJ (1982) Incidence of white spot formation after bonding and banding. *American Journal of Orthodontics* 81: 93–8.

Gregg TA, Boyd DH (1998) Treatment of avulsed permanent teeth in children. UK National Guidelines in Paediatric Dentistry. Royal College of Surgeons, Faculty of Dental Surgery. *International Journal of Pediatric Dentistry* 8: 75–81.

Gulabivala K, Searson LJ (1995) Clinical diagnosis of internal resorption: an exception to the rule. *International Endodontic Journal* 28: 255–60.

Gulsahi A, Gulsahi K, Ungor M (2007) Invasive cervical resorption: clinical and radiological diagnosis and treatment of 3 cases. *Oral Surgery Oral Medicine Oral Pathology Oral Radiology and Endodontics* 103: e65–72.

Gwinnett AJ, Ceen F (1979) Plaque distribution on bonded brackets: a scanning microscope study. *American Journal of Orthodontics* 75: 667–77.

Hamersky P, Weimar AD, Taintor J (1980) The effect of orthodontic force application on the pulpal tissue respiration rate in the human premolar. *American Journal of Orthodontics* 77: 368–78.

Hamilton RS, Gutmann JL (1999) Endodontic-orthodontic relationships: a review of integrated treatment planning challenges. *International Endodontic Journal* 32: 343–60.

Heide S (1991) The effect of pulp capping and pulpotomy on hard tissue bridges of contaminated pulps. *International Endodontic Journal* 24: 126–34.

Heithersay GS (1999) Clinical, radiologic, and histopathologic features of invasive cervical resorption. *Quintessence International* 30: 27–37.

Heithersay GS (2004) Invasive cervical resorption. *Endodontic Topics* 7: 73–92.

Heithersay GS, Moule AJ (1982) Anterior subgingival fractures: a review of treatment alternatives. *Australian Dental Journal* 27: 368–76.

Hicks MJ, Silverstone LM, Flaitz CM (1984) A scanning electron microscopic and polarized light study of acid etching of caries like lesions in human enamel treated with sodium fluoride in vitro. *Archives of Oral Biology* 29: 765–72.

Hicks MJ, Flaitz CM, Westerman GH, et al. (1995) Enamel caries initiation and progression following low fluence (energy) argon laser and fluoride treatment. *Journal of Clinical Pediatric Dentistry* 20: 9–13.

Hinckfuss SE, Messer LB (2009) An evidence-based assessment of the clinical guidelines for replanted avulsed teeth. Part I: Timing of pulp extirpation. *Dental Traumatology* 25: 32–42.

Hovland EJ (1992) Horizontal root fractures. Treatment and repair. *Dental Clinics of North America* 36: 509–25.

Hovland EJ, Dumsha TC, Gutmann JL (1983) Orthodontic movement of a horizontal root fractured tooth. *British Journal of Orthodontics* 10: 32–3.

Huang JC, King G, Kapila S (2005) Biologic mechanisms in orthodontic tooth movement. In: R Nanda (ed.) *Biomechanics and Esthetic Strategies in Clinical Orthodontics*. Elsevier, St Louis, MO, pp. 17–37.

Imazato S (2009) Bio-active restorative materials with antibacterial effects: new dimension of innovation in restorative dentistry. *Dental Materials Journal* 28: 11–19.

Ingber JS (1974) Forced eruption. I. A method of treating isolated one and two wall infrabony osseous defects-rationale and case report. *Journal of Periodontology* 45: 199–206.

Isaacson RJ, Strauss RA, Bridges-Poquis A, Peluso AR, Lindauer SJ (2001) Moving an ankylosed central incisor using orthodontics, surgery and distraction osteogenesis. *Angle Orthodontist* 71: 411–18.

Kayhan F, Küçükkeleş N, Demirel D (2000) A histologic and histomorphometric evaluation of pulpal reactions following rapid palatal expansion. *American Journal of Orthodontics and Dentofacial Orthopedics* 117: 465–73.

Kenny DJ, Barrett EJ (2001) Recent developments in dental traumatology. *Pediatric Dentistry* 23: 464–8.

Kerezoudis NP, Fried K, Olgart L (1995) Haemodynamic and immunohistochemical studies of rat incisor pulp after denervation and subsequent re-innervation. *Archives of Oral Biology* 40: 815–23.

Kidd EA (2004) How 'clean' must a cavity be before restoration? *Caries Research* 38: 305–13.

Kim E, Kim KD, Roh BD, et al. (2003) Computed tomography as a diagnostic aid for extracanal invasive resorption. *Journal of Endodontics* 29: 463–5.

Kinzinger GS, Jänicke S, Riediger D, et al. (2003) Orthodontic fine adjustment after vertical callus distraction of an ankylosed incisor using the floating bone concept. *American Journal of Orthodontics and Dentofacial Orthopedics* 124: 582–90.

Kling M, Cvek M, Mejare I (1986) Rate and predictability of pulp revascularization in therapeutically reimplanted permanent incisors. *Endodontics and Dental Traumatology* 2: 83–9.

Kocak MM, Ozcan S, Kocak S, et al. (2009) Comparison of the efficacy of three different mouthrinse solutions in decreasing the level of S. mutans in saliva. *European Journal of Dentistry* 3: 57–61.

Kofod T, Würtz V, Melsen B (2005) Treatment of an ankylosed central incisor by single tooth dento-osseous osteotomy and a simple distraction device. *American Journal of Orthodontics and Dentofacial Orthopedics* 127: 72–80.

Kokich VG (2002) The role of orthodontics as an adjunct to periodontal therapy. In: MG Newman, HH Takei, FA Carranza (eds) *Carranza's Clinical Periodontology*. Philadelphia, PA: WB Saunders, pp. 704–18.

Krishnan V, Davidovitch Z (2009) *Biologic Mechanisms of Tooth Movement*, 1st edn. London: Wiley-Blackwell.

Kudiyirickal MG, Ivancaková R (2008) Early enamel lesion part II. Histomorphology and prevention. *Acta Medica* 51: 151–6.

Küçükkeleş N, Okar I (1994) RME sonucu kök yüzeyinde oluşan rezorpsiyon alanlarının SEM ve ışık mikroskobu ile incelenmesi. *Journal of Marmara University* 2: 404–8.

Kurol J (2002) Early treatment of tooth-eruption disturbances. *American Journal of Orthodontics and Dentofacial Orthopedics* 121: 588–91.

Kurol J (2006) Impacted and ankylosed teeth: why, when, and how to intervene. *American Journal of Orthodontics and Dentofacial Orthopedics* 129: 86–90.

Kurol J, Koch G (1985) The effect of extraction of infraoccluded deciduous molars: A longitudinal study. *American Journal of Orthodontics* 87: 46–55.

Kurol J, Thilander B (1984) Infraocclusion of primary molars with aplasia of the permanent successor. A longitudinal study. *Angle Orthodontist* 54: 283–94.

Kvinnsland S, Heyeraas K, Ofjord ES (1989). Effect of experimental tooth movement on periodontal and pulpal blood flow. *European Journal of Orthodontics* 11: 200–5.

Kvint S, Lindsten R, Magnusson A, et al. (2010) Autotransplantation of teeth in 215 patients. *Angle Orthodontist* 80: 446–51.

Lagerström L, Kristerson L (1986) Influence of orthodontic treatment on root development of autotransplanted premolars. *American Journal of Orthodontics* 89: 146–50.

Larsen MJ (1990) Chemical events during tooth dissolution. *Journal of Dental Research* 69(Spec): 575–80.

Lee JY, Vann WF Jr, Sigurdsson A (2001) Management of avulsed permanent incisors: a decision analysis based on changing concepts. *Pediatric Dentistry* 23: 357–60.

Lee KJ, Joo E, Yu HS, et al. (2009) Restoration of an alveolar bone defect caused by an ankylosed mandibular molar by root movement of the adjacent tooth with miniscrew implants. *American Journal of Orthodontics and Dentofacial Orthopedics* 136: 440–9.

Leone A, Mauro A, Spatola GF, et al. (2009) MMP-2, MMP-9, and INOS expression in human dental pulp subjected to orthodontic traction. *Angle Orthodontist* 79: 1119–25.

Levander E, Malmgren O (1988) Evaluation of the risk of root resorption during orthodontic treatment: a study of upper incisors. *European Journal of Orthodontics* 10: 30–8.

Lim WH, Kim HJ, Chun YS (2008) Treatment of ankylosed mandibular first permanent molar. *American Journal of Orthodontics and Dentofacial Orthopedics* 133: 95–101.

Lima TJ, Ribeiro CCC, Tenuta LM, et al. (2008) Low fluoride dentifrice and caries lesions control in children with different caries experience: a randomized clinical trial. *Caries Research* 42: 46–50.

Linge L, Linge BO (1991) Patients characteristics and treatment variables associated with apical root resorption during orthodontic treatment. *American Journal of Orthodontics and Dentofacial Orthopedics* 99: 35–43.

Linton LJ (1996) Quantitative measurements of remineralization of incipient caries. *American Journal of Orthodontics and Dentofacial Orthopedics* 104: 590–7.

Liu L, Igarashi K, Haruyama N, et al. (2004) Effects of local administration of clodronate on orthodontic tooth movement and root resorption in rats. *European Journal of Orthodontics* 26: 469–73.

Lundberg T, Isaksson S (1996) A clinical follow-up study of 278 autotransplanted teeth. *British Journal of Oral and Maxillofacial Surgery* 34: 181–5.

Lustmann J, Ehrlich J (1974) Deep external resorption: treatment by combined endodontic and surgical approach. A report of 2 cases. *Journal of Dentistry* 24: 203–6.

Ma T, Marangoni RD, Flint W (1997) In vitro comparison of debonding force and intrapulpal temperature changes during ceramic orthodontic bracket removal using a carbondioxide laser. *American Journal of Orthodontics and Dentofacial Orthopedics* 111: 203–10.

Mackie IC, Warren VN (1988) Dental trauma: 3 splinting, displacement injuries, and root fracture of immature permanent incisor teeth. *Dental Update* 15: 332–5.

Mah J, Prasad N (2004) Dentine phosphoproteins in gingival crevicular fluid during root resorption. *European Journal of Orthodontics* 26: 25–30.

Malmgren B, Cvek M, Lundberg M, et al. (1984) Surgical treatment of ankylosed and infrapositioned reimplanted incisors in adolescents. *Scandinavian Journal of Dental Research* 92: 391–9.

Malmgren O, Levander E (2004) Minimizing orthodontically induced root resorption. In: TM Graber, T Eliades, AE Athanasiou (eds) *Risk Management in Orthodontics. Experts' guide to malpractice*. Hanover Park, IL. Quintessence.

Malmgren O, Goldson L, Hill C, et al. (1982) Root resorption after orthodontic treatment of traumatized teeth. *American Journal of Orthodontics* 82: 487–91.

Malmgren O, Malmgren B, Goldson L (1994) Orthodontic management of the traumatized dentition. In: JO Andreasen, FM Andreasen (eds) *Textbook and Color Atlas of Traumatic Injuries to the teeth*. Copenhagen: Munksgaard, pp. 587–633.

McCourt JW, Cooley RL, Huddleston AM (1990) Fluoride release from fluoride containing liners/bases. *Quintessence International* 21: 41–5.

McDonald F, Pitt Ford TR (1994) Blood flow changes in permanent maxillary canines during retraction. *European Journal of Orthodontics* 16: 1–9.

McNab S, Battistutta D, Taverne A, et al. (1999) External apical root resorption of posterior teeth in asthmatics after orthodontic treatment. *American Journal of Orthodontics and Dentofacial Orthopedics* 116: 545–51.

Medeiros PJ, Bezerra AR (1997) Treatment of an ankylosed central incisor by single tooth dento-osseous osteotomy. *American Journal of Orthodontics and Dentofacial Orthopedics* 112: 496–501.

Medeiros RB, Mucha JN (2009) Immediate vs late orthodontic extrusion of traumatically intruded teeth. *Dental Traumatology* 25: 380–5.

Meyer-Lueckel H, Paris S (2008) Improved resin infiltration of natural caries lesions. *Journal of Dental Research* 87: 1112–16.

Meyer-Lueckel H, Paris S, Kielbassa AM (2007) Surface layer erosion of natural caries lesions with phosphoric and hydrochloric acid gels. *Caries Research* 41: 223–30.

Miguel JA, Almeida MA, Chevitarese O (1995) Clinical comparison between a glass ionomer cement and a composite for direct bonding of orthodontic brackets. *American Journal of Orthodontics and Dentofacial Orthopedics* 107: 484–7.

Miller JR, Mancl L, Arbuckle G, et al. (1996) A three year clinical trial using a glass ionomer cement for the bonding of orthodontic brackets. *Angle Orthodontist* 66: 309–12.

Mizrahi E (1982) Enamel demineralization following orthodontic treatment. *American Journal of Orthodontics* 82: 62–7.

Mohandesan H, Ravanmehr H, Valaei N (2007) A radiographic analysis of external apical root resorption of maxillary incisors during active orthodontic treatment. *European Journal of Orthodontics* 29: 134–9.

Mostafa YA, Iskander KG, El-Mangoury NH (1991) Iatrogenic pulpal reactions to orthodontic extrusion. *American Journal of Orthodontics and Dentofacial Orthopedics* 99: 30–4.

Moule AJ, Moule CA (2009) Minor traumatic injuries to the permanent dentition. *Dental Clinics of North America* 53: 639–59.

Mullally BH, Blakely D, Burden DJ (1995) Ankylosis: an orthodontic problem with a restorative solution. *British Dental Journal* 179: 426–9.

Nishimura K, Amano S, Nakao K, et al. (2009) Orthodontic treatment including autotransplantation of a mature tooth. *Angle Orthodontist* 79: 387–93.

Nixon CE, Saviano JA, King GJ, et al. (1993) Histomorphometric study of dental pulp during orthodontic tooth movement. *Journal of Endodontics* 19: 13–16.

O'Reilly MM, Featherstone JD (1987) Demineralization and remineralization around orthodontic appliances: an in vivo study. *American Journal of Orthodontics and Dentofacial Orthopedics* 92: 33–40.

Ogaard B (1989) Prevalence of white spot lesions in 19-year-olds. A study on untreated and orthodontically treated persons 5 years after treatment. *American Journal of Orthodontics and Dentofacial Orthopedics* 96: 423–7.

Ogaard B (1990) Effects of fluoride on caries development and progression in vivo. *Journal of Dental Research* 69(Spec): 813–19.

Ogaard B (2001) Oral microbiological changes, long term enamel alterations due to decalcification, and caries prophylactic aspects. In: WA Brantley, T Eliades (eds) *Orthodontic Materials. Scientific and Clinical Aspects*. Stuttgart: Thieme, pp. 123–42.

Ogaard B (2008) White spot lesions during orthodontic treatment: mechanisms and fluoride preventive aspects. *Seminars in Orthodontics* 14: 183–93.

Ogaard B, Gjermo P, Rolla G (1980) Plaque inhibiting effect in orthodontic patients of a dentifrice containing stannous fluoride. *American Journal of Orthodontics* 78: 266–72.

Ogaard B, Rolla G, Arends J (1988) Orthodontic appliances and enamel demineralization. Part I. Lesion development. *American Journal of Orthodontics and Dentofacial Orthopedics* 94: 68–73.

Ogaard B, Larsson E, Henriksson T, et al. (2001) Effects of combined application of antimicrobial and fluoride varnishes in orthodontic patients. *American Journal of orthodontics and Dentofacial Orthopedics* 120: 28–35.

Ogaard B, Bishara SE, Duschner H (2004) Enamel effects during bonding-debonding and treatment with fixed orthodontic appliances. In: TM Graber, T Eliades, AE Athanasiou (eds) *Risk Management in Orthodontics:*

Experts Guide to Malpractice. Hanover Park, IL: Quintessence Publishing, pp. 30–2.

Ogaard B, Alm AA, Larsson E, et al. (2006) A prospective randomized clinical study on the effects of an amine fluoride/stannous fluoride toothpaste/mouthrinse on plaque, gingivitis and initial caries lesion development in orthodontic patients. *European Journal of Orthodontics* 28: 8–12.

Op Heij DG, Opdebeeck H, Steenberghe DV, et al. (2006) Facial development, continuous tooth eruption and mesial drift as compromising factors for implant placement. *International Journal of Maxillofacial Implantology* 21: 867–78.

Oulis C, Vadiakas G, Siskos G (1996) Management of intrusive luxation injuries. *Endodontic and Dental Traumatology* 12: 113–19.

Owman-Moll P, Kurol J (1998) The early reparative process of orthodontically induced root resorption in adolescents – location and type of tissue. *European Journal of Orthodontics* 20: 727–32.

Paris S, Meyer-Lueckel H (2009) Masking of labial enamel white spot lesions by resin infiltration- a clinical report. *Quintessence International* 40: 713–18.

Paris S, Meyer-Lueckel H, Kielbassa AM (2007) Resin infiltration of natural caries lesions. *Journal of Dental Research* 86: 662–6.

Paulsen HU, Andreasen JO, Schwartz O (1995) Pulp and periodontal healing, root development and root resorption subsequent to transplantation and orthodontic rotation: A long-term study of autotransplanted premolars. *American Journal of Orthodontics and Dentofacial Orthopedics* 108: 630–40.

Perinetti G, Varvara G, Festa F, et al. (2004) Aspartate aminotransferase activity in pulp of orthodontically treated teeth. *American Journal of Orthodontics and Dentofacial Orthopedics* 125: 88–92.

Pohl Y, Filippi A, Kirschner H (2005) Results after replantation of avulsed permanent teeth. I. Endodontic considerations. *Dental Traumatology* 21: 80–92.

Poi WR, Manfrin TM, Holland R, et al. (2002) Repair characteristics of horizontal root fracture: a case report. *Dental Traumatology* 18: 98–102.

Polat O, Karaman AI (2005) Pain control during fixed orthodontic appliance therapy. *Angle Orthodontist* 75: 214–19.

Popp TW, Artun J, Linge L (1992) Pulpal response to orthodontic tooth movement in adolescents: a radiographic study. *American Journal of Orthodontics and Dentofacial Orthopedics* 101: 228–33.

Proffit WR (1986) *Contemporary Orthodontics*. St Louis, MO: Mosby, pp. 191–92, 408–11.

Proffit WR (2000) *Contemporary Orthodontics*. St. Louis, MO: Mosby-Year Book Inc., pp. 615–73.

Rafter M (2005) Apexification: a review. *Dental Traumatology* 21: 1–8.

Raghoebar GM, Boering G, Jansen HW, et al. (1989) Secondary retention of permanent molars: a histologic study. *Journal of Oral Pathology and Medicine* 18: 427–31.

Ram D, Cohenca N (2004) Therapeutic protocols for avulsed permanent teeth: review and clinical update. *Pediatric Dentistry* 26: 251–5.

Rana MW, Pothisiri V, Killiany DM, et al. (2001). Detection of apoptosis during orthodontic tooth movement in rats. *American Journal of Orthodontics and Dentofacial Orthopedics* 119: 516–21.

Razdolsky Y, El-Bialy TH, Dessner S, et al. (2004) Movement of ankylosed permanent teeth with a distraction device. *Journal of Clinical Orthodontics* 38: 612–20.

Reitan K (1964) Effects of force magnitude and direction of tooth movement on different alveolar bone types. *Angle Orthodontist* 34: 244–55.

Reitan K (1974) Initial tissue behavior during apical root resorption. *Angle Orthodontist* 44: 68–82.

Reitan K (1985) Biomechanical principles and reactions. In: TM Graber, BF Swain (eds) *Orthodontics: Current Principles and Techniques*. St Louis, MO: Mosby, pp. 101–92.

Remington DN, Joondeph DR, Artun J, et al. (1989) Long-term evaluation of root resorption occuring during orthodontic treatment. *American Journal of Orthodontics and Dentofacial Orthopedics* 96: 43–6.

Ren W, Yang L, Chen X, et al. (2000) The effect of fibrin sealant in dental pulp capping in experimental dogs. *West China Journal of Stomatology* 18: 380–2.

Reynolds EC (1987) The prevention of sub-surface demineralization of bovine enamel and change in plaque composition by casein in an intra-oral model. *Journal of Dental Research* 66: 1120–7.

Reynolds EC (1997) Remineralization of enamel subsurface lesions by casein phosphopeptide-stabilized calcium phosphate solutions. *Journal of Dental Research* 76: 1587–95.

Reynolds EC, Cai F, Shen P, et al. (2003) Retention and remineralization of enamel lesions by various forms of calcium in a mouthrinse or sugarfree chewing gum. *Journal of Dental Research* 82: 206–11.

Roberts WE (2000) Bone physiology of tooth movement, ankylosis, and osseointegration. *Seminars in Orthodontics* 6: 173–82.

Robertson A, Andreasen FM, Andreasen JO, et al. (2000) Long-term prognosis of crown-fractured permanent incisors. The effect of stage of root development and associated luxation injury. *International Journal of Paediatric Dentistry* 10: 191–9.

Robinson PP (1983) An electrophysiological study of the reinnervation of reimplanted and autotransplanted teeth in the cat. *Archives of Oral Biology* 28: 1139–47.

Rosenberg B, Murray PE, Namerow K (2007) The effect of calcium hydroxide root filling on dentin fracture strength. *Dental Traumatology* 23: 26–9.

Rygh P (1977) Orthodontic root resorption studied by electron microscopy. *Angle Orthodontist* 44: 1–16.

Sameshima GT, Asgarifar KO (2001) Assessment of root resorption and root shape: periapical vs panoramic films. *Angle Orthodontist* 71: 185–9.

Sano Y, Ikawa M, Sugawara J, et al. (2002) The effect of continuous intrusive force on human pulpal blood flow. *European Journal of Orthodontics* 24: 159–66.

Schwartz O, Rank CP (1986) Autotransplantation of cryopreserved tooth in connection with orthodontic treatment. *American Journal of Orthodontics and Dentofacial Orthopedics* 90: 67–72.

Schwartz O, Bergmann P, Klausen B (1985) Resorption of autotransplanted human teeth: a retrospective study of 291 transplantations over a period of 25 years. *International Endodontic Journal* 18: 119–31.

Shaw WC, O'Brien KD, Richmond S, et al. (1991) Quality control in orthodontics: risk/benefit considerations. *British Dental Journal* 170: 33–7.

Silverstone LM (1983) Remineralization and enamel caries: significance of fluoride and effect on crystal diameters. In: I Leach, WM Edgar (eds) *Demineralization and Remineralization of the Teeth*. Oxford: IRL Press, pp. 185–205.

Simon S, Rilliard F, Berdal A, et al. (2007) The use of mineral trioxide aggregate in one-visit apexification treatment: a prospective study. *International Endodontic Journal* 40: 186–97.

Skaare AB, Jacobsen I (2003) Dental injuries in Norwegians aged 7–18 years. *Dental Traumatology* 19: 67–71.

Skoglund A, Tronstad L, Wallenius K (1978) A microangiographic study of vascular changes in replanted and autotransplanted teeth of young dogs. *Oral Surgery Oral Medicine Oral Pathology* 45: 17–28.

Skoglund A, Hasselgren G, Tronstad L (1981) Oxidoreductase activity in the pulp of replanted and autotransplanted teeth in young dogs. *Oral Surgery Oral Medicine Oral Pathology* 52: 205–9.

Smidt A, Nuni E, Keinan D (2007) Invasive cervical resorption: treatment rationale with an interdisciplinary approach. *Journal of Endodontics* 33: 1383–7.

Spurrier SW, Hall SH, Joondeph DR, et al. (1990) A comparison of apical root resorption during orthodontic treatment in endodontically treated and vital teeth. *American Journal of Orthodontics and Dentofacial Orthopedics* 97: 130–4.

Steiner DR, West JD (1997) Orthodontic-endodontic treatment planning of traumatized teeth. *Seminars in Orthodontics* 3: 39–44.

Stenvik A, Mjör A (1970) Pulp and dentine reactions to experimental tooth intrusion. A histological study of the initial changes. *American Journal of Orthodontics* 57: 370–85.

Sudjalim TR, Woods MG, Manton DJ (2006) Prevention of white spot lesions in orthodontic practice; a contemporary review. *Australian Dental Journal* 51: 284–9.

Susami T, Matsuzaki M, Ogihara Y, et al. (2006) Segmental alveolar distraction for the correction of unilateral open-bite caused by multiple ankylosed teeth: a case report. *Journal of Orthodontics* 33: 153–9.

Swift EJ Jr (1989) Effects of glass ionomers on recurrent caries. *Operative Dentistry* 14: 40–3.

Talic NF, Evans C, Zaki AM (2006) Inhibition of orthodontically induced root resorption with echistatin, an RGD containing peptide. *American Journal of Orthodontics and Dentofacial Orthopedics* 129: 252–60.

Temmerman L, De Pauw GA, Beele H, et al. (2006) Tooth transplantation and cryopreservation: state of the art. *American Journal of Orthodontics and Dentofacial Orthopedics* 129: 691–5.

Ten Cate JM, van Loveren C (1999) Fluoride mechanisms. *Dental Clinics of North America* 43: 713–42.

Thomas S, Turner SR, Sandy JR (1998).Autotransplantation of teeth: is there a role? *British Journal of Orthodontics* 25: 275–82.

Thong YL, Messer HH, Siar CH, et al. (2001).Periodontal response to two intracanal medicaments in replanted monkey incisors. *Dental Traumatology* 17: 254–9.

Torabinejad M, Anderson P, Bader J, et al. (2007) Outcomes of root canal treatment and restoration, implant-supported single crowns, fixed partial dentures, and extraction without replacement: a systematic review. *Journal of Prosthetic Dentistry* 98: 285–311.

Travassos RM, Caldas Ade F, de Albuquerque DS (2003) Cohort study of endodontic therapy success. *Brazilian Dental Journal* 14: 109–13.

Trope M (2002) Root resorption due to dental trauma. *Endodontic Topics* 1: 79–100.

Turley PK, Crawford LB, Carrington KW (1987) Traumatically intruded teeth. *Angle Orthodontist* 57: 234–44.

Unsterseher R, Nieberg L, Weimar A, et al. (1987) The response of human pulp tissue after orthodontic force application. *American Journal of Orthodontics and Dentofacial Orthopedics* 92: 220–4.

Uysal T, Eldeniz AU, Usumez S, et al. (2005) Thermal changes in the pulp chamber during different adhesive clean-up procedures. *Angle Orthodontist* 75: 220–5.

Vandevska-Radunovic V, Kristiansen AB, Heyeraas KJ, et al. (1994) Changes in blood circulation in teeth supporting tissues incident to experimental tooth movement. *European Journal of Orthodontics* 16: 361–9.

Veberiene R, Smailiene D, Danielyte J, et al. (2009) Effects of intrusive force on selected determinants of pulp vitality. *Angle Orthodontist* 79: 1114–18.

Vitale MC, Caprioglio C, Martignone A, et al. (2004) Combined technique with polyethylene fibers and composite resins in restoration of traumatized anterior teeth. *Dental Traumatology* 20: 172–7.

Vivaldi-Rodrigues G, Demito CF, Bowman SJ, et al. (2006) The effectiveness of a fluoride varnish in preventing the development of white spot lesions. *World Journal of Orthodontics* 7: 138–44.

Waggoner WF, Johnston WM, Schumann S, et al. (1989) Microabrasion of human enamel in vitro using hydrochloric acid and pumice. *Pediatric Dentistry* 11: 319–23.

White C Jr, Bryant N (2002) Combined therapy of mineral trioxide aggregate and guided tissue regeneration in the treatment of external root resorption and an associated osseous defect. *Journal of Periodontology* 73: 1517–21.

Wickwire NA, McNeil MH, Norton LA, et al. (1974) The effects of tooth movement upon endodontically treated teeth. *Angle Orthodontist* 44: 235–42.

Willmot DR (2004) White lesions after orthodontic treatment: does low fluoride make a difference? *Journal of Orthodontics* 31: 235–42.

Willmot DR (2008) White spot lesions after orthodontic treatment. *Seminars in Orthodontics* 14: 209–19.

Yagi M, Ohno H, Takada K (2009) Computational formulation of orthodontic tooth extraction decisions. Part II: Which tooth should be extracted? *Angle Orthodontist* 79: 892–8.

Yates JA (1992) Root fractures in permanent teeth: a clinical review. *International Endodontic Journal* 25: 150–7.

Yilmaz HG, Kalender A, Cengiz E (2010) Use of mineral trioxide aggregade in the treatment of invasive cervical resorption. *Journal of Endodontics* 36: 160–3.

Yüzügüllü B, Polat O, Ungör M (2008) Multidisciplinary approach to traumatized teeth: a case report. *Dental Traumatology* 24: e27–30.

Zach L, Cohen C (1965) Pulp response to externally applied heat. *Oral Surgery Oral Medicine Oral Pathology* 19: 515–30.

Zachrisson BU, Stenvik A, Haanaes HR (2004) Management of missing maxillary anterior teeth with emphasis on autotransplantation. *American Journal of Orthodontics and Dentofacial Orthopedics* 126: 284–8.

Zero DT (1999) Dental caries process. *Dental Clinics of North America* 43: 635–64.

17

Pre-Prosthetic Orthodontic Tooth Movement: Interdisciplinary Concepts for Optimizing Prosthodontic Care

Julie Holloway, Meade C Van Putten Jr, Sarandeep Huja

Summary

This chapter describes the effects of pre-prosthetic orthodontic treatment to improve and enhance restorative and prosthetic outcomes in adult patients. Also described is the use of orthodontic biomechanical concepts in patients with acquired defects of the maxilla. Three fixed prosthodontic cases and two maxillofacial prosthodontic cases illustrate the advantages gained through the inclusion of orthodontics in the treatment plan. The need for proper planning and collaborative approach as essential components in proper tooth position for improved prosthetic outcomes is emphasized. Finally, the use of orthodontic principles to preserve teeth in cases where significant oral structures have been removed is also demonstrated.

Introduction

The orthodontic profession is undergoing a rapid and enormous growing phase with expansion in its approach towards interactive care. The more progressive specialists in our specialty recognize the fact that if treatment with optimal long-term prognoses is to be provided, we should extend collaboration with other dental specialists too, without any hesitation. Except in cases of exodontia, the main purpose of our profession is restoration and maintenance of normal occlusion, which means that all teeth in one jaw occlude with teeth in the opposing jaw, so that the largest area of functional, masticatory surface is provided. There are many areas where orthodontists are in close collaboration with prosthodontic specialists such as prior to replacement of missing teeth, closure/consolidation of

spaces for esthetic and periodontal improvement, intrusion or extrusion of certain teeth, correction of axial inclination of teeth, space maintenance and management of impacted teeth. The rationale as well as procedures performed as part of pre-prosthodontic orthodontic treatment is the central theme of this chapter.

The restorative dentist will occasionally be confronted with complex treatment planning decisions resulting from the following (Miller, 1995):

- Unesthetic position of the anterior dentition caused by overcrowding or excessive spacing
- Poor position of posterior abutments due to malocclusion
- Supraeruption and occlusal plane discrepancies
- Mesial drift into edentulous areas
- Collapse of the occlusal vertical dimension due to loss of posterior teeth.

An interactive approach between orthodontists and restorative dentists is deemed necessary for effective management of these problems. While it is not our intention to identify and describe the entire range of indications for the use of pre-prosthodontic orthodontic treatment, the above five points provide examples of the major indicators for this interdisciplinary collaboration.

Dental professionals should always carefully consider tooth position in prosthodontic treatment to determine whether orthodontic treatment can improve prosthodontic treatment outcomes. Optimizing tooth position can improve periodontal health, reduce pathological occlusion, and conserve tooth structure; it also allows the dentist to create restorations that are more stable, functional, and esthetic (Evans and Nathanson, 1979; Spalding and Cohen, 1992; Boyd, 2009). Intrusion, extrusion, correction of tipped teeth, and reduction of crowding or excessive spacing are treatments that an orthodontist can provide. Implants can also be used for orthodontic anchorage to improve treatment outcomes (Goodacre et al., 1997). This chapter will describe several patient treatments where collaboration between orthodontists and prosthodontists was used to improve treatment outcomes. Finally there will also be a section highlighting the use of orthodontic principles in cases where maxillofacial structures have been lost due to cancer.

Case 1: Orthodontic intrusion

Diagnosis and etiology

A 46-year-old Caucasian man was referred to the practice of the first author for restoration of the anterior teeth. The patient was concerned about the shape, color, and worn-out incisal edges of the teeth, for which he requested the options for gaining length and change in the color. He reported regular medical and dental attendance and had a noncontributory medical/dental history other than localized anterior wear.

The extraoral examination revealed an orthognathic profile without facial asymmetry and the lips competent at rest (Figure 17.1). Intraoral examination revealed two full-coverage temporary crowns along with several amalgam and composite restorations. There was localized moderate attrition of the anterior teeth and compensatory supra-eruption, while the posterior teeth showed little wear. The periodontal examination revealed no significant pocket depths with absence of bleeding on probing and excellent dental hygiene. The patient was presented with the option to intrude the anterior teeth orthodontically, followed by restoration of both anterior segments.

The patient was referred to an orthodontist who diagnosed the case as Class II Division 2 malocclusion characterized by a 2 mm overjet, a 90% overbite, a 1 mm deviation of the lower dental arch midline to the right of facial midline, and significant unesthetic gingival height concerns secondary to tooth wear and resulting cementoenamel junction (CEJ) extrusion. Analysis of the cephalometric radiograph indicated harmonious sagittal and vertical skeletal relationships, while the panoramic radiograph showed no pathology (Figure 17.1d).

The two treatment options available were placement of crowns over the anterior teeth or orthodontic intrusion to gain necessary clearance for tooth build-up. In addition, the guide for intrusion included not only reduction of the deep bite but also differential leveling of the CEJ and gingival margins as required.

Orthodontic treatment

Fixed appliances (0.022 inch × 0.028 inch, preadjusted edgewise) were bonded on the maxillary teeth in order to level and align the dental arch using the CEJ as a reference (Figure 17.1e). The maxillary incisors were intruded and the dental arches aligned according to standard orthodontic protocols. Once the objectives were accomplished, the fixed appliances were removed in consultation with the restoring dentist. The supraerupted maxillary and mandibular teeth along with their altered gingival margins were leveled (Figure 17.1f). Full coverage maxillary and mandibular clear retainers were delivered following the end of orthodontic treatment, and the retention was modified as needed during the restorative therapy. Permanent retention was placed at the completion of the restorative therapy.

Prosthodontic treatment

A diagnostic wax-up was performed after the orthodontic treatment to plan the contours of the final restorations (Figure 17.1g), which was utilized to fabricate the provisional crowns for the anterior teeth after tooth preparation. All-ceramic full crown restorations (Empress Esthetic) were fabricated and cemented with a resin luting agent (Figure 17.1h,i). A post-insertion occlusal splint was fabricated.

Briefly, conservative rehabilitation of the patient was carried out by an orthodontic–prosthodontic interaction for restoring the maxillary anterior dentition. Although various other approaches, such as restoring the maxillary arch, and endodontic therapy with crowns on all anterior teeth are available, but the associated increase in financial burden and compromised esthetics were considered major drawbacks. Accordingly, the orthodontic treatment plan was felt to be the best option and the one which would provide an optimal result. The interactive approach that followed was the most logical one for the preservation of the dental occlusion and for the restoration of anterior function and esthetics (Figure 17.1j,k).

Case 2: Use of dental implants for anchorage and orthodontic tooth extrusion for implant site development

Diagnosis and etiology

A 58-year-old Caucasian man was referred to the graduate prosthodontics clinic at the Ohio State University for prosthodontic rehabilitation (Figure 17.2a–c). The patient's medical history revealed that he was allergic to penicillin with no systemic diseases and a negative smoking history. He was under no medications requiring dental precautions. He was categorized as American Society of Anesthesiologists (ASA) I (normal, healthy with no systemic disease).

The intraoral examination revealed several carious teeth, generalized attrition with an increased interocclusal space,

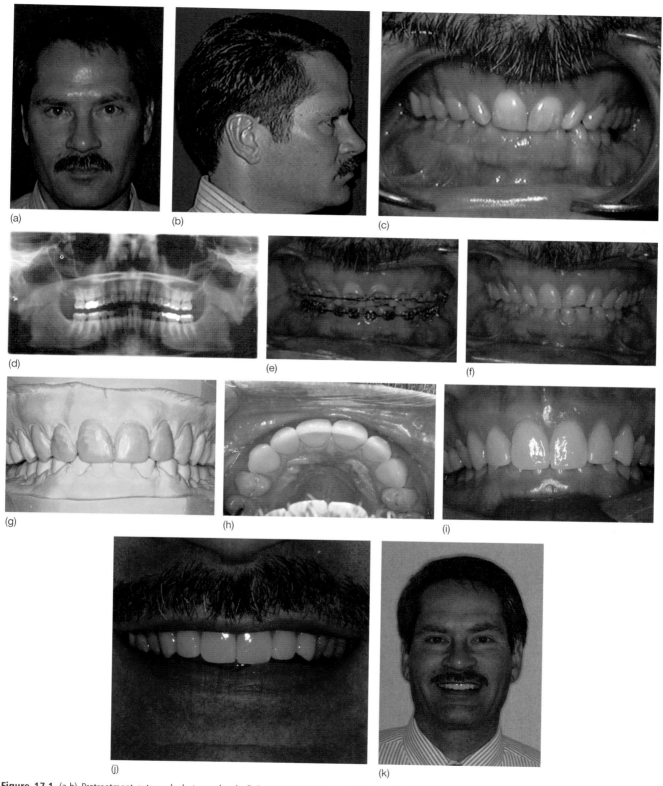

Figure 17.1 (a,b) Pretreatment extraoral photographs. (c,d) Pretreatment intraoral photograph and orthopantomogram. (e) Patient under fixed orthodontic treatment. (f) Post-orthodontic phase. (g) Diagnostic wax-up of anterior dentition for full ceramic crowns. (h,i) Final restorations: (h) occlusal view of anterior crowns; (i) frontal view. (j,k) Frontal photographs showing treatment results.

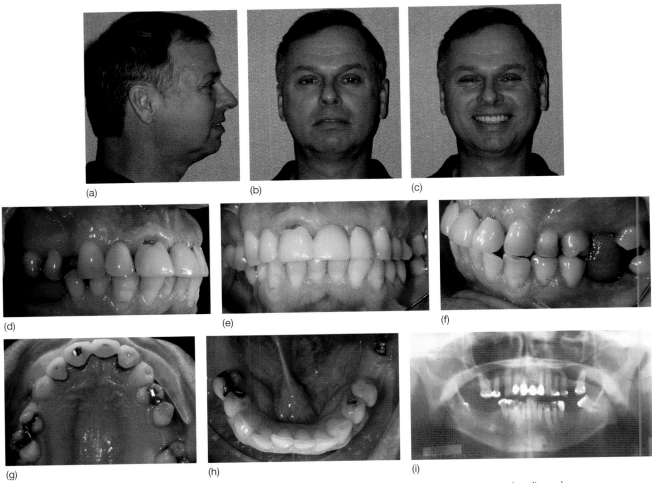

Figure 17.2 (a–c) Pretreatment extraoral photographs. (d–h) Pretreatment intraoral photographs. (i) Pretreatment panoramic radiograph.

tooth malpositions, and a loose fixed partial dental prosthesis on the upper central incisors and the upper left lateral incisor caused by the fracture of the left lateral incisor abutment tooth (Figure 17.2d–h). The upper left central incisor was lost at the age of 30 years due to trauma while playing basketball. The patient reported that his posterior teeth had been removed due to caries and provided history of sporadic dental care. There was 'edge-to-edge' occlusion in the anterior region, contributing to deleterious forces on the anterior fixed partial dental prosthesis causing the abutment tooth fracture. In addition, the left mandibular third molar was severely tipped, with no other mandibular molars present. This situation, most likely, caused the patient to primarily use his anterior teeth during masticatory function. The periodontal examination revealed generalized, plaque-induced mild gingivitis with localized pocketing. There was an absence of bleeding on probing with satisfactory dental hygiene.

A Cadiax electronic pantographic analysis (WhipMix Corp, Louisville, KY) was performed to assist in the diagnosis of occlusal parameters, and to determine the hinge axis location (Figure 17.2i). This provided clinical information for therapeutic decisions. Diagnostic casts were obtained and mounted with a kinematic facebow and standard centric relation records. An analysis of the casts and patient data revealed that even though the remaining dentition could be used, there was a need for extensive rehabilitation involving well-coordinated surgical, periodontal, orthodontic, endodontic and prosthodontic treatment procedures. Accordingly, the treatment plan included the following:

1. Extraction of the remaining mandibular third molar
2. Endodontic treatment of the left mandibular second premolar with a provisional crown
3. Dental implants in position of the mandibular right and left second molars to be used initially for orthodontic anchorage (Figure 17.2j)
4. Orthodontic treatment, repositioning of the maxillary and mandibular dentition
5. Extraction of the maxillary right central incisor and left lateral incisor

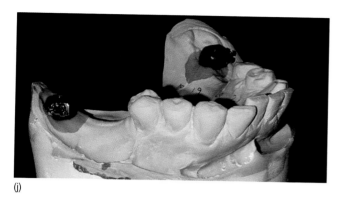

(j)

Figure 17.2 (j) Pre-orthodontic implant placement (treatment provided by Dr Brock Satoris). Implants were placed in the position of the mandibular right and left second molars for anchorage for the orthodontic therapy. Orthodontic brackets were attached to the abutments. Precise location of implants was obtained through a diagnostic set-up.

6. Periodontal free soft tissue graft surgery for both mandibular second premolars
7. Dental implants in positions maxillary right first premolar, right central incisor, left lateral incisor and left first molar, and mandibular right and left first molars (Zimmer Tapered Screw Vent, various lengths)
8. Single crowns for the maxillary right and left first molars, right and left first and right second premolars, and right lateral incisor and the mandibular right and left second premolars
9. Fixed partial dentures to replace the maxillary central incisors, left lateral incisor and mandibular right and left first and second molars.

The patient was then referred to the Graduate Periodontics and Orthodontics clinics for a consultation to determine whether the above-mentioned therapy was feasible.

Orthodontic consultation

The patient was first referred to the orthodontic clinic of the Ohio State University. The orthodontic resident and the third author determined that the mandibular anterior teeth needed to be retroclined to gain horizontal and vertical overlap of the anterior teeth in order to restore anterior guidance. The bony architecture around the maxillary left lateral incisor was not favorable for implant placement, so this root was to be orthodontically extruded in preparation for implant placement.

Analysis of the cephalometric radiograph revealed a skeletal Class I malocclusion (SNA = 82.3°, SNB = 80.3°), with normal facial divergence (SN-MP = 29.3°). The lower incisors were proclined (108° to mandibular plane), and were at 8.4 mm from the A-Po line. The panoramic radiograph demonstrated evidence of amalgam (tattoo), condensing osteitis, and mandibular tori (Figure 17.2i). Examination of the periapical radiographs confirmed the presence of pulp pathology in the maxillary right central incisor and the mandibular left second premolar.

An analysis of the dental casts revealed asymmetrical occlusion, with a mild Class III canine relationship on the right side, end-on Class II canine relationship on the left side and a maxillomandibular midline discrepancy of 3 mm. The occlusion was characterized by a 2 mm overjet and 2 mm overbite. There were generalized wear facets.

Orthodontic treatment

The primary objective of the orthodontic treatment was to provide adequate overjet so that the maxillary implants could be placed with proper axial inclination and allow for occlusion with the natural mandibular anterior teeth. Thus distalization of the mandibular arch was desired. Such en masse tooth movements require solid, reliable orthodontic anchorage. The patient had missing multiple posterior teeth, further complicating the desired posterior en masse movement. Endosseous implants were placed initially to provide anchorage for the orthodontic tooth movement and these same implants were later used for restoring some of the missing teeth, making implant placement a critical step. A diagnostic orthodontic wax-up was used to simulate tooth movements (e.g. the mandibular premolars were distalized and the mandibular anterior teeth were retracted). The space for future implants was estimated and the position of the terminal mandibular implants that were to serve as orthodontic anchors was accurately determined. Similarly, the positions of the maxillary teeth at the end of orthodontic treatment were also determined. There was a cant in the mandibular arch and the full correction of this was not attempted.

Dental implants in the positions of the mandibular right and left second molars were used as anchorage for the mandibular tooth movement. Special abutments were fabricated, each with an orthodontic bracket soldered to it. It was from these orthodontic attachments that the retraction mechanics were initiated. New provisional restorations were made for the maxillary right central and left lateral incisors and a pontic with an orthodontic attachment was fabricated for the left central incisor (Figure 17.2k–o).

Fixed orthodontic appliances (0.022 inch × 0.025 inch, Roth) were bonded on both arches for initial leveling and aligning. At first, the mandibular premolars were distalized and each posterior segment was then consolidated to the mandibular implants. This step allowed for the mandibular anterior teeth to be retracted en masse by using the premolars as the indirect anchors. In the maxillary arch, spaces were idealized for maxillary implants, and extrusion of the maxillary right central and left lateral incisors was achieved. The fixed appliances were removed after leveling, alignment, space redistribution, and distalization of the mandibular arch (Figure 17.2p–v). In addition extrusion of the maxillary incisors was achieved. Maxillary and mandibular

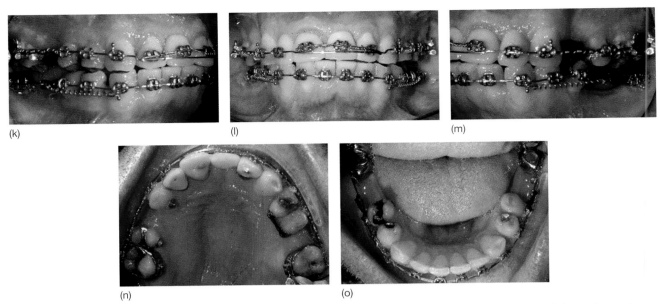

Figure 17.2 (k–o) Fixed orthodontic treatment. The maxillary posterior spaces were developed. In the mandible, coil springs are being used to produce en masse retraction of the mandibular incisors.

Essix retainers were delivered and prosthodontic rehabilitation was commenced immediately. Cephalometric superimposition of pre- and post-treatment radiographs demonstrated the en masse distalization of the mandibular arch by 2.5 mm.

Periodontal and preliminary restorative therapy

The patient was treated in the graduate periodontics clinic and his periodontal health was maintained throughout the surgical and orthodontic phase of the therapy. Extractions and several graft procedures were carried out, along with placement of several amalgam and composite dental restorations to re-establish oral health and to create the necessary base for the proposed crowns. Finally, implants were placed in the positions of the maxillary right central incisor, left lateral incisor and first molar, and mandibular right and left first molars in preparation for single crowns and fixed partial denture restorations.

This interactive case did not progress in a linear fashion. There were several changes in the treatment plan during the course of care. However, such changes are not unusual in the treatment of patients for whom several plan options are possible. Initially, the treatment plan called for the retention of the maxillary right central incisor. However, halfway into the plan it was determined that this tooth would not be of benefit and a decision was made to extract it (Figure 17.2k–o). Also several additional implants were added to the treatment plan after it was determined that adequate spacing would be achieved through orthodontic care (Figure 17.2p–v).

A definitive prosthodontic treatment plan was established after the surgical, periodontics, orthodontic, and restorative treatments. It should be stated that the orthodontic therapy provided additional conservative treatment options that allowed the practitioner to retain several of the patient's teeth.

When the above therapies were completed the patient's dentition was restored with conventional and implant-supported metal-ceramic restorations (Figure 17.2w–z). Screw-retained single crown implant restorations were placed on the maxillary right first premolar and the left first molar. Conventional single crown restorations were cemented on the maxillary right first molar, second premolar, and lateral incisor, left first premolar and the mandibular right and left second premolars. Screw-retained, implant-supported fixed partial dentures were placed on implant abutments in the positions of the maxillary central and left lateral incisors and the mandibular right and left first and second molars. An occlusal splint was fabricated after the completion of prosthodontic treatment, and the patient was instructed to use it at night. Instructions for maintenance care were given. The patient was also scheduled for long-term periodontal maintenance care in the graduate periodontics clinic.

In this case, a full mouth rehabilitation of the patient was achieved. Implants provided anchorage for tooth movement and were later used as abutments for the posterior restorations. Figure 17.2w–za shows the final treatment results. The interactive approach was necessary for the creation of adequate spacing for the fixed partial dentures, especially in the maxillary anterior area, as well as to manage

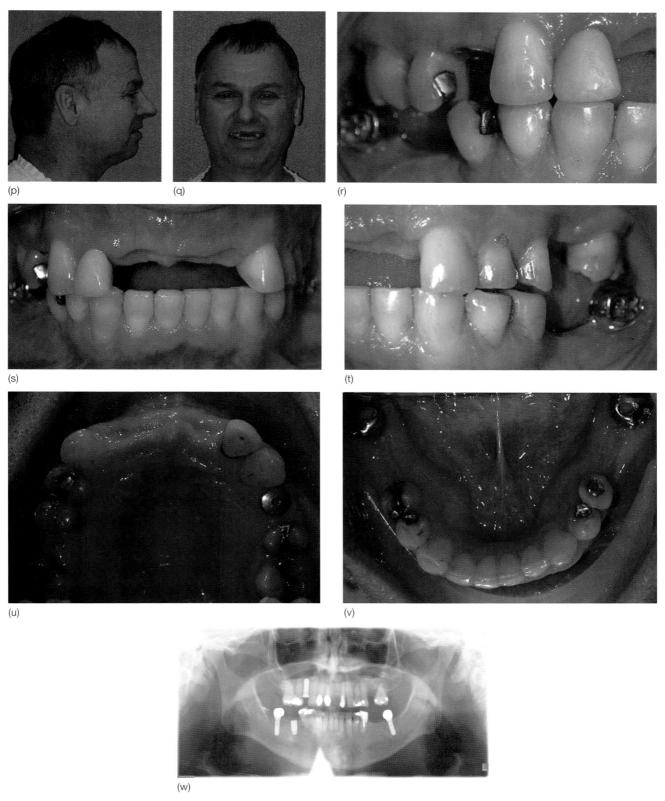

Figure 17.2 (p,q) Post-orthodontic extraoral photographs. (r–v) Post-orthodontic intraoral photographs. The maxillary anterior fixed partial denture was removed. Spaces were obtained for both anterior and posterior teeth for both arches. (w) Post-orthodontic panoramic radiograph.

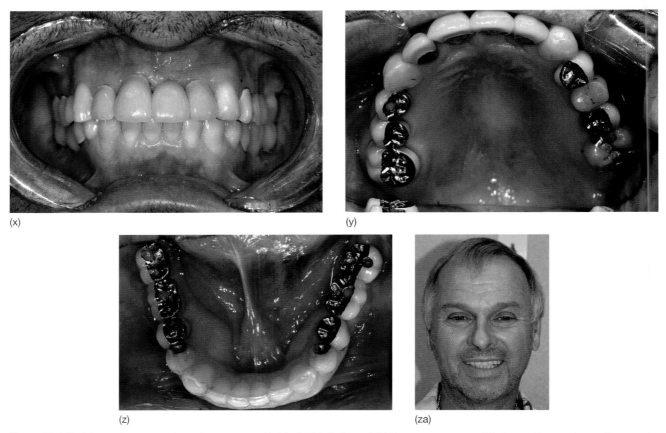

(x) (y)

(z) (za)

Figure 17.2 Final intraoral treatment photos (treatment provided by Dr Valerie Cooper). (x) Tissue contours were difficult to achieve on the maxillary anterior fixed partial denture. But the esthetic result was acceptable and was the best that could be accomplished considering the pretreatment scenario. (y,z) Occlusal views of the porcelain fused to metal restorations with gold occlusals. Orthodontic treatment allowed the prosthodontist to fabricate the restorations with proper crown contours. (za) Final extraoral view shows the smile line and anterior esthetic display.

the anterior bony architecture in preparation for dental implants in the esthetic zone.

Case 3: Minor tooth movement to gain canine guidance for full mouth rehabilitation

Diagnosis and etiology

A 63-year-old Caucasian man requiring rehabilitation was referred to the practice of the first author for a prosthodontic examination. The patient presented with moderate attrition and loss of teeth due to fracture. The patient's medical/dental history were noncontributory, other than the patient's account that his tooth loss was due to fracture of the maxillary right and left first premolars and the mandibular right second molar over the past decade. He had implants placed in these areas as teeth were extracted, however, they were not yet restored.

The extraoral examination revealed an orthognathic profile with slight facial asymmetry (Figure 17.3a,b). The intraoral examination disclosed moderate wear (Figure 17.3c,d) and the periodontal examination revealed no significant pocket depths with absence of bleeding on probing and satisfactory dental hygiene.

Orthodontic consultation

An analysis of the dental casts revealed a Class I malocclusion characterized by a 1 mm overjet and a 2.5 mm deviation of the lower dental arch midline to the left. The panoramic radiograph showed no pathology (Figure 17.3e). It was determined that minor tooth movement would be needed to close the diastema between the right canine and lateral incisor for two reasons:

- To help gain canine guidance
- To reduce tooth size discrepancies in the final restorations.

Orthodontic treatment

There was a discrepancy in the mesiodistal space of the edentulous areas of the maxillary right and left first premolars. Mesial movement of the maxillary right canine would help gain mesiodistal restorative space for the anticipated implant crown. Also, changing the position of this tooth would allow for the development of optimal crown contours and guidance. A fixed appliance was bonded to the buccal surfaces of the maxillary right canine and lateral incisor. A closed coil spring was used to tip/rotate the

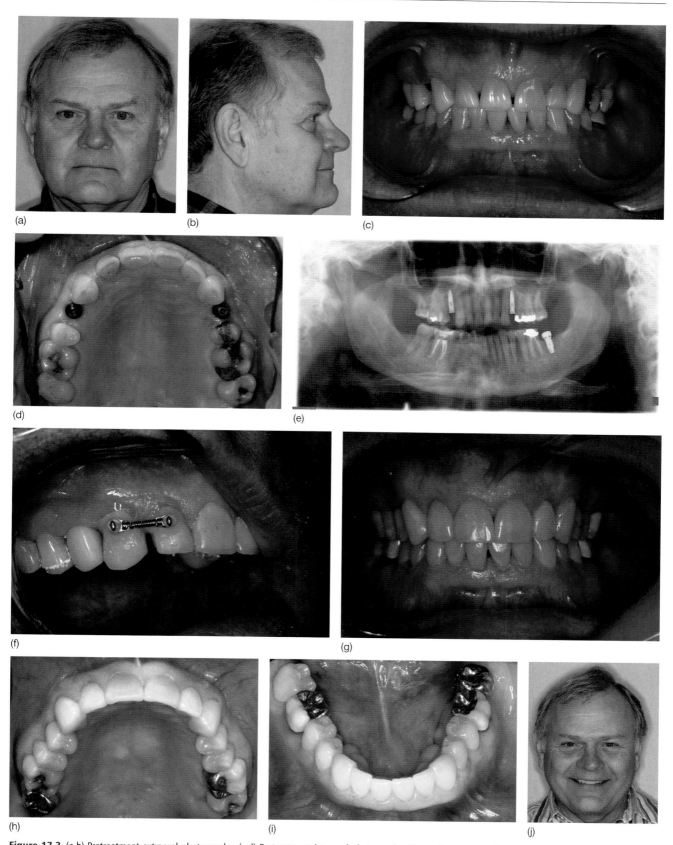

Figure 17.3 (a,b) Pretreatment extraoral photographs. (c,d) Pretreatment intraoral photographs. The patient presented with a well-maintained dentition with good oral hygiene. There was a 1.5 mm space distal to the left canine and inadequate space mesial to the left implant abutment. (e) Pre-orthodontic treatment panoramic radiograph. (f) Orthodontic treatment being carried out. (g–i) Post-orthodontic intraoral photographs. (j) Post-orthodontic extraoral photograph.

canine mesially about 1 mm (Figure 17.3f). The fixed appliance was removed after alignment of the canine and provisional restorations were used to stabilize the teeth for a 6-week period prior to final impressions for the fixed prostheses.

Prosthodontics

After orthodontic therapy was completed, the patient's dentition was restored with conventional and implant-supported metal-ceramic restorations (Figure 17.3g–i). In this case, full mouth rehabilitation was achieved. Implants were also used as abutments for the maxillary first premolar restorations and the mandibular left second molar. Figure 17.3j shows the final treatment results. An interactive approach was necessary for creating adequate spacing for the maxillary anterior restorations. An excellent functional and esthetic result was achieved with limited but necessary orthodontic treatment.

Orthodontic techniques in maxillofacial prosthodontics

Removable appliances are used extensively in orthodontics as retainers after fixed appliance therapy. They are also used for minor tooth movements, biteplates and as functional appliances for the correction of anterior and posterior crossbites (Hawley, 1919; Staley and Reske, 2001). The design of removable appliances varies considerably depending on the objectives of therapy. However, the fundamental design principles of orthodontic retainers have been found by the second author to be conceptually sound and useful for treating head and neck cancer patients. These appliances can be used to improve retention, support, and force distribution to the remaining maxillary dentition when a maxillectomy has been performed. They are especially beneficial in young cancer patients in whom long-term preservation of teeth is critical.

Removable orthodontic appliances

Hawley retainers are the most common type of removable appliance used in orthodontics. The components of a typical Hawley appliance are: an acrylic resin base, bilateral posterior retentive clasps, and an anterior labial bow. The circumferential clasps used are made from round orthodontic wire of various gauges. Adams, ball, and arrow-head clasps are also used.

The labial bow

The labial bow, a standard component of Hawley retainers is used to retain the anterior teeth along their labial surfaces. The labial bow can also function as a retentive element in patients wearing maxillofacial prosthesis (Berlocher and Mueller, 1986). The reason for considering their use is that

they reduce the force and weight distribution of the prosthesis to the anterior teeth and simplify placement and adjustment procedures (Figure 17.4a–d). The force an obturator exerts on the abutment teeth depends on its weight and the occlusal load. Obturator weight varies considerably and is dependent on its size and the materials used for fabrication. Surgical and interim obturators commonly have a resting weight of about 25 g. A definitive obturator can weigh considerably more due to its metal base.

Obturators are used by maxillectomy patients to facilitate basic speech and swallowing functions. They are used 8–10 hours/day since speech and fluid management is impossible when the obturator is removed. When clasps are placed on maxillary central or lateral incisors they can inadvertently function as orthodontic appliances due to their constant use and weight. Occlusal loads on obturators vary from patient to patient and depend on the distribution of the remaining natural dentition in the maxilla and mandible, the design and patient habits. A concerted effort is made to reduce the occlusal load on the side of the maxillectomy due to the lack of underlying support.

The labial bow allows the prosthodontist to use all available anterior teeth for retention but does not engage the undercut as aggressively as conventional cast clasp. The improvement in force distribution is essential to reducing abutment overloading. The resting weight of the prosthesis can place a force capable of moving anterior abutments over time. However, placing a bow in the middle to gingival third of the teeth allows it to disengage when the prosthesis is at rest. This disengagement is important since resting gravitational forces are significant and represent the major force acting on anterior abutments. Keeping the bow in the middle to gingival third of the teeth allows it to engage when an occlusal load is applied, improving retention. Consequently, placing the bow in the gingival third provides adequate retention without placing potential orthodontic forces on the anterior abutments. Since labial bows are commonly seen on orthodontic retainers they do not carry the stigma of clasps.

The clasp

Stainless steel clasps are also used in surgical and interim obturators due to ease of placement into the acrylic resin base and flexibility.

Surgical obturators are often placed at the time of the maxillectomy or postsurgically prior to discharge from the hospital. When placed after the surgery, the obturator is seated on postsurgical day 5–7 after the surgical sponge (bolster) has been removed. As the area heals the prosthesis is adjusted to maintain adequate obturation and to maintain retention within the mouth. Ball clasps are useful and effective clasps that are commonly used in orthodontic retainers. They are placed in the undercuts commonly found in posterior interproximal embrasures. It has been

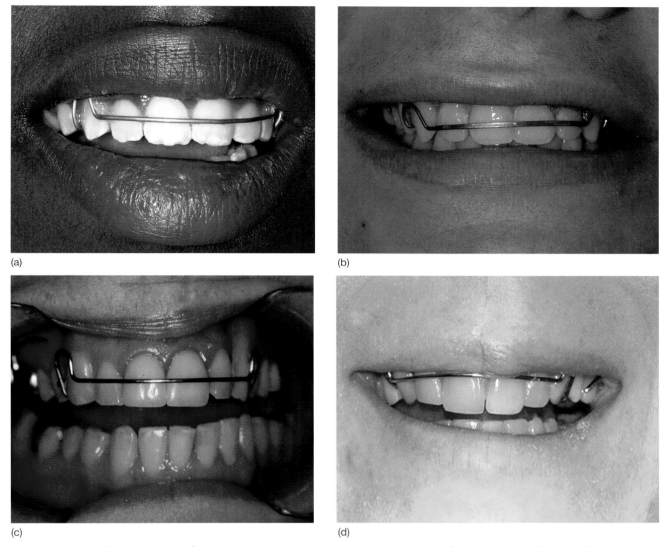

Figure 17.4 The use of labial bows is beneficial in obturator cases. The bow can be used in interim and definitive obturators. (a,b) Interim obturators in young patients with the bow serving as a retentive aid. (c,d) In definitive obturators the bow provides a more favorable distribution of the forces to the anterior teeth where a central or lateral incisor would have been used.

observed that ball clasps can also be used as a circumferential clasp where the ball provides a purchase point for easy removal by the patient (Figure 17.5a). This feature is especially important with elderly patients with poor to failing eyesight, poor dexterity, or arthritic hands. The ball on the end also provides protection to the cheek during placement of the prosthesis.

In addition, vertical loops are a useful adjunct to surgical and interim obturators. Vertical loops have been used extensively in fixed orthodontics appliances (Begg, 1956; Sims, 1972). Loops are generally used to improve the resiliency of wire appliances between teeth, improve control over tooth movements, and to simplify adjustment procedures. When placed just behind the shoulder portion of a circumferential clasp it can reduce placement problems for

obturators in situations where the patient's teeth are rotated, tipped or present with significantly divergent angulations (Figure 17.5b). Instead of adjusting the arm of the clasp, the width of the loop is closed or opened depending on the desired effect. Closing the loop tightens the clasp against the tooth and also tends to lift the prosthesis. Adjustments are simplified since only the loop is altered, and not the clasp arm.

Vertical loops are used in all obturator types. However, they are most useful in surgical obturators. Time for extensive preprosthetic treatment planning is usually not available due to the urgency of cancer treatment. Placing a vertical loop simplifies placement, which can be an important factor when the prosthesis is placed by the surgeon.

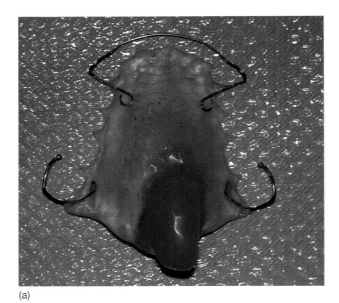

(a)

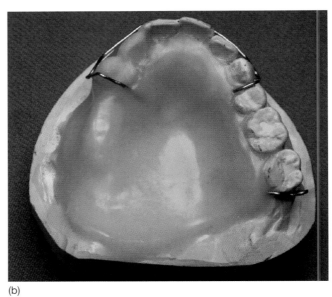

(b)

Figure 17.5 (a) An interim obturator where both a labial bow and ball clasps were used. The ball clasps provide a purchase point for the patient's finger for ease of removal. (b) An interim obturator where a vertical loop was used on the posterior clasp. This simplified placement and adjustment procedures.

Case 4: Restoration after a maxillectomy for osteomyelitis

The Division of Head and Neck Surgical Oncology at the James Cancer Hospital referred a 45-year-old Caucasian woman to the maxillofacial clinic for a postsurgical evaluation and prosthesis (Figure 17.6a). Medical diagnosis was consistent with chronic osteomyelitis involving the left posterior maxilla. Examination revealed no significant medical problems or systemic diseases. The referring physician had placed her on an antibiotic during her postoperative period. Vital signs were normal. The patient had no history of tobacco or alcohol abuse. The dental history revealed regular biyearly dental attendance. She had a full lower dentition in good repair. All of the maxillary posterior teeth had been removed except for the right first premolar. The left maxillary canine had been removed. The right first premolar had been endodontically treated and had been scheduled for a metal-ceramic crown by her local dentist. There were few restorations and her periodontal diagnosis was mild gingivitis on a reduced periodontium.

There was a 1 cm oval defect in the left buccal vestibule that communicated with the maxillary sinus. The defect was clean and well healed. The patient was to undergo a revision of the area distal to the left lateral incisor due to a sharp bony margin to be performed by her surgeon (Figure 17.6b). No other oral infections were noted at that time. Her speech was normal, however, she did complain of fluid regurgitation into the sinus and nose. She was planning to have the right first premolar extracted as a preventive

measure but the decision was discouraged by the second author. It was decided that an interim obturator would be prescribed followed by a definitive obturator after adequate healing had taken place.

Medical/dental history

The patient had an 11-year history of osteomyelitis of the left maxilla that started after endodontic treatment of the first maxillary molar (Figure 17.6c). The treatment was unsuccessful and the tooth was eventually extracted. However, the extraction site did not heal and the patient had intense pain in and around the exposed bony wound. After a course of antibiotics and closure of the site a fixed partial denture was placed. The pain continued and it was decided that the fixed partial denture should be removed. She was referred to an oral surgeon about a year later, who ordered a computed tomography (CT) scan of the maxilla. The scan showed an extensive area of infection around the extraction site and teeth. The diagnosis was confirmed by a bone biopsy of the site.

Several practitioners including general dentists, oral surgeons, an endodontist, primary care physicians, a neurologist, a pain management physician, an internist, and several otolaryngologists attempted various curative therapies during the 10-year period following diagnosis. The patient was placed on countless courses of antibiotics including at least six intravenous courses while in hospital. The remaining left posterior teeth were endodontically treated early in the process; however, the pain con-

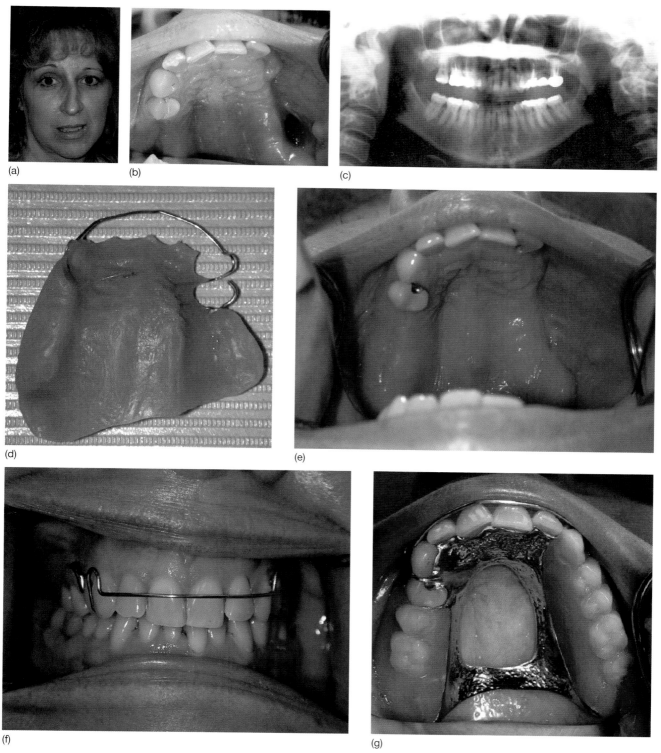

Figure 17.6 (a) Frontal photograph of a patient who underwent maxillectomy for osteomyelitis. (b) Occlusal intraoral photograph showing all the posterior teeth removed except for the right first premolar. The acquired defect communicated with the patient's maxillary sinus. (c) Panoramic radiograph showing patient's condition prior to the extraction of the maxillary posterior teeth and maxillectomy. The osteomyelitis had been present for over 10 years but was not visible on standard radiographic films. (d) The interim obturator. Since the patient was missing the left canine, a labial bow was used. (e) A full crown was fabricated on the right premolar. The acquired defect healed and closed improving the patient's overall prognosis. (f,g) Final result with the definitive obturator in place. The bow provided adequate retention and was esthetically acceptable to the patient.

tinued. Apicectomies were then performed, which also failed. At least three open surgical curettage procedures of the posterior maxilla had been done with some limited success. This course of treatment ultimately failed and the patient finally had the canine and all the other remaining posterior teeth extracted. She stated that this step had alleviated the pain for a short time. When the pain and related symptoms returned, her internist (an infectious diseases specialist) referred her to an otolaryngologist for a maxillectomy. The partial maxillectomy was performed and the pain and the related symptoms finally subsided.

Osteomyelitis

Osteomyelitis of the jaws is uncommon in developed countries but usually arises after an odontogenic infection or fracture of the jaws (Bouquot and LaMarche, 1999; Prasad et al., 2007). Chronic systemic diseases and disorders associated with decreased vascularity such as diabetes, acquired immune deficiency syndrome, malignancy and malnutrition can predispose people to this condition. An increased frequency has also been noted in patients who use tobacco, alcohol and intravenous drugs, and those who have undergone radiation therapy. Patients of all ages can be affected and there appears to be a strong male predominance. Most cases involve the mandible (Koorbusch et al., 1992; Neville et al., 2002).

Chronic osteomyelitis usually arises in cases where an acute episode has not resolved. The signs and symptoms mimic those of the more common dental infections, making it difficult to diagnose. There may be swelling, sinus pain, purulent discharge, tooth loss, pathological fracture, and sequestrum formation. Loss of an entire quadrant of the jaw has been reported in longstanding cases (Neville et al., 2002).

Even though a diagnosis was confirmed early, it is interesting to note the stubborn and resistant nature of this infection and the extensive therapeutic modalities needed to achieve a cure. The problem started as an ordinary dental infection that was treated following a standard dental protocol. However, later numerous therapeutic regimens were attempted by dental and medical providers without success.

Prosthodontic treatment

The interim obturator was waxed in pink baseplate wax (Truwax Baseplate Wax, Dentsply) with a labial bow, which was fabricated using 0.036 inch stainless steel orthodontic wire. The bow was placed high on the central incisors, due to their lingual-vertical angulations. A circumferential clasp was made for the right first premolar. The completed wax-up was flasked and processed in Palapress Vario Autocure Resin according to the manufacturer's

instructions (Heraeus Kulzer, Hanau, Germany) (Figure 17.6d). The patient was seen for the insertion of the interim obturator prosthesis, and was scheduled to return 1 week later for a post insertion follow-up evaluation. Healing was normal and it was noted that the defect was closing. She stated that she had made an appointment with her dentist for the fabrication of a crown on the right first premolar.

Fabrication of a definitive obturator was initiated after it was determined that the tissues had adequately healed (Figure 17.6e). A survey crown had been fabricated and cemented on the right first premolar. The final impressions were made in irreversible hydrocolloid (Jeltrate Fast Set Alginate, Dentsply Caulk) and poured in a die stone (Velmix, Whip Mix Inc.). The obturator framework was fabricated in Vitallium alloy (Austenal Corp.). A receptacle was made in the framework to retain the labial bow distal to the left canine.

The patient was seen a week later for a try-in of the framework, and intermaxillary and facebow records and selection of teeth (Ivoclar Vivadent Inc.). The maxillary and mandibular casts were mounted on a Hanau H2 articulator (Denar Corp.) and the teeth were set in a standard baseplate wax. After the teeth were set, the cast was sent to the laboratory for the fabrication of a labial bow. The bow was made similar to the one on the interim obturator and was placed in the upper middle third of the remaining anterior teeth. The patient was seen 2 weeks later for an esthetic try-in. The occlusion, esthetics, and the position of the labial bow were evaluated and verified. The wax-up was sent to the laboratory for processing.

The obturator was inserted and adjusted according to a standard prosthetic insertion protocol. The anterior esthetics of the prosthesis was evaluated and was considered acceptable by the clinician and patient (Figure 17.6f,g). The patient was given post-insertion instructions and scheduled for a 1-week post insertion follow-up, which was uneventful with minor adjustments needed to the obturator bulb labial bow and framework. The bow was tightened by reducing the width of the omega loop with standard orthodontic pliers.

Discussion

Osteomyelitis in the oral cavity can be difficult to diagnose, but once diagnosed its treatment involves removal of the infected bone. In this case, the partial maxillectomy removed the diseased tissues with subsequent cessation of all symptoms. With the insertion of the obturator, the communication between the maxillary sinus and oral cavity was closed. The patient has assumed an acceptable quality of life and is currently on a follow-up schedule that coincides with her appointments with her otolaryngologist.

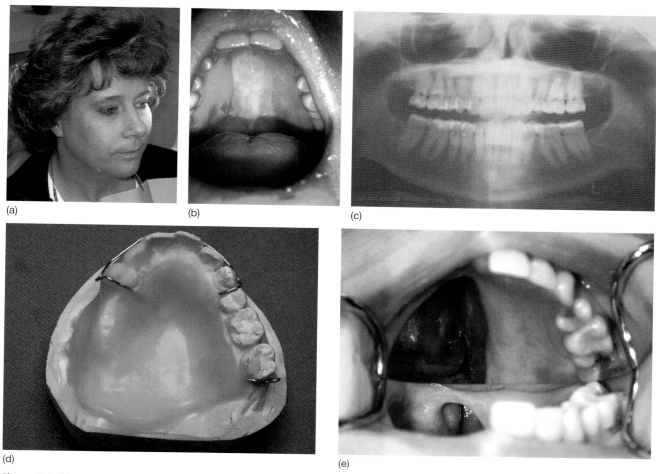

Figure 17.7 (a) Patient presents for presurgical evaluation for a right adenoid cystic carcinoma. (b) The lesion was located just in front of soft palate, in the depression over the greater palatine foramen. (c) The panoramic radiograph reveals a full dentition in good repair. (d) The cast was modified and a wax-up was performed. A labial bow was added for anterior retention. A circumferential clasp was created with a vertical loop was added to the clasp for ease of adjustment. Only two retentive elements were needed. (e) The acquired defect. This prosthesis was modified since a second surgery was necessary which extended the acquired defect to the left central incisor.

Case 5: Prosthetic restoration of maxillectomy due to adenoid cystic carcinoma

A 45-year-old Caucasian woman was referred to the maxillofacial clinic by the oncology division of otolaryngology in the James Cancer Hospital on August 6, 2001 for a presurgical evaluation and impressions. Her medical diagnosis was consistent with adenoid cystic carcinoma involving the soft tissue of the right posterior maxilla with extension into the palate and maxillary sinus (Figure 17.7a,b). The patient had been scheduled to have a right total maxillectomy and palatectomy. A decision on radiation therapy was to be made postsurgically.

An examination revealed no significant medical problems or medications. Vital signs were normal. The patient had no history of tobacco use or significant alcohol consumption. Dental history revealed regular bi-yearly dental attendance. She had a full dentition in good repair with a history of orthodontic treatment (Figure 17.7c). There were few restorations and no periodontal disease.

Irreversible hydrocolloid impressions were made of the upper and lower dental arches (Jeltrate, Fast Set, Dentsply Caulk) and poured in an American Dental Association (ADA) type III dental (Microstone, Whip Mix Corp.). Intra- and extraoral photographs were also taken at this time.

The initial surgery was performed in September 2001. She was visited by the second author at 3 days post-surgery to determine the extent of the ablation and to map the defect margins on the master cast. The surgeons had used an extraoral, Weber-Ferguson approach and removed the right maxilla, palate, and a portion of the maxillary sinus. The acquired defect extended to the hamular notch distally. The soft palate was spared. The area was lined with a full thickness skin graft from the patient's left thigh. All the posterior teeth and the canine were included in the resection. The right central incisor had been spared. The defect had been packed with a surgical sponge that was to be removed 7–10 days post surgery. The surgical prosthesis was placed at the same appointment as the removal of the surgical bolster (delayed surgical obturator) (Curtis and Beumer, 1996). The remaining maxilla was classified as an Aramany Cl II (Aramany, 1978a and b).

The cast was altered and the delayed surgical obturator was waxed in pink baseplate wax (Truwax Baseplate Wax, Dentsply Inc.). It was decided that the right lateral incisor and canine would be added for esthetic reasons due to the age of the patient. A labial bow was also used, and was fabricated using 0.036 inch stainless steel orthodontic wire. The canine and lateral incisors were fabricated from a provisional resin material, with a template made from the pre-surgical cast. The bow was placed in the gingival third of the central incisors to utilize the undercut present in this area. A circumferential clasp with a vertical loop was also made for the second molar as shown. The wax-up was completed, flasked and processed in Palapress Vario denture resin (Heareus Kulzer, Inc.) and processed in the Palapress Vario curing tank according to the manufacturer's instructions (Figure 17.7d–g).

The patient was seen in the maxillofacial prosthodontics clinic at 8 days post surgery for the insertion of the delayed surgical prosthesis. The prosthesis was placed, adjusted, and relined with Coe-Soft Resilient Denture Liner (GC America Inc.). The labial bow was tightened and the patient was instructed in the placement and care of the prosthesis and defect hygiene. She was told to purchase a WaterPik Oral Irrigator (WaterPik Technologies, Inc.) and to bring a tip on the next appointment for modification. She was scheduled for a 1-week post insertion check, when it was noted that healing was occurring normally. The obturator was reduced and relined again with Coe-Soft and the clasps readjusted. The patient was scheduled for a follow-up 3 weeks later. At this follow-up visit, the patient stated that she would need a second surgery due to a positive margin in the orbital region. She was also to receive a tumoricidal dose of radiation therapy after the second surgery. A topical fluoride regimen (Prevident Topical Fluoride, Serele Inc.) was prescribed along with custom trays for its application.

The second surgery was performed in October 2001. The patient was visited 3 days post surgery. The surgical margins had been extended to include the right central incisor, and superiorly to the floor of the orbit. The patient was seen in the maxillofacial clinic at 7 days postsurgery for modification and placement of the delayed surgical obturator. The right central incisor was added and the obturator relined with Coe-Soft. She was then scheduled for a 1-week recall appointment. The obturator was converted to the all-acrylic interim obturator 3 weeks later just before the radiation therapy was initiated (Figure 17.7h–k). The labial bow was positioned in the gingival third of the central incisors and was very retentive. The esthetics of the anterior bow was evaluated, and its appearance is similar to a typical orthodontic retainer. Placement of the bow in the gingival one-third of the central incisors maximizes retention and allows it to rotate deeper into the undercut as the prosthesis moves downward posteriorly. The small maxillary right lateral incisor was spared from being the primary anterior abutment, thereby improving its long-term prognosis.

The patient started radiation therapy 3 weeks postsurgery and received 6 weeks of radiation, bilateral, opposed parts to the affected area. She was scheduled for a follow-up during week 3 of the radiation therapy. At that time it was noted that she had a mild mucositis on the soft palate and was placed on palliative rinses (NaCl, $H(CO)^-_2$ 1–2 tsp/qt of H_2O). She was scheduled for another appointment at 3 weeks (sixth week of radiation therapy). The irradiated areas were allowed to heal for 5 months. During this period it was noted that the patient developed moderate postradiation trismus with an interincisal distance that ranged from 22 to 27 mm. Standard stretching exercises were prescribed.

Fabrication of a definitive obturator was initiated in October 2002. A final impression was made in irreversible hydrocolloid (Jeltrate, Fast Set, Dentsply Caulk) and poured in an improved stone (Velmix, Whip Mix Inc.). The obturator framework was fabricated in Vitallium alloy. A labial bow was incorporated into the framework design (Figure 17.7l,m). A loop was added to the ends of the bow and retained on the framework distal to the canines by acrylic resin.

At the framework try-in, an altered cast impression was performed of the acquired defect with impression compound (Kerr Impression Compound, Kerr USA) and polysulfide impression material (Coe Flex Type III Rubber Base, GC America). The impression was boxed and poured in an improved stone (Figure 17.7g,h). The patient was seen a week later for intermaxillary and facebow records and to select teeth. The casts were mounted on a Hanau H2 (Whip Mix Corp.) articulator. The teeth were waxed in a standard baseplate wax (Figure 17.7i). After the try-in, the obturator was processed in Characterized Lucitone Heat Polymerized Acrylic Resin (Dentsply Inc.), remounted, and finished. The obturator was inserted in October 2002. Figure 17.7n,o shows the final treatment result. The obturator was easy to place and was retentive. The simplicity of the design and reduction of clasping reduced potential deleterious stress on the one remaining central incisor. The patient was given post-insertion instructions and has been on active recall status since that time. She is still seen on a regular basis.

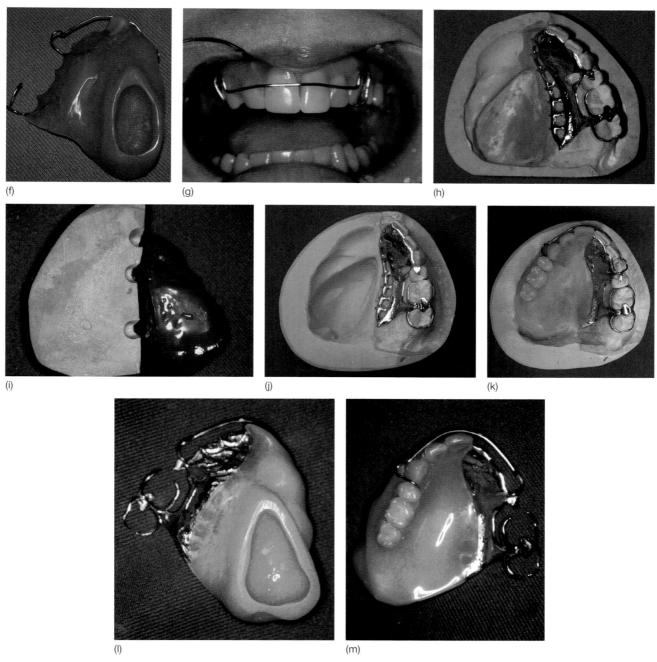

Figure 17.7 (f) The interim obturator. (g) The interim obturator seated in the patient's mouth. The patient used this prosthesis for the duration of radiation therapy. (h) The definitive obturator framework was designed and fabricated as shown. A receptacle was placed in the framework to receive and retain the labial bow. (i) An altered cast impression was made in polysulfide impression material and poured. (j) The altered cast was poured in improved stone and mounted from an intraoral registration and facebow. (k) The completed set-up and wax-up with the placement of the labial bow. (l) The intaglio surface of the processed definitive obturator prosthesis. (m) The occlusal surface is shown in this photo. Note that the labial bow is secured on both ends with acrylic resin.

Discussion

Adenoid cystic carcinoma is an aggressive tumor that tends to travel along the perineural sheath (Neville et al., 2002). It has a poor 5-year prognosis. Additional surgeries have been performed since 2002 in an attempt to control the disease. There has been significant morbidity from these surgeries with trismus being the most problematic from a prosthetic standpoint. However, the dentition has been stable and well maintained. The prosthesis has been modified to accommodate these problems and to allow its continued use. The labial bow is still a functional part of the prosthesis in spite of the morbidities.

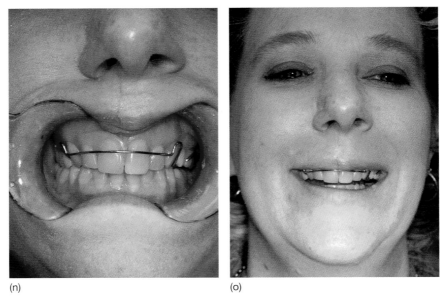

(n)   (o)

Figure 17.7 (n) The final esthetic result. Note that the labial bow is placed in the gingival third of the anterior teeth. (o) It was visible when smiling but was esthetically acceptable to the patient.

Conclusions

Cases 4 and 5 show the use of obturator designs where labial bows were of significant benefit. In Case 4, the bow was an esthetic and functional alternative that provided a transition into the obturator. It provided adequate retention where a canine had been lost. In Case 5, the labial bow was used as a retainer when few anterior maxillary teeth were available to use as abutments.

The biomechanical orthodontic concepts mentioned above were used in the designing of the surgical, interim and definitive obturators. The definitive obturator frameworks were altered to allow retention of the labial bow. However, the overall obturator designs were consistent with established prosthetic principles. The knowledge of biomechanical orthodontic concepts has been used successfully for over 10 years in the second author's practice in a variety of maxillofacial cases ranging from maxillectomy to extensive soft palatal defects and has proven to be a practical addition to the maxillofacial treatment armamentarium.

Acknowledgments

Graduate residents:

- Orthodontics: Drs Chad Webb, Misty Lenk and Darin Lunt
- Periodontics: Dr Natasha May
- Prosthodontics: Drs Brock Satoris and Valarie Cooper.

Periodontics faculty:

- Dr Dimitris Tatakis, Graduate Program Director

Orthodontic technician:

- James Rodriguez, CDT.

References

Aramany MA (1978a) Basic principles of obturator design for partially edentulous patients. Part 1: classification. *Journal of Prosthetic Dentistry* 40: 554–7.

Aramany MA (1978b) Basic principles of obturator design for partially edentulous patients. Part II: design principles. *Journal of Prosthetic Dentistry* 40: 656–62.

Begg PR (1956) Differential force in orthodontic treatment. *American Journal of Orthodontics* 42: 481–510.

Berlocher WC, Mueller BH (1986) Orthodontic procedures. In: KD Rudd, RM Morrow, JE Rhodes (eds) *Dental Laboratory Procedures: Removable Partial Dentures*. St. Louis, MO: Mosby, pp. 617–63.

Bouquot JE, LaMarche MG (1999) Ischemic osteonecrosis under fixed partial denture pontics: radiographic and microscopic features in 38 patients with chronic pain. *Journal of Prosthetic Dentistry* 81(2): 148–58.

Boyd RL (2009) Periodontal and restorative considerations with clear aligner treatment to establish a more favorable restorative environment. *Compendium of Continuing Education in Dentistry* 30(5): 280–2, 284, 286–8.

Curtis TA, Beumer J (1996) Restoration of acquired hard palate defects. In: J Beumer, TA Curtis, MT Marunick (eds) *Maxillofacial Rehabilitation: Prosthodontic and Surgical Considerations*. St Louis, MO: Ishiyaku EuroAmerica, Inc., pp. 245–6.

Evans CA, Nathanson D (1979) Indications for orthodontic-prosthodontic collaboration in dental treatment. *Journal of the American Dental Association* 99(5): 825–30.

Goodacre CJ, Brown DT, Roberts WE, et al. (1997) Prosthodontic considerations when using implants for orthodontic anchorage. *Journal of Prosthetic Dentistry* 77(2): 162–70.

Hawley CA (1919) A removable retainer. *International Journal of Orthodontics, Oral Surgery* 2: 291–8.

Koorbusch GF, Fotos P, Terhark K (1992) Retrospective assessment of osteomyelitis: etiology, demographics, risk factors, and management in 35 cases. *Oral Surgery Oral Medicine Oral Pathology* 74: 149–54.

Miller TE (1995) Orthodontic and restorative procedures for retained deciduous teeth in the adult. *Journal of Prosthetic Dentistry* 73(6): 501–9.

Neville BW, Damm DD, Allen CM, et al. (2002) Pulpal and periapical disease. In: BW Neville, DD Damm, CM Allen, et al. (eds) *Oral and Maxillofacial Pathology*, 2nd edn. Philadelphia, PA: WB Saunders, pp. 126–8, 426–8.

Prasad KC, Prasad SC, Mouli N, et al. (2007) Osteomyelitis in the head and neck. *Acta Otolaryngology* 127(2): 194–205.

Sims MR (1972) Loop systems – a contemporary reassessment. *American Journal of Orthodontics* 61: 270–8.

Spalding PM, Cohen BD (1992) Orthodontic adjunctive treatment in fixed prosthodontics. *Dental Clinics of North America* 36(3): 607–29.

Staley RN, Reske NT (2001) Treatment of Class I nonextraction problems, principles of appliance construction, and retention appliances. In: SE Bishara (ed.) *Textbook of Orthodontics*. Philadelphia, PA: WB Sanders, pp. 290–323.

18

Orthodontic Treatment in Patients Requiring Orthognathic Surgical Procedures

David R Musich

Summary

Orthodontists and oral/maxillofacial surgeons have been working as a team for several decades to treat patients with significant skeletal jaw imbalances. As described in the quote below by Atul Gawande, advances in our technology and know-how have the potential to create better medical and dental outcomes for our patients, but they also create situations in which avoidable failures occur. Therefore, in the management of patients with skeletal jaw imbalances in the horizontal, vertical and/or transverse plane will benefit from the use of a checklist. While many of the steps listed in the checklist are well known by many providers, some of the steps listed below and described in this chapter will serve as a reminder of their importance and will encourage implementation of each of the steps by orthognathic teams and their staff.

The following checklist has been used by the author and his orthognathic teams to help patients not only achieve functional balance of the intricate stomatognathic system which is generally the primary goal of therapy, but also to provide esthetic improvement. When treating patients with complex jaw imbalances, orthognathic teams also strive to achieve functional balance, using reliable methods that achieve realistic, esthetic outcomes that are economically feasible. In addition, the orthodontist's/surgeon's teamwork also strives to provide a stable, satisfactory relationship that enhances the overall orofacial health of the patient. The acronym **FRESH**, described in step II, has been useful as a guide to specifically describe the major goals of orthodontic/orthognathic treatment for patients considering this option.

Thus, creating an orthognathic team, identifying specific treatment goals for each patient, and focusing on each step in the sequence of treatment (*checklist*), presented in this chapter, will help accomplish the desired outcome of orthognathic treatment on a routine basis.

Here then is our situation at the start of the twenty-first century: We have accumulated stupendous know-how. We have put it in the hands of the most highly trained, highly skilled, and hardworking people in our society. And, with it, they have indeed accomplished extraordinary things.

Nonetheless, that know-how is often unmanageable. Avoidable failures are common and persistent, not to mention demoralizing and frustrating, across many fields – from medicine to finance, business to government. And the reason is increasingly more evident: the volume and complexity of what we know has exceeded our individual ability to deliver its benefits correctly, safely, or reliably. Knowledge has both saved us and burdened us.

That means we need a different strategy for overcoming failure: one that builds on experience and takes advantage of the knowledge people have but somehow also makes up for our inevitable human inadequacies. And there is such a strategy – though it will seem almost ridiculous in its simplicity, maybe even crazy to those of us who have spent years carefully developing ever more advanced skills and technologies.

It is the checklist.

Gawande (2010)

The importance of the sequence/checklist

While most people think that a successful orthognathic treatment starts with an interview and an examination of the patient with skeletal jaw imbalance, the most important steps in providing treatment take place long before the surgeon or orthodontist meets the patient. The feedback loop sequence (checklist) described in Table 18.1 identifies eighteen significant steps that provide both the patient and their doctors with an excellent means of achieving the desired treatment outcome when there is a significant dentofacial imbalance.

This chapter will highlight each of the steps needed to address every aspect of care for this special group of

Table 18.1 The preferred sequence of treatment for patients with significant dentofacial imbalances

Stage	Description	Stage	Description
Team preparation – Steps I and II		*Presurgical – Steps XI and XII*	
I	Multiple provider team selection	XI	Comprehensive orthodontic treatment (usually for 8–18 months before surgery)
	• Orthodontist • Periodontist • Restorative dentist • Oral surgeon • Psychologist • Physical therapist		• Orthodontic movement to decompensate tooth positions • Coordination of arches in anticipation of surgical repositioning • Alignment of teeth and correction of rotations
II	Goal clarification for team members	XII	Presurgical re-evaluation records
	• Functional occlusion • Reliable methods • Esthetics • Stability • Health		• Complete records (models, panoramic radiograph, cephalogram, and photos) • Prediction tracing (detailed movements planned) • Model surgery (reviewed by orthodontist and surgeon) • Determination of specific fixation needs • Patient–spouse/other review with orthodontist and surgeon
Diagnosis and patient care – Steps III – X		*Postsurgical – Steps XIII – XVI*	
III	Clinical awareness of dentofacial deformity	XIII	Orthognathic surgery
	• Self, general dentist, spouse/other		• Simplest procedure or procedures to achieve professional goals and satisfy patient's needs
IV	General assessment of patient	XIV	Postsurgical period
	• A good candidate? • Periodontal status • Temporomandibular joint status		• Early: 2–3 weeks of fixation • Late: 3–8 weeks of fixation • Re-evaluation of surgical procedure • Review outcome with patient • Assess need for physical therapy
V	Evaluation of preliminary records by the dental team	XV	Evaluation and surgical stability
	• Splint therapy for diagnosis of temporomandibular dysfunction, if needed		• Orthodontic finishing, occlusal adjustments, and retention procedures • Optimal continuation of contact with psychologist
VI	Completion of diagnostic records	XVI	Post-treatment records
	• May include lifestyle assessment by clinical psychologist • May require more sophisticated temporomandibular joint studies		• 1 year post-treatment • Treatment evaluation by patient and orthodontist
VII	Multidisciplinary review of dentofacial problem based on patient records	*Feedback – Steps XVII – XVIII*	
VIII	Explanation to patient of available treatment options	XVII	Re-evaluation of findings with dental team, especially oral surgeon and general dentist
	• Optimal treatment plan • Alternatives • New, less invasive techniques		• Problem solving • Re-evaluation of degree of success in achieving goals
IX	Consultation with patient and significant other by dental team providers	XVIII	Treatment experience to be used in management of future cases to enhance/refine *checklist*
	• Risk-benefit ratio • Fees and insurance coverage • Treatment time • Other concerns		• Re-evaluation of degree of success in achieving goals • Positive reinforcement
X	Patient acceptance of treatment plan		

patients. In the sequence of treatment for patients with major dentofacial imbalances, Steps I, II, XVII, and XVIII are most often *under*emphasized. It is recommended that the reader review Steps I, II, XVII, and XVIII carefully, to optimize the checklist approach to the management of orthognathic patients and to improve the care as

each orthognathic patient is treatment planned. In addition, Steps III through XVI are required to make sure that a uniform communication process is incorporated by each of the providers for all orthognathic patients; each step will be illustrated and reinforced through presentations of successfully treated case examples in this chapter.

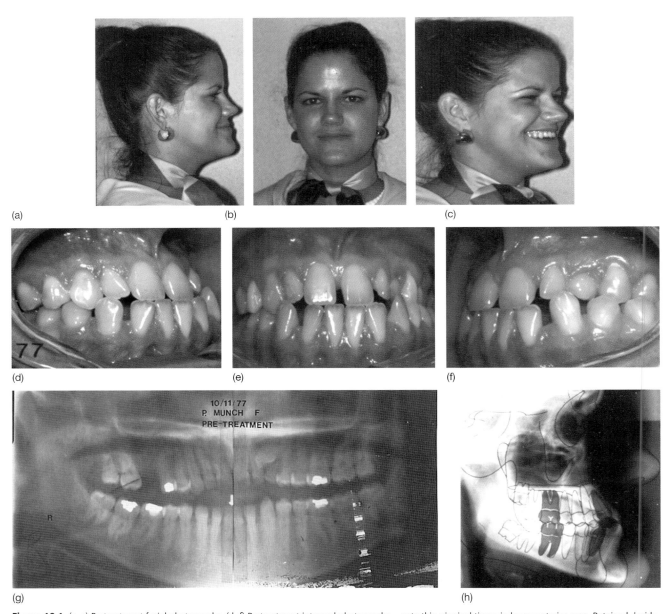

Figure 18.1 (a–c) Pretreatment facial photographs. (d–f) Pretreatment intraoral photographs – note thin gingival tissue in lower anterior area. Retained deciduous maxillary left canine and midline asymmetry. (g) Pretreatment panoramic radiograph. (h) Pretreatment cephalometric radiograph with Bolton template overlay. (Note the skeletal Class III malocclusion with significant mandibular excess.)

By following the general concepts stated in each step, the orthodontist, general dentist, and surgeon will spend the necessary time with the patient and be able to effectively address most of the patient's pre- and postsurgical concerns. Using this checklist, the orthodontist can explain the sequence of treatment steps to the patient and the general dentist through the use of a treatment conference report. Orthognathic patients often experience increased anxiety and ask extra questions about the surgery; these questions need to be addressed, to help maintain their confidence and

trust. The patient records in Figure 18.1 illustrate an adult patient with complex treatment requirements:

- Skeletal Class III with asymmetry of the mandible to the left
- Anterior crossbite
- Impacted maxillary left canine with retained deciduous canine
- Gingival deficiency in the lower anterior incisor area
- Missing maxillary right first molar (recently extracted)

- Patient's attitude about treatment and the longevity of her dentition (asked about the option of dentures during her initial interview).

Due to the complexity of the treatment planning for the patient seen in Figure 18.1, and the other patients with similar skeletal jaw imbalances, an individualized treatment plan is necessary. This will help to detail the sequence of the steps, so that all of the interdisciplinary providers and the patient understand the process, the timetable, and the specific sequence of steps (Figure 18.2).

The following explanations of each step in the sequence detail the rationales and strategies for providing careful treatment planning for patients with complex treatment requirements.

Team preparation – Steps I and II

Step I: Multiple provider team selection (Table 18.1)

- Orthodontist
- Periodontist
- Restorative dentist
- Oral surgeon
- Psychologist
- Physical therapist

Development of the interdisciplinary team is a deliberate step that requires judicious interaction (sometimes 'interviews') with other potential members of the team. The interaction can occur within continuing education

---

TREATMENT CONFERENCE REPORT

TO: Dr. General DDS	RE: Pam M.	DATE: 10-18-03

I. **Classification and diagnostic description of malocclusion:**
    Class III Skeletal Maxillary deficiency (mild) / Mandibular excess (severe) /
    Lower anterior spacing / Upper right posterior spacing

II. **List of dental problems: (mild / moderate / severe)**
    * Impacted #11 / Retained "H"
    * Gingival deficiency lower anterior
    * Impacted 3rd Molars
    * Missing #3

III. **Treatment sequence recommended at this time:**   **Provider:**
    1. Cleanings, decay control and preventative care at DDS   Dr. General DDS
       every 6 mos
    2. Consultation with Oral Maxillofacial Surgeon regarding: Dr. OMFS
       · Removal of 3rd Molars
       · Surgery - Single or double jaw surgery
       · Insurance issues
       · Impacted #11

    3. **Orthodontic Pre-surgery Plan:**   Dr. Musich /Dr. Busch
       · Full upper and lower braces
       · Extraction of "H" - Expose #11 at 4 to 5 months into upper treatment
       · Evaluate for adding lower left bicuspid to aid in long-term stability
         and prepare for surgery
       · Re-evaluate records at 12 to 16 months
       · Evaluate for lower gingival grafts   Dr. Periodontist
       · Dual consultation regarding jaw surgery   Musich/Busch/Oral surgeon

IV. **Overall problem severity: (0-10 scale, with 10 being most severe) 8.5/10**
    Due to complex Inner Disciplinary Therapy problem.

V. **Limiting factors in achieving "text book ideal" result:**
    1. Stability of space closure may require adding lower premolar on lower left.
    2. Jaw surgery is needed for correction of Class III problem.
    3. Bridge or implant is needed on upper right posterior.

VI. **Patient concerns and current paln of action:**
    1. Pam understands the above treatment plan.
    2. Pam will consult with the Oral Surgeon.
    2. Pam is excited to have problems corrected.

    Treatment Time: 20-26 months   Treatment Start Date: To be decided

        cc: **Oral Maxillofacial Surgeon**
            Periodontist
            Pam M
            Patients Chart

Figure 18.2 The *Treatment Conference Report*. For patients with interdisciplinary therapy requirements it is important to have the steps in the plan summarized for each of the providers and for the patient. The Treatment Conference Report provides the 'roadmap' for treatment and the approximate timing of the steps.

Box 18.1 Basic goals for interdisciplinary dentofacial teams

- Philosophy of treatment consistent to achieve desired goals
- Ability to recognize, prioritize, and address the patient's chief concern
- High-quality communication process between the doctors and treatment coordinators
- Logistic availability of office; office hours; method of doctor-to-doctor communication
- Compatible insurance coverage (in network – out of network)
- Patient's comfort and trust of the providers within the referral loop

professional study clubs or might evolve from the discussions of patient treatment planning (Box 18.1). As stated by Turpin (2010): 'Talking with current members of successful study clubs, I found that they share many traits. Historically, most study clubs had rather modest beginnings, but, with strong leadership, they can evolve into large organizations with lofty goals. No matter the size or the location, the secret of orthodontic study clubs is clear to me: you get out of them what you put into them.' Study clubs that include both orthodontists and surgeons as members, can develop effective interactions and an accelerated awareness of new, evidence-based insights regarding the type of care that is best suited for their patients with skeletal jaw imbalances.

An excellent book by Roblee (1994), *Interdisciplinary Dentofacial Therapy: A Comprehensive Approach to Optimal Patient Care*, advanced the concept of interdisciplinary dentofacial therapy and provided a strategy for developing predictable outcomes for patients with complex dentofacial situations:

The concept of Interdisciplinary Dentofacial Therapy (IDT) was developed to maximize treatment results by optimally synergizing the knowledge, skills, and experience of all the disciplines in dentistry and its associated fields, while minimizing the frustrating and problematic shortcomings typically associated with working as a team.

Roblee et al. (2009)

This book is recommended reading for any IDT team that is in its formative stages. Roblee et al. (2009) emphasized two key elements of the teamwork needed to consistently produce high quality results:

Regimental sequencing to insure that every procedure is performed in the order closest to ideal throughout the entire interdisciplinary process.

Extensive communication between providers, to optimize all aspects of IDT.

The dentist will refer patients (Figure 18.3) with skeletal malocclusion to the orthodontist, but only if he/she is con-

fident that the patient will receive appropriate state-of-the-art care. The orthodontist must then select surgeons who are experienced and well-trained in the spectrum of orthognathic procedures. A periodontist, psychologist, and physical therapist may become key team members in selected cases, as they may be required for certain types of orthognathic situations. With the advent of rigid fixation, patients seem to have less of a need for psychological intervention as the post-operative phase of depression has been less of a problem (Dolce et al., 2002).

However, there are patients with profound self-esteem issues, for whom presurgical counseling may better prepare them for the changes that may occur during the orthodontic/orthognathic treatment. This counseling may also help patients develop realistic expectations of the treatment outcome (Figure 18.4).

Step II: Goal clarification for team members (Box 18.2)

- **F** unction (optimal)
- **R** eliable/realistic
- **E** sthetic/economic
- **S** tability/satisfaction
- **H** ealth – dental/mental

The members of the provider team should share similar concepts of treatment goals. For example, functional occlusal goals, stability of outcome, and dental and facial esthetic goals can mean different things to different professionals. Periodic group meetings oriented to individual case analysis offer an opportunity for team members to discuss their concepts of the treatment goals that apply to the individual patient, and to establish consistency in pursuing treatment and treatment goals.

Borderline surgery Class II – case report (Figure 18.5)

Sometimes 'borderline' surgical patients are referred to oral and maxillofacial surgeons (OMS) to enhance informed consent and to help the patient develop better insights into the options of their care. There is value in considering all treatment goals as a group, using the acronym FRESH.

- Interdisciplinary consultation can improve dialog between the provider and the patient, so that prioritization becomes clearer to each. When one goal or several are prioritized over others, careful consideration should be given to which goals are being de-prioritized, so that the outcome of treatment is not undermined. For example, if the goal of economic treatment becomes a priority when the stability of the outcome is not factored into the treatment plan, the results will fail when the equilibrium requirements of the stomatognathic system cause the malocclusion to reoccur.

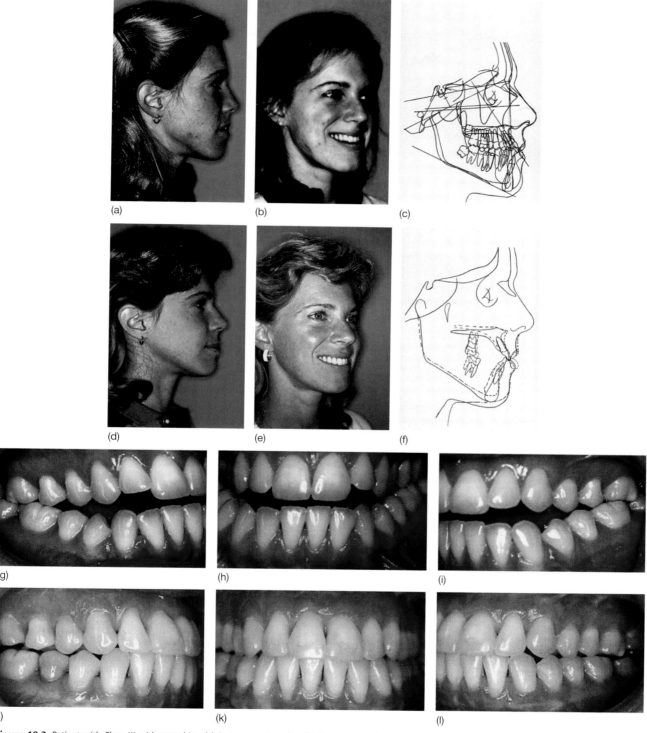

Figure 18.3 Patient with Class III with open bite. (a) Pretreatment profile. (b) Pretreatment three-quarter smile photograph. (c) Pretreatment tracing of cephalogram with Bolton template superimposed to provide a *template-guided treatment plan.* (d) Post-treatment profile. (e) Post-treatment three-quarter smile photograph after maxillomandibular surgery and orthodontics, and periodontal grafting to improve her overall dental health and functional environment. (f) Cephalometric superimposition of before and after tracings. (g–i) Pretreatment intraoral photographs. (j–l) Post-treatment intraoral photographs.

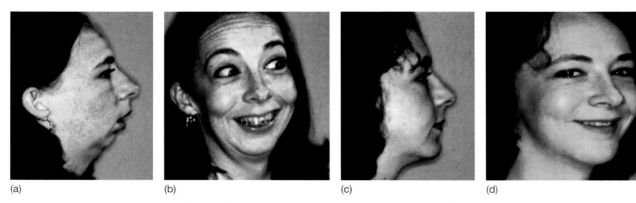

(a)   (b)   (c)   (d)

Figure 18.4 Patient with significant mandibular deficiency and chin deficiency. (a) Presurgical facial profile of (b) Presurgical three-quarter smile. (c) Postsurgical facial profile of same patient following orthodontics and bimaxillary surgery. (d) Postsurgical three-quarter smile of same patient – patient had mandibular advancement and maxillary impaction and genioplasty.

Box 18.2 F.R.E.S.H

- *Function* – The fundamental goal of improving occlusal relationship is paramount; it is desirable to establish optimal gnathological parameters for the stomatognathic system (incisal guidance, canine rise, and balanced, bilateral posterior occlusal support), temporomandibular joint (TMJ) health, and TMJ stability without symptoms.
- *Reliable* – Methods of treatment that have been scientifically verified to be highly successful in achieving correction of skeletal imbalances, and that are of lower risks than other available procedures for the improvement of a given condition, are utilized. Recent examples of techniques that have proven their reliability include rigid fixation approaches; jaw surgery to resolve sleep apnea; and use of microscrews as anchorage-to improve the range of nonsurgical treatment.
- *Realistic* – The plan of treatment has a high probability of correcting the patient's chief concern, and offers the best option to achieve an outcome with a high probability of meeting both the patient's and doctor's expectations.
- *Esthetics* – Issues of esthetics relate to both dental and facial appearance; facial esthetics requires assessment of both the profile and frontal views, to achieve soft tissue balance, as well as optimal symmetry. The facial balance should be present both statically and dynamically in speech and during facial expression, especially in smiling. The role of the 'aging process of the face' should also be integrated into the treatment planning process, especially when considering camouflage options.
- *Economic* – The cost of the proposed treatment requires consideration because most patients have a well-defined budget for their medical and dental needs. With limited insurance for orthodontic care, and reduced coverage for orthognathic surgical procedures, financial considerations frequently interfere with the optimal combined orthognathic/orthodontic treatment plan.
- *Stability* – A key part of the treatment outcome is ending with jaw and tooth positions that are reasonably stable. There are several dimensions to stability, and there are many adult orthodontic problems that require fixed retention to assure stability, especially of the lower and upper incisors.
- *Satisfaction* – Achieving both patient and provider satisfaction is important. This usually occurs when there is *open discussion*, prior to treatment, about the goals that both the doctor and the patient are striving to achieve in this individual situation. This would include a frank discussion from the doctor about the 'downside' or 'limits' of the accepted plan. This is particularly true in patients who have a skeletal diagnosis and are being considered for camouflage therapy when skeletal correction is more ideal. The use of visualized treatment objectives and computerized predictions can assist the patient and the providers.

- Interdisciplinary consultation allows restatement of the conditions of the disharmony that can successfully be treated and the ones that cannot.
- The use of *therapeutic diagnosis* with functional appliances is appropriately presented (Figure 18.6)
- Medicolegal issues will be less likely with this sort of full disclosure (Wheeler, 1992; Jerrold, 2000).

In addition to the above points, during the past decade, the treatment paradigm has changed with the effectiveness of newly developed modalities, such as the use of temporary anchorage devices (TADs) (Xun et al., 2007), surgically facilitated orthodontic treatment (SFOT) (Roblee et al., 2009), and periodontal accelerated orthodontic procedures (PAOP) (Murphy et al., 2009). As a result, there are several more treatment planning options available for the patient with borderline surgical problems.

Diagnosis and patient care – Steps III–X

Step III: Clinical awareness of dentofacial deformity (Figure 18.7)

- Self – through awareness of symptoms or intrinsic esthetic issues
- General dentist – through diagnostic process or increase of subjective and objective symptoms
- Spouse/other – through personal research and support
- Friend – who might have experienced an orthognathic correction and encourages the patient to pursue correction

Patients learn about their dentofacial imbalance through a variety of ways. Frequently, awareness of the problem starts with early diagnosis at the family dentist's practice. Some patients exhibit disproportionate growth patterns that will not show up until early adulthood. For example, the patient in Figure 18.8 only became aware of the need for orthog-

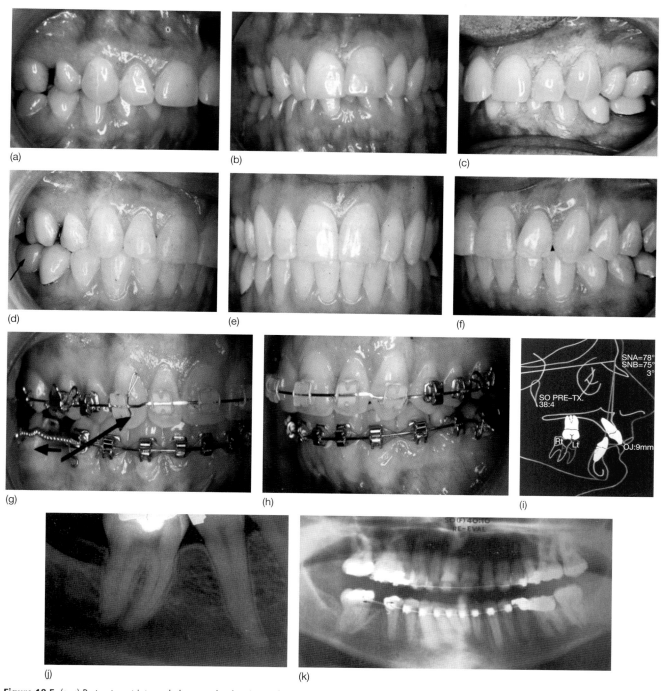

Figure 18.5 (a–c) Pretreatment intraoral photographs showing a Class II malocclusion with maxillary protrusion, with upper premolars missing, crowded lower anteriors and a significant overjet. (d–f) Post-treatment intraoral photographs with correction of overjet, crowding, and Class I canine relationship. (g,h) Progress intraoral photographs showing reversal of arch collapse due to early extraction of the mandibular right first molar. Longstanding arch collapse created the appearance of a skeletal malocclusion, when much of the overjet was a result of the collapsed mandibular arch, drifting of the right buccal segment, and collapsed lower incisor area secondary to lip entrapment. (i) Pretreatment cephalometric tracing; initial treatment plan by first orthodontist suggested a surgical approach to resolve the overjet. (j) Pretreatment periapical radiograph showing the collapsed area at the mandibular right first molar. (k) Progress panoramic radiograph showing space opening at mandibular right first molar that also advanced the lower anteriors, which reduced the overjet without surgical intervention. The space at the missing mandibular right first molar was stabilized with a fixed restoration.

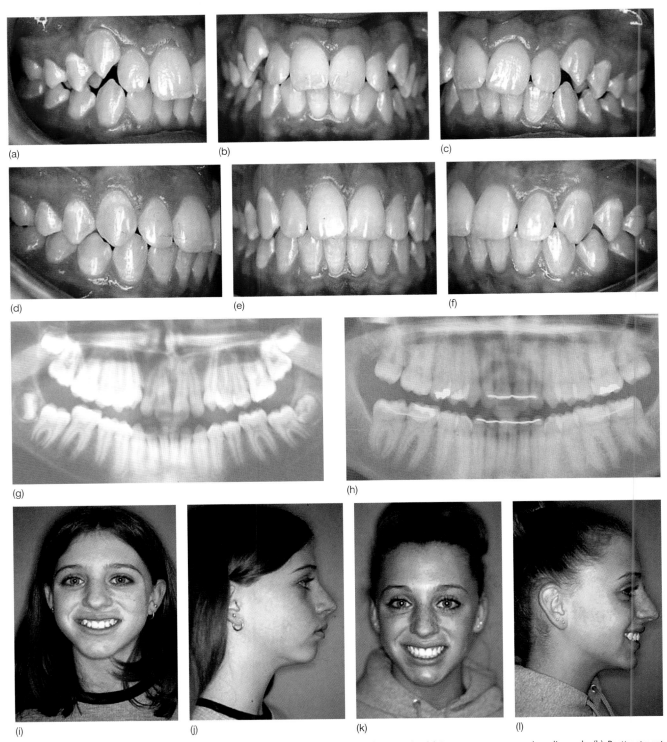

Figure 18.6 (a–c) Pretreatment intraoral photographs. (d–f) Posttreatment intraoral photographs. (g) Pretreatment panoramic radiograph. (h) Posttreatment panoramic radiograph. (i,j) Pretreatment facial photographs. (k,l) Post-treatment facial photographs.

nathic surgery after a robust adolescent growth spurt, which occurred after two years of full orthodontic treatment. Other factors that lead patients to consider orthognathic procedures are facial and/or jaw trauma, pain due to dysfunctional TMJ apparatus, inability to chew and digest food, periodontal breakdown, and combinations of the above conditions, frequently augmented by the patient's esthetic concerns. Tables 18.2–18.4 show the prevalence of skeletal jaw imbalances that would be significant enough to require surgery.

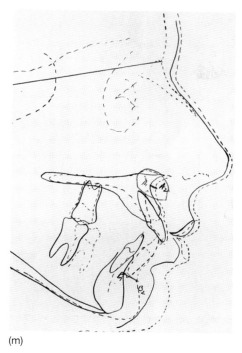

(m)

Figure 18.6 (m) Pretreatment and posttreatment cephalometric tracings superimposed, illustrating excellent growth response of the mandible through the use of the mandibular anterior repositioning appliance (MARA).

Step IV: General assessment of a patient

For all patients, periodontal diagnosis requires the attention of the orthodontist. One of the most overlooked considerations in the management of the adult patient considering combined orthodontic and orthognathic treatment is the impact of patient susceptibility to periodontal disease, coupled with the pre-existing habit of smoking. Up until 2003, many orthodontists did not include a question on the adult medical history form asking if the patient used tobacco products, nor did the form include a follow-up question about the frequency of tobacco use. In 1996, the American Academy of Periodontists published a position paper titled 'Tobacco use and the periodontal patient' (Ryder, 1996). In this well-researched paper, the American Academy of Periodontists referenced 97 published papers, which verify the following:

Clinical and epidemiological studies support the concept that tobacco use is an important variable affecting the prevalence and progression of periodontal diseases, such as adult periodontitis, refractory periodontitis, and ANUG [acute necrotizing ulcerative gingivitis]. Several studies have demonstrated that the severity of periodontal disease appears to be related to the duration of the tobacco use, smoking status, and amount of daily tobacco intake.

The orthodontist and the surgeon, through the patient's health history, should understand the patient's tobacco use

habits, and provide follow-up in which the patient is informed of the risk of accelerated bone loss and a poor prognosis for long-term health (Ryder, 1996). In addition, orthognathic outcomes may be affected if the patient smokes during the postsurgical healing period.

In summary, the orthodontist plays a key role in diagnosing a skeletal problem that may require surgery, a periodontal condition, which may worsen as a result of tooth movement, and a temporomandibular disorder, which requires its own differential diagnosis and plan. *Diagnostic* steps described previously lead the orthodontist and the team of dental providers to a comprehensive *treatment plan* *that* has the highest probability of achieving the desired *goals* of treatment. Figure 18.9 illustrates an adult patient who had previous orthodontic treatment with the extraction of four first premolars; however the transverse deficiency of the maxilla had not been diagnosed. In addition, the patient smoked heavily, resulting in gingival inflammation, and the smoking habit, in addition to the severe maxillary transverse skeletal discrepancy, aggravated her gingival recession. Through appropriate diagnosis, planning, and adherence to a smoking cessation program, the patient responded well to her comprehensive treatment.

Step V: Evaluation of preliminary records by the dental team

- Splint therapy for diagnosis of temporomandibular dysfunction, if needed
- Referral for more advanced TMJ imaging and/or treatment with physical therapist

Questions to be resolved at this stage of the assessment:

- What are all of the dentofacial problems to be addressed by the treatment plan?
- Is there temporomandibular stability and health?
- Is there periodontal stability and health?
- Are there restorative requirements due to missing or deteriorated teeth?
- Is there a skeletal discrepancy of maxilla and mandible in any or all of the three planes of space?
- Is the patient aware of the problems and the degree of severity of the problems?
- Will the treatment plan (i.e. problem solving) be required to proceed in phases with time intervals between steps, or can the plan be managed in a straightforward sequential pattern?
- Are other providers needed to answer additional questions or to diagnose new problems?

Step VI: Completion of diagnostic records

- May include lifestyle assessment by clinical psychologist
- May require more sophisticated TMJ studies

Many adult patients who have a dentofacial imbalance and seek treatment are unaware of the treatment requirements

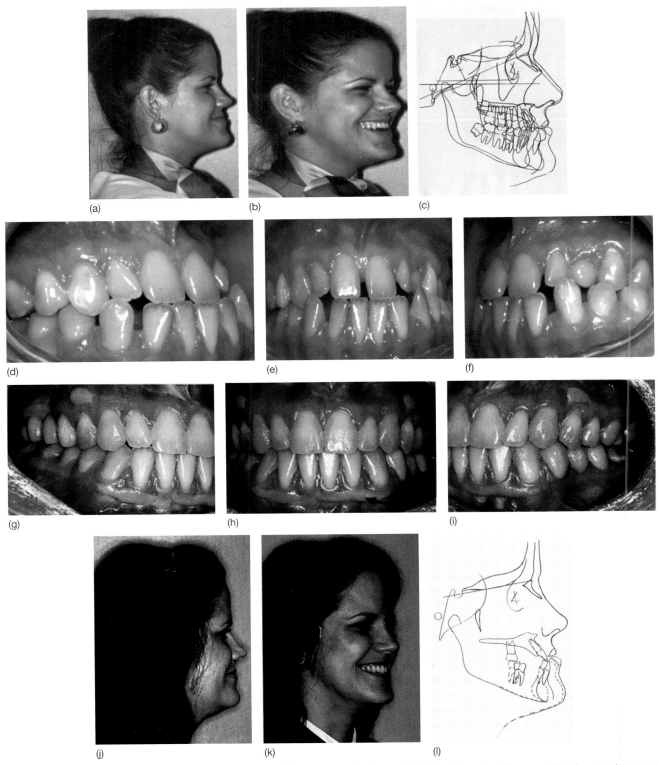

Figure 18.7 (a) Pretreatment facial photograph. (b) Pretreatment three-quarter smile photograph. (c) Template-guided diagnosis with Bolton template super-imposed on pretreatment cephalometric tracing of patient. (d–f) Pretreatment intraoral photographs. (g–i) Post-treatment intraoral photographs showing successful outcome of interdisciplinary dentofacial therapy, as illustrated in Figure 18.2. (j) Post-treatment facial profile photograph. (k) Post-treatment three-quarter smile photographs. (l) Superimposition of pretreatment tracing with post-treatment skeletal change demonstrated.

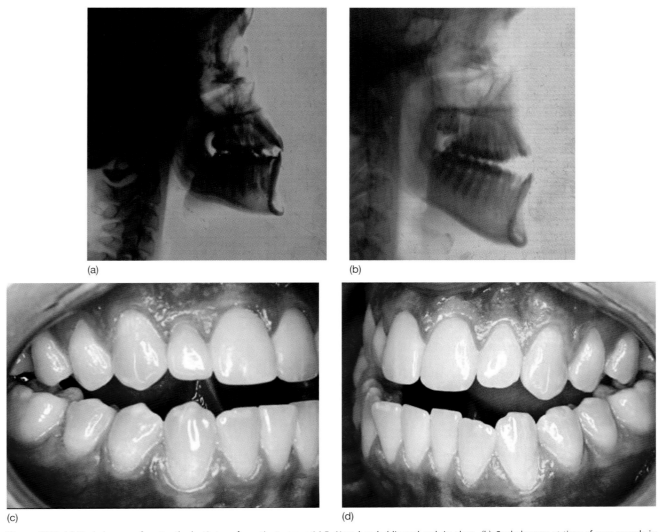

Figure 18.8 (a) Cephalogram of post-orthodontic transfer patient at age 14.5. Note bonded lingual arch in place. (b) Cephalogram at time of new records in new office following a robust adolescent male growth spurt, illustrating significant differential growth of maxilla and mandible which ultimately required orthodontic retreatment and bimaxillary surgery. (c,d) Intraoral photographs showing the degree of Class III malocclusion and the anterior open bite.

Table 18.2 Estimated prevalence of mandibular deficiency severe enough to indicate surgery

	Percentage	Number
Prevalence of skeletal Class II malocclusion	10[a]	31 000 000
At appropriate age for surgical treatment	68	21 125 000
Severe enough to warrant surgery	5	1 056 250
Mandibular advancement	70	739,375
Maxillary setback	10	105 625
Both	20	211 250
New patients added to the population yearly[b]	0.5	21 250

[a]Assuming US population of 325 million.
[b]Assuming 4.25 million live births per year.

Table 18.3 Estimated prevalence of Class III problems severe enough to indicate surgery

	Percentage	Number
Prevalence of skeletal Class III malocclusion	0.6[a]	1 950 000
At appropriate age for surgical treatment	65	1 267 500
Severe enough to warrant surgery	33	418 275
Mandibular setback	45	188 224
Maxillary advancement	35	146 396
Both	20	83 655
New patients added to the population yearly[b]	0.2	8 500

[a]Assuming US population of 325 million.
[b]Assuming 4.25 million live births per year.

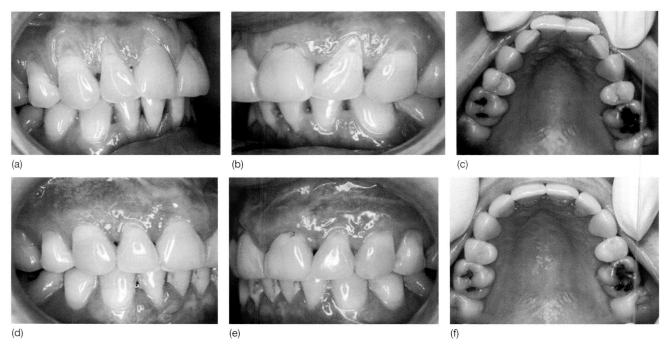

Figure 18.9 (a–c) Pretreatment right and left view of occlusal relationship; note significant degree of gingival recession. This patient had previous orthodontic treatment with four premolar extractions; in addition she was a heavy smoker. (d–f) Post-treatment right and left view of occlusal relationship. Due to significant degree of maxillary skeletal transverse deficiency, this patient required multiple treatment steps: surgically assisted rapid maxillary expansion; smoking cessation program; orthodontic treatment; and gingival grafting procedures.

Table 18.4 Estimated prevalence of long-face problems severe enough to indicate surgery

	Percentage	Number
Prevalence of severe anterior open bite	0.6[a]	1 950 000
At appropriate age for surgical treatment	65	1 267 500
Severe enough to warrant surgery (superior repositioning of the maxilla)	25	316 875
New patients added to the population yearly[b]	0.2	6375

[a]Assuming US population of 325 million.
[b]Assuming 4.25 million live births per year.

to accomplish an optimal outcome. Some patients have received preliminary information from their general dentists that treatment may require jaw surgery, and some have had previous orthodontic treatment that was unable to resolve the skeletal component of the problem effectively. Also, it must be noted that many patients appear to have more of a skeletal component to their malocclusion than is diagnosed by their records and fall into a *borderline surgical* category. The borderline surgical group frequently can be managed through judicious treatment planning, which may include an initial phase of therapeutic diagnosis to

determine the degree of functional shift in an adult Class III patient, and the additional step of strategic extraction to allow optimal dentoalveolar changes to camouflage the skeletal imbalance. While this approach does not always fulfill all of the treatment goals described in the FRESH paradigm (Box 18.2), it is frequently a satisfactory approach to creating a secondary treatment plan if surgery is not desired or not approved by the insurance plan. A key step in this scenario is clarifying what compromises (trade-offs) are to be expected and what measures will be needed to offset the residual skeletal imbalance.

Step VII: Multidisciplinary review of a dentofacial problem based on patient records

At this stage of the assessment, the preliminary work done to establish a compatible interdisciplinary team enhances the uniformity of the planning. The philosophy of care of the providers is harmonious, which allows the patient to make a discretionary decision regarding the treatment plan that has been recommended.

Diagnoses in the anteroposterior and vertical planes are typically completed using a variety of cephalometric analyses. Newer computerized software programs allow cephalograms to be digitized and analyzed, providing an abundant amount of numerical information about the patient's skeletal jaw relations. Frequently, cephalometric analyses generate confusing and, at times, conflicting information regarding the differential diagnosis of the patient's conditions (Jacobson, 1995).

In borderline surgical problems, we have found that differential diagnosis can be most easily accomplished through the use of *template-guided diagnosis* and the *treatment planning process*. Jacobson (1979) presented the use of a simplified approach to aid in the diagnosis of skeletal disproportions that might be evident on a patient's lateral cephalogram. This report demonstrated the value of using normative, composite templates to aid in diagnosis and treatment planning. Since that time, two of America's most respected orthodontic department chairs have made statements that have validated the use of templates to aid in differential diagnosis. Johnston (1987) observed that 'many clinicians stop tracing cephalograms at about the time their practices start to get busy. Ideally, a descriptive analysis should consist only of those measurements that are needed to illuminate the clinically significant idiosyncrasies of the patient at hand. Template analysis may seem an ideal solution.' Proffit and White (1990) pointed out that 'the template may appear to be somewhat less scientific than a table of cephalometric measurements with standard deviations, but the template is a visual analog of a table and is just as valid.' Proffit and White (1990) also state, 'What a template does is place the emphasis on the analysis itself; that is, deciding what the distortions are, rather than on an intermediate measurement that too often becomes an end in itself rather than just a means to an end'.

For the past 25 years, we have adopted a variation of the Jacobson template method of superimposition, and its use has been described as 'template-guided diagnosis and treatment planning' (Musich, 2005). The method that has been described in *Orthodontics: Current Principles and Practices* (Graber et al., 2005) incorporates the following concepts:

- Standardized templates (Figure 18.10) from the Broadbent/Bolton study (Broadbent et al., 1975) provide a proportionate soft and hard tissue comparison to predetermined norms of an age-matched, balanced profile that can be of diagnostic value when compared with the patient's cephalometric tracing (for adults, the 18-year-old standard is used). This superimposition technique acknowledges that the size of the patient's nose is a key factor in actual visualized, profile perceptions (e.g., a patient with a large nose and a mild mandibular deficiency may appear to have a severe mandibular deficiency when viewed in profile because of nasal dominance)
- The template method described in Figure 18.10 and illustrated in the clinical application in Figure 18.11 is

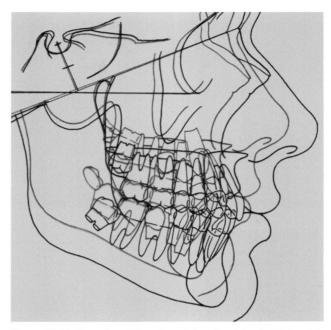

Figure 18.10 Illustration of Broadbent Bolton Templates (adult template superimposed on child at SN to illustrate normal growth amounts during adolescence). These templates can be incorporated to assist the differential diagnosis of maxillary and mandibular skeletal/dental problems. In addition the *template-guided diagnosis and treatment plan* approach is a useful concept for patient education of the nature of the skeletal problem that is affecting the occlusion.

very 'staff and patient friendly', as it allows rapid visualization of the skeletal discrepancy – which helps patients understand why surgical intervention may be needed in a variety of situations. *Template-guided diagnosis and treatment planning* provides an excellent orientation for the clinician to make decisions that will help guide both the skeletal and dental corrections to be made in the direction of balanced hard and soft tissue facial proportions.

Step VIII: Explanation to patient of available treatment options

- Optimal treatment plan
- Alternatives
- New, less invasive techniques
  - Collect data accurately
  - Analyze database
  - Develop problem list
  - Prepare tentative treatment plan
  - Interact with those who are involved; discuss plans and options (may include other providers); clarify sequence; acquire patient acceptance
  - Create final treatment plan (Figure 18.12)

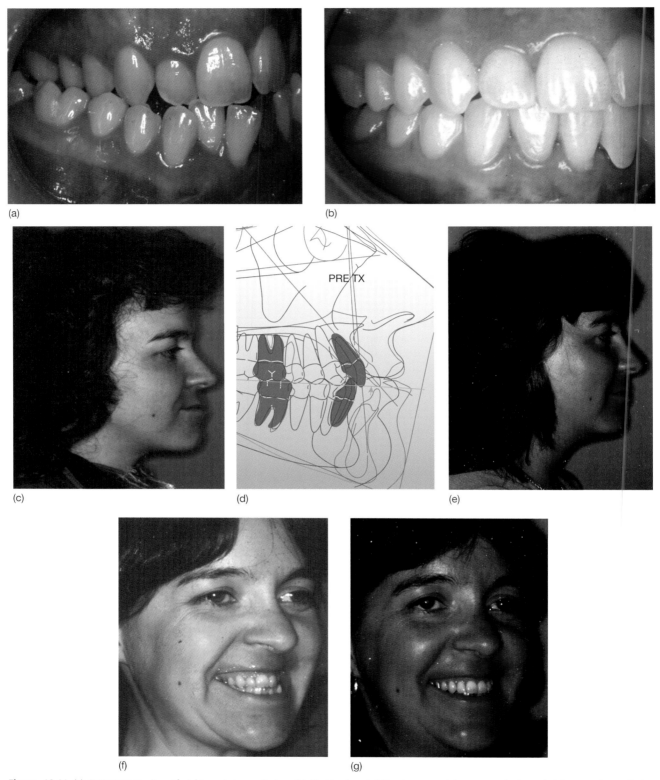

Figure 18.11 (a) Pretreatment view of right posterior occlusion. (b) Post-treatment (after braces and jaw surgery) view of right posterior occlusion. (c) Pretreatment view of facial profile. (d) Pretreatment Bolton superimposition on patient's cephalometric tracing to illustrate the effectiveness of template diagnosis and treatment planning. (e) Post- treatment view of facial profile. (f) Pretreatment view three-quarter smile. (g) Post-treatment view of three-quarter smile showing good facial balance in smile pose.

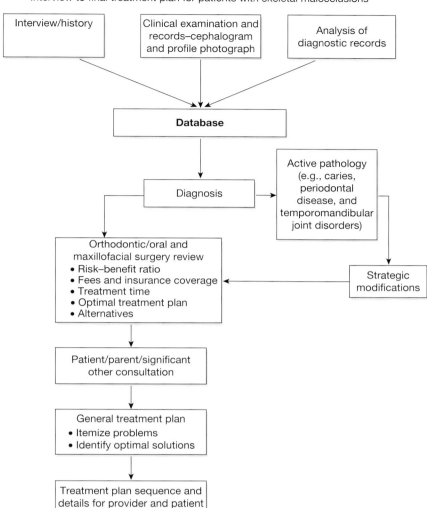

Interview to final treatment plan for patients with skeletal malocclusions

Figure 18.12 Treatment pathway for patients with significant skeletal malocclusions illustrating the many decisions that are required to accomplish an optimal treatment plan.

The correct skeletal differential diagnosis is the key responsibility of the orthodontic member of the interdisciplinary team. While the lateral cephalogram has been relied on for the skeletal diagnosis in the anteroposterior and vertical planes, the frontal or posteroanterior cephalogram has not been routinely used by orthodontists to make an appropriate three-dimensional (3D) diagnosis. As recently as 2001, the *Journal of Clinical Orthodontics* surveyed readers and found that only 8% of those responding to the survey routinely took a posteroanterior cephalogram, while 95% routinely took a panoramic radiograph and 90% routinely took a lateral cephalogram (Gottlieb et al., 1991). In a recent clinical assessment of adult patients who seek orthodontic re-treatment, I found and reported that 18% have a maxillomandibular skeletal discrepancy in the transverse dimension that requires jaw surgery. Usually surgically

assisted rapid palatal expansion (Figure 18.13) is required to achieve an optimal treatment outcome.

The patient illustrated in Figure 18.14 had previous treatment as an adolescent but did not wear retainers as directed, and her maxillary skeletal transverse deficiency was not treated in the basal bone as was necessary. As a result, she sought treatment as an adult, which required surgically assisted expansion and Class III maxillary distraction to correct her mild Class III malocclusion.

Step IX: Consultation with patient and significant other by dental team providers

- Risk–benefit ratio
- Fees and insurance coverage
- Treatment time
- Other concerns

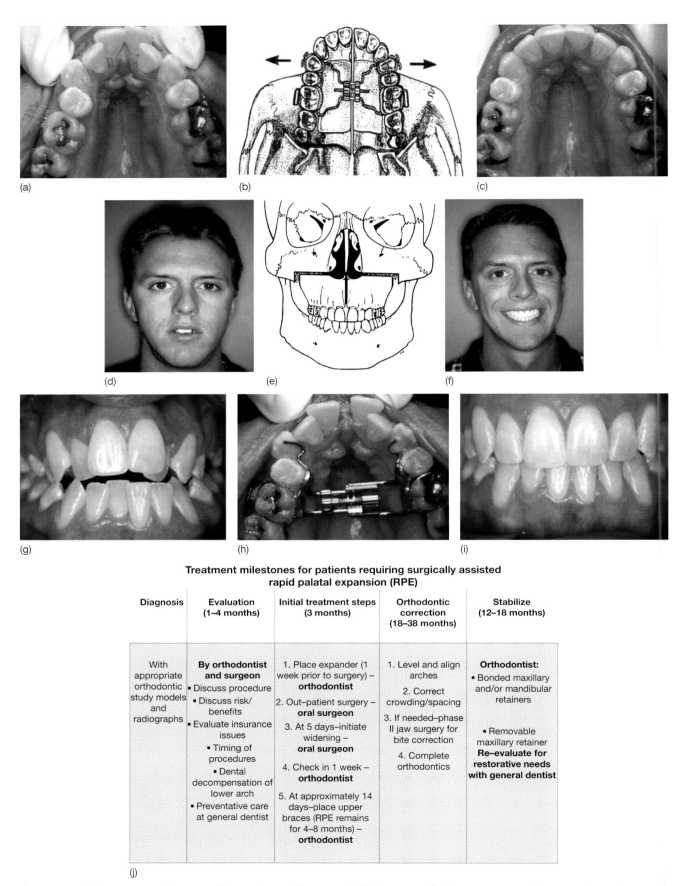

Treatment milestones for patients requiring surgically assisted rapid palatal expansion (RPE)

Diagnosis	Evaluation (1–4 months)	Initial treatment steps (3 months)	Orthodontic correction (18–38 months)	Stabilize (12–18 months)
With appropriate orthodontic study models and radiographs	**By orthodontist and surgeon** ▪ Discuss procedure ▪ Discuss risk/benefits ▪ Evaluate insurance issues ▪ Timing of procedures ▪ Dental decompensation of lower arch ▪ Preventative care at general dentist	1. Place expander (1 week prior to surgery) – **orthodontist** 2. Out–patient surgery – **oral surgeon** 3. At 5 days–initiate widening – **oral surgeon** 4. Check in 1 week – **orthodontist** 5. At approximately 14 days–place upper braces (RPE remains for 4–8 months) – **orthodontist**	1. Level and align arches 2. Correct crowding/spacing 3. If needed–phase II jaw surgery for bite correction 4. Complete orthodontics	**Orthodontist:** ▪ Bonded maxillary and/or mandibular retainers ▪ Removable maxillary retainer **Re–evaluate for restorative needs with general dentist**

(j)

Figure 18.13 (a,g) Pretreatment (re-treatment) intraoral view of patient who had previous orthodontic treatment and four premolar teeth extracted. (b,e,h) Illustration of maxillary expansion utilizing surgical assistance. (c,i) Post-treatment intraoral photographs. The patient underwent surgically assisted rapid maxillary expansion and full braces to correct a significant maxillary skeletal transverse deficiency. (d,f) Pre- and post-treatment (re-treatment) frontal facial view. (j) Treatment milestones for patients requiring basal bone correction of maxillary skeletal transverse deficiency.

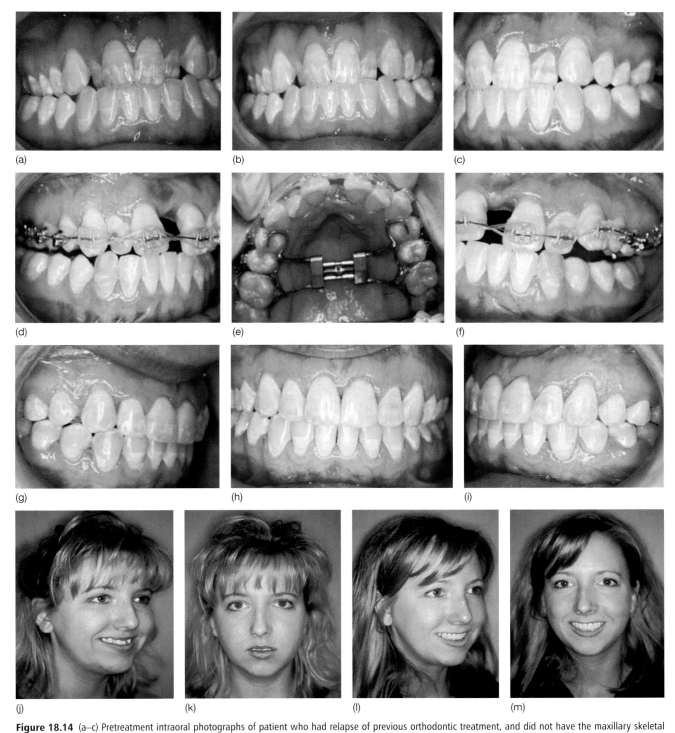

Figure 18.14 (a–c) Pretreatment intraoral photographs of patient who had relapse of previous orthodontic treatment, and did not have the maxillary skeletal deficiency diagnosed or treated. (d–f) Intraoral progress photographs illustrating the effective expansion and diastema creation during the first 3 weeks of maxillary expansion. (g–i) Intraoral photographs of patient following rapid maxillary expansion and full fixed appliance treatment. Correction of the skeletal deficiency of the maxilla allowed stable alignment of the incisors and some degree of anteroposterior correction of the Class III maxillary deficiency. (j,k) Pretreatment facial photographs. (l,m) Post-treatment facial photographs illustrating the improved upper lip support and fuller smile secondary to the correction of the skeletal and dental imbalances.

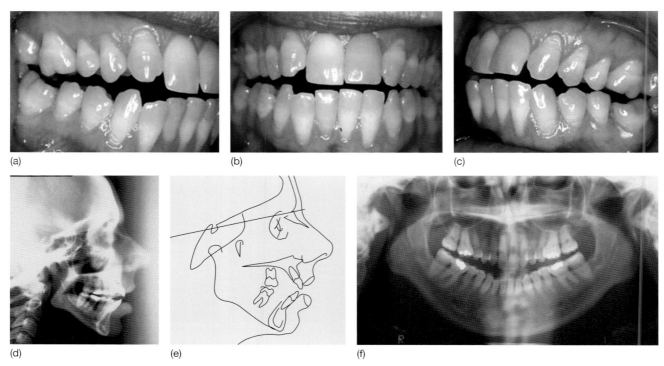

Figure 18.15 (a–c) Pretreatment intraoral photographs of patient who had previous orthodontic treatment, but had subsequent facial trauma and temporomandibular joint dysfunction. (d,e) Cephalogram and tracing of cephalogram, respectively. (f) Panoramic radiograph showing bilateral condylar resorption which is a factor in this patient's bite changes and occlusal instability.

Seeking and verifying coverage through certain US insurance companies and the degree of coverage for complicated procedures such as jaw surgery has added another hurdle in achieving high quality, reliable treatment outcomes for patients with skeletal jaw imbalances. Because of insurance denials, orthodontists and surgeons have had to attempt to achieve major occlusal changes without changing the basal bone relationship. Some of these attempts have failed and have led to results that are unfavorable (Figure 18.15).

Step X: Patient acceptance of treatment plan

When patients have skeletal imbalances in all three planes of space and have experienced an adolescent stage of orthodontics (Figure 18.16) that clearly failed, it is a challenge to convince them that there is a surgical solution to their malocclusion. At the consultation appointment, a thorough review of the records is used to outline the specific sequence for their problem. For such patients (e.g. the patient in Figure 18.16), who want the most reliable approach to solve their bite problems, a two-stage surgical procedure with orthodontic arch preparation is usually recommended.

Case summary for patient in Figure 18.16

- **Chief concern**: Jaw locks forward; poor jaw alignment; frequent muscle fatigue; difficulty chewing; jaw pain.
- **Dental history**: Several years of orthodontics as teenager; second molar removed; removable appliance tried

to correct bite; treated by general dentist. Recent opinion sought at other orthodontist.
- **Referral by oral surgeon**: For orthodontic/surgical treatment.
- **Medical history**: Mouth breather; nasal passages damaged by allergies.

The patient in Figure 18.16 was treated with phase I surgically assisted rapid palatal expansion, followed by orthodontic alignment and arch preparation for the second stage of surgical treatment, which included a Le Fort procedure with differential impaction of the maxilla. During the final assessment of the patient's outcome (Step XVII), this patient made the following comments about his treatment:

This letter is to reiterate the many benefits that this orthodontic treatment has provided for me. Of these, I have noted three significant categories: mechanical, digestive, and hygienic. Mechanical simply relates to the function of my jaw opening and closing. Before this treatment I would awake several mornings each week unable to open my mouth. This problem has now been alleviated and, with it, the pain, the discomfort, and the nights of poor sleep.

The category of digestion is somewhat more complex. Chewing used to be very fatiguing. For this reason I had a tendency to rush through meals. Eating was not an enjoy-

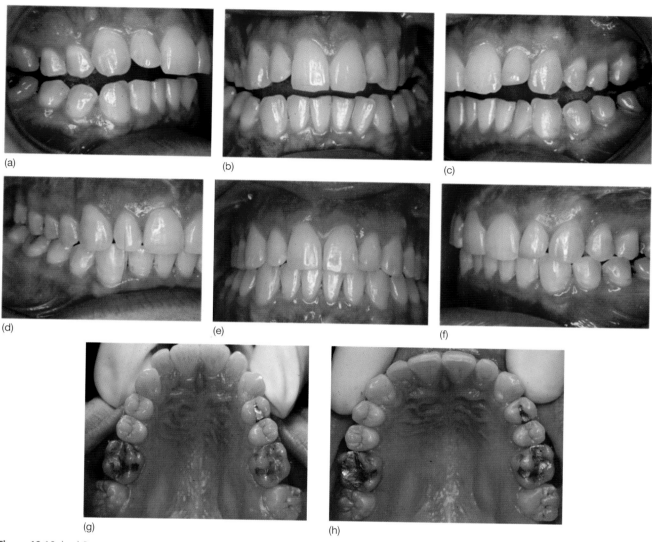

Figure 18.16 (a–c) Pretreatment intraoral photographs of patient who had previous orthodontic treatment and second molar extractions with additional treatment with a bionator by the family dentist. The maxillary skeletal transverse deficiency was not diagnosed or treated. (d–f) Post-treatment intraoral photographs of patient following surgical maxillary expansion treatment, full fixed appliance treatment and phase II surgery with a Le Fort osteotomy with differential impaction to allow mandibular autorotation to aid in bite closure. (g) Pretreatment intraoral occlusal view. (h) Post-treatment intraoral photograph of the occlusal view following surgically assisted rapid maxillary expansion and full fixed appliance treatment.

able experience. With little contact among my teeth and jaw too tired to chew, most of my food was swallowed nearly whole. I often suffered from a variety of ailments related to poor digestion and had difficulty gaining any weight. Presently, however, I am happy to say that eating is a pleasure – one which I must consciously make an effort to do more slowly because of my many years of previously necessitated habits. I suffer few digestive problems and have now gained a better weight for my size and age. As a result of this gain, I find myself generally healthier these days and much less prone to illness.

All these things I have mentioned make this treatment the single most significant step in the improvement in my

overall health that I have taken thus far in my life. I would like to thank both you and your staff for all the excellent care and professionalism I have received these past three years. All of my questions were met with patience and courtesy. Your scheduling was convenient and your office staff was always accessible and concerned.

Presurgical – Steps XI and XII

Step XI: Comprehensive orthodontic treatment (8–18 months before surgery)
- Orthodontic movement to decompensate tooth positions

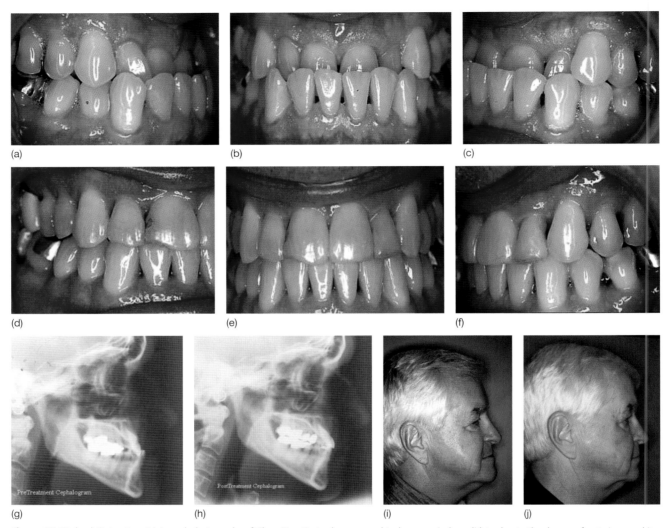

Figure 18.17 (a–c) Pretreatment intraoral photographs of Class III patient who appeared to be a surgical candidate due to the degree of anterior crossbite. (d–f) Post-treatment intraoral photographs; treatment included a phase I therapeutic diagnosis. A functional shift forward of the mandible made this patient's Class III problem appear more severe that it was. (g,i) Pretreatment cephalogram and profile photograph, respectively. (h,j) Post-treatment cephalogram and profile photograph, respectively.

- Coordination of arches in anticipation of surgical repositioning
- Alignment of teeth and correction of rotations

Some patients may still require an additional diagnostic step, termed *therapeutic diagnosis*, which allows the clinicians and the patients to make the final decision regarding plan and outcome. The patient in Figure 18.17 elected not to proceed with bite correction until later in life, because he was told that he would need surgery to correct his Class III malocclusion. A short therapeutic diagnosis phase of treatment indicated that his Class III problem was exaggerated by a mandibular functional shift. Once this shift was diagnosed, he opted for non-surgical camouflage treatment to create an occlusal scheme that was balanced and healthy.

Orthognathic patient preparation by the orthodontist for jaw surgery includes:

- Establish differential diagnosis as discussed previously – therapeutic diagnosis if necessary
- Integrate the periodontal treatment necessary to maintain a healthy periodontium throughout treatment
- Determine whether extractions are needed to properly prepare the patient for the skeletal changes required
- Outline the sequence of steps and a general timeline for patient and provider team awareness
- Level, align, and coordinate arches to provide a balanced postsurgical occlusal relationship. Interocclusal splints used postsurgically can create vertical and mandibular rotation variables; therefore, the orthodontist should try to avoid the need for their use through careful surgically simulated arch coordination. Note: surgical splints cannot be avoided if maxillary transverse discrepancies are resolved with multi-piece osteotomies to widen the maxilla.

Step XII: Presurgical re-evaluation records

- Complete records
- Prediction tracing (detailed movements planned)
- Model surgery (reviewed by orthodontist and surgeon)
- Determination of specific fixation needs
- Patient/parent/spouse/significant other review with orthodontist and surgeon

At the presurgical consultation (Step XII), the orthodontist and the surgeon must listen carefully to the patient and determine the patient's physical, dental, and emotional readiness for surgery (Kiyak et al., 1985; Kiyak and Bell, 1991; Broder et al., 2000; DeSousa, 2008). The surgeon should present a clear review of the surgical procedure and

the risks of surgery. The surgeon and the orthodontist must remember that most orthognathic patients have much to learn about their options, the recommended procedures, and the incumbent risks. The current trend to have a 'one-step consultation' for orthodontic patients generally does not apply to orthognathic patients. One must respect the individual patient's *learning curve* requirements and be supportive by providing needed information and patience. Therefore, the consultation process in orthognathic cases may involve multiple visits and discussions. The patient records in Figure 18.18 illustrate a protracted treatment of a growing patient with a Class II malocclusion. After phase II records were analyzed, it was decided that her malocclusion was beyond the range of orthodontics alone

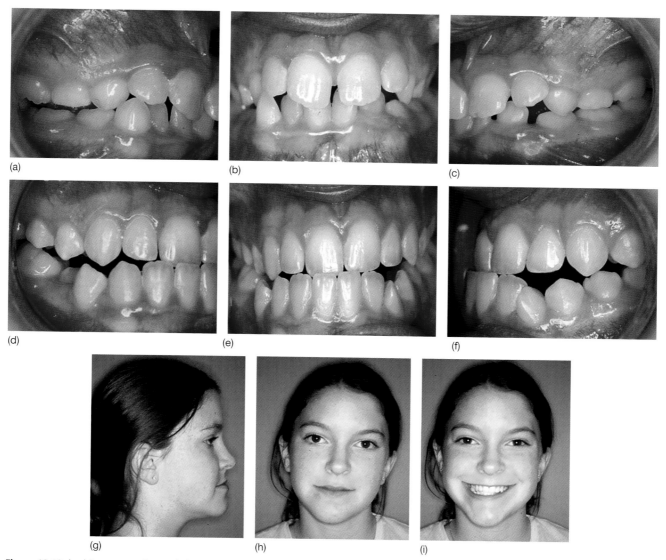

Figure 18.18 (a–c) Pretreatment intraoral photographs showing maxillary constriction and anterior crowding. Patient is 8 years old. (d–f) Intraoral photographs – several years after phase I treatment. The impact of differential mandibular growth is seen in the developing anterior cross bite and occlusal asymmetry to right. Patient is 14.5 years old. (g–i) Profile, frontal and frontal photograph with smile, respectively. Patient is 14.5 years old, but still growing. Note the degree of asymmetry that is evident in the smile photograph (18.19l).

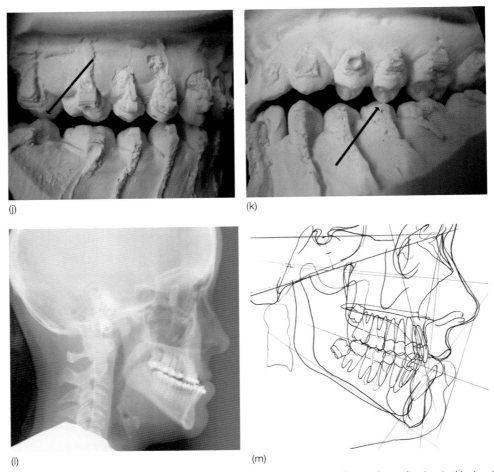

(j)   (k)

(l)   (m)

Figure 18.18 (j,k) Progress study models taken several months before the planned jaw surgery to evaluate arch coordination. In this situation the models were hand articulated anticipating the surgical movement. Note the second molar prematurity (arrow) in Figure 18.18j. Also note the buccolingual discrepancy (arrow) in Figure 18.18k. (l) Progress cephalogram showing degree of decompensation of lower incisors accomplished prior to surgery. These dental changes were needed to accomplish the surgical correction that was appropriate. (m) Bolton template superimposition used to plan the surgical movements needed to achieve the most optimal functional balance and facial balance.

(Figure 18.18). For younger patients with Class III growth vectors, not only do orthodontists help decide the optimal timing of surgical treatment as it relates to facial growth, but they must also periodically take progress study models (Figure 18.18j,k) to assess presurgical arch coordination, which is another important aspect of surgical timing.

Bellucci and Kapp-Simon (2007), Pavone et al. (2005), and Kiyak et al. (1981, 1982a,b, 1985) conducted numerous studies to assess patients' responses to current ortho/surgical treatment modalities. Bellucci and Kapp-Simon (2007) suggest:

Focus is on correcting the morphologic deformity, but assessment and planning should include psychosocial aspects of the patient. Adolescents and young adults who need psychological support should be followed closely from the beginning, until at least 1 year postsurgery. Success of surgical intervention should be measured both in terms of

the occlusal function and morphological improvement, and changes in psychosocial interaction and an improved quality of life for the patient.

Similarly to Belluci and associates, Pavone et al. (2005) in their case report concluded:

Orthognathic surgery involves more than the correction of a physical problem. The psychological needs of the patient must be recognized and acknowledged, and communication between surgeons and patients is essential. It is important to understand that any surgical treatment that modifies body image could generate psychological disorders for some patients. Early surgical intervention and referral for psychological counseling may reduce long-term morbidity.

For additional insights into understanding and integrating the psychosocial aspects of the management of

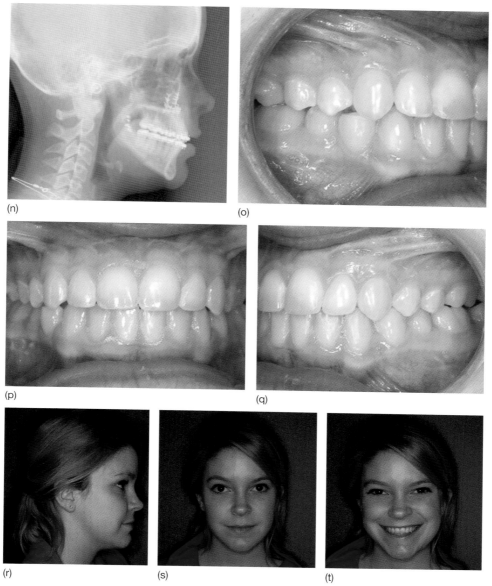

Figure 18.18 (n) Postsurgical cephalogram showing the results of maxillo/mandibular surgery. (o–q) Post-treatment intraoral photographs showing correction of multiple components of this patient's original Class III malocclusion with asymmetry and crowding. The patient is 18 years old. (r–t) Profile, frontal and frontal photograph with smile, respectively. Patient is 18 years old and has had a very successful orthodontic/surgical treatment which followed the steps in the 'checklist'. Compare each of these photos with the pretreatment facial photographs in Figure 18.18g–i.

the orthognathic patient, see Chapter 3 of Proffit et al. (2003). The chapter's authors, Phillips and Proffit, assess the psychosocial approach, which can be summarized as follows:

Recommendations for a psychosocial approach to interviewing and counseling patients are important to be aware of with specific comments about steps and points of emphasis. What counts in the long term, after all, is how the patient perceives the treatment outcome, not what the doctor thinks he or she ought to perceive. Fortunately, den-

tofacial problems now can be treated with a high probability of success in both objective (clinical measurement) and subjective (patient satisfaction) criteria. Appropriate management of the psychosocial aspects of treatment maximizes the chance of success in both areas.

The patient illustrated in Figure 18.19 delayed treatment until she was an adult, and neuromuscular symptoms began to interfere with her *quality of life,* secondary to the lack of a balanced occlusion. Orthodontic and surgical treatment planning was integrated according to the steps in

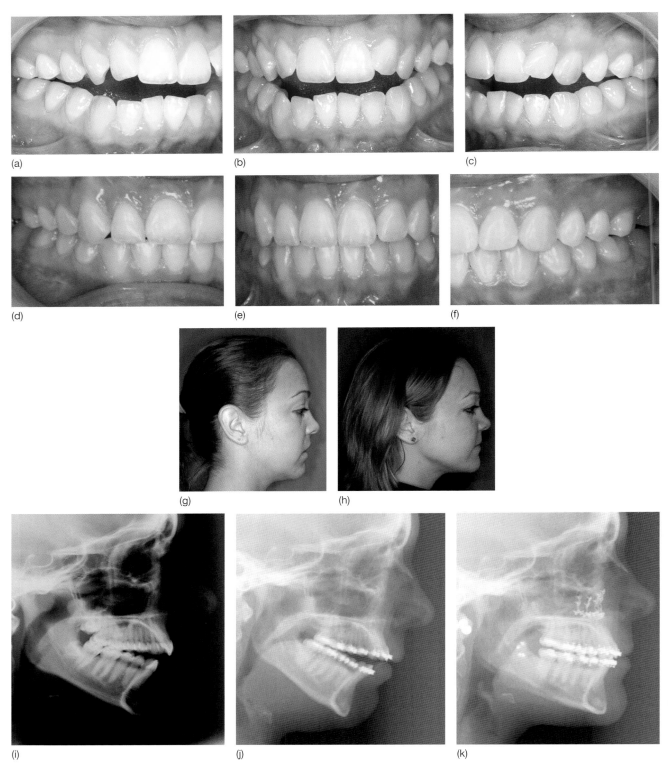

Figure 18.19 (a–c) Pretreatment intraoral photographs of the occlusal relationship showing progressive open bite from molar to molar. There is also mild incisor crowding. Post-treatment intraoral photographs of the occlusal relationship showing the result of combined orthodontic/orthognathic treatment steps according to the checklist described in Table 18.1. (g) Pretreatment profile facial photograph showing the results of downward and backward mandibular rotation during growth leading to the open bite seen in Figure 18.19a–c. Post-treatment profile facial photograph illustrating the facial change from a maxillomandibular surgical procedure that utilized the principles of occlusal plane change to close the open bite and optimize facial balance. (i–k) Pretreatment, re-evaluation, and post-treatment cephalogram, respectively. Note the miniaturized fixation devices (k) used to stabilize the orthognathic changes with occlusal plane change jaw surgery.

this checklist. Furthermore, it was decided that she would benefit most (i.e. achieve all the goals of treatment) through orthodontic leveling and aligning and presurgical arch preparation, followed by bimaxillary surgery with the incorporation of an *occlusal plane change* (Arnett and Bergman, 1993). As can be seen from the post-treatment photographs, very desirable occlusal and esthetic changes occurred for this patient, with the checklist serving as the guide for the surgeon and the orthodontist.

The orthodontist needs to consider the following questions for the Class II and Class III patients who may have a skeletal imbalance that appears to require jaw surgery.

- The need to decompensate through premolar extraction should have been decided early in the treatment planning process and generally should not be under consideration at this time unless there are unusual aspects of the patient's care, such as pulpal or periodontal deterioration that may generate a 'strategic extraction' .decision.
- Will this be a one-jaw surgery? This consideration should have been resolved in the initial treatment plan, but it still should be re-evaluated based on findings during the presurgical leveling and alignment stage. If there was any doubt due to vertical considerations or postsurgical chin position, it is always better to plan for bimaxillary surgery and reduce the number of osteotomies from an insurance management consideration.
- What are the horizontal, vertical, and transverse considerations? (see Figures 18.14 and 18.16)
- Are the patient's maxillary and mandibular incisors leveled adequately so that the mandibular anteroposterior repositioning can occur without leaving a large posterior open bite, incisor trauma, and a lower facial height increased beyond what is esthetically desirable?
- Will there be some requirement to rotate the mandible to resolve moderate to severe asymmetry?
- Is there a mandibular functional shift? Are there prematurities when the mandible is positioned into the correct postsurgical occlusion? (Some orthodontic presurgical alignment efforts do not take into consideration the need to put attachments on the second molars and level the posterior areas of both the maxillary arch and the mandibular arch. It is highly undesirable to leave the second molars (or third molars if erupted and part of the occlusal scheme) without orthodontic attachments when preparing a patient for orthognathic procedures).

Postsurgical – *Steps XIII–XVI*

Step XIII: Orthognathic surgery
- Minimize surgical risks
- Simplest procedure or procedures to achieve professional goals

- Simplest procedure or procedures to satisfy patient's needs

The diagnostic aspects of treatment planning in patients with maxillomandibular imbalances are critical. Frequently patients present with one aspect of their facial imbalance very obvious, while secondary components to the problem may require equal attention. For example, a Class III patient may have an obvious mandibular excess, but a mild open bite, mild asymmetry, and maxillary cant. All aspects of the patient's imbalance need proper assessment so that appropriate surgical steps can be taken to manage each aspect at the time of surgery.

A variety of predictable surgical procedures have been established for each skeletal disproportion that is diagnosed. Some of the more frequently used procedures are schematically illustrated in Figure 18.20. In our experience, showing illustrations of the surgical procedures to patients who are candidates for surgical correction can help visualize how the proposed surgery will allow the skeletal and dental changes to occur.

Step XIV: The postsurgical period
- Early: 2–3 weeks of fixation
- Late: 3–8 weeks of fixation
- Re-evaluation of surgical procedure
- Assess need for physical therapy

The reliability of rigid fixation procedures has reduced the necessity of psychological support that was required after intermaxillary fixation (Dolce et al., 2002). Before the universal use of rigid fixation, patients who required intermaxillary fixation seemed to feel a sense of 'being disabled' due to speech and eating difficulties. Patients who required intermaxillary fixation also lost a great deal of weight. The orthodontic and surgical specialties have now incorporated new procedures to help the patient understand and prepare for the facial change and the postoperative period. However, Williams et al. (2004) found that more can be done to prepare the orthognathic patients: 'A total of 327 patients (53% response rate) participated. Although most participants (n = 249, 76%) reported that symptoms of pain, swelling, or difficulty in eating that they experienced immediately post-operatively were worse than expected. A third also reported that it took them longer to recover from the operation than they anticipated. Patients undergoing orthognathic surgery in the south west of UK need more specific information about what to expect both immediately post-operatively and at home after discharge.'

While the outcomes of current orthognathic/orthodontic treatment result in very few complications (Bays and Bouloux, 2003), this should not invite complacency in any of the steps of the treatment process because complications do occur, and they can be very serious. Figure 18.21 shows a person in whom mandibular setback was done in such a

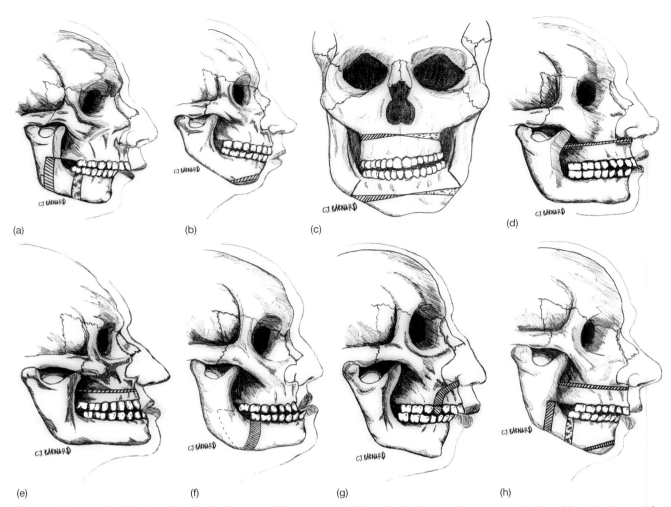

Figure 18.20 Anatomical sketches: (a) sagittal split surgery; (b) osteotomy used for vertical reduction, advancement genioplasty; (c) osteotomies used for correction of maxillomandibular asymmetry; (d) osteotomy used for correction of vertical maxillary excess – Le Fort osteotomy; (e) osteotomy (Le Fort) used in the correction of maxillary deficiency to allow maxillary advancement; (f) osteotomy (sagittal split) used for correction of skeletal Class III with mandibular excess; (g) maxillary segmental osteotomy for correction of maxillary dentoalveolar protrusion; and (h) osteotomies used to correct vertical maxillary excess and mandibular deficiency with chin deficiency.

way that her mild mandibular asymmetry to the left was unintentionally overcorrected to the right. This surgical error resulted in several additional months of orthodontic treatment to compensate the occlusion back to the left and to resolve the surgical overcorrection.

Complications related to orthognathics can be divided into the following categories: physical wellbeing, stomatognathic function, emotional wellbeing, and oral health sequelae.

Complications in physical wellbeing
- Excessive blood loss (Lanigan, 1990)
- Neurologic injury (anesthesia, paresthesia) (Walter and Gregg, 1979):
  - Hypoesthesia (decreased sensation) (Van Sickels et al., 2002)
  - Hyperpathia (increased sensation)
  - Dysesthesia (altered sensation that is painful)
- Allergic reaction to anesthetic, antibiotic, or anti-inflammatory drugs (Hegtvedt, 1990)
- Postoperative infections:
  - Surgical site
  - Skeletal fixation wires
  - Rigid fixation plates.

Current techniques for prevention of infection are discussed by Hegtvedt (1990). In addition, orthodontists can aid the surgeon in reducing potential iatrogenic incidence of nidi of infection by using soldered or slide-on surgical hooks, well-secured brackets, and stainless steel ligatures (not elastomeric modules because their force decays rapidly, and they are not radiopaque; if elastomeric ligatures inad-

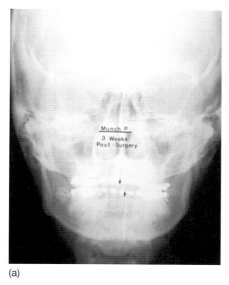
(a)

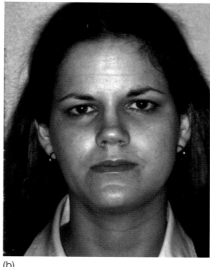
(b)

Figure 18.21 (a) Postsurgical frontal cephalogram. Note the asymmetry that was erroneously introduced as part of the surgical procedure. The surgeon significantly overcorrected an original mild asymmetry; this error created a true facial asymmetry of the mandible to the patient's right. (b) Frontal photograph of the patient 3 weeks following the surgery. Due to the surgical error, an effort was made to reduce the time in fixation and use elastics to generate corrective remodeling of the surgical site. This was possible (full records seen in Figure 18.7) because of the wire fixation that was used. Such occlusal and facial improvement from this surgical error would not be possible if rigid fixation were used. Obviously, it is very important to avoid surgical errors.

vertently fall into the surgical site, they can be difficult to locate and remove).

Bone fractures

There are reports in the literature of unfavorable surgical splits of the mandible including buccal plate fracture, associated with impacted third molar teeth that were extracted at the time of the mandibular osteotomy. When unfavorable splits occur, the stability of the procedure is jeopardized and the likelihood of neuropathies and facial deformities is greater. To help prevent these unfavorable results, when sagittal split procedures are planned for mandibular deficiency or mandibular excess, the third molars should be removed 6–12 months before the osteotomy (Reyneke et al., 2002). If an unfavorable split occurs, the surgeon must decide whether to proceed with the surgery or repair the fracture and redo the surgery at a later time.

Delayed healing and nonhealing

Delayed healing and nonhealing occur most often when unexpected microtrauma or macrotrauma occurs in the surgical and postsurgical periods. Intraoperative complications including unfavorable splits in the sagittal split or unfavorable down-fracture in the Le Fort osteotomy can result in incomplete bone healing (Van Sickels and Tucker, 1990).

Retrieval of rigid fixation devices

One of the few disadvantages of the mini-plates and screws used in rigid fixation is the need to remove them because of the potential risk of stress protection-induced osteo-

penia. Another concern is inflammatory reactions due to corrosion of these metallic devices (French et al., 1984). However, research is under way to assess the effectiveness of biodegradable (resorbable) plates and screws (Bos et al., 1989, 1990). Orthopedic repair materials of resorbable poly L-lactide, polyglycolide, and polydioxanon are being strength tested as maxillofacial surgery fixation devices. Improvements in the rate of resorption and the reliability of these materials may provide a means of fixation that is biologically absorbed over time.

Secondary surgery

A small percentage of orthognathic patients must return to the operating room for secondary surgery because of unexpected surgical outcomes. Some return before release from the hospital after the first surgery; others return months or years later. The most common reasons for secondary surgery include the following:

- Early relapse (condylar distraction) (Worms et al., 1980)
- Post-healing relapse
- Unfavorable split
- Patient dissatisfaction with the esthetic result (in the early years of the Le Fort procedure, the maxilla was impacted beyond an esthetic smile line in some patients).

Over impaction of the maxilla can occur for several reasons:

- Inappropriate treatment planning
- Removal of an excessive amount of bone from the lateral walls

- Presence of thin, concave maxillary bone that may collapse on loading
- Use of overly tight interosseous suspension wires that tend to pull the maxilla superiorly
- Excessive masticatory function that overrides the stability of the bony interfaces
- Lack of bony contact.

Correction of over impaction cannot be achieved short of surgically repositioning the maxilla inferiorly and returning the dentoalveolar portion to its original position. This would require interpositional bone grafting and rigid internal fixation and possibly concomitant mandibular surgery (West, 1990).

Sinus complications
Studies of postsurgical patients have found that a higher percentage than expected reported sinus problems after Le Fort procedures (Kiyak et al., 1985; Doyle, 1986). Other studies have indicated that postsurgical sinus disease is no greater than that in the general population (Nustad et al., 1986). Postsurgically, the maxillary sinus function may have been altered so that it interferes with proper drainage, causing sinus-type headaches. Sinuses may also congest more frequently, interfering with nasal breathing. Although this complication may seem relatively minor, it can have an adverse effect on the quality of life of patients who must deal with chronic sinus flare-ups.

Complications in stomatognathic function
- Decreased efficiency and discomfort during chewing as a result of:
  - Posterior open bites caused by overseating of condyles during mandibular surgery
  - Excessive superior positioning of the posterior maxilla, especially when posterior vertical stops are inadequate in the area of the osteotomy
- Temporomandibular dysfunction, discomfort, and pain.

Orthognathic surgery in some cases is justified because it has the potential to reduce temporomandibular dysfunction symptoms. Karabouta and Martis (1985) reported that temporomandibular dysfunction symptoms declined from 40% to 11% of the sample. However, 4% of previously asymptomatic patients developed temporomandibular dysfunction symptoms after surgery. In another study, Kerstens et al. (1989) and Kim et al. (2002) found a 66% reduction in temporomandibular dysfunction symptoms; they also found that 11.5% of preoperatively asymptomatic patients experienced symptoms after surgery. Many of these patients may have had latent temporomandibular dysfunction problems that were activated by the altered joint loading after jaw surgery.

Table 18.5 Reduction in maximal incisal opening following orthognathic surgery

Procedure	MIO reduction (mean percentage)
Sagittal split osteotomy (SSO)	29
Vertical subcondylar osteotomy (VSO)	10
Le Fort I	2
Le Fort I and SSO	28
Le Fort I and VSO	9

Limitation in range of motion
A program of physical therapy is prescribed for most orthognathic patients shortly after the release of fixation. If mandibular hypomobility is present after jaw surgery, it could have an intracapsular or an extracapsular cause. Intracapsular problems are characterized by a sharp pain localized in the TMJs. Extracapsular problems are characterized by less intense, dull pain that is generalized and diffuse and may or may not be aggravated by mandibular movements; often the pain is alleviated by biting (Epker and LaBlanc, 1990). A prospective study of 55 orthognathic patients by Aragon et al. (1985) found that the maximal incisal opening (MIO) decreased in most of these patients after surgery. The percentage of MIO decrease depended on the surgery performed (Table 18.5).

Complications in emotional wellbeing
Because orthognathic procedures can change facial appearance significantly, numerous studies have investigated patients' emotional response after surgery (Kiyak et al., 1981, 1982a,b, 1985; Kiyak and Bell, 1991; Broder et al., 2000; Motegi et al., 2003; Bellucci and Kapp-Simon, 2007). In our experience, negative emotional responses seldom occur with single-jaw mandibular advancement or mandibular setback procedures because these procedures mainly affect the patient's profile, and therefore the patient does not observe these changes readily. Changes that occur with single-jaw Le Fort procedures or Le Fort procedures along with mandibular advancement or setback alter the frontal facial appearance immediately, and the patient must adapt to the new look (Kiyak et al., 1982a,b).

Self-esteem changes caused by unexpected facial changes
In Jacobson's study (1984), most patients (80%) reported that the orthodontic-orthognathic treatment influenced their life positively, and 4% were of the opinion that the treatment had had a negative influence on social activities. The remaining 16% were neutral about the impact of surgery on their life. In a study of 55 patients, Kiyak et al. (1982b) found that 9 months postoperatively, patients' self-esteem declined significantly from the early postsurgical period as they adapted to the facial change and reconsidered the effort and challenges to accomplish the change.

The orthodontist and staff who follow such patients after surgery must be aware of the potential for emotional highs and lows during the postsurgical period. Being able to consult with a psychologist who is aware of the needs of orthognathic patients and who is able to intercept significant patient emotional problems is imperative.

Lack of preparation for changes in interpersonal relationships

As surgical technology has improved to allow more stable, functional results, so too has the capacity to alter a person's appearance and identity. Most orthognathic patients are women between the ages of 20 and 40 years. Many are married and have husbands and young children. When these patients return home from the hospital after a Le Fort osteotomy and genioplasty, they are swollen, black and blue (bruised), and may be in fixation, with limited speech and eating capacities. If the immediate family members in the support group are not prepared fully for them to return looking so different, significant stress and disruption of normal family functions will result. As one patient in the study by Kiyak et al. (1982b) said, 'I would not recommend this surgery to anyone without thorough counseling'. In fact, patients who have had the surgery have many good ideas about ways to enhance the recovery process. One patient reported that (Kiyak et al., 1982b): 'Much more time is needed to prepare the patient with facts and information. I was unprepared for the bleeding and earaches, leaving the hospital so soon – less than 24 hours after surgery. I lost more weight than expected and really suffered psychologically and felt little support during the fixation period. Maybe the patients could be invited to form a mutual support group.'

Depression

Postsurgical depression has received little attention in the orthognathic literature, and only recently has it been discussed as a legitimate complication of jaw surgery (Stewart and Sexton, 1986). Generally, dentists are not trained properly to handle depression medically, even if it is likely to be a transitory state of mind for the orthognathic patient. However, the orthodontic members of the healthcare team have the duty to recognize the symptoms of depression, discuss them with the patient and family, refer the patient when necessary, and interact with the psychologist to aid in the patient's recovery. In addition, the orthodontist should try to be aware of other stressful events in the patient's life that may add to the anxiety level during the 2–3 years these patients are followed. Although the current literature discusses the postsurgical sequela of depression (Kiyak et al., 1981, 1982a,b, 1985; Jacobson, 1984; Kerstens et al., 1989; Kiyak and Bell, 1991), our experience is that patients with rigid fixation show rapid psychological rebound and fewer signs of depression than patients who required intermaxil-

lary fixation for 6–10 weeks, as was necessary before rigid fixation was proven to be so effective.

Negative oral health sequelae

- Bone loss.
- Exacerbation of periodontal disease.
- Gingival deficiency with recession: Doyle (1986) reported that of his sample of 50 patients, only four required gingival grafts after jaw surgery. He indicated that 10 other patients were being monitored for inadequate attached gingiva. It was not clear whether the gingival problem existed before the osteotomy or caused the tissue deficiency, as can happen in the area of the lower incisors after genioplasty.
- Pulpal changes: The osteotomies that are done often approximate root apices, particularly Le Fort I procedures and segmental surgery. Occasionally, after an osteotomy, the affected tooth starts to change color and loses its vitality, and eventually it requires endodontic treatment.
- Tooth loss is an uncommon sequela, but it does warrant a brief discussion. When segmental procedures are done on the maxilla for leveling the occlusal plane, or to aid minor transverse corrections, there is a higher risk of tooth loss due to limited interproximal area for surgical cuts. The orthodontist can aid the surgeon by altering root proximity and creating ≥3 mm of root divergence for ease of segmental surgical cuts.

Step XV: Evaluation and surgical stability

- Orthodontic finishing, occlusal adjustments, and retention procedures
- Optimal continuation of any necessary treatments with a physical therapist

It is advisable for both the surgeon and the orthodontist to evaluate the patient's postsurgical recovery. A good time for the orthodontist to evaluate the patient is approximately 2 weeks after the surgery. The primary objectives of this evaluation are to:

- Assess the surgical outcome both clinically and cephalometrically
- Ensure that none of the surgical hooks are displaced, causing tissue irritation
- Ensure that there are no significant occlusal prematurities causing surgical site mobility or tooth mobility
- Ascertain that the patient is comfortable, and clarify future orthodontic steps.

This is also a good time for communication with the patient's general dentist to update them on the procedures and to give them an overview of the outcome. It is also a very important time to emphasize the anticipated timing of restorative therapy and periodontal treatment needed to finalize the stabilization of the outcome.

Step XVI: Post-treatment records

One year post-treatment: treatment evaluation by patient and orthodontist

By taking the step to collect post-treatment records, the dentofacial team has a chance to reassess each aspect of treatment and to determine if their overall approach has been as successful as desired. It is also helpful to collect input from the patient who had just completed the interdisciplinary treatment according to plan. While these steps take time, they are very helpful in advancing the team's capacity to improve their approach as they work together to manage other cases. One can think of taking Steps XVI, XVII, and XVIII as an 'in-house' continuing education course. Practitioners who take the time to add these steps to their management of patients with dentofacial imbalances who have gone through the recommended orthodontics and jaw surgery, will become the most effective dentofacial team in their community.

Feedback – Steps XVII–XVIII

Step XVII: Re-evaluation of findings with dental team, especially the oral surgeon and general dentist

- Problem solving
- Treatment evaluation by patient and all providers

Step XVII is not always incorporated in the routine part of the sequence in private orthodontic and surgical practices. To gain the most from this step, all team members should review the postsurgical records and discuss the positive and negative aspects of the overall treatment plan, the sequence of treatment, and provider interaction. Each completed case provides an opportunity for providers to consider feedback from one another and the patient. This step is the most powerful continuing education program in which a practitioner can participate. Having each orthognathic patient complete a post-treatment questionnaire also provides additional feedback and is an integral part of practice maturation.

Step XVIII: Treatment experience (used in management of future cases to enhance/refine the checklist)

- Re-evaluation of degree of success in achieving goals
- Positive reinforcement (Figures 18.22, 18.23)

The patients illustrated in Figures 18.22 and 18.23 both had mandibular deficiency problems, and both were treated with bimaxillary surgery to resolve their skeletal imbalance. Following their orthodontic/orthognathic experience, both patients were asked to chart their emotional 'highs and lows' during the course of treatment. Comparing the postsurgical period in the graphs in Figure 18.22a and 18.23a,

it is notable that the patient in Figure 18.22a had a very difficult time, and she actually became depressed during that healing period. In Figure 18.23a, the patient's graph of her emotional 'highs and lows,' especially following the jaw surgery, documents a very different experience from that seen in Figure 18.22a. Several factors may account for this difference, but it is believed that the intermaxillary fixation utilized for the patient in Figure 18.22a was a key factor in her discomfort and her emotional distress. The patient treated in Figure 18.23 was treated with rigid fixation methods. Having patients keep this type of 'log' or a simple graph as seen in the figures indicated above, can help them communicate their experience and assist orthognathic teams to become more informed and more sensitive to the experiences of their patients. When asked, patients will readily provide ideas for improving the steps in the orthodontic/orthognathic treatment experience.

Once treatment is complete and the patient's chief concerns have been resolved, the interdisciplinary team should meet again to discuss each of the steps in the checklist as they applied to the patient under consideration. Although this approach takes time, and specialists can seldom find the time to incorporate the last steps in this checklist into their treatment process, the rewards of doing so would be quickly recognized. Some of the advantages of incorporating these last steps are:

- The general dentist would develop better awareness of diagnostic and treatment planning steps for patients with skeletal imbalances
- The general dentist would be more confident in referring other patients with similar conditions for treatment since he or she would have a better understanding of the predictability of the orthognathic approach
- The surgeon and orthodontist would be more consistent in their treatment planning approach
- The surgeon's and orthodontist's staff would have an easier time providing patients with relevant information regarding insurance and the coordination of appointments between offices.

Every patient can be considered as a continuing education opportunity for all the treating doctors and staff. The greatest advantage of incorporating the *checklist* (Table 18.1) and taking the extra time that is needed for this step is that new patients seeking treatment for their skeletal imbalances will find an interdisciplinary team ready and capable of providing the highest available quality of care.

Conclusions

Frequently, patients with skeletal imbalances of the jaws are initially examined by orthodontists. It is up to the orthodontist to determine through an effective diagnostic protocol if the imbalances are minor, moderate, or major, and to what degree the imbalances affect the day-to-day function,

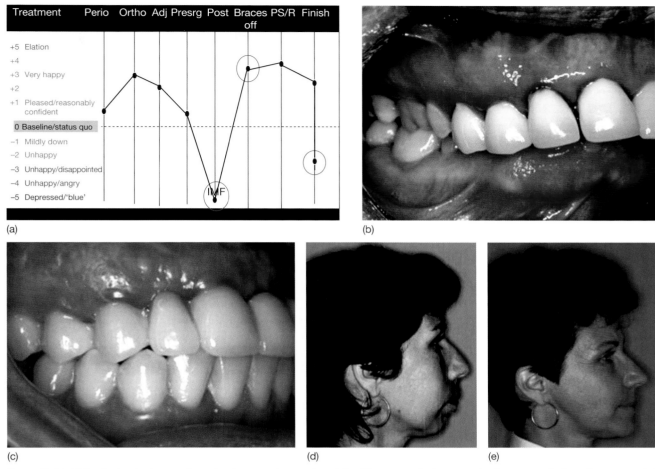

Figure 18.22 (a) Graph of patient's general emotional state as she experienced the different steps in the preparation for surgery; the immediate postsurgical period and the completion of treatment steps with restorative procedures. Note the severe drop in the sense of 'wellbeing' during the intermaxillary fixation period. Also note the indication of unhappiness at the end of treatment. Through the communication process generated by this graph mechanism, we learned of the patient's temporomandibular joint pain which she felt was exacerbated with the jaw surgery. Splint therapy and physical therapy were prescribed and her symptoms subsided. (b) Pretreatment right side view of the Class II malocclusion, with deep bite and telescoping crossbite. Also noted is the gingival inflammation with probable advanced periodontal disease. (c) Post-treatment view (periodontics, orthodontics, orthognathics and restorative dentistry) of the right side of the corrected malocclusion. Note correction of deep bite, periodontal issues and the 10 mm overjet). (d) Pretreatment profile. (e) Post-treatment profile showing very good facial balance.

long-term health, and quality of life of those patients. Before the evolution of the many technical advances described and documented in Bell et al.'s classic textbook (1985), orthodontic treatment plans stretched the limits of conventional orthodontic care to improve the function of the stomatognathic system through a variety of camouflage techniques. With four decades of success in advanced surgical techniques, anesthetic improvements, and risk reduction, this chapter has provided a *checklist* that will predictably help orthognathic teams provide the patients with optimal care.

This chapter emphasized the steps that are necessary to:

- Develop an orthognathic team
- Diagnose the problems and educate the patients regarding their conditions
- Implement presurgical care
- Implement effective postsurgical care
- Evaluate post-treatment patient and team feedback.

The clinical cases discussed in this chapter illustrated key concepts and emphasized and confirmed the value of implementing a checklist, so that all the members of the orthognathic team can optimize their role in helping patients attain outcomes that not only resolve their chief concerns, but also achieve all the goals that are feasible with the current technology, thereby improving the quality of life for all patients with a dentofacial imbalance. This protocol will undoubtedly continue to evolve and improve with advances in knowledge and expertise in biological fields such as tissue engineering and the recruitment of stem cells for altering craniofacial form and function.

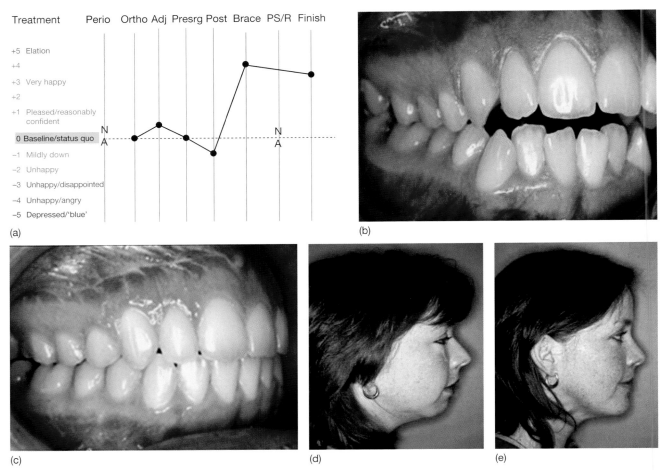

Figure 18.23 (a) Graph of patient's general emotional state in the different steps in the preparation for surgery, the immediate postsurgical period and the completion of treatment steps. Note the minimal postsurgical change in the sense of 'wellbeing' during the immediate postsurgical period. There are several differences between this patient and the one illustrated in Figure 18.22, but a key difference at this stage in treatment was that the patient in Figure 18.22 had 10 weeks of intermaxillary fixation, but the patient in Figure 18.23 had rigid fixation. The incorporation of rigid fixation has greatly facilitated healing and a healthier emotional state during recovery from surgery. (b) Pretreatment right side view of the Class II malocclusion, showing open bite and crowding in the anterior segments. (c) Post-treatment of the right side of the corrected malocclusion. Note correction of open bite, and due to the high risk of incisor relapse, this patient was fitted with fixed, bonded lingual arches for long-term retention. (d) Pretreatment profile. (e) Post-treatment profile showing exceptional facial balance. This patient had bimaxillary surgery with an occlusal plane change to optimize the chin position without a genioplasty and to create a more acute gonial angle to balance the mandibular appearance in profile view.

References

Aragon SB, Van Sickels JE, Dolwick MF, et al. (1985) The effects of orthognathic surgery on mandibular range of motion. *Journal of Oral and Maxillofacial Surgery* 43: 938–43.

Arnett GW, Bergman R (1993) Facial keys to orthodontic diagnosis and treatment planning. Parts I and II. *American Journal of Orthodontics and Dentofacial Orthopedics* 103: 299–312, 395–411.

Bays RA, Bouloux GF (2003) Complications of orthognathic surgery. *Oral and Maxillofacial Surgery Clinics of North America* 15(2): 229–42.

Bell WH, Proffit WR, White RP (1985) *Surgical Correction of Dentofacial Deformities*, vols I and II. Philadelphia, PA: WB Saunders.

Bellucci CC, Kapp-Simon KA (2007) Psychological considerations in orthognathic surgery. *Clinics in Plastic Surgery* 34(3): e11–16.

Bos RRM, Rozema FR, Boering G, et al. (1989) Bone plates and screws of bioabsorbable poly (L-lactide): and animal pilot study. *Journal of Oral and Maxillofacial Surgery* 27: 467.

Bos RRM, Rozema FR, Boering G, et al. (1990) Bioresorbable osteosynthesis in maxillofacial surgery: present and future. *Oral and Maxillofacial Surgery Clinics of North America* 2(4): 745.

Broadbent BH Sr, Broadbent BH Jr, Golden WH (1975) *Bolton Standards of Dentofacial Developmental Growth*. St. Louis, MO: Mosby.

Broder HL, Phillips C, Kaminetzky S (2000) Issues in decision making: Should I have orthognathic surgery? *Seminars in Orthodontics: Psychological Issues Related to Orthodontic Treatment and Patient Compliance* 6(4): 249–58.

DeSousa A (2008) Psychological issues in oral and maxillofacial reconstructive surgery. *British Journal of Oral and Maxillofacial Surgery* 46(8): 661–4.

Dolce C, Hatch JP, VanSickels JE, et al. (2002) Rigid versus wire fixation for mandibular advancement: skeletal and dental changes after 5 years. *American Journal of Orthodontics and Dentofacial Orthopedics* 121(6): 610–19.

Doyle MG (1986) Stability and complications in 50 consecutively treated surgical-orthodontic patients: a retrospective longitudinal analysis from private practice. *International Journal of Adult Orthodontics and Orthognathic Surgery* 1: 23–36.

Epker BN, LaBlanc JP (1990) Orthognathic surgery: management of postoperative complications. *Oral and Maxillofacial Surgery Clinics of North America* 2: 109.

French HG, Cook SD, Haddad RJ (1984) Correlations of tissue reaction to corrosion in osteosynthetic devices. *Journal of Biomedical Material Research* 18: 817–28.

Gawande A (2010) *Checklist Manifesto*. New York, NY: Metropolitan Books, Henry Holt and Company, LLC.

Gottlieb EL, Nelson AH, Bogel DS (1991) 1990 JCO study of orthodontic diagnosis and treatment procedures. *Journal of Clinical Orthodontics* 25(3): 145.

Hegtvedt AK (1990) Intraoperative and postoperative patient care. In: RA West (ed.) *Oral and Maxillofacial Surgery Clinics of North America*. Philadelphia, PA: WB Saunders.

Jacobson A (1979) The proportionate template as a diagnostic aid. *American Journal of Orthodontics* 75: 156–72.

Jacobson A (1984) Psychological aspects of dentofacial esthetics and orthognathic surgery. *Angle Orthodontist* 54: 18–35.

Jacobson A (1995) *Radiographic Cephalometry: From Basics to Videoimaging*. Chicago, IL: Quintessence Publishing Co, Inc.

Jerrold L (2000) Informed consent and the fourth dimension. *American Journal of Orthodontics and Dentofacial Orthopedics* 118(4): 476–7.

Johnston L (1987) Template Analysis. *Journal of Clinical Orthodontics* 87: 585–90.

Karabouta I, Martis C (1985) The TMJ dysfunction syndrome before and after sagittal split osteotomy of the ramus. *Journal of Maxillofacial Surgery* 13: 185–8.

Kerstens HC, Tuinzing DB, VanderKwast WA (1989) Temporomandibular joint symptoms in orthognathic surgery. *Journal of Oral Surgery* 17: 215–18.

Kim MR, Graber TM, Viana MA (2002) Orthodontics and temporomandibular disorder: a meta-analysis. *American Journal of Orthodontics and Dentofacial Orthopedics* 121: 438–46.

Kiyak HA, Bell R (1991) Psychological considerations in surgery and orthodontics. In: WR Proffit, PR White (eds) *Surgical Orthodontic Treatment*. St. Louis, MO: Mosby.

Kiyak HA, Hohl T, Sherrick P, et al. (1981) Sex differences in motives for outcomes of orthognathic surgery. *Journal of Oral Surgery* 39: 757–64.

Kiyak HA, McNeill RW, West RA (1982a) Predicting psychological responses to orthognathic surgery. *Journal of Oral and Maxillofacial Surgery* 48: 150–5.

Kiyak HA, West RA, Hohl T, et al. (1982b) The psychological impact of orthognathic surgery: a 9-month follow-up. *American Journal of Orthodontics* 81: 404–12.

Kiyak HA, McNeill RW, West RA (1985) The emotional impact of orthognathic surgery and conventional orthodontics. *American Journal of Orthodontics* 88: 224–34.

Lanigan DR (1990) Hemorrhage associated with orthognathic surgery. *Oral and Maxillofacial Surgery Clinics of North America* 2: 4.

Motegi E, Hatch JP, Rugh JD, et al. (2003) Health-related quality of life, and psychosocial function 5 years after orthognathic surgery. *American Journal of Orthodontics and Dentofacial Orthopedics* 123: 138–43.

Murphy KG, Wilcko MT, Wilcko WM, et al. (2009) Periodontal Accelerated Osteogenic Orthodontics: A description of the surgical technique. *Journal of Oral and Maxillofacial Surgery* 67(10): 2160–6.

Musich DR (2005) Orthodontic aspects of orthognathic surgery. In: TM Graber, RL Vanarsdall, KWL Vig (eds) *Orthodontics: Current Principles and Practices*. St. Louis, MO: Elsevier.

Nustad RA, Fonseca RJ, Zeitler D (1986) Evaluation of maxillary sinus disease in maxillary orthognathic patients. *International Journal of Adult Orthodontics and Orthognathic Surgery* 1: 195–202.

Pavone I, Rispoli A, Acocella A, et al. (2005) Psychological impact of self-image dissatisfaction after orthognathic surgery: a case report. *World Journal of Orthodontics* 6(2): 141–8.

Proffit WR, White R (1990) *Surgical-Orthodontic Treatment*. St. Louis, MO: Mosby.

Proffit WR, White RW Jr, Sarver DM (eds) (2003) *Contemporary Treatment of Dentofacial Deformit*. St. Louis, MO: Mosby.

Reyneke JP, Tasakiris P, Becker P (2002) Age as a factor in the complication rate after removal of unerupted/impacted third molars at the time of mandibular sagittal split osteotomy. *Journal of Oral and Maxillofacial Surgery* 60: 654–9.

Roblee RD (1994) *Interdisciplinary Dentofacial Therapy: A Comprehensive Approach to Optimal Patient Care*. Chicago, IL: Quintessence Books.

Roblee RD, Bolding SL, Landers JM (2009) Surgically facilitated orthodontic therapy: a new tool for optimal interdisciplinary results. *Compendium of Continuing Education in Dentistry* 30(5): 264–75.

Ryder MI (1996) Tobacco use and the periodontal patient. *Journal of Periodontology* 67: 51–6.

Stewart TD, Sexton J (1986) Depression: a possible complication of orthognathic surgery. *Journal of Oral and Maxillofacial Surgery* 44: 94.

Turpin DL (2010) Study clubs share their secrets. *American Journal of Orthodontics and Dentofacial Orthopedics* 137(5): 573–4.

Van Sickels JE, Tucker MR (1990) Management of delayed union and nonunion of maxillary osteotomies. *Journal of Oral and Maxillofacial Surgery* 48: 1039–44.

Van Sickels JE, Hatch JP, Colce C, et al. (2002) Effects of age, amount of advancement, and genioplasty or neurosensory disturbance after a bilateral sagittal split osteotomy. *Journal of Oral and Maxillofacial Surgery* 60: 1012–17.

Walter WM, Gregg JM (1979) Analysis of postsurgical neurologic alterations in the trigeminal nerve. *Journal of Oral Surgery* 37: 410–14.

West RA (1990) Vertical maxillary dysplasia: Diagnosis, treatment planning, and treatment response – a reappraisal. *Oral and Maxillofacial Surgery Clinics of North America* 2: 775.

Wheeler PW (1992) Risk preclusion. *American Journal of Orthodontics and Dentofacial Orthopedics* 101(2): 194–5.

Williams RW, Travess HC, Williams AC (2004) Patient's experiences after undergoing orthognathic surgery at NHS hospitals in the south west of England. *British Journal of Oral and Maxillofacial Surgery* 42(5): 419–35.

Worms FW, Spiedel TM, Bevis RR (1980) Posttreatment stability and esthetics of orthognathic surgery. *Angle Orthodontist* 50: 251–6.

Xun C, Zeng X, Wang X (2007) Microscrew anchorage in skeletal anterior open-bite treatment. *Angle Orthodontist* 77(1): 47–56.

19

The Role of Biomedical Engineers in the Design and Manufacture of Customized Orthodontic Appliances

William A Brantley, Theodore Eliades

Summary

Currently, there are numerous opportunities for biomedical engineers to interact with orthodontists to produce customized appliances, such as shape-memory polymer wires, self-healing materials, smart brackets with force-moment sensors, biomimetic adhesives, and self-cleaning materials. These exciting new applications are discussed in the second part of this chapter. The first part summarizes extensive past work performed by investigators with a biomedical engineering orientation, and also reviews important complementary publications, to gain insight into orthodontic appliances and develop new appliances.

Introduction

The broad scope of modern biomedical engineering (Box 19.1) is based on integration of engineering principles with biological sciences to develop devices, materials, and procedures that improve the health of people. To seek past examples of collaboration between biomedical engineers and orthodontists, a search of the biomedical literature using PubMed (www.ncbi.nlm.nih.gov/pubmed/), and the search terms 'orthodontic appliances' and 'biomedical engineering', was performed and revealed 42 publications since 1971 in the areas of: archwire-bracket friction; archwires; force measurements, including degradation of force-delivery modules; orthodontic appliances, including use of finite element analysis; and miscellaneous subjects, such as *Streptococcus mutans* and PCR (polymerase chain reaction), allergic reactions to materials, and mechanical behavior of the periodontal ligament. Examination of these publica-

tions revealed that authors typically had biomedical engineering and other engineering affiliations, which accounted for the indexing of the articles by PubMed, although there was generally no specific mention in the articles about the applications of biomedical engineering principles. While these publications are only a small subset of the many published articles in the aforementioned areas, they nonetheless provide excellent examples of how biomedical engineering principles have been applied in the past to orthodontic appliances. The first part of this chapter will summarize important past research activities involving collaborations between biomedical engineers and orthodontists, and the second part will describe current areas of research and potential future applications where there are highly promising new opportunities for such collaboration.

Past research activities

Archwire-bracket friction

The principal past research to understand the scientific basis of archwire-bracket friction and its applications to clinical orthodontic treatment was performed by the late Professor Robert Kusy and his group of graduate students. Professor Kusy was jointly appointed to the Department of Biomedical Engineering of the School of Medicine and in the School of Dentistry at the University of North Carolina at Chapel Hill.

Professor Kusy's initial study (Kusy et al., 1988) investigated the effects of surface roughness measured by laser

---

Integrated Clinical Orthodontics, First Edition. Edited by Vinod Krishnan, Ze'ev Davidovitch.
© 2012 Blackwell Publishing Ltd. Published 2012 by Blackwell Publishing Ltd.

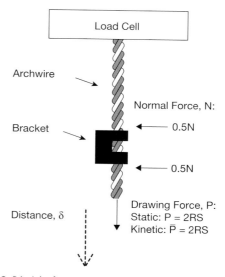

Figure 19.2 Principles for measurement of archwire–bracket friction, showing normal force (N) applied to multistrand archwire, drawing force (P), distance of movement (δ), and relationships of static and kinetic force to resistance to sliding (RS). (From Rucker and Kusy [2002a]. Reprinted with permission from Elsevier.)

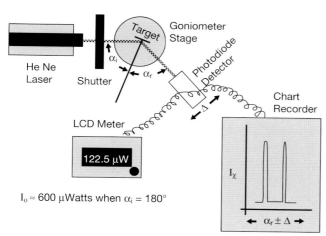

Figure 19.1 Schematic measurement of archwire surface roughness using laser reflectance spectroscopy. (From Kusy et al. [2004]. Reprinted with permission from Elsevier.)

specular reflectance (Figure 19.1) on the coefficients of static and dynamic friction in the dry state for model orthodontic systems that employed metallic archwires, lapped stainless steel, and as-received polycrystalline alumina surfaces to simulate brackets (Kusy and Whitley, 1990a). All-stainless steel couples of archwire and contacting surface had lower kinetic coefficients of friction than stainless steel-alumina couples, and beta-titanium had the highest coefficient of friction among archwires, although nickel-titanium archwires had the roughest surfaces. Scanning electron microscope (SEM) observations using energy-dispersive X-ray analyses revealed adhesion of beta-titanium archwires to stainless steel flat surfaces and abrasion of beta-titanium archwires by flat alumina surfaces that were microscopically rough due to the sharp facets of the fine grains of the material.

These pioneering studies with model systems were followed by an extensive series of investigations that evolved as new archwire and bracket products were introduced. Dry

state friction was measured for archwires in stainless steel and polycrystalline alumina bracket slots by Kusy and Whitley (1990b). The resistance to sliding of self-ligating brackets and conventional stainless steel twin brackets for second-order angulation in the dry and wet (saliva) states was studied by Thorstenson and Kusy (2001), followed by evaluation of sliding resistance of stainless steel archwires in self-ligating brackets having passive slides and active clips (Thorstenson and Kusy, 2002a). Thorstenson and Kusy (2002b) then examined four designs of self-ligating brackets coupled with four different nickel-titanium archwires varying in size and nickel-titanium phase (Brantley, 2001). In subsequent studies, Thorstenson and Kusy (2003a) first compared the resistance to sliding for polycrystalline alumina brackets and polycarbonate brackets, with and without stainless steel inserts with control stainless steel brackets with stainless steel archwires, and then investigated (Thorstenson and Kusy, 2003b, 2004) the resistance to sliding for stainless steel archwires coupled to conventional stainless steel brackets and new bracket designs. Figures 19.2 and 19.3 (Rucker and Kusy, 2002a) illustrate the principles, schematic apparatus, and typical results for friction measurements. This study compared the resistance to sliding, in the dry and wet (saliva) conditions, of multistrand stainless steel, single-strand stainless steel and nickel-titanium archwires. The coefficients of binding were not affected by saliva but were proportional to wire stiffness, and differences in the kinetic coefficients of friction for stainless steel and nickel-titanium archwires became unimportant shortly after binding occurred.

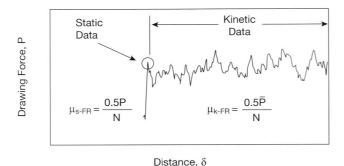

Figure 19.3 Schematic illustration of drawing force–distance data, showing determination of static and kinetic coefficients of friction ($\mu_{s\text{-FR}}$ and $\mu_{k\text{-FR}}$). (From Rucker and Kusy [2002a]. Reprinted with permission from Elsevier.)

In the final two studies of archwire-bracket friction from the Kusy laboratory, a more clinically oriented approach was employed to compare four conventional and four self-ligating brackets. Standardized archwires were drawn through quadrants of typodont models in dry and wet (saliva) states, and the drawing forces were measured for friction evaluation (Henao and Kusy, 2004). A small archwire simulated the earlier treatment stage, and two larger archwires simulated later stages; typodonts had quadrants with progressively increasing malocclusions. In their following study (Henao and Kusy, 2005) the same methodology was used to seek the optimal archwire-bracket system, using archwires and bracket designs from four manufacturers.

The foregoing laboratory studies by the Kusy research group has provided considerable fundamental understanding about the resistance to sliding for commercial archwires in commercial conventional and self-ligating brackets, along with the role of the critical angle for binding, the consequences of using inserts in brackets, the results from novel bracket designs, and use of different archwire materials and designs. Such information in principle provides the orthodontist with the ability to select the optimum archwires and brackets for a scientific approach to different patient treatment cases.

There is a prolific literature in this area in which biomedical engineers were not generally involved, with over 300 articles cited by PubMed, beginning with Andreasen and colleagues in 1969. The articles by the Kusy research group were selected to illustrate past interactions between biomedical engineers and orthodontists in the investigation of archwire-bracket friction.

In a recent review article, Burrow (2009) comments that clinical studies indicate a minimal role for archwire-bracket sliding friction in bodily tooth movement, which instead involves successive steps of archwire binding by the bracket and its release. He also notes that clinical studies to date do not indicate that treatment time is reduced with self-ligating

brackets because of lower friction. This important article stimulated several responses and replies in the Readers' Forum of the *American Journal of Orthodontics and Dentofacial Orthopedics* (July and December 2009). The reader is also directed to a classic article by Tidy (1989) on the *in vitro* measurement of frictional forces in fixed orthodontic appliances and a later article by Loftus et al. (1999) presenting an *in vitro* dentoalveolar model for measurement of frictional forces. Reznikov et al. (2010) have recently described a new system for measuring friction *in vitro* in a study that investigated stainless steel archwires and self-ligating brackets. These authors found that under certain clinical situations a firm passive bracket clip can adversely affect friction. However, none of these four pieces of research involved collaboration between orthodontists and biomedical engineers. New collaborations are needed for further progress in fundamental understanding of the sliding of the different types of archwires in the wide variety of commercially available brackets and how clinical treatment is affected by the complex archwire-bracket interactions that occur.

Fabrication and characterization of nonmetallic archwires

McKamey and Kusy (1999) created a polymer-polymer composite wire, designed for use as a ligature, by encasing ultra-high molecular weight polyethylene fibers in poly (n-butyl methacrylate) formulated from a polysol containing benzoin ethyl ether. Subsequently, Zufall and Kusy (2000a,b) created poly(chloro-p-xylylene)-coated glass fiber-reinforced composite archwires made by photo-pultrusion from S2-glass and a polymer formed from bisphenol-A diglycidyl methacrylate (Bis-GMA) and triethylene glycol dimethacrylate (TEGDMA), with benzoin ethyl ether as ultraviolet-light photoinitiator. Strength and force decay were measured for the polymer-polymer composite archwires, and the frictional and viscoelastic behavior of the fiber-reinforced polymer archwires was investigated extensively. Mathematical models were developed that described the *in vitro* behavior of the polymeric wires. Nonetheless, while laboratory results indicated that both polymeric wires would be suitable for their intended clinical applications, these wires were never introduced as commercial products, presumably because of the costs associated with developing the manufacturing techniques.

Besides the aforementioned articles published by the Kusy research group that involved collaborations between biomedical engineers and orthodontists, other similar collaborative research on nonmetallic archwires has also been reported. Based on collaboration between the orthodontic faculty at the Hokkaido University School of Dentistry and an engineering faculty member at the Chiba Institute of Technology in Japan, Imai et al. (1998) reported a study of fiber-reinforced polymeric archwires containing CaO–P_2O_5–SiO_2–Al_2O_3 glass fibers that were longitudinally oriented in a polymethyl methacrylate matrix using a hot-drawing method. The glass fiber surfaces of these wires were treated by a silane coupling agent to improve bonding with the polymer matrix. More recent collaboration between engineering mechanics, bioengineering, and orthodontics faculty at Tongji University in China and the National University of Singapore resulted in an article by Huang et al. (2003) on a tube-shrinkage technique that was used to fabricate longitudinally oriented glass fibers (E-glass) in an epoxy resin matrix. These authors noted that this novel technique did not have the problem of fiber damage or the limitation of a straight cylindrical geometry associated with the pultrusion (drawing) technique that had been previously used to fabricate unidirectional fiber-oriented composite archwires. Their work also led to a US Provisional Patent (60/436,466; December 27, 2002): 'Fiber-reinforced composite product with flexible longitudinal geometry'.

It is important to acknowledge the extensive past research by Goldberg and Burstone, which also represented collaboration between a bioengineer and an orthodontist, on the development of fiber composites for a variety of dental applications, including orthodontic archwires. The publica-tions from their past work can be easily found on PubMed, and at the time of going to press, an exciting new publication (Burstone et al., 2011) on polyphenylene polymer archwires appeared in the *American Journal of Orthodontics and Dentofacial Orthopedics.*

Fundamental studies of metallic archwires

Two important laboratory techniques that have been employed to investigate the mechanical properties and structures of nickel-titanium orthodontic archwires, where these relationships have enormous clinical importance (Brantley, 2001), are differential scanning calorimetry (DSC) (Lee et al., 1988; Khier et al., 1991) and dynamic mechanical analysis (DMA) (Kusy and Wilson, 1990; Kusy and Whitley, 2007). Schematic illustrations of the experimental set-ups for conventional DSC and DMA, along with schematic plots of the results from both techniques, are provided in Figures 19.4 and 19.5.

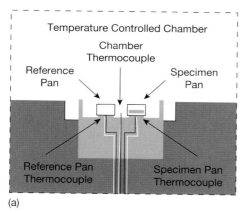

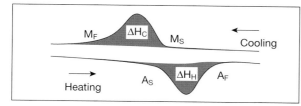

Figure 19.4 (a) Schematic experimental set-up for conventional differential scanning calorimetry (DSC). (b) Schematic DSC plot for nickel-titanium ortho-dontic wire, showing enthalpy changes for heating (ΔH_H) and cooling (ΔH_C), start (A_s) and finish (A_F) temperatures for transformation from martensite to austenite during heating, and start (M_s) and finish (M_F) temperatures for transformation from austenite to martensite on cooling. (From Kusy and Whitley [2007]. Reprinted with permission from Elsevier.)

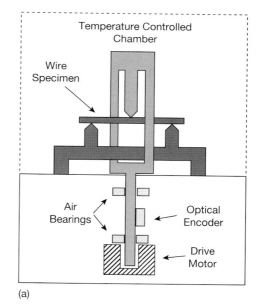

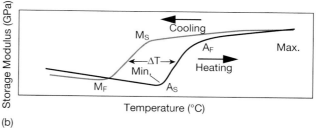

Figure 19.5 (a) Schematic experimental set-up for dynamic mechanical analysis (DMA). (b) Schematic DMA plot of changes in storage modulus for nickel-titanium orthodontic wire, showing effects of transformation from mar-tensite to austenite for heating and transformation from austenite to marten-site for cooling, start and finish temperatures for both transformations, and temperature difference (hysteresis) between heating and cooling curves in transformation temperature range. (From Kusy and Whitley (2007). Reprinted with permission from Elsevier.)

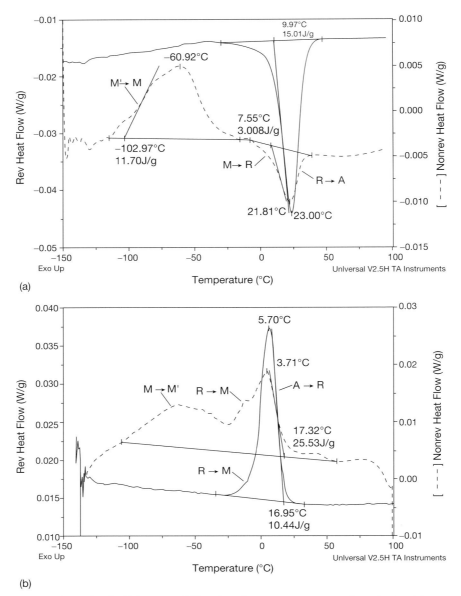

Figure 19.6 Temperature-modulated DSC plots for (a) heating and (b) cooling of 35°C Copper Ni-Ti. Transformations involving austenite (A), martensite (M) and R-phase (R) are designated by arrows. The R-phase transformation in many orthodontic wires is not detected by conventional DSC analysis. (From Brantley et al. [2003]. Reprinted with permission from Elsevier.)

Conventional DSC provides information about temperatures for transformations between higher-temperature austenite and lower-temperature martensite phases, along with enthalpy changes (ΔH), and clearly differentiates among wires having true shape memory *in vivo* and the superelastic and nonsuperelastic wires (Khier et al., 1991). Temperature-modulated DSC (Brantley et al., 2003), where a small sinusoidal thermal oscillation is superimposed on the linear heating/cooling ramp of conventional DSC, provides additional insight into transformations of nickel-titanium wires (Figure 19.6), including occurrence of

the intermediate R-phase and a low-temperature transformation within martensite, which was found to be twinning by transmission electron microscopy (Brantley et al., 2008).

With dynamic mechanical analysis, test specimens are subjected to an oscillating stress. Values are obtained for: (1) storage modulus corresponding to the strain component in-phase with stress (analogous to Young's modulus for tension or shear modulus for that loading mode), (2) loss modulus for the strain component 90° out-of-phase with stress, and (3) tangent delta (ratio of loss modulus and storage modulus), which indicates the level of viscoelastic (nonlinear elastic) behavior. While the dynamic mechanical properties of stainless steel and beta-titanium archwires did not vary over the DMA temperature range from −30°C to 80°C, differences in transformations observed by Kusy and Whitley (2007) for nonsuperelastic and superelastic archwires could have clinical significance. Values of transformation temperatures determined by DSC and DMA differ because the test specimens for the former technique are not subjected to stress during analysis, in contrast to the sinusoidal stress for DMA.

The mechanical properties of stiffness (elastic modulus), strength (force or stress for elastic limit, or maximum moment for elastic deformation) and range (extent of elastic deformation) are fundamental for the clinical performance of archwires. The relationship between these elastic properties and their measurement (which can be performed in tension, bending, or torsion) are discussed by Brantley et al. (2001), where previous research on measuring these properties by the Kusy group is also presented.

In more recent research, Rucker and Kusy (2002b) compared stiffness, strength, and range for three-strand and six-strand stainless steel wires with single-strand stainless steel and nickel-titanium leveling wires, as well as measuring the properties of wire segments in tension. They concluded that fabrication of multistrand stainless steel wires using alloys with enhanced tensile yield strength would allow these wires to compete better against conventional nickel-titanium wires. Rucker and Kusy (2002c) used bending and tension tests to investigate the properties of noncoated single-strand stainless steel and superelastic nickel-titanium wires, nylon-coated single-strand and multistrand stainless steel wires, and noncoated multistrand stainless steel and nickel-titanium wires. An important conclusion of this research was that few superelastic nickel-titanium wires are activated sufficiently *in vivo* to exhibit superelastic behavior, i.e. the superelastic plateau for unloading (Brantley, 2001).

In another important study, Kusy et al. (2004) investigated the composition, morphology, surface roughness, and sliding mechanics of six titanium-based archwires using an SEM with X-ray energy-dispersive analyses, laser specular reflectance, and a friction testing machine. Five wires were beta-titanium alloys with compositions similar to the original TMA (Ormco) product, and the sixth was an alpha-beta alloy containing 6 wt. % Al and 3 wt. % V. Beta-titanium alloys are of particular clinical interest because of their biocompatibility due to the absence of nickel (Brantley, 2001). A variety of surface morphologies were observed, and specular reflectance and optical roughness measurements divided these wires into two groups. For values of angulation covering passive and active regions of sliding, coefficients of friction varied narrowly and were independent of surface roughness.

Consequently, the authors suggested that from a clinical viewpoint, all six titanium-based archwire products were comparable.

A recent study by Walker et al. (2007), involving collaboration between an orthodontist, a dental biomaterials faculty member, and an engineering faculty member, employed the three-point bending test methodology in ANSI/ADA Specification No. 32. The elastic properties of 3M Unitek Beta III titanium and stainless steel archwires in distilled water, a neutral fluoride solution, and an acidulated phosphate fluoride solution were compared at 37°C. The two fluoride solutions caused decreases in the clinically relevant unloading mechanical properties of both the beta-titanium and stainless steel archwires, as well as changes in surface topography from corrosive attack. The important result from this study was that use of these fluoride solutions by patients could extend the time for orthodontic treatment.

Other studies on metallic archwires with a biomedical engineering focus reported relationships between surface condition and electrochemical behavior of nickel-titanium wires and the use of diamond-like coatings. Clarke et al. (2006) prepared a series of wires having a variety of surface conditions. Wires with very thick oxides contained high nickel contents in the oxide layer, and untreated samples with thicker oxides showed lower pitting potential values and greater nickel release in both long and short-term experiments. For long-term immersion tests in 0.9% NaCl solutions, breakdown potentials for the oxide layers increased. Results demonstrated that appropriate surface treatment of nickel-titanium wires is essential for optimum biomedical performance. Kobayashi et al. (2007) used an arc-discharge ion-plating process and deposited diamond-like coatings (DLC) on nickel-titanium orthodontic archwires. The wires were immersed in physiological saline at 37°C for 6 months, and the concentration of nickel ions released from DLC-coated wires was one-sixth that from non-coated wires. The growth rate of squamous carcinoma cells on DLC-coated wires was higher than that on non-coated wires. Wang and Zheng (2008) compared vacuum arc-melted, hot-rolled, quenched and annealed plate specimens of a nickel-titanium alloy containing 2.8% cobalt and the equiatomic nickel-titanium alloy in deaerated artificial saliva. Potentiodynamic and potentiostatic test results showed that the corrosion behavior of the two alloys was similar, and that with increasing electrolyte pH, both the corrosion potential and the breakdown potential for pitting decreased. X-ray photoelectron spectroscopy (XPS) revealed that the outermost passive film for the nickel-titanium-cobalt alloy consisted mainly of TiO_2, as found for nickel-titanium. Inductively-coupled plasma/optical emission spectroscopy (ICP/OES) indicated that nickel ion release from nickel-titanium-cobalt was very close to that from nickel-titanium, and neither titanium nor cobalt ions could be detected. This study emphasized the important *in vitro* relationship between corrosion behavior and pH underpinning the clinical use of nickel-titanium orthodontic wires.

Force measurements

With the recent improvements in technology, there has been much interest in orthodontic force measurements. Friedrich et al. (1999) described three-dimensional recording of orthodontic forces during treatment *in vivo* with fixed appliances, using brackets with a special design. Measurements were obtained by a six-axis force-torque sensor with strain gauge elements. Badawi et al. (2009) reported an *in vitro* method for three-dimensional measurements and analyses of orthodontic force systems. Their orthodontic simulator was based on a single dental arch containing 14 teeth, to which brackets could be bonded and wires ligated. Using transducers, it was possible to measure simultaneously the force systems applied on all teeth in the arch by orthodontic appliances and generate three-dimensional force displays. This article raised several controversies, with several comments subsequently appearing in the Readers' Forum of the *American Journal of Orthodontics and Dentofacial Orthopedics* (January and April 2010). It is evident that further research is needed to evaluate the biomechanics of conventional and self-ligating brackets and their clinical efficacy.

Other investigations have examined the behavior of polymeric force-producing modules. Stevenson and Kusy (1994) evaluated the effects of pre-stressing, environmental acidity, oxygen content, and temperature on polyurethane chains. Specimens were treated for 10 and 100 days, and mechanical properties were compared with untreated specimens, using stress-relaxation tests. Conditioning treatments affected the residual load after relaxation, with the largest effect due to pre-stressing. An increase in temperature significantly affected deterioration of mechanical properties, while acidity and oxygen content of the environment had no significant effects. *In vitro* force decay was described by a Maxwell-Weichert model that assumed one mechanism was responsible for the rapid initial force loss and another mechanism was responsible for the slow force loss at longer times. While this model would ideally allow the orthodontist to predict the force supplied by these polyurethane chains at initial activation and any subsequent time during treatment, the *in vivo* environment to which the chains are exposed during clinical use causes complex degradation processes (Eliades et al., 2001a). The force decay of 3/16-inch latex elastics (3M Unitek) was evaluated by Wang et al. (2007). All specimen groups showed rapid force loss during the first hour, which had been reported previously. At later times of 24 and 48 hours, there was highly significant force decrease *in vivo* and in artificial saliva, but no significant differences in a dry room. There was significantly more degradation for intermaxillary traction (where different times for wearing the elastics were important) than for intramaxillary traction, and for *in vivo* conditions compared with a dry room environment.

Another earlier force measurement study was reported by Katona and Chen (1994), who performed an engineering analysis of a popular tensile bond strength testing methodology at that time for brackets bonded to enamel. They proposed that use of a long harness (wire loop) around the bracket constructed from thin ligature wire, pre-stressing the harness, and lubrication may reduce effects of inevitable load-bracket misalignment. These authors and their colleagues subsequently conducted numerous other studies on orthodontic force measurements and biomechanics, involving collaborations between orthodontics, biomechanics and engineering faculty, and the corresponding publications can be found on PubMed.

Orthodontic appliances and finite element analysis

Finite element analysis has been extensively employed in orthodontic research for three decades, with over 340 articles in PubMed. This technique, which has been utilized extensively by Katona, Chen and their colleagues, is a common procedure for solving biomedical engineering problems and is particularly useful for orthodontic biomechanics. Recent publications by this group (Viecilli et al., 2008, 2009; Meyer et al., 2010) illustrate the methodology and orthodontic applications.

Finite element analysis is a computational process that requires special software. A computer model of the system is initially subdivided into meshes. Using knowledge of elastic constants (Young's modulus and Poisson's ratio), computerized loading of the model causes deformation of the meshes, with displacements of their intersection points (nodes) that are converted to three-dimensional strains and stresses using the special finite element analysis software. Nonlinear elastic behavior can also be incorporated into finite element analyses.

An example of a model ceramic bracket with a network of meshes in shown in Figure 19.7. In an important earlier study, Ghosh et al. (1995) applied finite element analysis to several commercial ceramic brackets, observed the resulting stress distributions, and emphasized the value of this technique for investigating bracket design.

Several miscellaneous articles on orthodontic appliances, involving finite element analysis and other sophisticated approaches in collaborations between biomedical engineers and orthodontists, were also retrieved using PubMed. Lewis et al. (1996) used finite element analysis to determine stresses in the adhesive layer of two-dimensional models of bonded brackets. PH Liu et al. (2004) used strain tensor analysis to investigate effects of chin cup therapy on the mandible in Class III malocclusions. Lin et al. (2004) used finite element analyses to study the effect of retainer thickness on posterior resin-bonded prostheses. Pilliar et al.

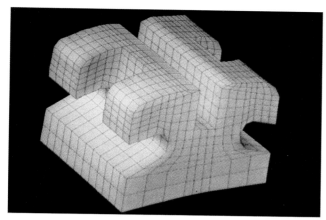

Figure 19.7 Example of bracket model with mesh pattern for finite element analyses of ceramic brackets. (From Ghosh et al. [1995]. Reprinted with permission from Elsevier.)

(2006) developed a finite element model to investigate crestal bone loss patterns around sintered porous-surface and machined threaded implants produced for orthodontic anchorage that were used in an animal study. Qi et al. (2007) measured the transmission of forces for a cast-metal, fixed, twin-block appliance used to achieve rapid correction of Class II malocclusions. The very wide scope of these articles illustrates the range of research that can be performed in this area and should encourage future collaboration between biomedical engineers and orthodontists.

Miscellaneous areas of research

In the first of three diverse articles, J Liu (2004) investigated genotypic stability of *Streptococcus mutans*, using plaque samples obtained from supragingival smooth surfaces of right maxillary teeth at four stages of orthodontic treatment. DNA was prepared from a large number of *S. mutans* strains, and strains were identified using polymerase chain reaction (PCR). PCR fingerprinting was applied to determine genotypes. The amount of *S. mutans* increased significantly after fixed appliances were bonded, and *S. mutans* clones were stable during orthodontic treatment.

In the second article, Kusy (2004) presented a theoretical bioengineering model that considered the influences of specific concentrations of allergens on their clinical effects, focusing on nickel and chromium for orthodontic patients. He noted clinical responses to these two allergens in a large number of patients. The practical application of his model involved a questionnaire, and in the patient reporting an allergy, a skin patch test would be administered to establish whether alternative alloys not containing these elements should be used during treatment.

The third article was by Toms et al. (2002), who investigated the stress-strain behavior of the periodontal ligament (PDL), using tissues obtained from cadaveric specimens of young and elderly adults. The schematic experimental set-up is shown in Figure 19.8, and a representative stress-strain curve for the PDL is presented in Figure 19.9. The stress-strain curves for both intrusion and extrusion loading had nonlinear behavior with distinct low-elastic-modulus toe and higher-elastic-modulus linear regions. The loading behavior of the PDL was found to be dependent on age, location (cervical margin, apex region and midroot region), and load direction (intrusion or extrusion). An important consequence from this study was the suggestion that computer simulations of orthodontic tooth movement should incorporate the nonlinear behavior of the PDL.

Current research activities and potential future applications

Advances in materials science and related fields have resulted in the introduction of materials and processes that create applications of unique properties in a wide range of biomedical disciplines. The purpose of this part of the chapter is to highlight advances (Box 19.2) that may have direct application to orthodontic materials from both the clinical and research perspectives. The majority of these advances have not yet been applied to orthodontic materials; in some areas preliminary data on experimental products have been published, although without current translation into commercial availability.

Shape-memory polymers – polymer wires

Shape-memory polymers are an emerging class of polymers with applications spanning various areas of everyday life. These polymers are dual-shape materials belonging to the group of 'actively moving' polymers that can change from one shape to another, the first being a temporary shape obtained by mechanical deformation and the second obtained from subsequent fixation of that deformation (Behl and Lendlein, 2007).

For shape-memory polymers, heat, light, infrared radiation, electrical and magnetic fields, and immersion in water have been used to induce this property. The shape-memory effect depends on the molecular architecture and does not require a specific chemical structure in the repeating units. In essence, application of external stimuli to these materials introduces a departure from the as-received shape to a new configuration that is reversible. This cycle of programming and recovery can be repeated several times, with different temporary shapes in subsequent cycles. In comparison with metallic shape-memory alloys, the shape-memory 'cycle' for these polymers can take place in much shorter time and at much higher deformation rate between shapes. An example of a biomedical application of shape-memory polymers is a laser-activated device for the mechanical

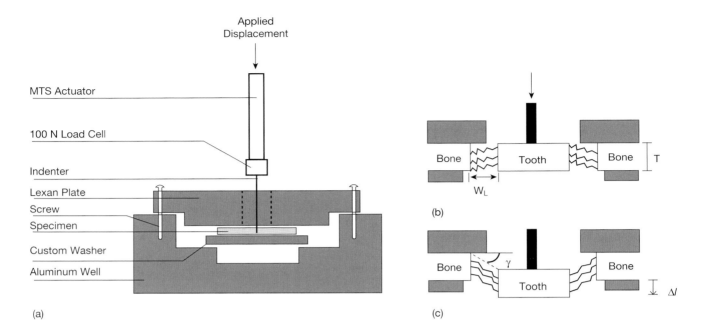

(a)

(b)

(c)

Figure 19.8 (a) Schematic experimental set-up used to investigate stress-strain behavior of periodontal ligament (PDL). Schematic illustrations of clamped specimen for loading in extrusion (b) before and (c) after application of load. From Toms et al. [2002] Reprinted with permission from Elsevier.)

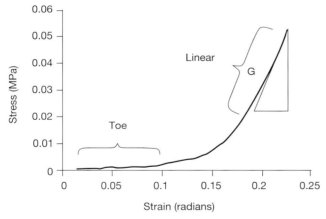

Figure 19.9 Nonlinear stress-strain curve for the periodontal ligament (PDL) at low stress. Toe modulus was calculated for toe region, beginning at origin, and linear modulus was calculated in linear region shown. Modulus values were calculated for intrusion and extrusion. (From Toms et al. [2002] Reprinted with permission from Elsevier.)

Box 19.2 Recent advances in materials science and engineering areas with application to orthodontics

- Shape-memory polymers for archwires
- Self-healing materials
- Smart brackets with force-moment sensors
- Biomimetic adhesives
- Self-cleaning materials
- Other smart biomaterials

parent wires with minimum stiffness, which could then be transformed into archwires of predetermined elastic modulus upon exposure to a stimulus such as light or heat. Therefore, aesthetics along with a preferable stiffness would be attained during intraoral application of these materials.

Self-healing materials

The design and manufacturing of 'smart' synthetic systems that can mimic the behavior of biological systems that heal themselves has been an objective of intense research during the past decade. Hybrid materials have been recently created, where micrometer-scale conduits extend throughout the material and contain healing fluids or dissolved healing agents (Balazs, 2007). When a crack appears near the network, the fluid can flow to the damaged region and

removal of blood clots. The device is inserted by minimally invasive surgery into the blood vessel, and upon laser activation the shape-memory polymer coils into its permanent shape, enabling the mechanical removal of the clot.

In orthodontics, the potential application of these materials involves the manufacturing of polymeric trans-fill the fissure. The simplest form to achieve this behavior might be the incorporation of bubbles of a material/substance/precursor in the raw material. This reservoir, upon exposure to air, polymerizes as a result of crack formation and spontaneously closes the crack, thus maintaining the structural integrity of the material.

The orthodontic application of this concept may involve polymer brackets and archwires. The integration of nano-sized bubbles filled with autopolymerized monomer in these materials may result in reduction of wire and bracket breakages. Fracture of the bracket or wire would induce bursting of the nano-bubbles and exposure of the monomer to air, thereby resulting in polymerization and filling of the crack-induced gap.

Brackets with force-moment sensors

Estimation of force and moment magnitudes applied during standard mechanotherapeutic configurations in orthodontics has been the focus of many *in vitro* studies during the past two decades. These efforts have employed numerous devices and techniques, as described by Bourauel et al. (1992) and Badawi et al. (2009), to measure forces applied to teeth. Limitations of the *in vitro* environment, however, have imposed a substantial burden on the clinical relevance of the results.

A recent research perspective on this topic, which has been long sought in the orthodontic materials and biomechanics fields, has provided a breakthrough in developments in monitoring the variation of force applied to teeth *in vivo* under real-time conditions (Lapatki et al., 2007). These researchers, who are from Departments of Orthodontics and Microsystems Engineering at the University of Freiberg in Germany, have manufactured an orthodontic bracket with an integrated microelectronic chip equipped with multiple piezo-resistive stress sensors capable of quantitatively determining forces in three dimensions (Figure 19.10). A study assessing the accuracy of this sensor-integrated bracket demonstrated good agreement between measured and reference values with standard deviations in the differences of 0.037 N for forces and 0.985 N·mm for moments. This bracket will be of major service to both the clinician and researcher, allowing applications of low-force bracket-wire configurations and providing the means to perform research on this subject in humans.

Biomimetic adhesives

The issue of an enamel-friendly bonding mechanism for orthodontic appliances has been the subject of investigations since the original introduction of the acid-etching technique. This intense interest derived from the description of alterations of enamel color and structure associated with acid-etched-mediated bonding (Eliades et al., 2001b). Although glass-ionomer adhesives have offered an alternative, their applications remain limited, probably because of the higher failure rates.

The introduction during the past 15 years of a new class of materials that adopt the paradigms of nature has gradually established the category of biomimetic materials. This term derives from Greek 'bio' (living) and 'mimetic' (imitating or resembling), and refers to how creatures ingenuously employ natural elements to solve problems in the environment (Lee et al., 2007; Hamming et al., 2008; Bilic et al., 2010).

For example, geckos are lizards that belong to the species of *gekkonidae* and are characterized by a remarkable ability to sustain their weight while upside down. The strong but temporary adhesion employed by a gecko comes from a mechanical principle known as 'contact splitting'. The foot of a gecko has a flat pad which is densely packed with very fine hairs that are split at the ends, resulting in a greater number of contact points than if the hairs were not split. More contact points between these hairs and a surface result in a significant increase in adhesion. Researchers have discovered that this special nature of the foot pads allows the gecko to stick to surfaces through the formation of localized van der Waals forces. This mechanism has been employed for high-friction microfibers or carbon nanotubes, which are sprayed on a surface. Because of their enormous number per unit area, the physical forces developed mimic the ability of a gecko to attach firmly to surfaces without the use of a chemical substance.

While this mode of bonding may be suitable for dry environments, it fails to provide reliable performance with wet surfaces (Lee et al., 2007). This problem inspired researchers to adopt another natural example of bonding: that of mussels. Combining the important elements of gecko and mussel adhesion, the new adhesive material, called 'geckel', functions like a sticky note and exhibits strong yet reversible adhesion in both air and water. Mussel-mimetic polymers have an amino acid called L-3,4-dihydroxyphenylalanine (DOPA) found in high concentrations in the 'glue' proteins of mussels (Hamming et al., 2008). Analogous to the gecko-based approach, pillar arrays (400–600 nm in diameter and length) coated with the mussel-mimetic polymer improved wet adhesion by 15-fold over uncoated pillar arrays. One of the first applications of this new material has involved fetal membrane defects, which pose a serious risk for leakage of amniotic fluid that can result in premature birth or termination of pregnancy. A sealant inspired by the ability of mussels to stick to surfaces under wet conditions has shown promise for repairing defects in human fetal membranes (Bilic et al., 2010).

There is a vast scope for orthodontic application of this innovation. Brackets having bases with pads mimicking the gecko foot and covered with a layer of DOPA would provide adequate bond strength to sound enamel without prior enamel conditioning and with minimal color and

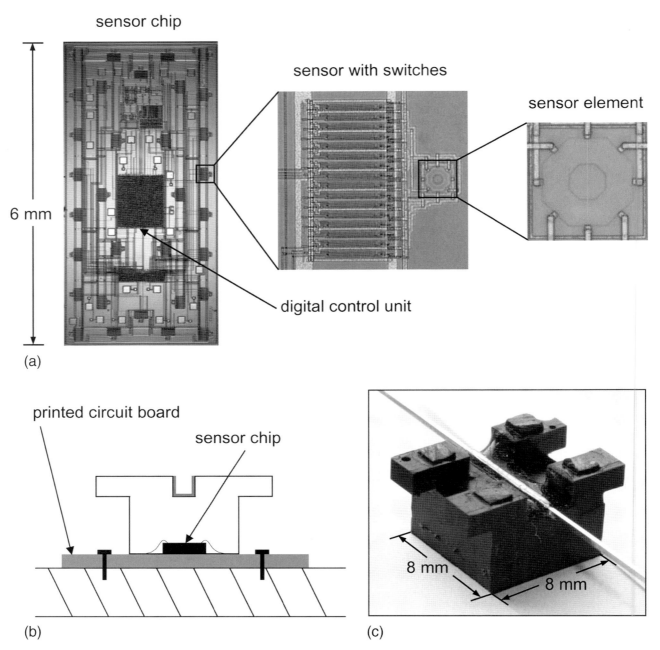

Figure 19.10 Smart bracket (a) Micrograph of sensor chip, showing individual sensor with switches and sensor element. (b) Schematic cross-section of smart bracket model, with sensor chip wire-bonded to printed circuit board and encapsulated in plastic bracket. (c) Photograph of manufactured smart bracket with base of $8\times8\,mm^2$ (approximate scale 2.5:1 compared with normal bracket). (Reprinted from Lapatki et al. [2007] with permission from Sage Publications.)

structural alterations to the enamel. To the best of our knowledge, the use of this type of biomimetic adhesive has not yet been adapted by manufacturers of orthodontic brackets.

Self-cleaning materials

The issue of plaque retention on brackets and microbial attachment onto these calcified biofilms has been a major concern from an enamel prophylactic perspective. The development of a material that could clean itself of not only inorganic (mainly), but also organic, precipitations is an attractive prospect in the materials science areas involving biomedical, industrial, and aeronautical applications. Early research in this field adopted the paradigm of microscopic bumps on a lotus leaf, which transform its waxy surface into an extremely water repellent, or superhydrophobic, material (Forbes, 2008). Synthetic self-cleaning materials have been developed, some of which are based on this 'lotus effect', whereas others employ the opposite property of 'superhydrophilicity' as well as catalytic chemical reactions.

The use of titanium oxide nanocoatings has been found to increase the safety of aircraft by preventing the build-up of ice and other contaminants. This process creates self-cleaning 'superhydrophobic' surfaces, and involves the application of a hydrofluoric acid coating on the titanium alloy substrate. A substantially self-cleaning superhydrophobic surface is created when exposure to ultraviolet light causes the titanium oxide layer to undergo photocatalytic reaction with oxygen to oxidize any organic contaminants that may be present. Since superhydrophobic surfaces resist soiling by water-borne contaminants, they are easily cleaned and useful in directing flow in microfluidic devices.

Polyoxometalates (POM) have a rich and promising photochemical behavior. Upon illumination corresponding to the OMCT (oxygen-metal-charge transfer) band (i.e. in the ultraviolet and near-visible areas), POM become powerful oxidizing reagents able to oxidize a wide variety of organic compounds (Papaconstantinou et al., 2003). In the process, the POM undergo stepwise reduction, accumulating electrons that can be subsequently delivered via thermal reactions to different oxidants. In this way a wide variety of organic compounds are oxidized and mineralized to carbon dioxide, water, and inorganic anions. Several organic and inorganic compounds can be reduced via a photocatalytic process in which the POM serve as electron relays. Thus, in principle, POM can serve as decontamination photocatalysts of aquatic media, removing both organic pollutants and metal ions.

Photocatalytic activity from the reaction of titanium oxide with ultraviolet light has recently gained attention in orthodontic materials (Horiuchi et al., 2007). In particular, there is scientific interest in inducing photocatalytic reactions on the nickel-titanium archwire alloy. By thickening the titanium oxide film with electrolytic treatment and then applying heat treatment, the surface film on nickel-titanium was modified from an amorphous structure to crystalline rutile (TiO_2).

Other smart biomaterials

Other 'smart biomaterials' are described in an article by Anderson et al. (2004). For example, some polymeric biomimetic materials that utilize nanofibers formed from peptides and proteins have the ability to self-assemble into three-dimensional structures. Such materials may be able to control cellular behavior and enable production of multiple lineages from a single stem cell type. Hydrogels containing matrix metalloproteinase (MMP) degradable sites and growth factors such as bone morphogenetic proteins (BMP) may find application for healing of bony defects.

Implant biomaterials are being developed that can be converted from the liquid state to the solid state at desired sites *in vivo*, using light, temperature or pH changes. Other biomaterials with 'smart surfaces' are being developed that can reversibly switch between hydrophilic and hydrophobic character with the application of an electrical potential, and such coatings would enable the production of devices with digitally responsive surfaces. All of these materials might potentially find applications in orthodontics, provided that continued laboratory developments are successful and these innovations are communicated to orthodontists and biomedical engineers. This exciting new field of smart biomaterials lies at the intersection of cell biology, tissue engineering, and materials science, which are major domain areas for modern biomedical engineering.

Conclusions

These are exciting times for the development of customized orthodontic materials and appliances, and interactions with biomedical engineers will accelerate the pace of improvements. Smart biocompatible materials and brackets will become part of the armamentarium in the future. Important domains of biomedical engineering, particularly use of nanotechnology for device fabrication, continued development of nanostructured and biomimetic materials, and application of tissue engineering principles for hard and soft tissues, should be prominent areas of forthcoming research.

Based on our experience, orthodontic faculties in research-oriented institutions need to approach faculty in biomedical engineering or bioengineering departments and point out the opportunities that are available for collaboration. While such collaborations have occurred in a few universities in the past, there is a critical need for much greater mutual interaction, which can be fostered by joint departmental appointments. Innovative research that translates into fruitful relationships between *in vitro* laboratory studies and the *in vivo* clinical environment will require considerable dialog between researchers with disparate orthodontic and biomedical engineering viewpoints to frame the appropriate protocols. In the USA, novel research proposals on the applications of biomimetic materials and smart materials, and the interaction between biomechanical and biological processes for orthodontics, may be considered favorably for support by the National Institutes of Health.

References

Anderson DG, Burdick JA, Langer R (2004) Smart biomaterials. *Science* 305: 1923–4.

Badawi HM, Toogood RW, Carey JP, et al. (2009) Three-dimensional orthodontic force measurements. *American Journal of Orthodontics and Dentofacial Orthopedics* 136: 518–28.

Balazs AC (2007) Modeling self-healing materials. *Materials Today* 10: 18–23.

Behl M, Lendlein A (2007) Shape-memory polymers. *Materials Today* 4: 20–8.

Bilic G, Brubaker C, Messersmith PB, et al. (2010) Injectable candidate sealants for fetal membrane repair: bonding and toxicity in vitro. *American Journal of Obstetrics and Gynecology* 202: 85.e1–9.

Bourauel C, Drescher D, Thier M (1992) An experimental apparatus for the simulation of three-dimensional movements in orthodontics. *Journal of Biomedical Engineering* 14: 371–8.

Brantley WA (2001) Orthodontic wires. In: WA Brantley, T Eliades (eds) *Orthodontic Materials: Scientific and Clinical Aspects.* Stuttgart: Thieme, pp. 79–97.

Brantley WA, Eliades T, Litsky AS (2001) Mechanics and mechanical testing of orthodontic materials. In: WA Brantley, T Eliades (eds) *Orthodontic Materials: Scientific and Clinical Aspects.* Stuttgart: Thieme, pp. 33–6.

Brantley WA, Iijima M, Grentzer TH (2003) Temperature-modulated DSC provides new insight about nickel-titanium wire transformations. *American Journal of Orthodontics and Dentofacial Orthopedics* 124: 387–94.

Brantley WA, Guo W, Clark WAT, et al. (2008) Microstructural studies of 35°C Copper Ni–Ti orthodontic wire and TEM confirmation of low-temperature martensite transformation. *Dental Materials* 24: 204–10.

Burrow SJ (2009) Friction and resistance to sliding in orthodontics: a critical review. *American Journal of Orthodontics and Dentofacial Orthopedics* 135: 442–7.

Burstone CJ, Liebler SAH, Goldberg AJ (2011) Polyphenylene polymers as esthetic orthodontic archwires. *American Journal of Orthodontics and Dentofacial Orthopedics* 139: e391–8.

Clarke B, Carroll W, Rochev Y, et al. (2006) Influence of Nitinol wire surface treatment on oxide thickness and composition and its subsequent effect on corrosion resistance and nickel ion release. *Journal of Biomedical Materials Research A* 79: 61–70.

Eliades T, Eliades G, Watts DC, et al. (2001a) Elastomeric ligatures and chains. In: WA Brantley, T Eliades (eds) *Orthodontic Materials: Scientific and Clinical Aspects.* Stuttgart: Thieme, pp. 173–87.

Eliades T, Kakaboura A, Eliades G, et al. (2001b) Comparison of enamel color changes associated with orthodontic bonding using two different adhesives. *European Journal of Orthodontics* 1: 85–90.

Forbes P (2008) Self-cleaning materials. *Scientific American* 299: 88–95.

Friedrich D, Rosarius N, Rau G, et al. (1999) Measuring system for in vivo recording of force systems in orthodontic treatment-concept and analysis of accuracy. *Journal of Biomechanics* 32: 81–5.

Ghosh J, Nanda RS, Duncanson MG Jr, et al. (1995) Ceramic bracket design: An analysis using the finite element method. *American Journal of Orthodontics and Dentofacial Orthopedics* 108: 575–82.

Hamming LM, Fan XW, Messersmith PB, et al. (2008) Mimicking mussel adhesion to improve interfacial properties in composites. *Composite Scientific Technology* 68: 2042–8.

Henao SP, Kusy RP (2004) Evaluation of the frictional resistance of conventional and self-ligating bracket designs using standardized archwires and dental typodonts. *Angle Orthodontist* 74: 202–11.

Henao SP, Kusy RP (2005) Frictional evaluations of dental typodont models using four self-ligating designs and a conventional design. *Angle Orthodontist* 75: 75–85.

Horiuchi Y, Horiuchi M, Hawana T, et al. (2007) Effect of surface modification on the photocatalysis of Ti-Ni alloy in orthodontics. *Dental Materials Journal* 26: 924–9.

Huang ZM, Gopal R, Fujihara K, et al. (2003) Fabrication of a new composite orthodontic archwire and validation by a bridging micromechanics model. *Biomaterials* 24: 2941–53.

Imai T, Watari F, Yamagata S, et al. (1998) Mechanical properties and aesthetics of FRP orthodontic wire fabricated by hot drawing. *Biomaterials* 19: 2195–200.

Katona TR, Chen J (1994) Engineering and experimental analyses of the tensile loads applied during strength testing of direct bonded orthodontic brackets. *American Journal of Orthodontics and Dentofacial Orthopedics* 106: 167–74.

Khier SE, Brantley WA, Fournelle RA (1991) Bending properties of superelastic and nonsuperelastic nickel-titanium orthodontic wires. *American Journal of Orthodontics and Dentofacial Orthopedics* 99: 310–18.

Kobayashi S, Ohgoe Y, Ozeki K, et al. (2007) Dissolution effect and cytotoxicity of diamond-like carbon coatings on orthodontic archwires. *Journal of Materials Science: Materials in Medicine* 18: 2263–8.

Kusy RP (2004) Clinical response to allergies in patients. *American Journal of Orthodontics and Dentofacial Orthopedics* 125: 544–7.

Kusy RP, Whitley JQ (1990a) Effects of surface roughness on the coefficients of friction in model orthodontic systems. *Journal of Biomechanics* 23: 913–25.

Kusy RP, Whitley JQ (1990b) Coefficients of friction for arch wires in stainless steel and polycrystalline alumina bracket slots. I. The dry state. *American Journal of Orthodontics and Dentofacial Orthopedics* 98: 300–12. Erratum (1993) in *American Journal of Orthodontics and Dentofacial Orthopedics* 104: 26.

Kusy RP, Whitley JQ (2007) Thermal and mechanical characteristics of stainless steel, titanium-molybdenum, and nickel-titanium archwires. *American Journal of Orthodontics and Dentofacial Orthopedics* 131: 229–37.

Kusy RP, Wilson TW (1990) Dynamic mechanical properties of straight titanium alloy arch wires. *Dental Materials* 6: 228–36.

Kusy RP, Whitley JQ, Mayhew MJ, et al. (1988) Surface roughness of orthodontic archwires via laser spectroscopy. *Angle Orthodontist* 58: 33–45.

Kusy RP, Whitley JQ, de Araújo Gurgel J (2004) Comparisons of surface roughnesses and sliding resistances of 6 titanium-based or TMA-type archwires. *American Journal of Orthodontics and Dentofacial Orthopedics* 126: 589–603.

Lapatki BG, Bartholomeyczik J, Ruther P, et al. (2007) Smart bracket for multi-dimensional force and moment measurement. *Journal of Dental Research* 86: 73–8.

Lee H, Lee BP, Messersmith PB (2007) A reversible wet/dry adhesive inspired by mussels and geckos. *Nature* 448: 338–41.

Lee JH, Park JB, Andreasen GF, et al. (1988) Thermomechanical study of Ni-Ti alloys. *Journal of Biomedical Materials Research* 22: 573–88.

Lewis G, Manickam S, Wharton D (1996) Effect of debonding forces on bonded orthodontic brackets: finite element study. *Biomedical Materials Engineering* 6: 113–21.

Lin TS, Lin CL, Wang CH, et al. (2004) The effect of retainer thickness on posterior resin-banded prostheses: a finite element study. *Journal of Oral Rehabilitation* 31: 1123–9.

Liu J, Bian Z, Fan M, et al. (2004) Typing of mutans streptococci by arbitrarily primed PCR in patients undergoing orthodontic treatment. *Caries Research* 38: 523–9.

Liu PH, Chang CH, Chang HP, et al. (2004) Treatment effects of chin cup appliance on mandible in Class III malocclusion: strain tensor analysis. A pilot study. *Quintessence International* 35: 621–9.

Loftus BP, Årtun J, Nicholls JI, et al. (1999) Evaluation of friction during sliding tooth movement in various bracket-arch wire combinations. *American Journal of Orthodontics and Dentofacial Orthopedics* 116: 336–45.

McKamey RP, Kusy RP (1999) Stress-relaxing composite ligature wires: formulations and characteristics. *Angle Orthodontist* 69: 441–9.

Meyer BN, Chen J, Katona TR (2010) Does the center of resistance depend on the direction of tooth movement? *American Journal of Orthodontics and Dentofacial Orthopedics* 137: 354–61.

Papaconstantinou E, Hiskia A, Troupis A (2003) Photocatalytic processes with tungsten oxygen anion clusters. *Frontiers in Bioscience* 8: s813–25.

Pilliar RM, Sagals G, Meguid SA, et al. (2006) Threaded versus porous-surfaced implants as anchorage units for orthodontic treatment: three-dimensional finite element analysis of peri-implant bone tissue stresses. *International Journal of Oral and Maxillofacial Implants* 21: 879–89.

Qi J, Tan ZR, He H, Pan D, Yeweng SJ (2007) A preliminary report of a new design of cast metal fixed twin-block appliance. *Journal of Orthodontics* 34: 213–19.

Reznikov N, Har-Zion G, Barkana I, et al. (2010) Measurement of friction forces between stainless steel wires and 'reduced-friction' self-ligating brackets. *American Journal of Orthodontics and Dentofacial Orthopedics* 138: 330–8.

Rucker BK, Kusy RP (2002a) Resistance to sliding of stainless steel multistranded archwires and comparison with single-stranded leveling wires. *American Journal of Orthodontics and Dentofacial Orthopedics* 122: 73–83.

Rucker BK, Kusy RP (2002b) Elastic flexural properties of multistranded stainless steel versus conventional nickel titanium archwires. *Angle Orthodontist* 72: 302–9.

Rucker BK, Kusy RP (2002c) Elastic properties of alternative versus single-stranded leveling archwires. *American Journal of Orthodontics and Dentofacial Orthopedics* 122: 528–41.

Stevenson JS, Kusy RP (1994) Force application and decay characteristics of untreated and treated polyurethane elastomeric chains. *Angle Orthodontist* 64: 455–64; discussion: 465–7.

Thorstenson GA, Kusy RP (2001) Resistance to sliding of self-ligating brackets versus conventional stainless steel twin brackets with second-order angulation in the dry and wet (saliva) states. *American Journal of Orthodontics and Dentofacial Orthopedics* 120: 361–70.

Thorstenson GA, Kusy RP (2002a) Comparison of resistance to sliding between different self-ligating brackets with second-order angulation in the dry and saliva states. *American Journal of Orthodontics and Dentofacial Orthopedics* 121: 472–82.

Thorstenson GA, Kusy RP (2002b) Effect of archwire size and material on the resistance to sliding of self-ligating brackets with second-order angulation in the dry state. *American Journal of Orthodontics and Dentofacial Orthopedics* 122: 295–305.

Thorstenson GA, Kusy R (2003a) Influence of stainless steel inserts on the resistance to sliding of esthetic brackets with second-order angulation in the dry and wet states. *Angle Orthodontist* 73: 167–75.

Thorstenson GA, Kusy RP (2003b) Effects of ligation type and method on the resistance to sliding of novel orthodontic brackets with second-order angulation in the dry and wet states. *Angle Orthodontist* 73: 418–30.

Thorstenson GA, Kusy RP (2004) Resistance to sliding of orthodontic brackets with bumps in the slot floors and walls: effects of second-order angulation. *Dental Materials* 20: 881–92.

Tidy DC (1989) Frictional forces in fixed appliances. *American Journal of Orthodontics and Dentofacial Orthopedics* 96: 249–54.

Toms SR, Lemons JE, Bartolucci AA, et al. (2002) Nonlinear stress-strain behavior of periodontal ligament under orthodontic loading. *American Journal of Orthodontics and Dentofacial Orthopedics* 122: 174–9.

Viecilli RF, Katona TR, Chen J, et al. (2008) Three-dimensional mechanical environment of orthodontic tooth movement and root resorption. *American Journal of Orthodontics and Dentofacial Orthopedics* 133: 791. e11–26.

Viecilli RF, Katona TR, Chen J, et al. (2009) Orthodontic mechanotransduction and the role of the P2X7 receptor. *American Journal of Orthodontics and Dentofacial Orthopedics* 135: 694.e1–16.

Walker MP, Ries D, Kula K, et al. (2007) Mechanical properties and surface characterization of beta titanium and stainless steel orthodontic wire following topical fluoride treatment. *Angle Orthodontist* 77: 342–8

Wang T, Zhou G, Tan X, Dong Y (2007) Evaluation of force degradation characteristics of orthodontic latex elastics in vitro and in vivo. *The Angle Orthodontist* 77(4): 688–93.

Wang QY, Zheng YF (2008) The electrochemical behavior and surface analysis of $Ti_{50}Ni_{47.2}Co_{2.8}$ alloy for orthodontic use. *Dental Materials* 24: 1207–11.

Zufall SW, Kusy RP (2000a) Sliding mechanics of coated composite wires and the development of an engineering model for binding. *Angle Orthodontist* 70: 34–47.

Zufall SW, Kusy RP (2000b) Stress relaxation and recovery behaviour of composite orthodontic archwires in bending. *European Journal of Orthodontics* 22: 1–12.

20

Tissue Engineering in Orthodontics Therapy

Nina Kaukua, Kaj Fried, Jeremy J Mao

Summary

The impact of tissue engineering on orthodontics is clearly visible in experimental studies, but it only represents the beginning of a process. Recent advances in the regeneration of anatomically correct teeth and periodontal ligament/bone are among examples of biological regeneration in the field of orthodontics. Regenerative therapies are already being utilized in the clinic, including enamel matrix extracts and platelet-derived growth factors for periodontal regeneration. Clinical orthodontics provides ample opportunities for tissue engineering including segmental tooth movement, cleft lip and palate, orofacial deformities, temporomandibular joint regeneration, and congenital craniofacial anomalies. Regeneration of multiple dental, oral and craniofacial tissues by bioscaffolds, bioactive factors, tissue engineering and/or stem cells offers unprecedented challenges and opportunities for orthodontics.

Introduction

Orthodontics and dentofacial orthopedics is 'the branch of dentistry that specializes in the diagnosis, prevention and treatment of dental and facial irregularities. The practice of orthodontics requires professional skills in the design, application and control of corrective appliances to bring teeth, lips and jaws into proper alignment and to achieve facial balance.' (American Association of Orthodontists, www.aaomembers.org). Contemporary orthodontics is widely considered to have originated in the early years of the twentieth century, when Edward Hartley Angle began to practice fixed appliance treatment, by dragging and/or pushing malaligned teeth into esthetic positions with metallic bands and brackets cemented to the teeth. Over the past century, orthodontics, or the field later named as orthodontics and dentofacial orthopedics (ODO), has witnessed few fundamental innovations, although many diagnostic and therapeutic refinements have been instituted (Mao et al., 2010).

Tissue engineering is defined as 'the application of the principles and methods of engineering and life sciences toward the fundamental understanding of structure/function relationships in normal and pathological mammalian tissues and the development of biological substitutes to restore, maintain, or improve functions.' This definition was crafted by a joint task force organized by the National Institutes of Health and the National Science Foundation in 1988. Thus, tissue engineering is a much younger field in comparison with orthodontics, but has nonetheless witnessed robust growth in the fields of tissue healing and organ defects that are currently deemed incurable by contemporary medicine.

Orthodontics and tissue engineering are two separate fields of studies, and yet with multitude of unrealized common threads. Both ODO and tissue engineering strive to improve tissue functions. Tissue engineering has evolved drastically from its inception, and today's tissue engineering is very different from that in the early days of late 1980s and early 1990s. ODO is considered to be at a pivotal point of transformation, with one of the key contributing factors being tissue engineering (Mao et al., 2010). This chapter attempts to identify potential interactions between ODO and tissue engineering, including situations in which ODO may generate translational and clinical motivations for tissue engineering.

Integrated Clinical Orthodontics, First Edition. Edited by Vinod Krishnan, Ze'ev Davidovitch.
© 2012 Blackwell Publishing Ltd. Published 2012 by Blackwell Publishing Ltd.

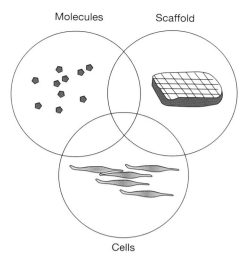

Molecules   Scaffold

Cells

Figure 20.1 The tissue engineering principle. The key components are cells, signaling molecules, and biomaterials.

Tissue engineering principles

Many challenges remain for tissue engineering of dental, oral and craniofacial structures. Considerations such as high demand for esthetics, appropriate vascularization, the complex environment, the need for accommodating multiple tissue phenotypes, and the need to be taken into account when dental, oral and craniofacial tissues are candidates for tissue engineering, are major determinants. A number of approaches have been explored to determine and accommodate the needs for regenerating craniofacial tissues. For tissue engineering to be successful, one must understand the structure and function of the tissue to be regenerated, and then apply this knowledge in the design of tissue engineering strategies. The basic tenets of tissue engineering have been to incorporate cells and scaffold and signaling molecules into *in vitro* analogs of tissues that are to functionally replace diseased or lost tissues (Figure 20.1) (Langer and Vacanti, 1993; Rahaman and Mao, 2005; Scheller et al., 2009).

Stem cells basics

In postnatal life, stem cells are generally those rare cells with potential to differentiate into multiple cell types. Usually, stem cells are quiescent in the body and serve as reserve cells. Under physiological conditions, stem cells periodically replenish themselves in a process known as cycling or self-renewal, to maintain a renewable stem cell pool (Watt and Hogan, 2000; Verfaillie, 2002). Self-renewal is fundamental for biological tissues, not only to replace dead or aged cells, but also to repair pathological defects or trauma (National Institutes of Health, 2009). With the great deal of interest in regeneration of dental, oral, and craniofacial tissues, one should not overlook the role of

stem cells in maintaining tissue homeostasis. Tissue turnover is exemplified most obviously by epithelial cells of the skin, and by bone cells. Skin and bone, as well as many other tissues, undergo physiologically necessary turnover throughout life.

Stem cells are unspecialized cells, and have the potential to become one or more specialized cell types. For example, mesenchymal stem cells are capable of differentiating into cells such as osteoblasts, fibroblasts, chondrocytes, and myocytes (Figure 20.2) and can give rise to bone, cartilage, bone marrow stroma, interstitial fibrous tissue, skeletal muscle, tendons, ligaments, as well as adipose tissue (Jiang et al., 2002; Mezey et al., 2003; Alhadlaq et al., 2005; Sonoyama et al., 2005; Marion and Mao, 2006; Stosich and Mao, 2007; Lee et al., 2010a). Upon injury or in diseases, adult stem cells are activated to repair tissue and organ defects. Whereas the ability to maintain homeostasis is physiological, wound healing and tissue regeneration represent interventional therapies of stem cells that are being pursued in virtually all tissues and organs (Watt and Hogan, 2000; NIH, 2009). Mesenchymal cells continue to reside in various tissues and are the sources of adult mesenchymal stem cells (MSCs).

Bone marrow is the source of at least two stem cell populations: MSCs and hematopoietic stem cells (HSCs). Isolation of MSCs from bone marrow was first described by Friedenstein and collaborators (1974). MSCs isolated by adherence to culture plates are heterogeneous. Only a fraction of cells among typical MSC preparations are stem cells (Lee et al., 2010b). Several studies have explored the potential of MSCs in the regeneration of craniofacial tissues, such as alveolar bone, periodontium, and even ectomesenchymal-based tooth structures (Kawaguchi et al., 2004; Maria et al., 2007; JY Kim et al., 2010; K Kim et al., 2010). HSCs are co-inhabitants of bone marrow with the MSCs and the MSCs and osteoblasts serve as stromal cells for HSCs. HSCs give rise to and replenish all blood cell lineages. The osteoclasts, the bone-resorbing cells during bone turnover and orthodontic tooth movement, derive from this hematopoietic lineage (Kyba, 2005).

Cranial neural crest cells are essential for the development of craniofacial structures. The head is formed through an interaction between mesodermal and cranial neural crest cells. The neural crest arises from the ectoderm-derived neural tube during prenatal development at approximately day 20 in the human embryo (Bhattacherjee et al., 2007). These cells migrate to the presumptive face, and possess the ability to self-renew and differentiate into multiple cell types for the genesis of teeth, bone, and cartilage. How neural crest cells differentiate into craniofacial tissues is only partially understood. The cranial neural crest cells migrate into the pharyngeal arches, disperse throughout this region, and give rise to the ectomesenchyme, which will interact with its surroundings to form the diverse tissues mentioned above as well as other tissues such as the

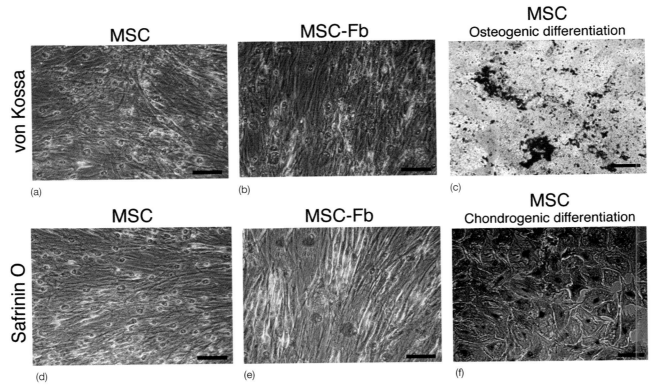

Figure 20.2 Mesenchymal stem cells (MSC) (a,b). (c) MSCs subjected to osteogenic stimulation readily differentiate into osteogenic cells that elaborated minerals. (d–f) Safranin O staining is negative in connective tissue growth factor (CTGF)-treated MSCs (e), just as in MSCs without CTGF treatment (d). (f) In contrast, MSCs subjected to chondrogenic stimulation readily differentiated into Safranin O positive chondrogenic cells. MSC-fb, MSC differentiated into fibroblasts. Scale bars: 100 μm (Lee et al., 2010). (Courtesy of the American Society for Clinical Investigation.)

neurons and glia of cranial ganglia (Chai et al., 2000; Graham and Smith, 2001; Le Douarin et al., 2008). Craniofacial bones are further developed by intramembranous ossification or deposition of bone matrix by osteoblasts. Tooth morphogenesis occurs via a series of complex signaling interactions between the oral epithelium (dental lamina) and the underlying ectomesenchyme (Olsen et al., 2000; Tucker and Sharpe, 2004). In comparison, the bones of the rest of the body form by mesoderm-derived mesenchymal cells, through endochondral ossification where there is a chondrogenic template, before bone matrix is laid down (Vaglia and Hall, 1999; Olsen et al., 2000; Noden and Trainor, 2005).

Neural crest cells differentiate into ectomesenchymal progenitor cells in the cap stage of the dental follicle. The dental follicle surrounds the dental papilla and dental epithelium, and gives rise to cementum, periodontal ligament, and alveolar bone. Specifically, interactions between Hertwig's epithelial root sheath and dental follicle lead to the differentiation of cementoblasts, osteoblasts, and fibroblasts. Important regulators of alveolar bone development include Runx2, Dlx 5/6, and Msx1 (Saito et al., 2009; Fleischmannova et al., 2010).

On completion of tooth morphogenesis, stem cells have been identified in several dental and periodontal structures including the dental pulp of both deciduous and permanent teeth, the papillae, periodontal ligament, dental follicles, and dental-derived epithelial stem cells (Gronthos et al., 2000; Miura et al., 2003; Seo et al., 2004; Honda et al., 2007; Sonoyama et al., 2008; Yao et al., 2008). It should come as no surprise when stem cells are discovered in any biological tissues, given the fundamental roles of stem cells to maintain tissue homeostasis and participate in tissue repair following trauma or pathological insults.

Dental pulp stem cells are among the most studied dental stem cells. When transplanted into mice ectopically *in vivo*, dental pulp stem cells form a dentin–pulp complex (Huang et al., 2009). Besides osteogenic/dentinogenic differentiation, clones of dental pulp stem cells differentiate into myogenic cells, and on *in vivo* infusion, participate in the healing of muscle defects (Yang et al., 2010). Whether stem cells from deciduous dental pulp are more potent as a putative therapeutic cell source than stem cells from permanent dental pulp is not known. Deciduous dental pulp stem cells express some of the pluripotent markers, such as Oct4, Nanog, and SSEA 3/4, and several neuronal markers, probably due to their neural crest origin (Kerkis et al., 2006). Periodontal ligament stem cells express STRO-1 and CD146, and when transplanted in immunocompromised mice, give rise to cementum- and periodontal ligament-like structures (Huang et al., 2009).

Biomaterials

Biomaterials are frequently, but not always, needed for tissue engineering and tissue regeneration. For example, stem cells are infused for the repair of cardiac infarcts and can be delivered into cardiac muscle defects typically without biomaterials as scaffolds. In contrast, a scaffold is frequently required for the regeneration of most dental, oral and craniofacial structures, because they are three-dimensional structures of functional and esthetic importance. A variety of scaffolds have been developed as extracellular matrix analogs, capable of supporting cells. At least, biomaterial scaffolds should be biocompatible, non-toxic, and promote tissue regeneration (Box 20.1). Biodegradable materials are frequently desirable, given their predesigned purpose to undergo controlled degradation, while tissue genesis takes place (Scheller et al., 2009).

Biomaterials can be of native origin, synthetic, or hybrids. The natural polymers, such as collagen, have the advantage of biocompatibility, whereas synthetic polymers allow precise control of the physicochemical properties such as mechanical properties, degradation rate, porosity, and microstructures (Sharma and Elisseeff, 2004). Some of the

popular synthetic biomaterials include co-polymers of polylactic-glycolic acid collagen, poly-phosphazenes, poly-urethanes, polycaprolactone, polyethylene glycol (PEG), poly (propylene fumarate), starch-based materials, alginate, silk, bioactive glasses and glass ceramics, calcium-phosphate ceramics, calcium-phosphate and collagen blends and synthetic polymer/apatite composites (Scheller et al., 2009).

Poly (D,L-lactide-co-glycolide) (PLGA) is a synthetic material, that can be fabricated into various kinds of structures, to better mimic the extracellular matrix environment (Figure 20.3). They are widely used as scaffolding materials for several biomedical applications in humans as part of tissue engineering (Athanasiou et al., 1996; Agrawal and Ray, 2001; Fu et al., 2008). Human MSCs (hMSCs)

Box 20.1 Design requirements of biomaterials

- Biocompatible
- Promote attachment and proliferation of cells and production of extra-cellular matrix
- Ability to integrate signaling factors to direct and enhance tissue growth
- Support vascular integration for oxygen and biomolecule transport
- Mechanical integrity to support load at the implant site
- Controlled rate of degradation into nontoxic products that are easily metabolized or excreted
- Easy and cost-effective processing into three-dimensional shapes of sufficient size to fill clinically relevant defects

---

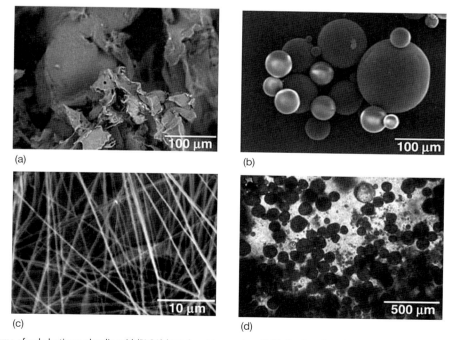

(a) (b)

(c) (d)

Figure 20.3 Various forms of poly-lactic-co-glycolic acid (PLGA) based matrices and scaffolds for dental, oral, and craniofacial tissue engineering (Moioli et al., 2007). (a) Porous PLGA sponge fabricated using salt-leaching techniques. (b) PLGA microspheres encapsulating growth factors showing smooth spherical surface and wide range of diameters. (c) PLGA nanofibers fabricated using electrospining techniques. (d) PLGA microspheres in chitosan-based gels for advanced controlled delivery and cell interaction. (a–c) Scanning electron microscopy (SEM). (d) Phase contrast image. (Courtesy of Elsevier.)

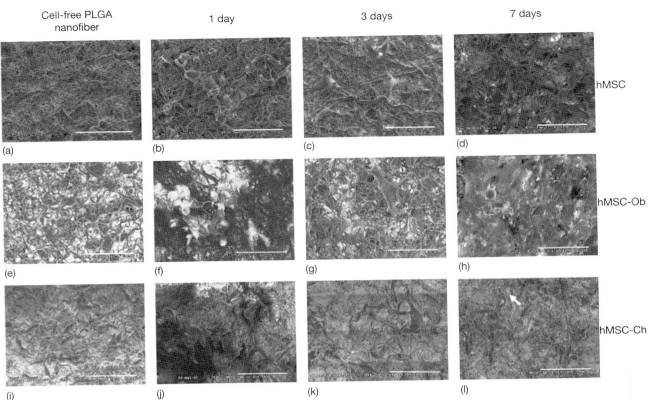

Figure 20.4 Electrospun PLGA nanofibers and the seeding of human mesenchymal stem cells (hMSCs), as well as hMSC-derived osteoblasts and hMSC-derived chondrocytes (Xin et al., 2007). (a,e,i) Prior to cell seeding, three randomly selected PLGA nanofiber scaffolds showed similar characteristics. On seeding of hMSCs (b–d), various extracellular matrices were apparently synthesized among PLGA nanofibers over time. By 7 days following hMSC seeding, the seeded cells apparently have attached to nanofiber surface and penetrated into the pores of PLGA nanofiber scaffolds (d), in comparison with 1 and 3 days after cell seeding (b and c, respectively). The morphology of hMSC-derived osteoblasts seeded in PLGA nanofibers also varied between 1 and 3 and 7 days following cell seeding (f, g, and h, respectively). By 7 days following cell seeding, hMSC-Ob apparently synthesized a substantial amount of extracellular matrices (h), in comparison with 1 and 3 days after cell seeding (f and g, respectively). Human MSC-derived osteoblasts apparently attached to nanofiber substrates. Human MSC-derived chondrocytes revealed characteristic features after seeding in PLGA nanofibers (j–l). Most PLGA nanofibers were still visible at 7 days following the seeding of hMSC-Ch (l), in comparison with the characteristics of hMSC-Ob seeded in PLGA nanofiber scaffolds after 7 days (h). A number of seeded hMSC-Ch apparently were located in lacunae-like structures, see arrow (l) (scale bar = 100 mm) (Xin et al., 2007). (Courtesy of Elsevier.)

proliferate and maintain differentiation characteristics towards osteoblasts and chondrocytes when seeded in PLGA nanofibers (Xin et al., 2007) (Figure 20.4). Another widely used nanofiber is poly (ε-caprolactone) (PCL), which has been used for the differentiation of hMSCs into adipogenic, osteogenic, and chondrogenic cells (Li et al., 2005).

Tissue engineering of tooth and periodontal tissues have frequently used multiple polymer biomaterials, which includes collagen, polyglycolic acid (PGA), peptides, gelatin-chondroitin-hyaluronan tri-copolymer, silk and polycaprolactone (Scheller et al., 2009; K Kim et al., 2010; JY Kim et al., 2010).

Signaling molecules

Cells that are delivered for tissue regeneration frequently need guidance signals to perform desired functional roles. Signaling molecules control multiple and complex cellular

processes, including cell migration, growth, differentiation, and matrix synthesis. One of the key issues in the delivery of signaling molecules is their premature diffusion; they get denatured after *in vivo* injection and thereby fail to induce the intended effects at the site of delivery. Furthermore, premature diffusion of delivered signaling molecules may cause side effects in other unintended tissues and organs (Moioli et al., 2007). Controlled release is an effective approach that prolongs the bioactivity of signaling molecules by encapsulation of signaling molecules in polymer material shells. Only upon gradual degradation of the polymer material shell is the encapsulated signaling cue released in a small amount at a time.

Impact of tissue engineering on orthodontics

Reconstruction of oral and craniofacial defects frequently involves multiple and complex issues, and has a high

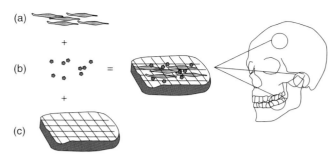

Figure 20.5 Traditional application of tissue engineering. Appropriate cells such as stem cells (a), bioactive molecules (b), and a compatible scaffold (c) are mixed together for the correct tissue formation of the craniofacial area such as teeth, periodontium, temporomandibular joints, and calvarial bone.

demand for the sake of improving both function and esthetics. Current approaches for facial reconstruction suffer from several intrinsic deficiencies. For example, autologous tissue grafts necessitate donor site morbidity; prostheses may not fully integrate with host tissues; allogeneic and other grafts are associated with immune incompatibility and potential pathogen transmission. Clinicians and scientists have aspired to restore facial defects with the patient's own cells, in approaches that minimize current deficiencies, such as donor site morbidity, immuno-rejection, pathogen transmission, and suboptimal repair. A number of recent studies have demonstrated the proof of principle of using stem cells in the reconstruction of dental, oral, and craniofacial defects (Mao et al., 2006). Tissue engineering is constituted by multiple disciplines that utilize biomaterials, mechanical stresses, bioactive factors, and/or stem cells for tissue regeneration (Figure 20.5).

Large-scale tissue engineering research in the craniofacial region or elsewhere began to take place in the early 1990s. Thus far, substantial advances have been made in tissue engineering due to advances from several seemingly unrelated disciplines, such as cell and molecular biology, polymer chemistry, molecular genetics, materials science, robotics and mechanical engineering, converged into the self-assembling field of tissue engineering (Nerem, 1991; Langer and Vacanti, 1993; Mao et al., 2006).

Cell delivery has been the predominant approach in orofacial regeneration. Disassociated cells of porcine or rat tooth buds in biomaterials yielded putative dentin and enamel organ (Young et al., 2002; Duailibi et al., 2004). Tooth bud cells and bone marrow osteoprogenitor cells in collagen, PLGA or silk-protein scaffolds induced putative tooth-like tissues, alveolar bone and periodontal ligament (Young et al., 2005; SE Duailibi et al., 2008; Kuo et al., 2008). Embryonic oral epithelium and adult mesenchyme, together up-regulate odontogenesis genes on mutual induction, and yielded dental structures on transplantation into adult renal capsules or jaw bone (Ohazama et al., 2004). Similarly,

implantation of E14.5 rat molar rudiments into adult mouse maxilla has been shown to produce tooth-like structures with surrounding bone (Modino and Sharpe, 2005; Mantesso and Sharpe, 2009). Multipotent cells of the tooth apical papilla in tricalcium phosphate in swine incisor extraction sockets were shown to generate soft and mineralized tissues resembling the periodontal ligament (Sonoyama et al., 2006). E14.5 oral epithelium and dental mesenchyme were reconstituted in collagen gels and cultured *ex vivo* (Nakao et al., 2007), and when implanted into the maxillary molar extraction sockets in 5-week-old mice, tooth morphogenesis took place and was followed by eruption into occlusion (Ikeda et al., 2009). Several studies have begun to tackle an obligatory task of scale-up towards human tooth size (Xu et al., 2008; Abukawa et al., 2009).

Cell transplantation, including its role in the regeneration of dental, oral and craniofacial tissues, is a valid and meritorious scientific concept and approach. However, there are hurdles in the translation of cell-delivery-based tooth regeneration into therapeutics. Autologous embryonic tooth germ cells are inaccessible for human applications (Modino and Sharpe, 2005; Nakao et al., 2007; Ikeda et al., 2009). Xenogenic embryonic tooth germ cells (from nonhuman species) may elicit immuno-rejection and tooth dysmorphogenesis. Autologous postnatal tooth germ cells (e.g. third molars) or autologous dental pulp stem cells are of limited availability. Regardless of cell source, cell delivery for tooth regeneration, similar to cell-based therapies for other tissues, encounters translational barriers (Maeda et al., 2008). Excessive cost of commercialization and difficulties in regulatory approval have precluded, to date, any significant clinical translation of tooth regeneration.

Recently, an anatomically correct tooth was regenerated with a periodontal ligament, and integrated into native alveolar bone orthotopically *in vivo* in a rat model (K Kim et al., 2010). As an initial attempt to regenerate teeth, we first fabricated an anatomically shaped and dimensioned scaffold from biomaterials, using our previously reported approach (Lee et al., 2009; Stosich et al., 2009). Scaffolds with the shape of the human mandibular first molar (Figure 20.6a) were fabricated. The composite consisted of PCL and hydroxyapatite (HA) with interconnecting microchannels (Figure 20.6b) (K Kim et al., 2010).

K Kim et al. (2010) infused a blended cocktail of SDF1 and BMP7 into the scaffold's microchannels. SDF1 was selected for its effects to bind to CXCR4 receptors of multiple cell lineages, including mesenchymal stem/progenitor cells (Belema-Bedada et al., 2008; Kitaori et al., 2009). BMP7 was selected for its effects on dental pulp cells, fibroblasts, and osteoblasts, in elaborating mineralization (Rutherford, 2001; Vaccaro et al., 2008). A rat mandibular incisor was regenerated with periodontal ligament and newly formed alveolar bone. The rat mandibular central incisor was extracted, followed by implantation of the

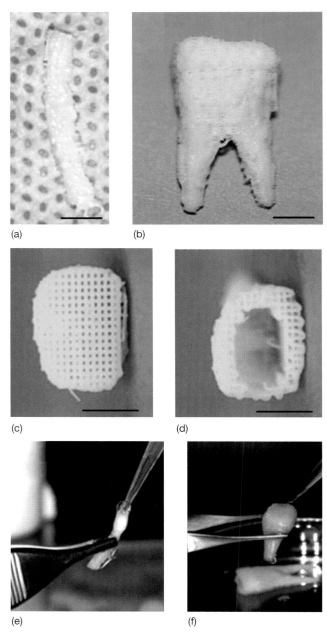

(a)   (b)

(c)   (d)

(e)   (f)

Figure 20.6 Design and fabrication of anatomically shaped human and rat tooth scaffolds by three-dimensional bioprinting. Anatomical shape of the rat mandibular central incisor (a) and human mandibular first molar (b) were used for three-dimensional reconstruction and bioprinting of a hybrid scaffold of poly-ε-caprolactone and hydroxyapatite, with 200 μm microstrands and interconnecting microchannels (diam., 200 μm), which serve as conduits for cell homing and angiogenesis (c,d). A blended cocktail of stromal-derived factor-1 (100 ng/mL) and bone morphogenetic protein-7 (100 ng/mL) was delivered in 2 mg/mL neutralized type I collagen solution and infused in scaffold microchannels for rat incisor scaffold (e) and human molar scaffold (f), followed by gelation (K Kim et al., 2010). (Courtesy of Sage Publications.)

anatomically shaped mandibular incisor scaffold (data not shown but available in K Kim et al., 2010) into the extraction socket. Combined SDF1 and BMP7 delivery homed significantly more cells and elaborated more blood vessels into the microchannels of the human molar scaffolds than without growth-factor delivery ($p < 0.05$). Scaffolds in the shape of the rat mandibular incisor integrated with surrounding tissue, clearly showed multiple tissue phenotypes including the native alveolar bone, newly formed bone, and a fibrous tissue interface reminiscent of the periodontal ligament (Figure 20.7) that integrated with the host alveolar bone.

These findings, which are described in detail in K Kim et al. (2010), represent the first report of regeneration of anatomically shaped tooth-like structures *in vivo*, and by cell homing, without cell delivery. The potency of cell homing is substantiated not only by cell recruitment into scaffold's microchannels, but also regeneration of a putative periodontal ligament and newly formed alveolar bone (K Kim et al., 2010). The observed putative periodontal ligament and newly formed alveolar bone suggest that SDF1 and/or BMP7 have the ability to recruit multiple cell lineages. Here, SDF1 likely has homed mesenchymal and endothelial stem/progenitor cells in native alveolar bone into porous tooth scaffolds in rat jaw bone, and connective tissue progenitor cells in dorsal subcutaneous tissue into human molar scaffold (Alhadlaq and Mao, 2004; Steinhardt et al., 2008; Crisan et al., 2009). Enamel is not formed due to the fact that ameloblasts, which normally form the enamel matrix or their progenitors, do not exist in the adult tissue. It is the one true challenge yet left to explore. BMP7 plays important roles in osteoblast differentiation (Itoh et al., 2001). Here, BMP7 likely is responsible for newly formed, mineralized alveolar bone in the rat extraction socket, and ectopic mineralization in a human tooth scaffold implanted in the dorsum. Cell homing is an underrecognized approach in tissue regeneration (Mao, 2009), and offers an alternative to cell-delivery-based tooth regeneration. Omission of cell isolation and *ex vivo* cell manipulation may accelerate regulatory, commercialization, and clinical processes. The costs related to tooth regeneration by cell homing are not anticipated to be nearly as excessive as for cell delivery. One of the pivotal issues in tooth regeneration is to devise economically viable approaches that are not cost-prohibitive, and can translate into therapies for patients who cannot afford expensive treatments, or are contraindicated for dental implants. Cell-homing-based tooth regeneration may provide a tangible pathway toward clinical translation (Mao, 2009).

Protein-based therapies are being developed or are now available for the regeneration of multiple dental, oral, and craniofacial tissues, including the periodontal bone. Enamel matrix derivatives (EMDs) are a mix of amelogenins and metallo-endoproteases and serine proteases. EMDs have been shown to improve the healing of human periodontal

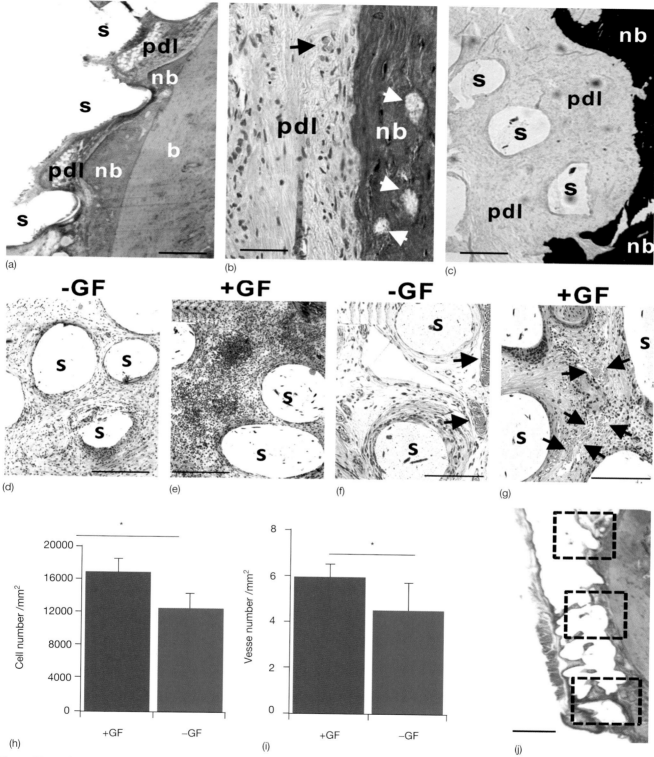

Figure 20.7 Orthotopic tooth regeneration. (a) The rat mandibular incisor scaffold integrated with surrounding tissue, showing tissue ingrowth into scaffold microchannels and multiple tissue phenotypes, including the native alveolar bone (b), newly formed bone (nb), and a fibrous tissue interface reminiscent of the periodontal ligament (pdl). The newly formed bone (nb) showed ingrowth into microchannel openings and inter-staggered with scaffold microstrands (s). (b) Newly formed bone (nb) has bone trabeculae-like structures (arrows) and embedded osteocyte-like cells, immediately adjacent to a putative periodontal ligament (pdl) consisting of fibroblast-like cells and collagen buddle-like structures. (c) Newly formed bone (nb) is well-mineralized (von Kossa preparation), in contrast to the adjacent unmineralized, putative periodontal ligament (pdl). (d) Cells populated the scaffold's microchannels even without growth-factor delivery. Remarkably, SDF1 and BMP7 delivery yielded substantial cell homing in microchannels (e). (f) Combined SDF1 and BMP7 delivery homed significantly more cells into microchannels than without growth-factor delivery ($p < 0.01$; $n = 11$). Angiogenesis took place in scaffolds' microchannels without growth-factor delivery (g), but was more substantial with growth-factor delivery (h). (i) Combined SDF1 and BMP7 delivery elaborated significantly more blood vessels than without growth-factor delivery ($p < 0.05$; $n = 11$). (j) The numbers of recruited cells and blood vessels were quantified from three different locations along the entire root length of the rat mandibular incisor scaffold: the superior region of alveolar ridge and the inferior region of root apex, with a midpoint in between. s, scaffold; GF, growth factor(s). Scale: 100 μm (K Kim et al., 2010). (Courtesy of Sage Publications.)

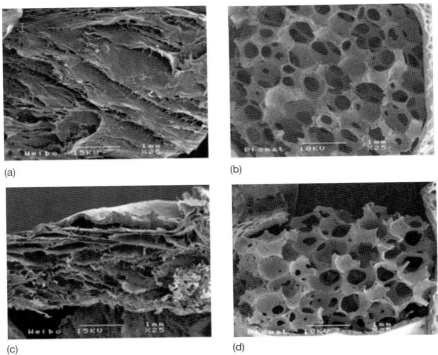

Figure 20.8 Scanning electron micrographs of different scaffolds (magnification ×25) (a) Collagen scaffold surface structure; (b) collagen scaffold cross-section; (c) HA/TCP ceramic surface structure; (d) HA/TCP ceramic cross-section (Zhang et al., 2006). (Courtesy of Elsevier.)

infrabony defects (Tonetti et al., 2002; Esposito et al., 2009). The first clinical trial on Emdogain's role in periodontal regeneration was carried out in 1997. Additional studies have further shown the clinical efficacy of Emdogain in the regeneration of periodontium structures. Emdogain is primarily used in repairing infrabony defects, frequently with a grafting material (Palmer and Cortellini, 2008; Lyngstadaas et al., 2009). Platelet-derived growth factor (PDGF) promotes alveolar bone repair in periodontal defects as a chemoattractant and proliferative factor for mesenchymal cells (Hollinger et al., 2008). PDGF promotes osteogenesis and angiogenesis at the site of periodontal bone repair (Hollinger et al., 2008). GEM21s is a commercial product that contains PDGF-BB for the treatment of periodontal infrabony and furcation defects (Pellegrini et al., 2009).

Bone morphogenetic proteins (BMPs) induce ectopic bone formation, especially BMP-2 and BMP-7 (Krebsbach et al., 2000; Nakashima and Reddi, 2003). When fibroblasts were transduced to release greater amounts of BMP-2 and BMP-7, a significant increase was noted in the amount of bone in critical-sized calvarial defects (Krebsbach et al., 2000; Shin et al., 2010), and both additionally also promote cementogenesis (Moioli et al., 2007). There is also a commercially available INFUSE bone graft, which consist of BMP-2 and a collagen sponge for the following conditions: tibial fractures, spinal fusions, sinus augmentation, and alveolar ridge defects due to tooth extractions (Bessa et al., 2008).

Basic fibroblast growth factor (bFGF or FGF-2) promotes the formation of bone, cementum, and the periodontal ligament (Nakahara et al., 2003; Sato et al., 2004). FGF-2 delivered topically with gelatinous carriers in furcation defects in dogs induces increase in new bone formation rate, trabecular bone formation, as well as cementum (Murakami et al., 2003). Multiple scaffolds have been exploited to enhance periodontal regeneration, including cell occlusive barrier membranes, collagen membranes, bioglasses, β-tricalcium phosphates (Figure 20.8), PLGA, and enamel matrix derivatives, with varying successful results (Moioli et al., 2007).

Orthodontics and dentofacial orthopedics as clinical motivation for tissue engineering

A newly regenerated periodontal ligament will surely have impact on orthodontics. Experimental approaches are also being explored towards the regeneration of cementum, dentin, dental pulp, and even the entire tooth (Mao et al., 2006; Mao, 2008). What would be the impact of these regenerated tooth structures or entire teeth, on orthodontic treatment as we know it today? If it takes 1.5–2.5 years for orthodontic treatment, would there be motivation for the placement of dental implants in esthetically pleasing positions, or one day to have whole teeth regenerated in esthetically pleasing positions? Would bioengineered cementum and/or dentin be a solution for root resorption? Even the decision of tooth extraction versus non-extraction may be impacted by recent interest from the general public to have dental stem cells from their extracted teeth 'banked' or cryopreserved (Mao, 2008). Would a patient more likely be receptive to tooth extraction, since extracted teeth are sources of their stem cells? For cleft lip or cleft palate, and craniofacial or temporomandibular anomalies, what is the impact of bioengineered bone and soft tissue grafting, which shows promise of becoming standard practice in surgical approaches related to orthodontics (Alhadlaq and Mao, 2003; Moioli et al., 2008; Stosich et al., 2009). Separate approaches are being explored for tissue engineering of skin and soft tissues such as adipose and muscle fibers (Egles et al., 2010; Mao et al., 2010; Stosich et al., 2007; Yang et al., 2010).

Bone grafts are typically autografts, allografts, xenografts, and alloplastics. Autografts are bone grafting materials taken from the same individual, whereas allografts are taken from a different individual of the same species. Xenografts are taken from a different species, whereas alloplastics are synthetically made bone grafting materials. Osteo-conductive grafts indicate that they only have the capacity to guide new bone growth. Osteo-inductive grafts, on the other hand, promote differentiation of progenitor cells to form bone. Teeth have been shown to move into areas where bone has been augmented with β-tricalcium-phosphate, hydroxyapatite, bovine bone graft material, PGLA/gelatin sponges with BMP-2, and bioglass (Eichhorn et al., 2009; Reichert et al., 2009). Allografts in combination with different materials, such as bioglass or enamel matrix derivatives, have also been shown to be successful in augmenting alveolar defects before moving teeth into that area. Hydroxyapatite alone as a filling material is another successful approach. Furthermore, in one case report, teeth were moved into bone grafts formed from a synthetic alloplast with a bioglass (Yilmaz et al., 2000), as well as into bovine bone grafts (Reichert et al., 2009). A collagen bovine bone mineral (bio-Oss) has also been used for augmenting periodontal defects with a subsequent successful orthodontic tooth movement (Cardaropoli et al., 2006). Barrier membranes have been used to block ingrowth of gingival epithelium into the periodontal ligament. After control of periodontitis, the area around the cemento-enamel junction is treated with e-PTFE membrane (expanded polytetrafluoroethylene), a synthetic polymer better known by its brand name Gore-Tex, followed by orthodontic tooth movement (Reichert et al., 2009). There are at least two case reports of successful orthodontic tooth movement into tissue-engineered bone in alveolar cleft defects, treated with a synthetic alloplast or HA. Here, tissue engineering principles have successfully shown that they are applicable in the craniofacial area with the potential for normal function and have the capability to work synergistically in conjunction with orthodontic treatment.

Conclusions

Orthodontics and tissue engineering, by their independent definitions, are two separate disciplines of learning but nonetheless have a great deal in common. Tissue engineering represents an opportunity that orthodontics should capture, incorporate, and individualize. Tissues of interest to orthodontics are those that are being regenerated by stem cells, scaffolds, and bioactive cues in experimental studies. Currently, several bioactive cues have been developed into products for periodontal regeneration, and novel technologies that regenerate bone modules, periodontal ligament, cementum, cartilage and soft tissue, will inevitably have impact on orthodontics in the near future.

Acknowledgments

We thank our colleagues whose work we cited and those whose work could be not cited due to space limitations, for their scientific work that has inspired our thinking process. We are grateful to the remaining members of the Tissue Engineering and Regenerative Medicine Laboratory for their dedication and hard work. We thank Ms Qiongfen Guo and Ms Kening Hua for administrative and technical assistance. This work is funded by NIH/NIDCR grant DE018248 to JJM.

References

Abukawa H, Zhang W, Young CS, et al. (2009) Reconstructing mandibular defects using autologous tissue engineered tooth and bone constructs. *Journal of Oral and Maxillofacial Surgery* 67: 335–47.

Agrawal CM, Ray RB (2001) Biodegradable polymeric scaffolds for musculoskeletal tissue engineering. *Journal of Biomedical Materials Research* 55: 141–50.

Alhadlaq A, Mao JJ (2003) Tissue-engineered neogenesis of human-shaped mandibular condyle from rat mesenchymal stem cells. *Journal of Dental Research* 82: 951–6.

Alhadlaq A, Mao JJ (2004) Mesenchymal stem cells: isolation and therapeutics. *Stem Cells and Development* 13: 436–48.

Alhadlaq A, Tang M, Mao JJ (2005) Engineered adipose tissue from human mesenchymal stem cells maintains predefined shape and dimension: implications in soft tissue augmentation and reconstruction. *Tissue Engineering* 11: 556–66.

Athanasiou KA, Niederauer GG, Agrawal CM (1996) Sterilization, toxicity, biocompatibility and clinical applications of polylactic acid/polyglycolic acid copolymers. *Biomaterials* 17: 93–102.

Belema-Bedada F, Uchida S, Martire A, et al. (2008) Efficient homing of multipotent adult mesenchymal stem cells depends on FROUNT-mediated clustering of CCR2. *Cell Stem Cell* 2: 566–75.

Bessa PC, Casal M, Reis RL (2008) Bone morphogenetic proteins in tissue engineering: the road from laboratory to clinic, part II (BMP delivery). *Journal of Tissue Engineering and Regenerative Medicine* 2: 81–96.

Bhattacherjee V, Mukhopadhyay P, Singh S, et al. (2007) Neural crest and mesoderm lineage-dependent gene expression in orofacial development. *Differentiation* 75: 463–77.

Cardaropoli D, Re S, Manuzzi W, et al. (2006) Bio-Oss collagen and orthodontic movement for the treatment of infrabony defects in the esthetic zone. *International journal of periodontics and restorative dentistry* 26: 553–9.

Chai Y, Jiang X, Ito Y et al. (2000) Fate of the mammalian cranial neural crest during tooth and mandibular morphogenesis. *Development* 127: 1671–9.

Crisan M, Chen CW, Corselli M, et al. (2009) Perivascular multipotent progenitor cells in human organs. *Annals of the New York Academy of Sciences* 1176: 118–23.

Duailibi MT, Duailibi SE, Young CS, et al. (2004) Bioengineered teeth from cultured rat tooth bud cells. *Journal of Dental Research* 83: 523–8.

Duailibi SE, Duailibi MT, Zhang W, et al. (2008) Bioengineered dental tissues grown in the rat jaw. *Journal of Dental Research* 87: 745–50.

Egles C, Garlick JA, Shamis Y (2010) Three-dimensional human tissue models of wounded skin. *Methods in Molecular Biology* 585: 345–59.

Eichhorn W, Blessmann M, Pohlenz P, et al. (2009) Primary osteoplasty using calvarian bone in patients with cleft lip, alveolus and palate. *Journal of Cranio-Maxillofacial Surgery* 37: 429–33.

Esposito M, Grusovin MG, Papanikolaou N, et al. (2009) Enamel matrix derivative (Emdogain(R)) for periodontal tissue regeneration in intrabony defects. *Cochrane Database of Systematic Reviews* 4: CD003875.

Fleischmannova J, Matalova E, Sharpe PT, et al. (2010) Formation of the tooth-bone interface. *Journal of Dental Research* 89: 108–15.

Friedenstein AJ, Deriglasova UF, Kulagina NN, et al. (1974) Precursors for fibroblasts in different populations of hematopoietic cells as detected by the in vitro colony assay method. *Experimental Hematology* 2: 83–92.

Fu YC, Nie H, Ho M, et al. (2008) Optimized bone regeneration based on sustained release from three-dimensional fibrous PLGA/HAp composite scaffolds loaded with BMP-2. *Biotechnology and Bioengineering* 99: 996–1006.

Graham A, Smith A (2001) Patterning the pharyngeal arches. *Bioessays* 23: 54–61.

Gronthos S, Mankani M, Brahim J, et al. (2000) Postnatal human dental pulp stem cells (DPSCs) in vitro and in vivo. *Proceedings of the National Academy of Sciences of the United States of America* 97: 13625–30.

Hollinger JO, Hart CE, Hirsch SN, et al. (2008) Recombinant human platelet-derived growth factor: biology and clinical applications. *Journal of Bone and Joint Surgery American* 90: 48–54.

Honda MJ, Shinohara Y, Hata KI, et al. (2007) Subcultured odontogenic epithelial cells in combination with dental mesenchymal cells produce enamel-dentin-like complex structures. *Cell Transplantation* 16: 833–47.

Huang GT, Gronthos S, Shi S (2009) Mesenchymal stem cells derived from dental tissues vs. those from other sources: their biology and role in regenerative medicine. *Journal of Dental Research* 88: 792–806.

Ikeda E, Morita R, Nakao K, et al. (2009) Fully functional bioengineered tooth replacement as an organ replacement therapy. *Proceedings of the National Academy of Sciences of the United States of America* 106: 13475–80.

Itoh F, Asao H, Sugamura K, et al. (2001) Promoting bone morphogenetic protein signaling through negative regulation of inhibitory Smads. *EMBO Journal* 20: 4132–42.

Jiang Y, Jahagirdar BN, Reinhardt RL, et al. (2002) Pluripotency of mesenchymal stem cells derived from adult marrow. *Nature* 418: 41–9.

Kawaguchi H, Hirachi A, Hasegawa N, et al. (2004) Enhancement of periodontal tissue regeneration by transplantation of bone marrow mesenchymal stem cells. *Journal of Periodontology* 75: 1281–7.

Kerkis I, Kerkis A, Dozortsev D, et al. (2006) Isolation and characterization of a population of immature dental pulp stem cells expressing OCT-4 and other embryonic stem cell markers. *Cells Tissues Organs* 184: 105–16.

Kim JY, Xin X, Moioli EK, et al. (2010) Regeneration of dental-pulp-like tissue by chemotaxis-induced cell homing. *Tissue Engineering Part A* 16: 3023–31.

Kim K, Lee CH, Kim BK, et al. (2010) Anatomically shaped tooth and periodontal regeneration by cell homing. *Journal of Dental Research* 89: 842–7.

Kitaori T, Ito H, Schwarz EM, et al. (2009) Stromal cell-derived factor 1/CXCR4 signaling is critical for the recruitment of mesenchymal stem cells to the fracture site during skeletal repair in a mouse model. *Arthritis and Rheumatism* 60: 813–23.

Krebsbach PH, Gu K, Franceschi RT, et al. (2000) Gene therapy-directed osteogenesis: BMP-7-transduced human fibroblasts form bone in vivo. *Human Gene Therapy* 11: 1201–10.

Kuo TF, Huang AT, Chang HH, et al. (2008) Regeneration of dentin-pulp complex with cementum and periodontal ligament formation using dental bud cells in gelatin-chondroitin-hyaluronan tri-copolymer scaffold in swine. *Journal of Biomedical Materials Research Part A* 86: 1062–8.

Kyba M (2005) Genesis of hematopoietic stem cells in vitro and in vivo: new insights into developmental maturation. *International Journal of Hematology* 81: 275–80.

Langer R, Vacanti JP (1993) Tissue engineering. *Science* 260: 920–6.

Le Douarin NM, Calloni GW, Dupin E (2008) The stem cells of the neural crest. *Cell Cycle* 7: 1013–19.

Lee CH, Marion NW, Hollister S, et al. (2009) Tissue formation and vascularization of anatomically shaped human tibial condyle in vivo. *Tissue Engineering Part A* 15: 3923–30.

Lee CH, Cook JL, Mendelson A, et al. (2010a) Regeneration of the articular surface of the rabbit synovial joint by cell homing: a proof of concept study. *Lancet* 376: 440–8.

Lee CH, Shah B, Moioli K, et al. (2010b) CTGF directs fibroblast differentiation from human mesenchymal stem/stromal cells and defines connective tissue healing in a rodent injury model. *Journal of Clinical Investigation* 120: 3340–9.

Li WJ, Tuli R, Huang X, et al. (2005) Multilineage differentiation of human mesenchymal stem cells in a three-dimensional nanofibrous scaffold. *Biomaterials* 26: 5158–66.

Lyngstadaas SP, Wohlfahrt JC, Brookes SJ, et al. (2009) Enamel matrix proteins; old molecules for new applications. *Orthodontics and Craniofacial Research* 12: 243–53.

Maeda S, Ono Y, Nakamura K, et al. (2008) Molar uprighting with extrusion for implant site bone regeneration and improvement of the periodontal environment. *International Journal of Periodontics and Restorative Dentistry* 28: 375–81.

Mantesso A, Sharpe P (2009) Dental stem cells for tooth regeneration and repair. *Expert Opinion on Biological Therapy* 9: 1143–54.

Mao JJ (2008) Stem cells and the future of dental care. *New York State Dental Journal* 74: 20–4.

Mao JJ (2009) Stem cells and dentistry. *Journal of Dental Hygiene* 83: 173–4.

Mao JJ, Giannobile WV, Helms JA, et al. (2006) Craniofacial tissue engineering by stem cells. *Journal of Dental Research* 85: 966–79.

Mao JJ, Stosich MS, Moioli EK, et al. (2010) Facial reconstruction by biosurgery: cell transplantation versus cell homing. *Tissue Engineering Part B: Reviews* 16: 257–62.

Maria OM, Khosravi R, Mezey E, et al. (2007) Cells from bone marrow that evolve into oral tissues and their clinical applications. *Oral Diseases* 13: 11–16.

Marion NW, Mao JJ (2006) Mesenchymal stem cells and tissue engineering. *Methods in Enzymology* 420: 339–61.

Mezey E, Key S, Vogelsang G, et al. (2003) Transplanted bone marrow generates new neurons in human brains. *Proceedings of the National Academy of Sciences of the United States of America* 100: 1364–9.

Miura M, Gronthos S, Zhao M, et al. (2003) SHED: stem cells from human exfoliated deciduous teeth. *Proceedings of the National Academy of Sciences of the United States of America* 100: 5807–12.

Modino SA, Sharpe PT (2005) Tissue engineering of teeth using adult stem cells. *Archives of Oral Biology* 50: 255–8.

Moioli EK, Clark PA, Xin X, et al. (2007) Matrices and scaffolds for drug delivery in dental, oral and craniofacial tissue engineering. *Advanced Drug Delivery Reviews* 59: 308–24.

Moioli EK, Clark PA, Sumner DR, et al. (2008) Autologous stem cell regeneration in craniosynostosis. *Bone* 42: 332–40.

Murakami S, Takayama S, Kitamura M, et al. (2003) Recombinant human basic fibroblast growth factor (bFGF) stimulates periodontal regeneration in class II furcation defects created in beagle dogs. *Journal of Periodontal Research* 38: 97–103.

Nakao K, Morita R, Saji Y, et al. (2007) The development of a bioengineered organ germ method. *Nature Methods* 4: 227–30.

Nakahara T, Nakamura T, Kobayashi E, et al. (2003) Novel approach to regeneration of periodontal tissues based on in situ tissue engineering: effects of controlled release of basic fibroblast growth factor from a sandwich membrane. *Tissue Engineering* 9: 153–62.

Nakashima M, Reddi AH (2003) The application of bone morphogenetic proteins to dental tissue engineering. *Nature Biotechnology* 21: 1025–32.

National Institutes of Health (2009) *Stem Cell Basics*. Available at: http://stemcells.nih.gov/info/basics/basics4 (accessed 13 July 2011).

Nerem RM (1991) Cellular engineering. *Annals of Biomedical Engineering* 19: 529–45.

Noden DM, Trainor PA (2005) Relations and interactions between cranial mesoderm and neural crest populations. *Journal of Anatomy* 207: 575–601.

Ohazama A, Modino SA, Miletich I, et al. (2004) Stem-cell-based tissue engineering of murine teeth. *Journal of Dental Research* 83: 518–22.

Olsen BR, Reginato AM, Wang W (2000). Bone development. *Annual Review of Cell and Developmental Biology* 16: 191–220.

Palmer RM, Cortellini P (2008) Periodontal tissue engineering and regeneration: Consensus Report of the Sixth European Workshop on Periodontology. *Journal of Clinical Periodontology* 35: 83–6.

Pellegrini G, Seol YJ, Gruber R, et al. (2009) Pre-clinical models for oral and periodontal reconstructive therapies. *Journal of Dental Research* 88: 1065–76.

Rahaman MN, Mao JJ (2005) Stem cell-based composite tissue constructs for regenerative medicine. *Biotechnology and Bioengineering* 91: 261–84.

Reichert C, Deschner J, Kasaj A, et al. (2009) Guided tissue regeneration and orthodontics. A review of the literature. *Journal of Orofacial Orthopedics* 70: 6–19.

Rutherford B (2001) BMP-7 gene transfer to inflamed feret dental pulps. *European Journal of Oral Sciences* 109: 422–4.

Saito M, Nishida E, Sasaki T, et al. (2009) The KK-Periome database for transcripts of periodontal ligament development. *Journal of Experimental Zoology Part B, Molecular and Developmental Evolution* 31: 495–502.

Sato Y, Kikuchi M, Ohata N, et al. (2004) Enhanced cementum formation in experimentally induced cementum defects of the root surface with the application of recombinant basic fibroblast growth factor in collagen gel in vivo. *Journal of Clinical Periodontology* 75: 243–8.

Scheller EL, Krebsbach PH, Kohn DH (2009) Tissue engineering: state of the art in oral rehabilitation. *Journal of Oral Rehabilitation* 36: 368–89.

Seo BM, Miura M, Gronthos S, et al. (2004) Investigation of multipotent postnatal stem cells from human periodontal ligament. *Lancet* 364: 149–55.

Sharma B, Elisseeff JH (2004) Engineering structurally organized cartilage and bone tissues. *Annals of Biomedical Engineering* 32: 148–59.

Shin JH, Kim KH, Kim SH, et al. (2010) Ex vivo bone morphogenetic protein-2 gene delivery using gingival fibroblasts promotes bone regeneration in rats. *Journal of Clinical Periodontology* 37: 305–11.

Sonoyama W, Coppe C, Gronthos S, et al. (2005) Skeletal stem cells in regenerative medicine. *Current Topics in Developmental Biology* 67: 305–23.

Sonoyama W, Liu Y, Fang D, et al. (2006) Mesenchymal stem cell-mediated functional tooth regeneration in swine. *PLoS One* 1: e79.

Sonoyama W, Liu Y, Yamaza T, et al. (2008) Characterization of the apical papilla and its residing stem cells from human immature permanent teeth: a pilot study. *Journal of Endodontics* 34: 166–71.

Steinhardt Y, Aslan H, Regev E, et al. (2008) Maxillofacial-derived stem cells regenerate critical mandibular bone defect. *Tissue Engineering Part A* 14: 1763–73.

Stosich MS, Mao JJ (2007) Adipose tissue engineering from human adult stem cells: clinical implications in plastic and reconstructive surgery. *Plastic and Reconstructive Surgery* 119: 71–83.

Stosich MS, Moioli EK, Wu JK, et al. (2009) Bioengineering strategies to generate vascularized soft tissue grafts with sustained shape. *Methods* 47: 116–21.

Tonetti MS, Lang NP, Cortellini P, et al. (2002) Enamel matrix proteins in the regenerative therapy of deep intrabony defects. *Journal of Clinical Periodontology* 29: 317–25.

Tucker A, Sharpe P (2004) The cutting-edge of mammalian development; how the embryo makes teeth. *Nature Reviews Genetics* 5: 499–508.

Vaccaro AR, Lawrence JP, Patel T, et al. (2008) The safety and efficacy of OP-1 (rhBMP-7) as a replacement for iliac crest autograft in posterolateral lumbar arthrodesis: a long-term (>4 years) pivotal study. *Spine* 33: 2850–62.

Vaglia JL, Hall BK (1999) Regulation of neural crest cell populations: occurrence, distribution and underlying mechanisms. *International Journal of Developmental Biology* 43: 95–110.

Verfaillie CM (2002) Adult stem cells: assessing the case for pluripotency. *Trends in Cell Biology* 12: 502–8.

Watt FM, Hogan BL (2000) Out of Eden: stem cells and their niches. *Science* 287: 1427–30.

Xin X, Hussain M, Mao JJ (2007) Continuing differentiation of human mesenchymal stem cells and induced chondrogenic and osteogenic lineages in electrospun PLGA nanofiber scaffold. *Biomaterials* 28: 316–25.

Xu WP, Zhang W, Asrican R, et al. (2008) Accurately shaped tooth bud cell-derived mineralized tissue formation on silk scaffolds. *Tissue Engineering Part A* 14: 549–57.

Yang R, Chen M, Lee CH, et al. (2010) Clones of ectopic stem cells in the regeneration of muscle defects in vivo. *PLoS One* 5: e13547.

Yao S, Pan F, Prpic V, et al. (2008) Differentiation of stem cells in the dental follicle. *Journal of Dental Research* 87: 767–71.

Yilmaz S, Kiliç AR, Keles A, et al. (2000) Reconstruction of an alveolar cleft for orthodontic tooth movement. *American Journal of Orthodontics and Dentofacial Orthopedics* 117: 156–63.

Young CS, Terada S, Vacanti JP, et al. (2002) Tissue engineering of complex tooth structures on biodegradable polymer scaffolds. *Journal of Dental Research* 81: 695–700.

Young CS, Abukawa H, Asrican R, et al. (2005) Tissue-engineered hybrid tooth and bone. *Tissue Engineering* 11: 1599–610.

Zhang W, Walboomers XF, van Kuppevelt TH, et al. (2006) The performance of human dental pulp stem cells on different three-dimensional scaffold materials. *Biomaterials* 27: 5658–68.

21

Corticotomy and Stem Cell Therapy for Orthodontists and Periodontists: Rationale, Hypotheses, and Protocol

Neal C Murphy, Nabil F Bissada, Ze'ev Davidovitch, Simone Kucska

Summary

This chapter is about Professor EO Wilson's *Consilience: the Unity of Knowledge* – it synthesizes periodontics and orthodontics, academics and practice, making the ideal practical. The dental specialties, divided by culture, are inseparable in science and justified by art, like the relationship between architects and structural engineers. The interface between these two disciplines focuses on two aspects: what can orthodontics do for periodontology and what can periodontics do for orthodontics? This chapter first reviews salient points of joint management that may have eluded prior papers on the subject and go into some more depth. So orthodontists can use periodontal knowledge and periodontists can answer the needs of the orthodontist. Safe methods of recognizing and avoiding attachment loss are described along with the use of asymmetric eruption when using forced eruption or molar uprighting. The concept of bone morphing is introduced and a rationale is presented that explains gingival recession as a bacterial infection, not tooth movement complication. Finally, a method of quantizing infection, probing efficiently, and assigning infection control management tips is briefly and succinctly presented.

Expanding on this theme, the second part introduces a variation on surgical orthopedics of the alveolus, a previously ignored dental 'organ'. Then it goes further to describe the theories, rationale, and protocol for stem cell therapy. This pioneering work is an attempt to enlarge the dental arch foundation more quickly, painlessly, and with less tissue morbidity than alternative methods. Finally, the chapter discusses novel ways of thinking that reduce the risk of foundering on the intimidating shoals of new ideas, ideas which seek to eliminate the need for extraction methods.

Then the chapter describes the basic science of stem cell therapy, viz. the introduction of living stem cells in graft form and then moving teeth into the graft with conventional biomechanical protocols. The simplicity of the procedure is explained in step-by-step terms as a synthesis or orchestration of conventional themes in a new and variable score. This takes both specialties into existing biology and new frontiers promised by the twenty-first century. The professional bridge is thus novel and effective, but fortified with logic and taught with helpful themes and analogies. All the while, these data stand firmly on the stable firmament of both traditional and emerging biological science and timeless themes of art.

Introduction

The effects of orthodontic tooth (root) movement on the alveolar bone (at the gross anatomical level) have been well documented in the periodontal literature since the 1970s (Brown, 1973; Ingber, 1974, 1976) and summarized by Mihram in 1997. Recent investigations were conducted in numerous venues, both clinical (Ducker, 1975; Merrill and Pedersen, 1976; Generson et al., 1978; Mostaza et al., 1985; Anholm et al., 1986; Yoshikawa, 1987; Matsuda, 1989; Liou and Huang, 1998; Owen, 2001; Wilcko et al., 2001; Fulk, 2002; Hajji, 2002; Kacewicz et al., 2004; Iseri et al., 2005; Ahlawat et al., 2006; Dosanjh et al., 2006) and experimental (Bell and Levy, 1972; Nakanishi, 1982; Gantes et al., 1990; Kawakami et al., 1996; Twaddle, 2001; Machado et al., 2002; Navarov et al., 2004; Ferguson et al., 2006; Kelson et al., 2005; Oliveira et al., 2006; Sebaoun et al., 2006). Specifically, later papers documented the efficacy of selective alveolar decortication (SAD) to accelerate orthodontic tooth movement, and bone grafts to add volume. An influential clinical description of this successful surgical manipulation was published by Kole in 1959. Interestingly, after the original description by Cunningham in 1894, iterations appeared in the scientific literature (Cohn-Stock, 1921; Bichlmayr, 1931; Ascher, 1947; Neuman, 1955) mostly in German.

The aim of this chapter is to demonstrate how this evolution has opened a frontier to tissue engineering and epigenetic manipulation of the alveolar phenotype. However, first a background summary will build context under the rubric of orthodontic 'OldThink' so the unfolding story of twenty-first-century orthodontic theory can evolve with relevance.

Integrated Clinical Orthodontics, First Edition. Edited by Vinod Krishnan, Ze'ev Davidovitch.
© 2012 Blackwell Publishing Ltd. Published 2012 by Blackwell Publishing Ltd.

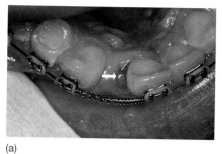
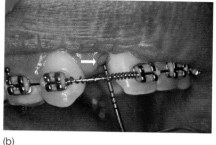
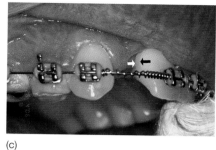

(a) (b) (c)

Figure 21.1 Patient VM. (a,b) The red patch (white arrows) noted by British orthodontist JD Atherton (1970). The orthodontist or the assistant usually sees the lesion from perspective (b). (c) Closer inspection reveals a point of vulnerability, or 'disease-health nexus', between the white and black arrows. The white arrow marks the coronal extent of a receded periodontal attachment apparatus and the black arrow marks the position it should normally assume in health. (Source:www.UniversityExperts.com. Used with permission.)

Twentieth-century 'OldThink'

Bone and attachment level in health and disease

The periodontium consists of the gingival unit and apical to that, the periodontal attachment apparatus. The gingival unit generally moves with the tooth and contains, when not bleeding on probing, a sulcus of 1–3 mm in health. If everted (prolapsed) by orthodontic force, a sulcus appears as the proverbial 'red patch of Atherton' (Figure 21.1). The so-called 'red patch' is an eversion (prolapse) of the gingival sulcus, exposing the thin, nonkeratinized epithelium and subjacent connective tissue of the periodontal ligament. This is a potential source of periodontal attachment loss. If the bacterial biofilm around the recession is benign, the everted red patch will mature into marginal gingiva because the marginal gingiva derives from the periodontal ligament and will move with a tooth upon eruption or therapeutic extrusion in health. As Figure 21.1 suggests, recession during tooth movement is caused proximately by the negligence of a patient (despite being well informed) and not necessarily by tooth movement per se. Aleo et al. (1974) showed that destructive endotoxins in dental plaque can inhibit fibroplasia in cell culture. This kind of recession is permanent in the orthodontic patient in the presence of virulent endotoxins and represents the *in vivo* analog of Aleo et al.'s observation.

From an orthodontist's usual incisal and labial views, the everted (prolapsed) sulcus distal to the mesially moving lateral incisor appears curiously benign. But a good clinical scientist *cum* orthodontist looks beyond the obvious as illustrated in Figure 21.1c. While the clinical recession anteriorly is usually obvious, recession around posterior teeth is not and leads to infected periodontal pockets and permanent bone loss. A vigilant orthodontist will be proactive in looking for such lesions where rapid tooth movement is anticipated and will monitor the patient for any future attachment loss at this vulnerable point. Red patches in posterior sextants are less obvious and thus more pernicious.

These unapparent iatrogenic pockets conceivably would be obscured by hypertrophy and hyperplasia and mark the beginning of progressive periodontitis in the patient's second or third decade of life. Postoperative periodontal charting and necessary periodontal therapy should therefore routinely follow fixed bracket removal. Moreover, the patient should be followed for 1–2 years to ensure orthodontic and periodontal stability. This subtle but notable phenomenon should be actively looked for in orthodontic cases where sliding or retraction mechanics are aggressively employed and where rapid palatal expansion separates the maxillary incisors rapidly. Recession and progressive disease may be precluded with early diagnosis by the vigilant clinician.

This attachment loss is viewed as 'bone loss' in radiographs when about 40% of the alveolar crest bone is decalcified. After decalcification by infection, the organic matrix is lost, usually permanently. The latter event is conveniently called 'bone loss' or more correctly, 'attachment loss'. Sometimes a long junctional epithelial attachment is observed when bone loss has occurred but tissue tonus is firm enough, like a tight collar, to hold onto the root tightly.

Sometimes clinicians are fooled into believing that regeneration has occurred and pockets have disappeared due to gain in regeneration. But actually firm tissue tone and a long junctional epithelium (JE) is only *an illusion of regeneration*. A long junctional epithelium is faulty because it breaks down suddenly during orthodontic fixed appliance therapy, often to the chagrin of the hapless orthodontist, who believes it may be caused by inferior supportive care or, more naïvely, the orthodontic tooth movement per se. Such 'unzipping' can reveal a true pocket that had preexisted but was treated with 'deep cleaning', a nonscientific term for subgingival root planing. Orthodontists should not be fooled into thinking that they are periodontally safe enough to ignore interactive supportive care from professional team members (including the patient). Tooth movement can indeed exacerbate progressive active attachment loss that is uncontrolled.

A shallow sulcus after 'cleaning' can be misleading because diagnostic probing of the 'bottom' of the sulcus is never achieved with the recommended diagnostic probing force of 20–25 g. (As a practical guide the Hu-Friedy Michigan-O probe weighs about 17 ± 3 g, so excessive force to negotiate a pocket is rarely necessary.) The 'long JE attachment' is thought by some periodontists to be less resistant to bacterial breakdown because the root–epithelial interface, a mucopolysaccharide, and hemidesmosomal attachment, is a less formidable defense to bacterial toxins. Other clinicians view it as an acceptable, albeit compromised, anatomical entity which should be maintained as esthetic compromises for surgery around anterior teeth. In health, the crest of the alveolar bone is usually about 1.3–2 mm apical to the bottom of the sulcus; this is called 'biologic width', an inviolable anatomical landmark. If the biologic width is encroached upon by an orthodontic band, the level of the bone will re-establish the width as the gingivae recede in response to the new bone level and that can form a nidus for future periodontal pocket formation. Therefore all orthodontic bands should be festooned. The bone crest will follow the movement of the teeth and its gingival unit when the periodontium is healthy.

In disease, however, the tooth moves independent of the crestal bone. Because of this relationship, orthodontic therapy can inadvertently extrude a tooth out of an infected socket and accelerate attachment loss if periodontal infection is not treated (Sanders, 1999). This is why periodontal health is essential during orthodontic therapy and also explains why recession is often evident when inflammation is resolved after debonding. The hypertrophy of tissue edema during therapy often hides the attachment loss and latent recession. This is why the orthodontist's index of suspicion should always make the entire staff vigilant to occult attachment loss and supportive of collaborative therapy by a periodontist or referring dental professional.

Morphing bone with orthodontic tooth movement

The orthodontist usually sees fixed appliances simply as ortho-*dontic* apparati for moving tooth crowns for cosmetic advantage. But, increasingly, they are seen as ortho-*pedic* devices for restructuring the malleable alveolus bone to more physiological form. This second use is employed for so-called 'crown lengthening', i.e. the exposure of more anatomical crown and/or root to facilitate restorative care. This therapy makes use of the independent movement of roots out of the bone. Crown lengthening is achieved in a healthy periodontal attachment apparatus if transseptal, gingival, and superficial crestal periodontal fibers are periodically severed during tooth extrusion. However, this can be a complicated protocol and deserves some concentrated study.

Note that when a molar is uprighted to evert a mesial periodontal pocket, an iatrogenic distal pocket can be created if the molar is not extruded symmetrically and the coronal surface reduced in the process (Figure 21.2). When Ingber (1974) first published the idea of 'forced eruption' in 1974, little was known about how to manage the mesial and distal bone level when a pocket appeared on one interproximal side and the other was healthy. That is, how can one unilaterally (e.g. distally) extrude a root orthodontically while maintaining periodontal attachment on the opposite proximal surface. This was explained in subsequent articles and illustrated by Mihram and Murphy (2008). This relationship of the crestal alveolar bone to the root is a critical concept to understand, because it allows correct intuitive judgments by the orthodontist about periodontal health when challenged by a full day of patient demands and biomechanical problems.

Psychosocial compliance issues unique to orthodontic offices, especially in an adolescent-based practice, are often more daunting in this regard than the pastoral environment

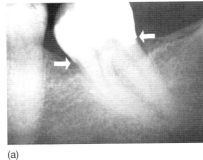
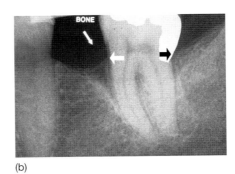

(a)   (b)

Figure 21.2 Note how the attachment level (white arrows) on the mandibular second molar stays at the cementoenamel junction in health (a) but transforms to a gingival (pseudo) pocket of pathological depth on the distal aspect when the mesial pocket (white arrow, (a)) is eliminated by orthodontic uprighting (white arrows, (b)). (Courtesy of Elsevier. Source: Dr William L. Mihram, Santa Ana, CA USA in *Seminars in Orthodontics*, December, 2008. Used with permission.)

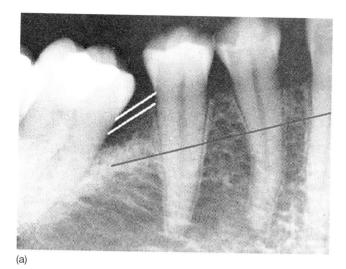

(a)

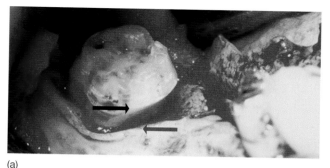

(a)

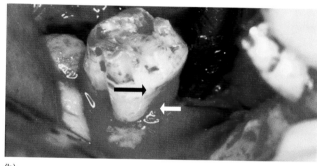

(b)

Figure 21.4 (a,b) This image is the clinical correlate of the radiographs in Figures 21.3 and 21.5. Note how the mesial aspect (black arrow (b)) of the molar is now clinically available for preparation, instead of hidden by bone (black arrow (a)). Caries on the mesial surface is often subgingival, even apical to the alveolar crest (blue arrow in (a)) which makes restoration impossible without facilitative (prerestorative) orthodontic therapy. The surgical flap was replaced at the white arrow in b. (Courtesy of Elsevier. Source: Dr William L. Mihram, Santa Ana, CA USA in *Seminars in Orthodontics*, December, 2008. Used with permission.)

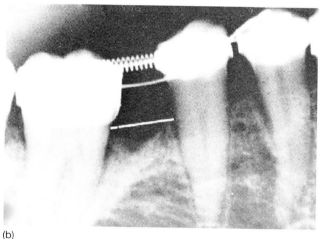

(b)

Figure 21.3 No treatment better exemplifies the need for so-called 'integrated clinical orthodontics' than molar uprighting. If orthodontic therapy is not employed in a conservative treatment plan, then unnecessarily excessive amounts of bone must be removed during periodontal osseous surgery. Bone coronal to the red line in (a) represents the amount of bone that is removed by standard osseous resection when no orthodontic treatment is used to upright the molar. The coronal and apical white lines in (a) and (b) represent the cementoenamel junction and alveolar osseous crest. The dramatic alteration of alveolar bone phenotype in this iconic representation shows how simple orthodontic aligning and leveling can eliminate the need for osseous surgery. This forms the conceptual basis for alveolar phenotype modification by selective alveolar decortication, periodontally accelerated osteogenic orthodontics, human mesenchymal stem cell placement or viable cell allograft surgical manipulation of the future.

of a surgeon's office. In the orthodontic clinical environment, maintaining a quick wit, born of serious study, is paramount in cases that have asymmetrical bone loss. With a pocket on one proximal side and healthy sulci on the other, only an 'asymmetrical forced eruption' can produce a symmetrically 'lengthened' crown, and the key to successful molar uprighting. Figures 21.3–21.5 illustrate this phenomenon nicely.

The interdisciplinary synergy between the periodontal and orthodontic specialties has made this low morbidity treatment feasible. The vertical (or angular) bony defect that forms the periodontal pocket on the schematic second premolar must be surgically recontoured (reshaped by removal of healthy bone) if orthodontic forced eruption is not performed. This unnecessary removal of healthy adjacent alveolar bone can be most dramatic. The pathological alveolar crest topography (architecture or shape) is represented by the dotted line in Figure 21.3b. Surgical bone removal must involve four teeth (solid line) to blend the architecture of the alveolar crest into a physiological shape because any abrupt change in the topography of the alveolar crest can cause coronal gingival 'rebound' after surgical apical positioning. When the crestal topography is gently sloping, the gingiva stays at its physiological position next to the bone crest and periodontal pockets do not re-form. The morbidity of extraction of the second premolar or periodontal osseous surgery is much greater than simple orthodontic forced eruption as illustrated in Figure 21.3. Another example of asymmetrical forced

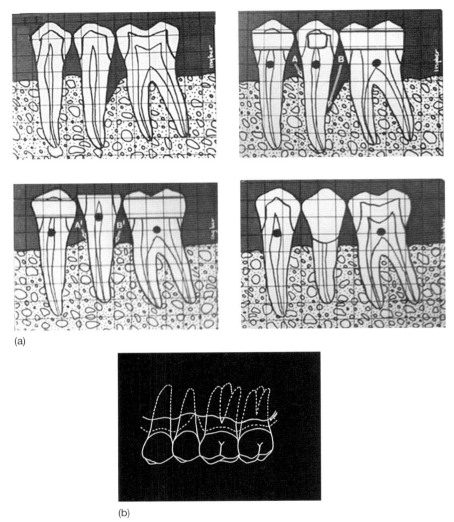

(a)

(b)

Figure 21.5 (a) Illustrations from JS Ingber's definitive articles (1974) demonstrating the relationship between the alveolar crest attached to the root in a one-walled infrabony defect (vertical or angular bone loss) and the effect of facilitative extrusion (upper left panel). In the upper right panel, A indicates normal side and B indicates the side with vertical bone loss. In the lower left panel A¹ indicates the area where there was no bone loss before and B¹ indicates the symmetrical bone level obtained after facilitative extrusion of teeth (combined with fiberotomy or subsequent osseous surgery as needed). Note the occlusal equilibration carried out on the tooth to maintain the occlusal plane. The lower right panel shows the prosthetic crown *in situ*. The interdisciplinary synergy between the periodontal and orthodontic specialties has made this low morbidity treatment feasible. (b) To eliminate the vertical defect (dotted line) the surgery must involve four more teeth (solid line) to blend the architecture. (Courtesy of Elsevier. Source: Dr William L. Mihram, Santa Ana, CA USA in *Seminars in Orthodontics*, December 2008. Used with permission.)

facilitating proper restoration of the tooth, is shown in Figure 21.6.

In summary, where infrabony periodontal defects present, asymmetrical forced eruption, producing symmetrical crown lengthening, can also be seen as the simple use of partial fiberotomies. A partial fiberotomy on opposite proximal surfaces keeps bone at consistent level (Figure 21.6, red arrows). The reader is encouraged to read about further techniques and complications by consulting the original journal article by Mihram and Murphy in *Seminars in Orthodontics*, December 2008, where more orthodontic–periodontic treatments and complications are discussed.

Asymmetrical forced eruption is achieved by periodically severing the attachment on the healthy side of the root, say the distal, while merely scaling and root planing the tooth surface on the side of the infrabony defect, in our example, the mesial in Figure 21.6. Asymmetrical forced eruption therapeutically everts the periodontal pocket on coronal movement of the bone and the creation of an artifactual infrabony defect on the other proximal side, e.g. in Figure 21.6, the mesial and distal aspects, respectively.

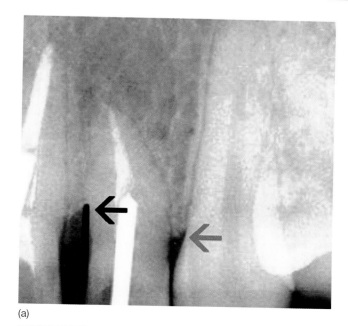

(a)

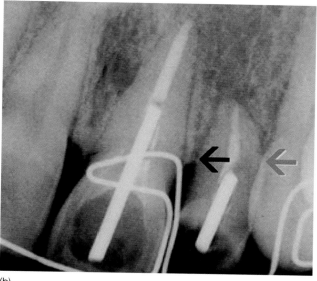

(b)

Figure 21.6 Note how the arrows match in (b) but are asymmetrical in (a) before asymmetrical forced eruption. As the lateral incisor was forcibly erupted with fixed orthodontic appliances, the soft tissue fibers were severed periodically to the crest of the alveolar bone between the canine and the lateral incisor distal surface. This allowed full eruption of the attachment apparatus (black arrow, (a)) fixed to the mesial surface of the lateral incisor while the distal root surface was therapeutically moved 'out of the bone' to provide symmetrical levels of attachment prior to restoration of the lateral incisor. All this complicated treatment could be obviated by the Holy Grail of attachment gain to the cementoenamel junction by stem cell reconstructive surgery *in situ* at the lateral incisor mesial surface. (Courtesy of Elsevier. Source: Dr William L. Mihram, Santa Ana, CA USA in *Seminars in Orthodontics*, December 2008. Used with permission.)

The infected orthodontic patient

The essence of periodontal–orthodontic management comes down to understanding alveolus physiology and managing infection even if that management is as mundane as recommending a modern floss holder designed for orthodontic patients (see www.platypusco.com). But the periodontal–orthodontic interface is often more complicated than that and the modern, erudite orthodontist ignores this scientific realm only to his or her detriment since excellent reviews of salient issues are replete in the literature and have been authoritatively summarized as recently as 2008 by Palomo et al. (2008). What these particular authors implicitly argued was that the human mouth is impossible to sterilize, so in the spirit of 'universal precaution', *all patients* are considered *always infected,* more or less. So the most important issue is this: given the ubiquitous and constant field of infected tissue in which the orthodontist operates, how does one minimize irreversible tissue damage? Since the authors published their survey, a number of pharmacological agents and periodontal 'friendly' accoutrements have become more widely accepted by practicing orthodontists.

The *in situ* pharmacologic agents are particularly noteworthy. When used *prudently* they are legitimate and effective, but short-acting, therapeutic adjuncts to scaling and root planing. Over time they represent an excellent investment, because they are effective in preventing or mitigating severe exacerbations of latent disease. When using any pharmacological anti-infective medium, it is critical to remember that the ultimate goal of any antibacterial therapy is to make a niche for commensal organisms which will 'crowd out' more virulent pathogens. But long-term reliance on pharmaceuticals risks the development of bacterial strains resistant to any pharmaceutical. Because of this limitation, most periodontists prefer that patients use mechanical methods of dental plaque (bacterial biofilm) removal, daily and assiduously.

Benign commensal bacteria are relatively welcomed residents when they limit their reversible damage to the gingival unit. But virulent pathogenic forms and commensal organisms cannot be well distinguished in oral bacterial biofilms. Therefore, it is argued that universal precaution, similar to that used in other infection-prone environments should be employed with all orthodontic patients. The key to success is to keep *bleeding on probing* (BOP) to a minimum. Since the task of infection control rests on undependable patient compliance, every orthodontic patient should be informed of the risks of periodontal damage and explicitly encouraged to participate in 'infection control' by a periodontist, dentist, dental hygienist, and other trained para-professionals during fixed appliance therapy. Even prior to bracket placement an 'oral *infection* control' consultation should be made with an informed and competent professional for scaling and root planing, comprehensive charting, continually supportive oral hygiene instructions and the application of a labial fluoride varnish. (*Note how the word 'infection' is used instead of trivializing euphemisms such as 'a little inflamed' or 'slight swelling'.*)

During all orthodontic treatment with fixed appliances, fluoride therapy should continue every 3–6 months depending on the degree of infection and fluoride varnish should be reapplied every 6 months around the bracket perimeters. Also, there is little need to remove archwires if the treating professional is well trained and experienced. Generally, taking off archwires and replacing them just for oral hygiene prophylaxis or oral hygiene method instruction is inconvenient to patients and interferes with compliance. To modulate infection control, usually a bleeding index (percentage of provoked sulci that bleed on probing) of less than 25% will keep patients safe.

Bone loss, or technically attachment loss, is the hallmark of periodontitis and may not be amenable to regeneration depending on the pattern of destruction, the patient's individual biological capacity for regeneration, preference, and personal compliance. Individual patients may demonstrate sudden bone damage during orthodontic care so periodontal probing should be done every 6 months, but preferably not by a preoccupied orthodontist as illustrated in Figure 21.7.

A common error, which misses the craters, is measuring at the line angle of the tooth and not advancing the probe far enough interproximally, directly apical to the contact point. The periodontal probe is 'walked' on the bottom of the sulcus or pocket and angled approximately 20–30° from the vertical axis (Figure 21.7b) between the teeth. This allows the clinician to follow the attachment around the tooth and reach the depth of the pocket that may be more clinically occult and dangerous to future periodontal health. Probing error is 1 mm, making an interexaminer calibration necessary, periodically. For the busy orthodontist, a screening by probing only interproximal surfaces will take less than 2 minutes, enjoys a high correlation with comprehensive probing techniques, and lends a laudably sober note to any orthodontic regimen.

Gingival enlargement

Orthodontists should take a collaborative approach to treatment planning, to achieve periodontal health and maximum esthetic outcomes, because altered passive eruption, hypertrophy, gingival hyperplasia, and true attachment loss may conspire to complicate treatment in the presence of inflammation and compromise the final esthetic result. Note that even a pseudopocket (gingival pocket) produced by gingival enlargement is a pathological entity that can lead to true attachment loss and periodontal bone loss, long after an adolescent is dismissed from orthodontic therapy. Therefore, the orthodontist should delegate a 'post-debonding inspection' to a responsible colleague or

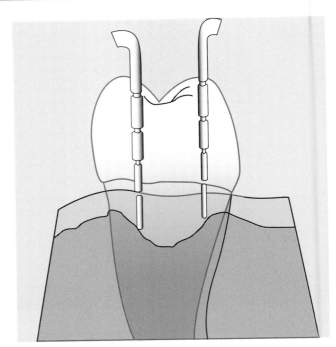

(a)

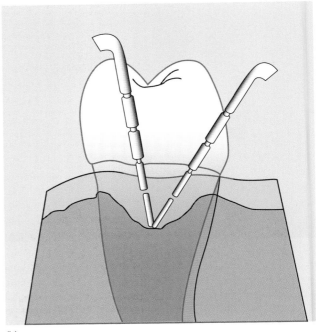

(b)

Figure 21.7 Probing at arbitrary points such as line angles (a) may miss defects such as two-walled infrabony defects, commonly referred to as 'craters' (b). (Courtesy of Elsevier. Source: Palomo L, Palomo JM, Bissada NF [2008] Salient periodontal issues for the modern biologic orthodontist. *Seminars in Orthodontics* 14: 229–45. Used with permission.)

scrutinize the orthodontic patient's periodontal health during the retention period. Although the patient often does not make the connection between gingival pocket formation as a teenager and bone loss in the late 20s–30s, the ethical obligation remains with the referring doctor, the orthodontist and the periodontist to maintain periodontal and gingival health as best as possible during and after fixed appliance therapy.

Increased public awareness and the introduction of clear aligners have helped reduce iatrogenic risk in the child and adolescent in recent years. But at the very least, the orthodontist has both an ethical and legal duty to inform the patient of the risks. Then the proximate cause of any attachment loss is the patient's negligence in not following directions. To this end, the American Board of Orthodontics (ABO) under the visionary leadership of Dr Grubb (2008), recommended a full periodontal charting and radiographic diagnostic series for patients of 18 years or older, in order to pass the board certification examination. In some American regions, managed care companies even compete by also requiring orthodontists to record periodontal and gingival pocket depth before, during, and after orthodontic therapy, in children, adolescents, and adults. Despite the criticism about the incursion of corporate insurance companies into traditional diagnostic and treatment prerogatives of orthodontists, they can hardly be criticized when such forward-thinking policies are established by the managed care stakeholders. But such leadership and visionary standards should rightfully be initiated by orthodontists, not corporations.

In a recent landmark study, Waldrop (2008) assessed the prevalence of gingival enlargement (altered passive eruption, hypertrophy, and hyperplasia), a harbinger of pocket formation in orthodontic patients. The same patients were studied 5 years after treatment, and the need for periodontal plastic surgery and esthetic crown lengthening was documented. Waldrop discovered over 60% of treated patients had inferior smiles due to gingival enlargement.

When the gingival margin fails to secure the cementoenamel junction of all teeth, surgical correction should be employed with a flap procedure. We contend that the case illustrated in Figure 21.8 is not finished according to twenty-first century standards of periodontics or even orthodontics until the gingival problems are addressed. In this case, one cannot distinguish whether the gingival enlargement is due to a transient hypertrophy, permanent hyperplasia, or altered passive eruption (gingiva and alveolar bone crest). Moreover, the gingival pockets created by this enlargement cannot be distinguished from the incipient attachment loss (even with radiographs) that follows it. Even negligent patients, concerned only about superficial cosmetics, can understand that cases such as Figure 21.8 are not finished and will commonly complain about 'showing too much gum'. With sophisticated twenty-first century

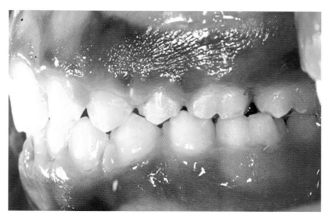

Figure 21.8 An unfinished finished case from an orthodontic as well as a periodontic perspective. Please note that the occlusion is not well settled and there are inconsistent gingival margins along with hypertrophic areas. (Courtesy of Elsevier. Source: Waldrop TC (2008) Gummy smiles: The challenge of gingival excess, prevalence and guidelines for clinical management. *Seminars in Orthodontics* 14: 260–71. Used with permission.)

patients making such observations, it is necessary for the modern orthodontist to treat with a team of supporting professionals during mechanotherapy. That is the essence of multidisciplinary care and 'integrated orthodontics', both administratively and intellectually. The case is 'finished' when the gingival margin approximates the cementoenamel junction (Figure 21.9). Only then is the patient fully informed of all treatment options and collaborative supportive therapy.

Naïve, but well-intentioned, doctors may use a gingivectomy to solve this problem, but even with hand-held lasers, this is unwise because few understand how ablative a gingivectomy really is. Laser therapy relies on ill-conceived notions that only soft tissue is redundant or misplaced. However, one cannot know for sure if the enlargement is a singular hyperplastic phenomenon or combined with altered passive eruption. In the latter case, lasers cauterize, can destroy biological width, and even alveolar crestal bone. Then pockets or recession can manifest years after debonding.

As a matter of fact, gingivectomies have very little role in modern periodontology, especially with infrabony defects, and have not been routinely used by enlightened periodontists for over 50 years. This is because of reconstructive limitations and the ablative nature of the surgery. The wise orthodontist is ill-advised to undertake such surgeries, to 'remove redundant tissue' or 'take off scar tissue', without first consulting a certified periodontist familiar with these biological phenomena, and fully informing patients. Shared knowledge ensures shared risk. Once these salient periodontal–orthodontic issues are realized and well managed, the twenty-first century orthodontist is competent to enter the stage of dentoalveolar tissue

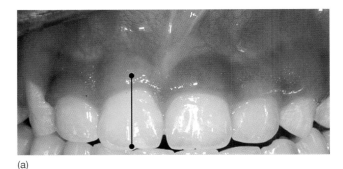

(a)

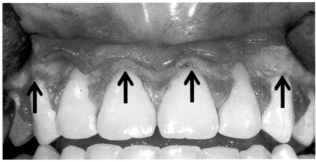

(b)

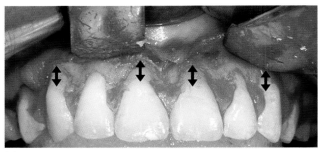

(c)

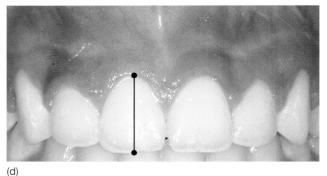

(d)

Figure 21.9 (a–d) The proper method of re-establishing the physiological biological width and reducing gingival enlargement associated with orthodontic fixed appliance therapy. This precise tissue manipulation and management of underlying bone tissue cannot be achieved with a laser. (Courtesy of Elsevier. Source: Waldrop TC (2008) Gummy smiles: The challenge of gingival excess, prevalence and guidelines for clinical management. *Seminars in Orthodontics* 14: 260–71. Used with permission.)

engineering and the burgeoning realm of stem cell and gene therapy.

Orthodontic 'NewThink': the age of the stem cell

In the past decade, professional societies and international academic workshops have witnessed advancements in both genetics and cell biology, which, conjoined, open spectacular vistas for biologists and clinicians alike. The entire human species is producing a kind of 'perfect storm' of intellectual growth with a plethora of historic opportunities, literally the dream of humankind. The new generation of orthodontists is positioned perfectly to become the specialists of facial tissue engineering, carrying on the legacy bequeathed to us by selfless educators and financial patrons. It is within this vision that the proposals for stem cell therapy are posited, the protocols are explained, and a new legacy is dedicated.

Definitions

Stem cells are generally defined as primitive cells that mature into specific-function cells. They are components of the viable cell-allograft, discussed in this chapter, with other types of bone forming cells in a processed bone matrix. The collection of precursor cells in the matrix provides many types of potentials which in fact contribute to a collective 'stem cell' function. While the definitions below are generally accepted, stem cell therapy (SCT) is young and definitions may take on new connotations in the future. So the astute clinician should be intellectually vigilant to the nuances of meaning.

The term 'stem cell', like the words 'love' and 'nice' has, unfortunately been so over-used that it has lost precise universal meaning. In one strict sense, the only 'true' stem cell is the fertilized ovum or one subjected to parthenogenesis. And more informally, a preosteoblast is, in a sense, a 'stem cell' because it can differentiate further into an irreversibly mature osteoblast. So, one must make a distinction between cells that undergo maturation and those which can give rise to more daughter cells as well as differentiated forms. Given this state of syntactical affairs, for the purpose of this reading, the terms of 'stem cell' therapy will be used as follows:

- **Totipotent** is the ability to give rise to *all the cell types* of the body *plus* all of the cell types that make up the *extraembryonic tissues* such as the *placenta*.
- **Pluripotent** is the ability to give rise to *all* of the *various cell types of the body except* extra-embryonic tissues such as placenta components.
- **Multipotent** is the ability to develop into *more than one cell type* of the body.
- **Stem cells** are cells with the ability to divide to produce a fully functional mature cell capable of specific func-

tions in tissue. Generally stem cells have the ability to divide to give rise to both daughter cells and more specialized function cells. In contrast, osteocytes and fibroblasts do not change into more specialized cells naturally. SCT can be local or systemic.

- **Mesenchymal stem cells** (MSCs) are non-blood adult stem cells from a variety of tissues. Although it is not clear that MSCs from different tissues are the same, they are multipotent for mesenchymal tissues derived embryologically from mesoderm. hMSCs are human MSCs.
- **Osteoprogenitor cells** (OPCs) are cells dedicated to producing osteoblasts but with more surface markers that allow them to be distinguished from MSCs.

Background and rationale

SCT rests upon methods of alveolar bone preparation that induce a temporary, reversible, non-pathological osteopenic state. These are collectively referred to with the term 'surgically-facilitated orthodontic therapy' (SFOT). It specifically refers to alveolar surgery that achieves an optimal response to orthodontic therapy, by selective decortication and grafting.

This is a temporary reduction of the organic and mineral content of the alveolus around the moving tooth root. Generally this alveolus manipulation will safely ensure that the tooth moves 200–400% faster than with conventional orthodontic methods, with more stability, and less inflammation. The exact nature of histological, cytological, and intracellular orthopedic effects from SFOT in the alveolus

remained enigmatic until controlled studies of tissue behavior appeared in the 1980s. Further validations of historical anecdotal claims of efficacy were added at the beginning of the twenty-first century and continue to emerge in the osteology literature.

Critical analysis of selective alveolar decortication (SAD) was formally published through the pioneering work of the gifted Professors Wilcko and Ferguson at Case Western Reserve University, St Louis University and Boston University at the turn of the twenty-first century. Then, by the addition of a bone graft to selective alveolar decortication (SAD), periodontally accelerated osteogenic orthodontics (PAOO) extended the scope of orthodontics into the world of clinical tissue engineering (note: where periodontal considerations are not relevant, the truncated term accelerated osteogenic orthodontics (AOO) is often substituted for PAOO. PAOO and AOO are trademarks of Wilckodontics Inc., Erie, Pennsylvania, USA.). PAOO demonstrates that one may re-engineer a stable alveolar bone phenotype to accommodate dental arch expansion with impunity. We translate this legacy into the science of hMSC therapy merging the clinical biomechanics of SFOT with the mechano-biologics of modern osteology and medical orthopedics.

Figure 21.10 demonstrates how progressive improvement in engineered facial growth can have dramatic effects with simple periodontal surgery even when orthognathic surgery is rejected for mandibular retrognathism. Although it is doubtful that the mandibular corpus has been altered, tissue engineering changed the form of the alveolus bone. These surgeries provided not only more stable dental

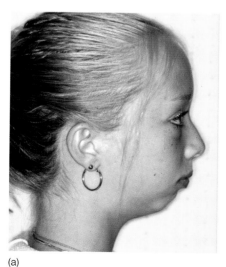 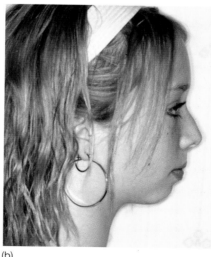 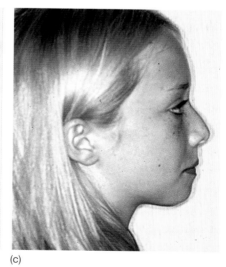

(a) (b) (c)

Figure 21.10 (a–c) Patient MK demonstrates progressive improvement with engineered facial growth. *Orthognathic surgery was rejected* as an alternative for this case of mandibular retrognathism. (Source: Images courtesy of the surgeon, Professor M Thomas Wilcko, Case Western Reserve University, School of Dental Medicine, Cleveland, Ohio, USA. Used with permission.)

alignment but also satisfactory facial form alternation. The patient was treated with two PAOO surgeries sequentially over a total treatment time of 18 months. The surgery did not involve orthognathic surgery, hospitalization, or general anesthesia, but rather outpatient periodontal surgery under intravenous sedation.

PAOO protocols reduce the need for premolar extraction with phenotype alteration but can also alter facial form without orthognathic surgery. This is done by epigenetic manipulation, effectively validating the tenets of the functional matrix hypothesis (FMH) (Moss, 1997a–d). The FMH explains that the root of a tooth acts as a template or 'functional matrix' for neo-morphogenesis of the alveolus bone.

After pioneering research at Loma Linda University, worldwide popularity of the Wilcko–Ferguson–Moss theses in the first decade of the twenty-first century had grown so quickly that the periodontal departments of some American universities, such as Case Western Reserve University in Cleveland, Ohio, and the University of Southern California, in Los Angeles, California, have incorporated PAOO into their standard postdoctoral curricula. This scholastic elevation challenged established therapies with a more cost-effective, healthier, and more benign outpatient science. By extrapolating these data and clinical impressions, what the future holds is not merely faster, better, and safer smile design, but rather nothing less than the intraoral, scarless, designer 'face engineering'.

Epistemological issues: choice and clinical styles

Slowly, as the dogma of alveolar immutability surrenders to modern concepts of phenotype plasticity, the alveolus is emerging as a malleable entity requiring new theories of morphogenesis and mechano-transduction. This paradigm is defined by the dynamics of bone healing and genetic expression to a pre-selected form, depending on root position (Murphy, 2006). This 'NewThink', a novel way of studying what orthodontics may become, evokes doubts in the minds of some who defend categorical mandates for premolar extraction. In contrast, other contemporary clinicians propose that the rationale for routine premolar extraction should be seriously reassessed. In many North American orthodontic practices, the percentage of extraction cases is dropping to less than 10%. Besides providing good science to non-extraction treatment plans, other biological advantages to PAOO and SCT are the reduction of bacterial damage caused by prolonged orthodontic care, and the notorious relapse potential of fixed appliance therapy (Little, 1993; Little et al., 1998; Oliveira et al., 2006).

Since conventional biomechanics does not alter bony phenotype, innovations are slowly replacing old paradigms with a new epistemology. Conventional dental techniques will always have their place, but cannot totally define the specialty due to the severe limitations mentioned above.

SCT prevents or mitigates the severity of side effects and thus earns its place in the pantheon of legitimate care. Even modern periodontal regeneration cannot match these achievements of orthodontic SCT. Periodontal bone grafting merely re-establishes the original phenotype, passively. But, orthodontic tissue engineering and SCT achieve permanent phenotypic change, pro-actively with viable cell dynamics and local immunosuppression. Thus, the challenges of molecular biology are making the study of orthodontic tooth movement at one time more difficult and yet vastly more interesting. Regardless of the perceived difficulties, SCT at least minimizes the unfortunately narrow 'arts and crafts' stigma carried by many orthodontic practices.

The ideas in this chapter are a natural extension of ongoing research efforts, and a synthesis of both manifest clinical need and contemporary hMSC science. Ironically, despite the sophisticated rationale, the actual procedures necessary to attain these vaunted goals can be achieved with a simple periodontal surgery, which is often performed by first-year postdoctoral dental students.

The key to success lies not in a particular material or surgical procedure, but rather in the *orchestration and timing* of traditional protocols, *viz.* simply moving dental roots in a field of healing tissues and mechanically strained bone. In wound healing, it appears that strained bone reacts differently from the steady-state bone, which the orthodontist usually encounters. Healing wounds recapitulate regional ontogeny and that ontogeny responds to local environmental (epigenetic) perturbations, e.g. optimal orthodontic force, to define phenotype change *via* stem cell differentiation. Some orthodontists may criticize SCT as unnecessarily morbid. However, considering the ablative nature of tooth extraction and its deforming effects on facial form, the minor side effects of superficial periodontal surgery (1–2 mm beneath the mucosal surface) compare most favorably for facial esthetics enhancement as in Figure 21.10.

Interestingly, the evolution of thought driving the synthesis of orthodontic tissue engineering is not the dogma of new autocratic professional authorities, but rather sensitivity to patient preference, respect for modern dental standards, and contemporary global definitions of facial esthetics. Specifically the use of living stem cells to regenerate original phenotype damaged by infection or to change phenotypic form and mass, presents new evidenced-based and positive options to any prudent clinician who contemplates dental arch advancement or expansion. Hence it is an educational imperative (Nowzari et al., 2008).

Progress by case study analysis

Specifically we aim to direct attention, by case study methods, to the practicality of redesigning alveolar bone through surgical manipulation and augmenting the mass of available bone by moving roots into a living (viable) hMSC allograft. This stem cell/graft matrix has been generally employed with notable success in thousands of patients undergoing spinal fusion and other kinds of orthopedic surgery (Brosky et al., 2009); herein we apply it intraorally. The tissue fate of the stem cells depends on the interaction of local environmental elements such as the interaction of growth factors with mechanical stimuli. However, the exact biochemical mechanisms and the pathways of architectural transcription factors have not yet been clearly defined. In the 'real world' of clinical orthodontic practice, this high-quality scholarship employing cell biology is matched only by the popularity of SCT with patients and the commercial purveyors' sensitivity to issues of safety and efficacy.

Yet, prudence dictates that final evaluations of any orthodontic innovation should be withheld until longitudinal studies document efficiencies in many population cohorts and subsets. Any grafted bone should be studied to full maturity with many analytic techniques, including the requisite computed tomography; our proposal is no exception. In this regard, any absolute certitude about the effects of orthodontic tooth movement or SFOT on the alveolus bone must be delayed 3–4 years because that is the amount of time alveolar bone needs to achieve a 'steady-state' equilibrium (Fuhrmann, 2002).

Figure 21.11 demonstrates dramatically the foolishness of making impetuous but definitive statements about how orthodontic tooth movement affects alveolar bone. Note that alveolar bone returns to the pretreatment steady state only after 3 years. In Figure 21.11b the bone is simply less calcified due to the regional acceleratory phenomenon (RAP) of Frost (Epker and Frost, 1965; Melsen, 2001) Figure 21.11c shows the situation 3 years into retention. The alveolar bone on the patient's left canine has returned to the cementoenamel junction and the alveolar bone on the lateral incisor has calcified coronally. Only the central incisors show evidence of bony dehiscence, the limit of individual phenotypic plasticity. Thus, evaluation of final alveolar crest position after orthodontic therapy cannot be made prior to the achievement of 'steady-state' equilibrium in bone, 3 or more years after debonding.

Nonetheless, conceptual imperatives and documentation of the protocol should sustain interest in living stem cells among clinicians who are already captivated by the merits of conventional alveolar tissue engineering with demineralized bone matrix grafts. We hypothesize, as demonstrated with the 'whole bone' model, that hMSCs will respond more effectively to strain gradients mediated through the osteocyte syncytium, as reported by a number of research-oriented clinicians (Yokota and Tanaka, 2005; Zhang et al., 2006, 2007).

A consilience of sciences

These 'internal strain hypotheses' and 'whole bone' model (Murphy, 2006; Williams and Murphy, 2008) posit the important mechano-biological notion that the alveolus

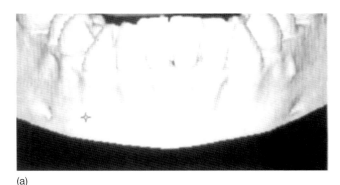

(a)

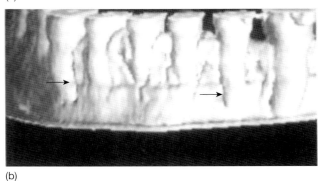

(b)

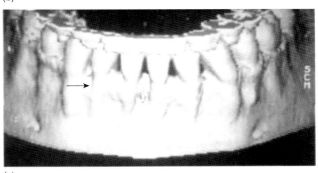

(c)

Figure 21.11 (a) The alveolar crest is at the cementoenamel junction (arrows). (b) After orthodontic treatment, there is dehiscence of the labial alveolar bone, where the alveolar crest seems to have retreated to the apex of each anterior tooth (arrows) and moved 'off the alveolar housing'. Note: this is an illusion. The bone is still present but is less calcified than in its original pre-orthodontic state. (c) Apparent regeneration of bone coronally but this is merely recalcified anatomy. (Courtesy of Elsevier. Source: Fuhrmann RAW (2002) *Seminars in Orthodontics*. Elsevier. Used with permission.)

osteocyte–canaliculi syncytium (during the initial short-term production of 'streaming potentials'), and cytoskeletal deformation in the entire alveolus (during alveolus 'bone bending') are significant biological events at the cellular level (similar to the Damon rationale.). Both appear to act in concert as significant transduction mechanisms (Ingber, 1998). This response to mechanical stress may be a universal phenomenon since these characteristic force transductions can be applied to cytoskeleton behavior in distraction osteogenesis and many other organs (Ingber, 2006). Thus, this chapter attempts to present a fusion of new and myriad ways of scientific thinking, in addition to a new clinical protocol.

Extrapolating from general osteology and medical distraction osteogenesis, it appears that when teeth are moved through a healing stem cell graft, the resultant pressure gradients stimulate hMSCs to differentiate and 'reprogram' genetic expression. In contrast, non-viable bone or even robustly inductive rhBMP-2 used in periodontal regeneration must rely on relatively effete endogenous hMSCs. Since viable cell allografts are often donated by individuals under the age of 30, their hMSCs appear to stimulate a more robust potential than a recipient's own bone (autografts), the presumptive 'gold standard' of regional bone augmentation (Zaky and Cancedda, 2009).

Moreover, stability is enhanced since conventional orthodontic treatment, even with extractions or circumferential fiberotomies, does not ensure dental stability. However, PAOO has shown better stability with equal quality as illustrated in Figure 21.12. It is proposed that, following the same surgical protocol with hMSC allografts will produce identical results, faster, and with fewer surgical complications, side effects, or sequelae, e.g. erythema, inflammation, or edema. The thesis this image demonstrates is that thicker bone, makes orthodontic clinical outcomes faster, safer and more stable by altering genetic expression to redefine the limits of the phenotypic spectrum. Independent experts contend that thicker alveolar bone (Roth et al., 2006) lends stability to clinical outcomes. When engineered painlessly and predictably, thicker bone

does indeed seem to be more stable according to postsurgical orthodontic analysis (Dosanjh et al., 2006; Oliveira et al., 2006). And, stem cell allografts, so far, seem to do it faster and better.

Interestingly, a viable cell allograft demonstrates less postoperative erythema and local inflammation than conventional DFDBA or decortication alone. Figure 21.13 illustrates the 'OldThink' claim that in case of incisor

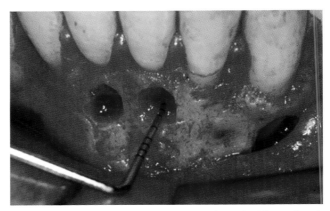

Figure 21.12 Moving roots into demineralized freeze-dried bone allograft (DFDBA) produces a thick labial mass of cortical and cancellous bone indistinguishable from native architecture, a blinded evaluation by an oral pathologist. (Source: Professor M. Thomas Wilcko, Case Western Reserve University School of Dental Medicine, Cleveland, Ohio USA 44106. Used with permission.)

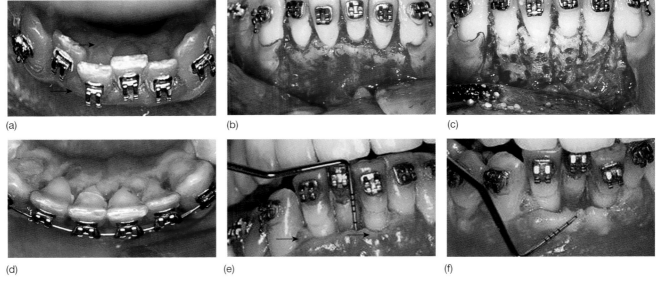

Figure 21.13 Patient AA (a–d) a 22-year-old man, presented with mandibular incisor crowding as defined by the 'OldThink' 'arch length deficiency' that can dictate premolar extraction. The 'NewThink' method uses the most facial dimension of the alveolus, the space between the black arrows in (a) as the landmark for 'available space' into which teeth may be moved. (e,f) Patient EO. (e) The new attachment is visible behind a matured incision line (arrowed). (f) The dark tissue accretion in the tooth is the periodontal surgical dressing. (Source: Neal C. Murphy, Departments of Orthodontics and Periodontics, Case Western Reserve University School of Dental Medicine, Cleveland, Ohio USA. Used with permission.)

crowding the alveolus is immutable, suggesting that 'too many teeth' are present for such a small arch. This, we contend, is no longer a tenable conclusion. This text demonstrates that *available arch length* should not necessarily be defined by the crowded dentition, but rather by *the labial-most dimension of the alveolus into which teeth may be moved or into which bone augmentation is possible, as illustrated in Figure 21.13a.*

The patient opted for SAD (a more precise term than "corticotomy") (Figure 21.13b,c). He was appointed for postoperative inspection 10 days later. At the postoperative visit, the patient reported that his teeth were 'perfectly straight in 4 days'. Stem cell grafting with hMSCs would have improved this outcome by reducing the amount of marginal inflammation seen postoperatively (Figure 21.13d). In another patient (Figure 21.13e,f), the absence of an inflamed surgical margin in Figure 21.13e is characteristic of the rapid healing seen in the stem cell graft and the rapid regeneration in Figure 21.13f. More rapid healing with less inflammation is characteristic of hMSC grafts and the reasons may be related to the secretion of cytokines and other factors that suppress a local immune response, 'rejection' responses, and graft-versus-host disease.

We also attribute this response to the proactive nature of the stem cells and their curious 'homing' mechanisms with which they 'seek out' damaged tissue and suppress local inflammation. The homing behavior is evident even when cells are injected systemically but the mechanism is still elusive and remains one of the intriguing characteristics of stem cell tissue engineering.

A consilience of style

The terms human mesenchymal stem cells, osteoprogenitor cells, and preosteoblasts present a conundrum for classification because viable hMSCs, OPCs, osteoblasts, and allografts (DBM or DFDBA) all combine to provide patients, especially those compromised by age, with a veritable cocktail of safety and efficacy. An investigation into government regulatory agencies revealed a startling degree of safety. Thousands of viable cell allografts have been placed by medical clinicians with no reports of adverse reactions, immunologic rejections or graft-versus-host disease.

The graft material demonstrated in this chapter does not contain a 100% hMSC population, so many purists feel the term 'stem cell allograft' is misleading. Since the graft is alive, they prefer to use the term 'viable cell allograft'. Yet, interestingly, many periodontists and patients who disdain conventional DBM or DFDBA as 'cadaver bone' and disparage it per se, actually prefer a living graft. Therefore, orthodontists must hold a place for each patient's preference in their informed consent forms. Grafts have been tested to show that a *minimum* of 50 000–250 000 viable cells/mL are available for healing. And, since healing is a tissue-forming-cell 'numbers game', more cells means better and faster healing. Moreover, all stem cell grafts are tested for cell count, osteogenicity, and viability. While technically, each commercialized cubic centimeter of graft cannot be tested for its osteo-inductive capacity, examinations for the 'three golden Os', osteo-*conductive*, osteo-*inductive* and osteo-*genic* capacities are made of each lot randomly.

The specific osteoinductive potential of most grafts is also arrived at deductively from the history of DFDBA as demonstrated decades ago. Other reasons for SCT success rest on logical scrutiny that demands new styles of practice and academic presentations. Indeed, employing strict epistemological tests of causation (Moss, 2004); while any one part of the surgical 'whole' may be necessary for bone growth, none is individually sufficient. In terms of new bone phenotype engineering, the proximate, or Aristotelian 'efficient cause', of the final epigenetic result, is the stem cell component. All the other components of the procedure, while *sine qua non*, are predisposing or 'formal' and necessary causal elements.

In this case, remember that SCT is more than just another graft material, ligand, or catalyst; SCT replicates natural phenomena more comprehensively than adding elements here and there, as an educated trial and error approach. SCT, through the replication of daughter cells can place millions of 'bone-forming factories' in the wound, not just a few necessary ingredients. As an analogy, this is tantamount to 'putting more cooks in the kitchen' instead of just a few more 'ingredients'. Probably, only a unique orchestration of healing conditions and elements, a highly individualized formula for each patient, is the key to success. The stem cells can address that challenge where other materials cannot. They become what the local environment tells them to become so each cell seeks and secures its own mode of differentiation and activity. That is the fundamental basis of stem cell activity. SCT does not add new 'parts', it induces new 'physiologies'.

When a patient's own bone grafts are used to augment alveolus bone mass lost to infection or to enhance alveolar development, the graft is termed *autograft*. In contrast, an *allograft* is tissue from another individual of the same species. The latter graft evokes issues of immunology. Because of the embryologically primitive nature of the hMSC, rejection and graft–host disease have not been noted in tens of thousands of cases in which hMSC allografts have been used. In fact, there is even some evidence that the hMSC itself may help regulate the activity of a recipient's T-cell subtypes, and antibody production by B-cells, and immune tolerance of allogeneic transplants (Patel et al., 2008). Experts generally acknowledge that one of the remarkable attributes of hMSCs is that they express neither human leukocyte antigen (HLA) class II markers, nor the accessory molecules (CD40, CD80, CD86) necessary to activate a cellular immune response. This is why graft-versus-host disease is not an issue and why donor–recipient matching for these cells is not required in medical orthopedic cases and ours. Thus, hMSC and

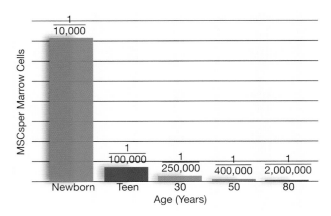

Figure 21.14 The concentration of stem cells diminishes rapidly with age. (Source: Images Compliments of Orthofix, Inc. San Diego, CA USA. Used with permission.)

viable cell allografts appear as safe as they are effective. hMSCs, we posit, are ideal for PAOO because late adolescent or young adult patients have endogenous stem cells which are later depleted by infirmity or age per se (Figure 21.14).

Since the healing potential, and more importantly the degree of stromal regeneration, is related to the concentration of stem cells in the wound, local augmentation of stem cells is entirely compatible with other bone grafts and regenerative materials, e.g. autograft, osteo-conductive extenders, DFDBA, and rhBMP-2. However, there is no compelling evidence that so-called 'extenders' or 'enhancers' that provide extra mass or biochemical supplements are necessary. In the absence of data to the contrary, the hMSC graft may be considered a singularly sufficient monotherapy.

A consilience of cognition

Given these recent findings, it is no longer fitting to present only outdated paradigms from the early 1900s to students and patients. Admittedly, the convenient pressure-tension model of Sandstedt and Oppenheim (1904–1911) might work well as a simplistic fiction to satisfy curious but uninitiated patients. But the PDL and spongiosa of bone are complex viscoelastic gels, so pressure, as in any closed hydraulic fluid system, is distributed evenly throughout the phase while stresses and strains are multidirectional and variable in magnitude. Moreover, old pressure-tension models and their derivatives do not subsume either streaming potentials or alveolus bone bending phenomena wherein *shear* forces may define the transduction element better than hyalinization and vascular infarction. Therefore, we suggest that in the professional lexicon of orthodontic theory, we speak in terms of 'fields of multi-directional

strain gradients' rather than pressure and tension. Baumrind (1969) reported that the latter, only weakly relevant, concept ignores the environment of an anisotropic complex gel that defines the PDL and spongiosa. In this physical system, trabeculae act as 'inclusions bodies' that complicate the flux of strain vector dynamics.

Regulatory imperatives

Despite the dramatic effects of hMSCs *in vivo*, it is important to realize that the human cellular bone matrix must conform to extremely rigorous standards promulgated by the United States Food and Drug Administration (FDA) (21 CFR part 1271) and should be used only with a sterile (aseptic) technique. Regardless of the commercial source, the best formulation for carrying stem cells to the surgical site is in cryopreserved cancellous fragments, viable cancellous matrix, and ground bone. The best test of a stem cell graft is its ability to differentiate, *in situ*, to any cell of mesenchymal origin and, ultimately, its organization, indistinguishable from the native architecture.

Criteria for hMSC graft donation

All hMSC donors must be screened to eliminate the chance of communicable disease agents. For example, the best laboratories will exclude donors who have had any xenograft or *even cohabited with a xenograft recipient*. In addition, tests for the following should be negative or nonreactive: human immunodeficiency virus (HIV) 1 and 2 antibody, hepatitis C virus (HCV) antibody and B surface antigen or B core antibody, syphilis rapid plasma reagin or treponemal specific assay, human T-cell lymphotropic virus type I and II antibody, and HIV/HCV nucleic acid test. Test kits must be approved by the FDA, which regulates donor eligibility as well.

Tissue recovery techniques

Recovery or 'harvest' of the bone graft is performed by licenced tissue bank personnel using aseptic techniques. Records review is collected at the time of recovery and reviewed again as part of the donor eligibility determination by the company selling the hMSC graft. In the case studies presented here (Figures 21.15–21.19), hMSC graft strict processing standards were confirmed. After harvest from a selected donor, the graft was processed in a proprietary manner that included disinfection, cryopreservation, and antibiotics. As a fail-safe redundancy, the MSC graft manufacturer (NuVasive, Inc, San Diego, California, USA) physically inspected a random sample of each lot to test for destructive microbiological organisms and ensure that the results showed 'no growth' after 14 days' incubation. Each lot was tested with an *in vitro* assay for viable osteogenic cells and osteoinductive potential.

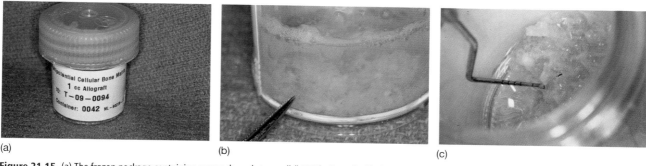

(a) (b) (c)

Figure 21.15 (a) The frozen package containing mesenchymal stem cell (hMSC) allograft. (b) The supernatant, which acts as cryopreservative. This cryopreservative also acts as the minimal essential medium (MEM) which maintains the viability of living cells (viable osteoprogenitor and stem cells) after chairside thawing. The allograft (at the level of the tip of the clinical instrument) has settled at the bottom of the container. (c) After the supernatant is poured off, the MSC allograft is soaked in a 'bath' of clindamycin 150 mg/mL. (Source: www.UniversityExperts.com.)

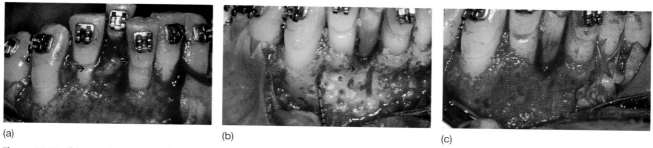

(a) (b) (c)

Figure 21.16 This case demonstrates that the so-called 'compromised periodontium' is no less amenable to orthodontic tooth movement, selective alveolar decortication, periodontally accelerated osteogenic orthodontics, or hMSC grafts than a healthy dentition, given that all infective elements on the roots are eliminated. (a) The appearance prior to decortication and infected tissue elimination. (b) Note how punctate and linear decortication frees endogenous mesenchymal cells with about 2–3 mm penetration into the spongiosa including the periodontal infrabony defect (arrow). (c) Active bleeding should be evident before the MSC allograft is placed on the recipient bed of decorticated labial alveolar bone. (Source: www.UniversityExperts.com.)

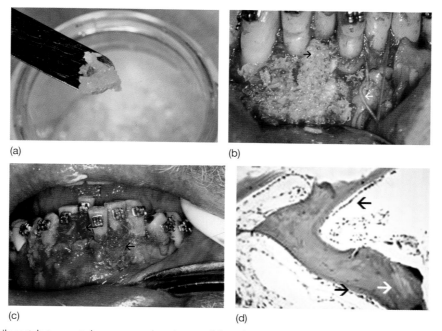

(a) (b)

(c) (d)

Figure 21.17 (a) The sterile spatula transports human mesenchymal stem cell (hMSC) allografts. (b) The stem cell allograft is molded to the prepared recipient site (black arrow) and tucked under the loosely sutured mucoperiosteal flap. The continuous locking suture (white arrow) is then drawn over the MSCs like a purse string. (c) After suturing has coronally positioned the surgical flap for patient EO and held the graft against the decorticated labial alveolar bone, a covering of cyanoacrylate (black arrows) ensures that the flap is immobilized and sutures are secure. (d) Histological analysis confirms normal healing of bone de novo with viable bone lining cells (black arrows) and remnants of the viable stem cell matrix (white arrow). (Source: www.UniversityExperts.com.)

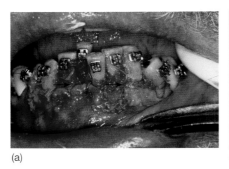
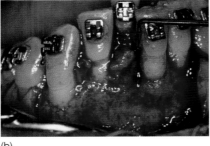
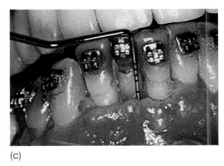

(a) (b) (c)

Figure 21.18 (a) The sutured flap is secured with a blanket (black arrow) of tissue adhesive (cyanoacrylate) when buccal-lingual primary closure is not possible. (b,c) The gain in attachment documents the efficacy of the techniques (note the new elevated position of the periodontal probe in Figure 21.18c). (Source: www.UniversityExperts.com.)

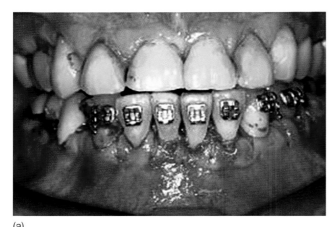

(a)

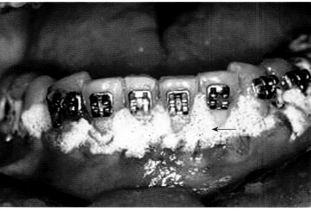

(b)

Figure 21.19 (a) Suture position between the lower right incisors is ideal to protect the growing stem cells. The suture position between the lower left incisors was repositioned prior to a cyanoacrylate 'blanket' placement. Some viable graft has extruded from the containment flap (white arrow). (b) Final position of sutures and cyanoacrylate blanket (black arrow) prior to patient dismissal. The cyanoacrylate will discolor over the following 2–3 weeks and fall off the teeth, just like a natural scab, when the subjacent tissue matures. (Source: www.UniversityExperts.com.)

Surgical protocol

Preparation

The following guidelines are found to be effective. After being interviewed and screened for surgery, co-signed and initialed an informed consent form, sedated and anesthetized with block injections and local infiltration, the patient is draped for the surgical procedure, which commences immediately after all brackets are secured on the teeth to be treated. Surgery is usually limited to only those areas where orthodontic tooth movement is compromised by insufficient alveolar bone. This insufficiency can be visualized on three-dimensional replicates of computed tomographs (Figure 21.20), but the density of dentin and thin alveolar bone often obscure the exact location of the alveolar crest even with modern imaging machines. So, obscurity itself may be used as an indication for stem cell allograft augmentation. In our protocol, archwires are placed immediately after the last suture is secured, so that standard orthodontic tooth movement can immediately begin stimulating the stem cells by straining the graft. This is a critical step that creates the new phenotype, as the surgery overcomes tissue stability or what Waddington (1957) called 'epigenetic buffering'. Once this is fully conceptualized by the clinician, periodic transmucosal perturbations can extend the time of a locally induced osteopenia, viz. the so-called RAP.

Graft delivery

After the hMSC is removed from cold storage, it is placed in a sterile saline bath at $37 \pm 2°C$ (95–102°F) to thaw/melt slowly over 15–30 minutes. This temperature must not be exceeded; otherwise the cell viability is compromised. The cells will maintain viability up to 2 hours post-thaw when left in their cryopreservative, and up to 6 hours when cryopreservative is decanted and replaced with sterile saline or 5% dextrose lactated Ringer's solution (D5LR).

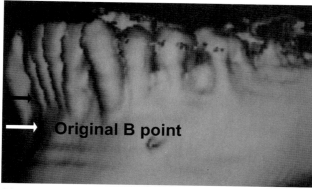

(a)

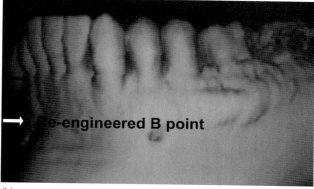

(b)

Figure 21.20 (a,b) This figure demonstrates a kind of re-engineering to a novel phenotype, but still within a spectrum of genotypic potential and newly designed to contain tooth root position. This exemplifies the validity of Moss's functional matrix hypothesis, which explains how the roots of the teeth are the 'functional matrix' (template) for new alveolus bone, new B point (white arrow) and a coronally repositioned alveolar crest (black arrow). (Source: Professor M. Thomas Wilcko, Case Western Reserve University School of Dental Medicine, Cleveland Ohio USA 44106. Used with permission.)

Some political regulations (e.g. New York State) demand that the graft be used within 4 hours, even though scientific data shows longer cell viability. What makes this viable allograft interesting and valuable is the fact that it can be stored for future use and simply defrosted. In storage between −45° and −75°C, the cells maintain viability for 90 days. Stored at −80°C the cells will remain alive for *5 years*!

Owing to the septic field, a final clindamycin lavage is done for 5 seconds immediately prior to graft placement. The graft flows freely upon inversion of the container when ready for transfer to the patient. After the graft has settled to the bottom of the liquid preservative and prior to use, the supernatant liquid cryopreservative (decant) is carefully discarded. In our particular case, after the antibiotic lavage, excess clindamycin was poured off the graft leaving only the clindamycin-soaked hMSC ready for immediate placement

(Figure 21.15) on the recipient bed of decorticated alveolus. This antibiotic rinse is commonly employed with outpatient periodontal regeneration using demineralized bone matrix (DBM/DFDBA) to reduce bacterial contamination. Postoperative histological analysis confirms that clindamycin lavage is safe for cell viability.

In medical orthopedic cases, the antibiotic concentrations associated with bone cements may have skeletal cell toxicity above certain thresholds. This toxicity can be seen *in vitro* by noting differences in cellular morphology. Antoci et al. (2007) found that ciprofloxacin doses greater than 100 µg/mL and vancomycin or tobramycin doses greater than 2000 µg/mL can severely decrease cell proliferation. Therefore, striking a therapeutic balance between antimicrobial effects and hMSC toxicity is a profound question that must be a part of clinical heuristics for each practitioner in the absence of compelling controlled studies.

Flap surgery

The surgical flap necessary is termed a 'full thickness' or mucoperiosteal flap of mucosa that encompasses the soft tissue over the alveolus from the surface oral loose (areolar) connective tissue and attached gingival mucosa, all the way through to the periosteum. Submarginal incisions with AOO cases, uncomplicated by periodontal considerations, may be helpful to preclude unesthetic embrasure opening. However, in cases with periodontitis, PAOO is employed because osseous defects must be managed in conjunction with the induced osteopenia. In such circumstances that involve a periodontal correction, sulcular incisions should be used. Surgical flap design guidelines are general and can be modified by patient preferences and each surgeon's objectives, experience, and style. The mucoperiosteal flaps are reflected in a conventional manner for inspection of the labial and lingual alveolar cortices, and vertical tension-releasing incisions are made where necessary at the end of the sulcular incision to allow coronal positioning of the flap without tension or graft spillage. Maintaining grafts distant from the vertical tension-releasing incisions also aids in stability since micro-movement of graft material may limit full engraftment, i.e. integration of the graft to the decorticated alveolus.

Because the graft increases the mass of bone covered by the flap, all tension in the replaced flap must be eliminated. A flap under tension will result in necrosis of the edge or even regression to the vestibular depth and exposure of a healing granulation mass. Surprisingly, such a dramatic clinical complication may not necessarily result in complete graft slough; however, the secondary intention healing resulting from exposure of the graft may delay total engraftment and extend the healing time by three to five times that seen in primary intention healing.

Before the alveolar bone is decorticated to receive the hMSC allograft in the PAOO procedure, all granulation tissue from periodontal defects and root accretions should be removed with definitive periodontal scaling and root planing (S/RP) (Figure 21.16). Orthodontic tooth movement can be achieved for patients with active infection, presenting so-called 'hot lesions', if comprehensive root debridement is done just prior to decortication and stem cell placement. Protracted initial periodontal therapy, such as S/RP, informally known as 'deep cleaning', produces a 'cold lesion' that is less receptive to regeneration or phenotype change. Ironic as it may seem, 6–8 weeks of S/RP can actually inhibit regenerative potential by eliminating high concentrations of growth factors that accompany local inflammation. It is helpful to note that the patient is in a 'healthy state', well prepared for regeneration or tissue engineering, merely seconds after the last root accretion is removed. Meanwhile, the soft issue is the flap loaded with growth factors ready to aid the healing wound.

Also, a healthy dentition with less than normal support is no more vulnerable to premature tooth loss than a fully supported dentition. Bone loss must never be conflated with its cause, active disease. They are two separate intellectual entities that may or may not be related. Just as a limping weak leg is not poliomyelitis but rather the result of the infection, so bone loss per se is not the disease but rather the result of the infection.

In this particular case (Figure 21.16), once the periodontal 'hot' lesion on the lower right central incisor is debrided and grafted, orthodontic therapy begins immediately. Although the periodontal literature preaches against graft 'micro-movement', the principles of regeneration are not necessarily compromised by induced internal bone strain when new phenotypes are regenerated through root movement, e.g. PAOO. So, infrabony regeneration and alveolar phenotype alteration can occur concomitantly. Orthodontists commonly make a mistake by failing to draw a distinction between stable (inactive) attachment loss and the actual infectious disease process itself. Integrated orthodontists solve this problem which insular orthodontists must live with to their detriment.

Stem cells from the marrow of the patient thrive in a field of copious bleeding so the virtue of traditional surgical homeostasis is questionable in some cases. Figure 21.16 shows a debrided and decorticated infrabony pocket on an incisor specifically treated to elicit copious bleeding. This is encouraged where *in situ* stem cell grafts are placed or when a mixture of so-called 'viable cell allografts' is used.

For the sake of syntactical clarity, a technical distinction must be made between this kind of *in situ* stem cell therapy or 'viable cell allograft' shown here and intravascular stem cell therapy used in other disciplines. Nonetheless one should not view this procedure as tantamount to traditional DBM or DFDBA regeneration. That common protocol only re-establishes a pre-existing phenotype. This 'stem cell therapy' engineers a new phenotype, better designed for tooth movement and responding epigenetically to it.

The guiding maxims are: 'wound healing recapitulates regional ontogeny' and 'stressed bone wounds heal differently than bone in steady state equilibrium'. Instead of seeking immobilization to preclude what medical orthopedists would call an osteopenic 'malunion' we intentionally deliver internal strain gradients to the wound in order to 're-program' or, in more correct biological terms, 'imprint' the hMSCs, OPCs, and osteoblasts in this viable cell allograft.

We propose that clinical phenotype change is achieved at the cytoskeletal level by re-engineering the delivery of novel architectural transcription factors to the nucleus of the stem cell. This cell level engineering is not possible with standard bone grafts such as DBM and DFDBA, and is manifestly not happening with conventional orthodontic mechanotherapy (Murphy, 2006).

The punctuate and linear decortication (about 2–3 mm into the spongiosa as demonstrated in Figures 21.13c and 21.16b, frees endogenous mesenchymal stem cells from the marrow of the patient. It is important that copious bleeding is evident before the MSC allograft is placed on the recipient bed. Generally the traditional standard for periodontal surgery is strict hemostasis, but that is encouraged for visibility during resective or ablative surgical procedures. Stem cell grafting is different, where fragile graft viability depends on a specific nutrient source, so bleeding is encouraged with hMSCs. Because the rigid allograft matrix binds the hMSC graft tightly and the physical handling of the graft is so easy, containment in a bloody field is usually not a problem. In contrast, other nonviable grafts (DFDBA or synthetic materials) tend to drift out of the graft site making stability and containment more difficult.

After sutures have been loosely placed, the graft is taken directly to the donor site from the sterile bottle with a sterile spatula and molded to the contour of the decorticated alveolar cortices (see Figure 21.17b,c), into which the clinician may anticipate root movement that needs new bone formation as demonstrated in Figure 21.17d. Prior to hMSC allograft placement, the labial cortex must be decorticated according to the standard protocol published earlier for periodontal regeneration with DFDBA (Wilcko et al., 2008) and the clinician must ensure that all infected root surfaces are thoroughly debrided of infectious elements, calcific accretions, necrotic cementum, and infected granulomatous tissue. Reiterating, where the alveolus is healthy and periodontal support is not compromised, simple AOO protocols can be employed with submarginal incisions for predictable success.

Figure 21.17 shows how a simple sterile spatula can transport hMSC allografts and how a covering of cyanoacrylate ensures that the flap is immobilized and the sutures are secure. Hardening of cyanoacrylates acts like an artificial 'scab', and ensures stability of the flap and sutures. In this process, the roots of the teeth act as a frame or 'functional matrix' of the newly designed alveolar bone, to create a larger bone mass and better form. The cyanoacrylates often fall off the graft site when healing is sufficient to hold the graft, usually in 2–5 days. A 0.018 inch nickel-titanium round archwire was placed immediately after the curing of cyanoacrylate, so that tooth movement could be commenced immediately into the graft, providing therapeutic strain gradients on the decorticated bone and hMSCs.

As wound healing recapitulates regional ontogeny (Murphy, 2006), it is hypothesized that these physiological strain gradients, estimated at 500–1000 μS will allow the stem cells to differentiate into daughter cells and osteoblasts, move labially to redefine local phenotype and increase labial alveolar bone mass. This can be confirmed by histological analysis as shown in Figure 21.17d and is the logical synthesis of work of Wilcko et al. (2003) and clinical tissue engineering and the Utah paradigm, a fundamentally new approach to clinical orthopedics (see Suggested reading). The movement of the lower right central incisor labially has genetically reprogrammed a new supporting phenotype that lends a more stable outcome than conventional orthodontic treatment and a better overall quality even when compared with standards of the ABO. This is an historical mandate for change.

However, when the patient presents with periodontal infection, PAOO should be the protocol of choice. Changing phenotypic design can be combined with standard periodontal regeneration. In this way, three objectives are achieved and the patient needs only to recover from one surgical procedure that maximizes therapeutic goals. The alternative of three procedures would be logically untenable as sequential treatments, i.e. opening embrasures with fixed appliances, regenerative surgery, and phenotype remodeling. With SCT, they are all done more efficiently with one treatment, in less time, and under one fee. That makes PAOO and SCT therapy a value at any cost.

In periodontal disease cases (as with our PAOO case study) the bases of all infrabony defects should be thoroughly decorticated prior to graft placement. Timid attempts to minimize decortication in an effort to reduce bleeding or postoperative morbidity are an ill-conceived notions; comprehensive decortication will not necessarily produce more postoperative pain or edema. The decortication is rarely deeper into the spongiosa than 2–3 mm and replacement of the mucoperiosteal flap with efficient surgery is better assurance of postoperative patient comfort than ineffectual decortication.

Poor technique causes pain. The PAOO protocol is indeed technique sensitive so one must strike a rational balance between aggressive tissue manipulation and prudent restraint. For example, ecchymosis, a physiologically insignificant event commonly seen in very elderly patients is admittedly a psychosocial liability. Yet this can be minimized even in patients with friable integument, if flap reflection is not pushed far beyond the mucogingival junction. The continuous locking suture just prior to graft placement allows rapid stem cell placement and bone coverage by providing a pouch-like recipient site. Once the allograft is secure, the flap can be tethered over the graft by simply tightening the continuous locking suture and leaving the graft and donor site exposed for no more than 3 minutes (Figure 21.17b).

Postsurgical evaluation

The total graft mass is not necessarily an accurate predictor of clinical outcome. So there is no need to overfill the site. The need is more physiological potential, not more bone per se. As the graft matures, it will resorb partially as teeth are moved. Yet, this does not justify minimal grafting either. The regression and reshaping of the stem cell allograft is not a measure of failure as it would be with filing a periodontal infrabony pocket. Rather it represents a natural redefinition of form, a new phenotype engineered by the body appropriate for the specific type of tooth movement and the final position of the teeth relative to the labial alveolar cortex. The final mass and labial contour of the new alveolus will be determined by the angle between the tooth and the cortex.

Specifically, at the anterior sextants of the alveoli, convetites, appearing immediately after grafting, evolve during healing to a specific labial concavity, termed the 'Wilcko curve' after its namesake. Surgeons new to the concepts of SCT may erroneously think that the graft is being overly resorbed as incisors are moved. They should be reassured that the curve is an important landmark in the study of this unique type of engineered bone wound healing because it redefines A point and B point. It is also an important concavity because the final curvature serves as a reliable marker of morphogenetic homeostasis. After 2–3 years' maturity, the anatomical form (phenotype) and clinical 'success' are documented with tomography (Figure 21.20) and defined, not by the amount of original bone graft, but rather the angulation of the lower incisors to a fixed anatomical landmark, e.g. the mandibular plane.

Figure 21.20 demonstrates an interesting phenomenon that applies to all orthodontic treatments but is especially germane in this discussion of tissue engineering. Periodontal regeneration merely re-establishes original form, while tissue engineering is seemingly re-engineering to a novel phenotype. It is still within a spectrum of genotypic potential, but newly designed to contain tooth root position. A new concavity forms at B point, after maturation of PAOO/AOO bone graft, which represents a stable morphotype known as the Wilcko Curve (Figure 21.20). The curve has a morphogenetic significance because it defines the mature labial convexity at B point. At this point in time, if orthodontic stress is not applied to the bone and Frost's RAP (Epker and Frost, 1965) is not employed through the original convexity, a clinical 'bulge' relapses back to the original B point curvature as the entire bone graft resorbs. The standard rationalization for such previous failures is 'You cannot grow bone on a flat surface'.

However, using PAOO with a stem cell component, the original clinical bulge and convexity can model to a new phenotype appropriate to the teeth in a treated position. This is why PAOO is so stable. But the treating orthodontist must be patient because the final Wilcko Curve may not fully define itself until 3 years into the retention phase. When it finally does, it serves as both a radiographic landmark for a histologically 'steady-state' equilibrium for the new labial bone. Note the different radius from B point in Figure 21.20 (white arrows). The linear distance between the white and black arrows demonstrates new attachment apparatus and alveolar bone support that was engineered as appropriate to the roots in a more physiological position. Stem cell allografts can make this surgical engineering safer, faster, and better.

Cell rejuvenation with transmucosal penetration

Tensional stress 'felt' by the alveolus must be constant but not to the point of resonance. It is the nature of bone to adapt to predictable changes in stress by remodeling its architecture (Wolff's law), but intermittent and random (stochastic) stimuli (adjustments every 1–2 weeks) keep the bone osteopenic; that is the objective of SCT. The intermittent nonresonant stresses that roots transfer to bone during mastication and fixed appliance activation perpetuate the osteopenic state of the RAP. When patients do not have archwire adjustments every 2 weeks, the alveolus may lose RAP and revert to a more calcified steady state.

However, the best protocols are meaningless unless they can adapt to real-world exigencies such as patient noncompliance, excessive expense, or scheduling conflicts. So a method of adaptation must accommodate these predictable complications. The best tool for this contingency is a kind of transmucosal penetration (TMP) into the alveolus as an intentional, controlled and therapeutic wounding (Figure 21.21).

While the acronym TMP usually stands for a clinical 'transmucosal penetration', to truly understand the dynamics of alveolar tissue engineering one should use it for 'transmucosal perturbation', *viz.* epigenetic perturbation of morphogenetic trajectory to prevent canalization. TMP is an attempt to reinvigorate the tissue healing dynamics, after the regional osteopenia (or RAP) has extinguished. The mechanically induced RAP, usually lasting only 6–9 months, can often be prolonged by the addition of viable stem cells. Because orthodontic mechanotherapy may last longer than the RAP, a kind of TMP 'booster' is sometimes needed to reassert the induced osteopenic state without resorting to a second surgery. TMP is also an epigenetic perturbation as hMSCs are re-stimulated to continue a novel trajectory to predesigned alveolus morphology on the epigenetic landscape of Waddington. Hence, RAP, the production of 'daughter cells' (conceivably for 6–9 generations), and stem cell differentiation must be sustained by constantly stressing the alveolus by appliance manipulation (Figure 21.21). Figure 21.22 illustrates the epigenetic landscape of Waddington, a visual metaphor and pedagogical tool to explain the interplay of genetic potential, ultimate genetic expression, and environmental

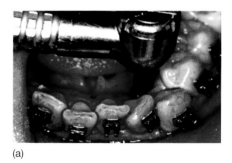 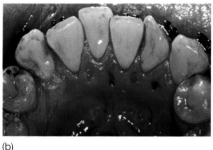 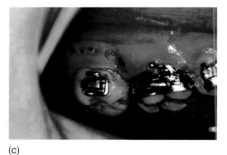

(a)   (b)   (c)

Figure 21.21 Transmucosal perforation/penetration (TMP) where one merely drills holes around the tooth to be moved, into the alveolus, approximating the depth of the center of rotation with an irrigated high speed #2 round bur. Reactivation of the regional acceleratory phenomenon (RAP) and a rejuvenation of stem cell viability can be accomplished by making these punctate penetrations/perturbations directly through the alveolus without flap reflection). (a) The technique employs a high speed surgical length #2 round bur with external irrigation. It is driven into the alveolus just past the center of rotation of the lower lateral incisor roots. This is repeated every 1–2 mm circumferentially. (b) The punctate divots in the attached gingiva represent TMP of the lingual cortex of the alveolus to facilitate rapid tipping movement of the incisors. Lower incisor crowding can be treated to completion in about a week. (c) TMP also has great utility in accelerating second molar eruption. Sometimes a case is finished only to have a malaligned eruption of second molars, which delay the debonding. Holding all the treated teeth hostage to a recalcitrant second molar is not good practice because it strains patient compliance and increases a time-sensitive bacterial load. So eruption of the second molar should be accelerated easily with TMP. (Source: Neal C. Murphy I Associate Case Western Reserve University School of Dental Medicine, Departments of Orthodontics and Periodontics, Cleveland, Ohio USA Used with permission.)

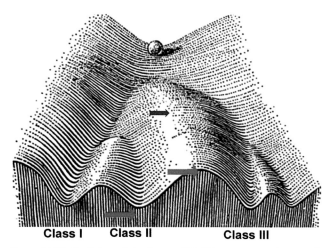

Figure 21.22 The Epigenetic Landscape of Waddington. Arrows show canalization (red) and buffering (blue) schematics that represent phenotype stabilization and the environmental perturbation (energy gradient) necessary to change it, respectively. The clinical analog to the blue arrow is periodontally accelerated osteogenic orthodontics (PAOO) and the red arrow represents the clinical stability of the PAOO result. (Source: Waddington CH, The Strategy of the Genes. *See* Suggested Reading.)

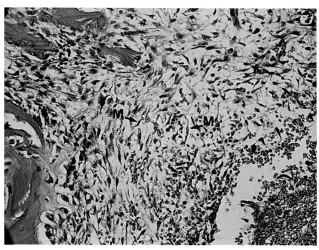

Figure 21.23 New stem cell healing in an animal model on day 4. Undifferentiated mesenchymal cells (M) stained with hematoxylin and eosin. Original magnification ×320). (Image courtesy of Dr A. Bakr Rabie, University of Hong Kong, Republic of China. Used with permission.)

'perturbations'. The ultimate fate of morphogenesis is generally dismissed as 'interplay between nature and nurture', but only the epigenetic landscape illustrates exactly how ultimately genetic expression and phenotype are realized. The ball, representing genetic potential, motivated by developmental factors (in health or disease) moves toward various fates (e.g. Class I, II, or III) within stable creases on the landscape. Ridges represent what Waddington called 'buffers' to change. The depth of each crease represents a kind of 'energy well' (canalization) that affords stability while the height of the ridges represent a kind of 'energy of activation' or energy gradient threshold necessary to overcome canalization and achieve new phenotypic fates.

Applying this conceptualization to conventional orthodontics, one would note that traditional biomechanics manifestly cannot overcome the energy gradient necessary for treatment stability. Thus, skeletal and dentoalveolar deformities may be described as the end products of simple genetic expression or epigenetic dynamics. Conventional treatment cannot quite get the 'ball over the ridge' (Figure 21.22). Where conventional biomechanics are insufficient, surgical intervention, such as SAD, PAOO, and TMP (or 'epigenetic perturbations') can indeed overcome 'buffering'. This achieves new canalizations necessary for a stable change in phenotype. Clinically, a phenotypic change is expressed as a 'stable treatment outcome', e.g. Angle's class I. The distance between the red arrows in Figure 21.22 represents the energy of activation that is necessary to rest secure in metaphorical 'energy wells', a process called 'canal-

ization' which is Waddington's term for the quantum amount of epigenetic perturbation necessary to change from one phenotype to another. The phenotype stability is said to be 'buffered' against change unless canalization can be overcome. Epigenetic influences may be heritable or non-heritable. However, no claim is made herein to Lamarckian concepts because we claim non-heritability to the epigenetic changes.

Corroborative clinical and histological data

Contraindications for the use of stem cells are the relative age and preferences of the patient and the potential for full natural regeneration due to stem cell populations *in situ*. The absolute number of stem cells at the site of the wound decreases as a function of age in the human and the absolute number of hMSCs correlates positively with the degree of regeneration potential, hence the rationale for MSC grafts instead of simple DBM. Overall, the excellent basic science is seen in Figure 21.23, the safety demonstrated by the test is illustrated in Figures 21.24–21.26, the clinical efficiency is shown in Figures 21.27–21.28 and finally, the product integrity is shown by Figures 21.29 and 21.30. Moreover, independent replication of histological evidence is seen in Figure 21.31; all combine with a reasonable cost, and patient aversion to 'dead cadaver bone' to make viable stem cell allografts a very promising material for PAOO and the development of orthodontic art into surgical orthopedics.

The evidence illustrated in Figures 21.23–21.31 defies the periodontal theory that one 'cannot grow bone on a flat

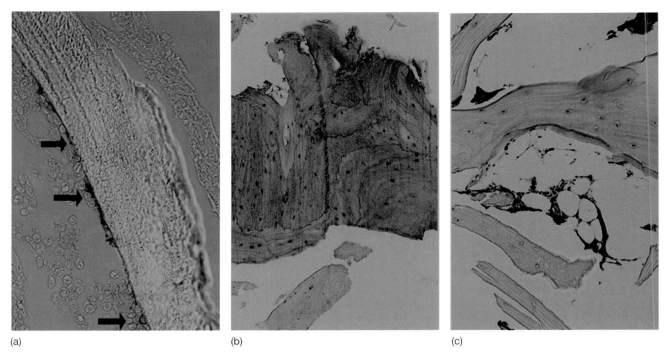

(a) (b) (c)

Figure 21.24 CD stands for 'cluster of differentiation' or 'cluster of designation' laboratory tests of quality which are consistent with and can even exceed the standards of the US Food and Drug Administration. This figure demonstrates the presence of (a) mesenchymal stem cells (MSCs) (marker CD 166 positive), (b) osteoprogenitor cells (OPCs) (osteocalcin stain), and (c) the absence of hematopoietic cells (marker CD 45 negative), components of human bone marrow that are selectively eliminated during allograft processing. (Images courtesy of Dr Ray Linovitz, Orthofix Inc., Lewisville, TX, USA. Used with permission.)

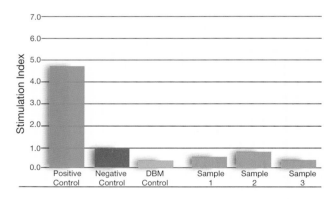

Figure 21.25 An illustration of how commercial sources can ensure that the cells are indeed viable in an allograft matrix. (Image courtesy of Dr. Ray Linovitz, Orthofix Inc., Lewisville, TX, USA. Used with permission.)

surface'. Thus, in this chapter we propose new hypotheses to explain the manifest tissue behavior. These hypotheses are posited to explain what conventional dental theory could not. To our knowledge this is the first publication of successful stem cell-enhanced alveolar orthopedic therapy in the dental literature orthodontic tissue engineering (OTE) (Murphy, 2006). This clearly opens interesting vistas for clinical practice since the surgical procedure was executed as an outpatient procedure with only light anxiolytic medication given orally and local anesthesia (lidocaine).

Figure 21.28 shows, with more pedagogical skill, the root of the lower right central incisor (see Figure 21.27) moved labially into the viable cell allograft, reduced clinical attachment loss, and presumably induced complete, anatomically normal and functional, periodontal attachment apparatus regeneration ('new attachment'). Immediately after the last suture was tied over the living cell allograft, mandibular incisors were moved anteriorly into the graft with the full engagement of a 0.018 inch nickel-titanium round archwire. The layer of bone forming cells (arrows) should not be conceived as a line, but rather as a kind of 'blanket' that covers the entire plane of new bone. Figure 21.28 shows a section of the viable stem cell allograft demonstrating bone matrix, viable osteocytes, and peripheral cells that may be characterized as possibly being stem cells. The viability of the cells accounts for the different images. Most cadaver bone after transplant *in vivo* looks very much like it does in the original container.

Although Popper's falsification principle (Williams and Murphy, 2008) is the best test of scientific truth,

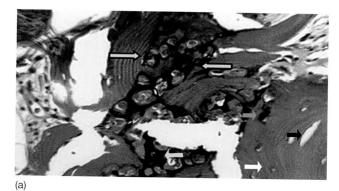

(a)

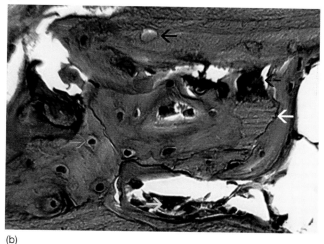

(b)

Figure 21.26 Note the nearly identical histological architecture of an orthopedic spine fusion model (a,b) with a specimen taken from a PAOO patient to ensure proper bone maturation. Each image demonstrates the empty lacunae of DBM (black arrows), reversal lines (white arrows), differentiated osteoblasts (yellow arrows) and viable bone de novo (green arrows). Thus, beyond the merits which stem cells contribute to alveolus phenotype alteration, the alveolus may also serve as a reasonable proxy for long bone and spine surgery analysis. (Images courtesy of Dr Ray Linovitz, Orthofix Inc., Lewisville, TX, USA.)

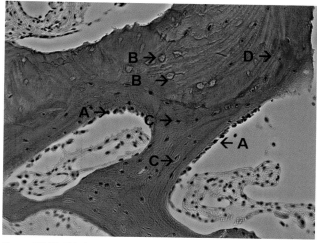

Figure 21.27 This human specimen was taken from the labial cortical bone, directly labial to the trajectory of lower incisor tooth movement (0.018 inch nickel-titanium round wire 2 months after patient EO was treated with PAOO surgery). A = a blanket of bone lining cells covering the surface and generating bone; B = empty lacunae from the human mesenchymal stem cells matrix; C = new bone de novo; D = a reversal line after 2 months of healing. (Source: www.UniversityExperts.com.)

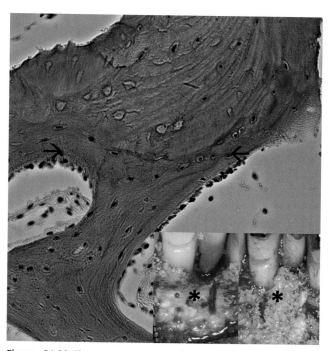

Figure 21.28 The composite image demonstrates the location from which the tissue sample was taken (asterisks) 2 months after commencement of labial movement of the mandibular incisors. (Source: www.UniversityExperts.com.)

another more common, albeit less robust, test of scientific veracity is independent corroboration. Figure 21.31 illustrates that the introduction of stem cell therapy is a *fait accompli* in other areas of clinical dentistry by pioneering clinical researchers in the USA and Canada. Note the consistent and similar histological picture in these histological sections, taken from a human maxillary sinus augmentation site after 3.5 months, in comparison with those in Figures 21.27 and 21.28, taken after 2 months.

Contraindications

Despite how well viable stem cell grafts work, one must not ignore contraindications, including immunocompromised patients, vascular pathoses, uncontrolled diabetes mellitus,

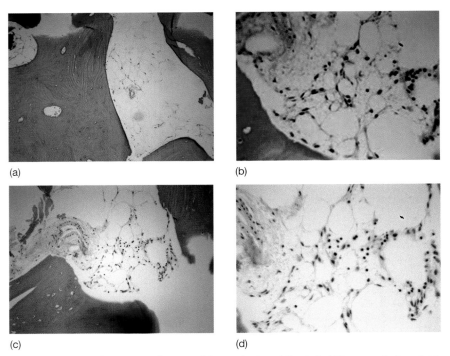

(a)

(b)

(c)

(d)

Figure 21.29 (a–d) A standard hematoxylin and eosin-stained section of the non-implanted (*in vitro*) viable stem cell allograft taken directly from the cryop-reserved container. (Source: www.UniversityExperts.com.)

fever, degenerative bone disease, bone infection, osteomy-elitis, pregnancy, and standalone weight-bearing sites, e.g. fremitus. An absolute contraindication presents when patients are allergic to any component in the graft or anti-biotic lavage. This is often indeterminate but should be included in all informed consent forms and reinforced with verbal inquiry of patient and responsible family agents. Signs of unanticipated allergic reaction include marked erythema at the surgical site beyond that usually seen during the immediate postoperative course, cutaneous urti-caria, rash, hives, or laryngeal edema ('fullness', 'tightening', or 'constriction' feeling in the area of the patient's throat). The latter obviously demands immediate emergency medical attention.

Practical considerations

The grafts are manufactured with the intention of single patient use only. hMSCs should never be refrozen after the initial defrosting because refreezing causes intracellular crystallization and cell death. Besides killing cells, refreezing or reusing the MSC graft for a second patient poses unten-able risk of cross-infection and a serious ethical breach. Obviously the expiration date on the container must be respected and strict adherence to storage temperature is necessary. The common household refrigerator freezing compartment cannot be reduced to this temperature

and, because of the critical nature of the material, even storage in commercial, hospital, or scientific lab freezers should be monitored to eliminate the chance of tempera-ture fluctuations.

A significant advantage to processed stem cell grafts is the fact that the amount of graft by volume is virtually unlimited, whereas autographs produce a second surgical wound at the harvest site, and prolonged surgical time can cause increased pain and swelling in the postoperative course. Slow, prolonged surgery dehydrates reflected tissue and often compromises the blood supply to the graft. Consequently, expedient execution of the graft surgery is encouraged and larger areas of stem cell grafts should be avoided if they require great dehydration of tissue or long exposure to air. This is not an absolute contraindication however because every surgeon possesses a unique style that should not be compromised if it is manifestly success-ful. Stepwise sextant surgery is recommended for the neophyte.

The periodontal theory justifying a presurgical 'initial therapy', also called 'the hygienic phase' of treatment, suggests that extensive wound debridement is necessary through extensive scaling and root planing before a lesion is operated. This has been taught traditionally as an important requirement for periodontal surgical success. But the rationale has become confounded over the years.

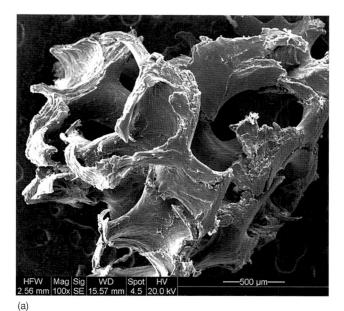

(a)

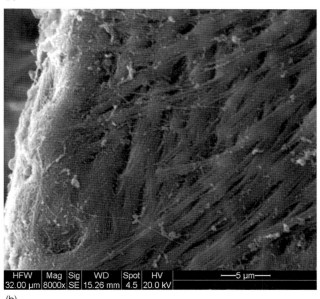

(b)

Figure 21.30 (a,b) Scanning electron microscopy of the viable cell matrix with stem cells and osteoprogenitor cells. (Source: Nuvasive, Inc. San Diego,California, USA. Used with permission.)

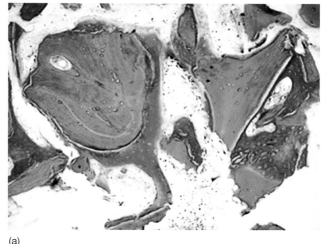

(a)

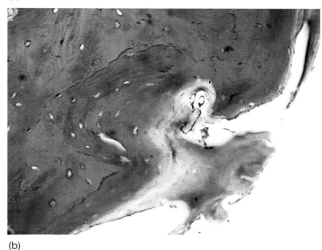

(b)

Figure 21.31 (a,b) The red-stained tissue is mineralized allograft, with the lighter red being the nonvital bone. The newly regenerated maxillary subantral bone is darker red, with visible cell nuclei. The green-stained tissue in (b) is demineralized allograft, containing neither viable bone, nor cells. (Images courtesy of Dr Aron Gonshor, Private practice in Montreal, Quebec, Canada and Brad McAllister Private Practice, Portland, OR, USA. Used with permission.)

The principal reasons for initial therapy are to reduce the inflammatory component of a periodontal infection so surgery may be minimized, and provide convenience and visibility to the surgical site. This is acceptable for resection surgery, and in some highly inflamed cases of horizontal bone loss, it may suffice for complete pocket elimination. However, for regeneration and SCT it may be counterproductive since inflammation, by its very nature, can carry a great deal of tissue elements that facilitate regeneration and phenotype modification.

The counterpoint suggests that highly inflamed but relatively uninfected soft tissue (in the flap) is the best recipient of graft material, irrespective of stem cell components. The defining notion is that inflamed tissue contains more endogenous growth factors that will be lost after 6–8 weeks of root debridement. Certainly a clean wound or so-called 'cold lesion' facilitates expedient surgery. On the other hand, operating in highly inflamed tissue surfeit with growth factors has led the senior author to startlingly successful regeneration.

Despite the use of inflamed soft tissue in the surgical flap, all root surfaces should be free of debris, calculus, and necrotic cementum, and infrabony defects should be extensively degranulated and decorticated. Some latitude for the individual doctor's style that deviate from strict compliance with this protocol should be respected. Moskow (1987) showed that many forms of periodontal therapies are effective and that many cases demonstrate active disease in as little as 5% of patients at any one time. And the ability of acutely inflamed tissue to heal as well as or better than chronically inflamed tissue has been general knowledge for over 100 years. So we are not historically alone with our contentions.

Specific surgical contraindications do not differ from those connected to any standard periodontal osseous or regenerative surgery. Yet, special attention should be paid to diabetic patients who, if their diabetes is uncontrolled, present serious problems to the periodontal surgeon. Where the diabetes is controlled, most authorities agree that healing is no different than in a non-diabetic patient. However, where serum glucose levels are erratic, as measured by glycosylated hemoglobin (A1C), exuberant granulation tissue may form at the graft site, demanding postoperative intervention and reducing the amount of healthy engraftment. Until specific literature explicates the exact relationship between medically compromised patients and predictable clinical outcomes, the elective surgery discussed herein should be considered only on responsible consultation with the patient's physician. Smokers, often problematic patients for dental implant procedures, are also notoriously poor candidates for regenerative periodontal surgery and should be selected for SCT with caution. For reasons unknown, clinical experience has indicated that empirically, smokers and poorly controlled diabetic patients seem to recover quite well from conservative, non-regenerative facilitative procedures such as TMP (see Figure 21.21).

Future research needs

Future research needs to define the precise optimal strain for alveolus subperiosteal osteogenesis. Yokota and Tanaka (2005) reported that, compared with no load controls in mice, osteogenesis was markedly induced with strains approximating 30 μS, well under the minimum effective strain of ~1000 μS, a threshold range thought necessary to evoke bone formation in *ex vivo* mouse femurs. Moreover, there seemed to be a correlation with streaming potentials and fluid flow speed in the medullary cavity of the bone. These findings reinforce our hypothesis that bone bending changes genetic expression (Murphy, 2006), and Baumrind's 1969 attack on the conventional pressure tension model. Mao et al. (2003) have also studied bone responses beyond the ligament and reported that one needs a bone strain threshold of approximately 500 μS for inducing sutural osteogenesis. Interestingly, a regimen of '20 000 μS, 10 times a day', has been documented for distraction osteogenesis of the mandibular corpus (Meyer et al., 2004).

Little do biologists really know which bench-top science project will ultimately prove useful? Since Urist (1965) first identified bone morphogenetic proteins as the critical growth factor in bone repair, the fields of molecular, cell, and developmental biology have become increasingly important in dentofacial orthopedics and have defined gross anatomical landmarks and clinical guidelines with increasingly greater refinement.

Not every case, however, will follow a predictable path. Bilateral asymmetries and various latent periods are the norm in all human cases to a greater or lesser degree. Even if orthodontic appliances deliver 'optimal force' one must consider that the individual biodiversity will render an unpredictable bone response in clinical environments. So, any additional scientific knowledge, even seemingly unrelated data concerning cell behavior can only fortify and improve our predictive powers and minimize treatment morbidities. For example, Wong and Rabie (1999) and Rabie et al. (2000) have reported that using intramembranous bone grafts can result in 166% more new bone than endochondral bone, when grafted into standard skull models of experimental animal defects and, importantly, bone, which SCT forms, is intramembranous. However this kind of subtle knowledge and its clinical application is virtually unknown to average clinicians.

Conclusions

A consilience of styles is clearly evident among clinicians such as Damon (Murphy, 2006), Williams and Murphy (2008), and Wilcko et al. (2008) when an open-minded approach to literature interpretation is employed. This is true for academics also, since all seemingly disparate terms such as 'compensatory appositional osteogenesis' (a paraphrase of Reitan's work, first proposed by Burch [1997]), 'osteogenesis at a distance', 'osteoblastic recruitment', and 'bone matrix transportation' can be seen as attempts to explain observed phenomena in terms of universal biologic principles. While each may not capture the entire domain of reactive bone physiology, an open-minded approach and patience with clinicians' observations promotes synergistic collaboration. This is the stuff of progress in any discipline.

Since the 1950s, when Reitan refined the theories of Sandstedt (1904–1905), Oppenheim (1911–1912), and Schwartz (1932), orthodontists have been seeking to uncover mechanisms that explain or predict tissue behavior and only time can determine which will prevail. By looking beyond the ligament and noting a 'whole bone' perspective, one does not deny events in the periodontal ligament, but rather sees them as part of a larger holistic system of cells and organs, (the alveolus 'organ' being the principal focus). As we enter what has been called 'the century of the biologist', many old paradigms have fallen and many more should be redefined. Even the concepts of frontal and rear resorption and periodontal ligament capillary pressure as therapeutic guides are questionable models for SCT. The idea that orthodontic force should be less than internal capillary pressure in the periodontal ligament is challenged by the observation that at the tissue and cell level, capillary pressure differentials can approach zero. Therefore, perhaps all orthodontic tooth movement has an 'undermining' component in its resorption pattern, especially when we realize the periodontal ligament is only about 0.25 mm wide.

Once the bacteriologist's concept of 'host response', the cell biologist's respect for 'streaming potential' and the molecular biologist's quest for a cytoskeletal 'architectural transcription factor' are all fully integrated into the conceptual framework of dentofacial orthopedics, the specialty will meet twenty-first century challenges and thrive. When the bench-top–chairside connection is fully envisioned, from intracellular cytoskeletal events to the psychosocial behavioral challenges of clinical practice, all theories and empirical data will be seen as mere parts of an integrated whole and all observers through time will be seen as generally correct for some cases.

This chapter has discussed contemporary, evolving clinical science, intending to synthesize and solidify new professional frontiers that are available to orthodontists who wish to expand the scope of their specialty further into areas of legitimate scientific province, an embellishment of the traditional best. Gross anatomical observations of functional orthopedics, viewed through prisms of cellular and molecular events, reveal how all levels of empirical inductive inference can work in harmony with the deductive logic of theory. Then dentofacial orthopedics or more specifically alveolar orthopedics, be it surgical or nonsurgical, can fully exploit the emerging opportunities in twenty-first century biology. Meanwhile, only time and the imagination of dedicated bench-top scientists collaborating freely with industry and astute clinicians can form the kind of synergy that delivers scientific progress and the 'consilience of intellect' that Harvard's Wilson (1998) has implored us to seek, create, and nurture.

For example, when epidemiologists found more periodontal attachment loss in minority adolescents than is normally acknowledged (Cappelli et al., 1994), a closer look at periodontal effects of orthodontic therapy was initiated. When the *New England Journal of Medicine* noted that oral infection causes endothelial damage in coronary arteries (Tonetti et al., 2007) orthodontists responded (MacLaine et al., 2010) and the report of a full-term fetus death caused by hematogenous infection from the mother's mouth (Han et al., 2010) will no doubt initiate investigations about the relationship between oral infection and systemic health in children. It is this kind of scholastic interaction that defines the family of global scientists, as clinical orthodontists cast a broader net of biological inquiry to find truth. In this quest we invite all colleagues, globally, be they in basic science, education or clinical practice, medical or dental, to join our consortium of progress. This spirit of biological enterprise is the requisite mindset for orthodontic stem cell therapy and that is EO Wilson's consilience, indeed.

Carpe diem!

Acknowledgment

This treatise is dedicated to the noble and selfless inspiration of our friend and mentor Dr Donald Enlow, Professor Emeritus, Case Western Reserve University, and the abiding scholastic legacy which he left and we are privileged to sustain.

What nobler employment, or more valuable to the state, than that of the man who instructs the rising generation?

Marcus Tillius Cicero (106–43 BC)

References

Ahlawat A, Ferguson DJ, Wilcko WM, et al. (2006) Influence of DI on orthodontic outcomes following selective alveolar decortication. *Journal of Dental Research* 85(Spec Iss A): abstract 0779.

Aleo JJ, DeRenzis FA, Farber PA, et al. (1974) The presence and biologic activity of cementum-bound endotoxin. *Journal of Periodontology* 45: 672–5.

Anholm JM, Crites DA, Hoff R, et al. (1986) Corticotomy facilitated orthodontics. *Journal of the California Dental Association* 14: 7–11.

Antoci V Jr, Adams CS, Hickok NJ, et al. (2007) Antibiotics for local delivery systems cause skeletal cell toxicity in vitro. *Clinical Orthopaedics and Related Research* 462: 200–6.

Ascher F (1947) Zur Spaetbehandlung der Prognathie des Oberkiefers. *Deutsche Zahnarztliche Zeitschrift* 2: 218–26.

Atherton JD (1970) The gingival response to orthodontic tooth movement. *American Journal of Orthodontics* 58: 179–86.

Baumrind S (1969) A reconsideration of the propriety of the 'pressure-tension' hypothesis. *American Journal of Orthodontics* 55: 12–22.

Bell WH, Levy BM (1972) Revascularization and bone healing after maxillary corticotomies. *Journal of Oral Surgery* 30: 640–8.

Bichlmayr A (1931) Ckirurgische Kieferothopaedie und das Verhalten des Knochens un der Wurzelspitzen nach derselben. *Deutsche Zahnaerztl Woschenschrift* 34: 835–42.

Brosky TA 2nd, Menke CR, Xenos D (2009) Reconstruction of the first metatarsophalangeal joint following post-cheilectomy avascular necrosis of the first metatarsal head: a case report. *Journal of Foot and Ankle Surgery* 48: 61–9.

Brown IS (1973) The effect of orthodontic therapy on certain types of periodontal defects. *Journal of Periodontology* 44: 742–56.

Burch JG (1997) Periodontal responses and problems in orthodontics. Chapter 21: Orthodontic and dentofacial orthopedic section. In: J Hardin (ed.) *Clarks Clinical Dentistry*, Vol 2. St. Louis, MO: Mosby-Yearbook.

Cappelli DP, Ebersole JL, Kornman KS (1994) Early-onset periodontitis in Hispanic-Americans adolescents associated with A. actinomycetemcomitans. *Community Dentistry and Oral Epidemiology* 22: 116–21.

Cohn-Stock G (1921) Die chirurgische immediatregulierung der Kiefer Speziell die Chirurgische Behandlung der Prognathie. *Vierteljahrsschrift fur Zahnheilkunde* 37: 320–54.

Cunningham G (1894) Methode sofortiger Regulierung von anomalen Zahnstellungen. *Oesterreichisch-Ungarische Vierteljahrsschrift fur Zahnheilkunde* 10: 455–7.

Dosanjh MS, Ferguson DJ, Wilcko WM, et al. (2006) Orthodontic outcome changes during retention following selective alveolar decortication. *Journal of Dental Research* 85(Spec Iss A): abstract 0768.

Ducker J (1975) Experimental animal research into segmental alveolar movement after corticotomy. *Journal of Maxillofacial Surgery* 3: 81–4.

Epker BN, Frost HM (1965) Correlation of bone resorption and formation with the physical behavior of loaded bone. *Journal of Dental Research* 44: 33–41.

Ferguson DJ, Sebaoun JD, Turner JW, et al. (2006) Anabolic modeling of trabecular bone following selective alveolar decortication. In: *Joint Symposium of the American Dental Education Association, American Association of Dental Research, California Association of Dental Research*, Paper 0768, Orlando, Florida, March 9–11.

Fuhrmann RAW (2002) Three-dimensional evaluation of periodontal remodeling during orthodontic treatment. *Seminars in Orthodontics* 8: 22–8.

Fulk L (2002) Lower arch decrowding comparing corticotomy-facilitated, midline distraction and conventional orthodontic techniques. Master's thesis, St. Louis University, MO, USA.

Gantes B, Rathbun E, Anholm M (1990) Effects on the periodontium following corticotomy-facilitated orthodontics, Case reports. *Journal of Periodontology* 62: 234–8.

Generson RM, Porter JM, Zell A, et al. (1978) Combined surgical and orthodontic management of anterior open bite using corticotomy. *Journal of Oral Surgery* 36: 216–19.

Grubb JE, Greco PM, English JD, et al. (2008) Radiographic and periodontal requirements of the American Board Of Orthodontics: A modification in case display requirements for adults and periodontally involved adolescents and preadolescent patients. *American Journal of Orthodontics and Dentofacial Orthopedics* 134: 3–4.

Hajji SS (2002) The influence of accelerated osteogenic response on mandibular decrowding, Master's thesis, St. Louis University, MO, USA.

Han YW, Fardini Y, Chen C, et al. (2010) Term stillbirth caused by oral fusobacterium nucleatum. *Obstetrics and Gynecology* 115: 442–5.

Ingber DE (1998) Cellular basis of mechanotransduction. *Biological Bulletin* 194: 323–7.

Ingber DE (2006) Cellular basis of mechanotransduction: putting all the pieces together again. *FASEB Journal* 20: 811–27.

Ingber JS (1974) Forced eruption as a method of treating one and two wall infrabony defects – a rationale and case report. *Journal of Periodontology* 45: 199–206.

Ingber JS (1976) Forced eruption Part II A method of treating isolated one and two wall infrabony osseous defects – rationale and case report. *Journal of Periodontology* 47: 203–16.

Iseri H, Kisnisci R, Bzizi N, et al. (2005) Rapid canine retraction and orthodontic treatment with dentoalveolar distraction osteogenesis. *American Journal of Orthodontics and Dentofacial Orthopedics* 127: 533–41.

Kacewicz MJ, Ferguson DJ, Wilcko WM (2004) Characterization of tooth movement in corticotomy-facilitated, non-extraction orthodontics. *Journal of Dental Research* 83(Spec Iss A): abstract 1289.

Kawakami T, Nishimoto M, Matsuda Y, et al. (1996) Histologic suture changes following retraction of the maxillary anterior bone segment after corticotomy. *Endodontics and Dental Traumatology* 12: 38–43.

Kelson CL, Ferguson DJ, Wilcko WM (2005) Characterization of maxillary tooth movement in corticotomy-facilitated orthodontics. *Journal of Dental Research* 84(Spec Iss A): abstract 1299.

Kole K (1959) Surgical operations of the alveolar ridge to correct occlusal abnormalities. *Oral Surgery, Oral Medicine, Oral Pathology* 12: 515–29.

Liou EJW, Huang CS (1998) Rapid canine retraction through distraction of the periodontal ligament. *American Journal of Orthodontics and Dentofacial Orthopedics* 114: 372–82.

Little RM (1993) Stability and relapse of dental arch alignment. In: CJ Burstone, R Nanda (eds) *Retention and Stabilty in Orthodontics*. Philadelphia, PA: WB Saunders, pp. 97–106.

Little RM, Riedel RA, Artun J (1998) An evaluation of changes in mandibular anterior alignment from 10 to 20 years post-retention. *American Journal of Orthodontics and Dentofacial Orthopedics* 93: 423–8.

Machado I, Ferguson DJ, Wilcko WM (2002) Root resorption following orthodontics with and without alveolar corticotomy. *Journal of Dental Research* 81: abstract 2378.

MacLaine J, Rabie ABM, Wong R (2010) Does orthodontic tooth movement cause an elevation in systemic inflammatory markers? *European Journal of Orthodontics* 32: 435–40.

Mao JJ, Wang X, Mooney MP, et al. (2003) Strain induced osteogenesis of the craniofacial suture upon controlled delivery of low-frequency cyclic forces. *Frontiers in Bioscience* 8: a10–17.

Matsuda Y (1989) Effect of two stage corticotomy on maxillary protraction. *Journal of the Japanese Orthodontic Society* 48: 506–20.

Melsen B (2001) Tissue reaction to orthodontic tooth movement – A new paradigm. *European Journal of Orthodontics* 23: 671–81.

Merrill RG, Pedersen GW (1976) Interdental osteotomy for immediate repositioning of dental-osseous elements. *Journal of Oral Surgery* 34: 118–25.

Meyer U, Kleinheinz J, Joos U (2004) Biomechanical and clinical implications of distraction osteogenesis in craniofacial surgery. *Journal of Cranio-Maxillofacial Surgery* 32: 140–9.

Mihram WL (1997) Dynamic biologic transformation of the periodontium: a clinical report. *Journal of Prosthetic Dentistry* 78: 337–40.

Mihram WL, Murphy NC (2008) The orthodontists role in 21st century periodontic-prosthodontists therapy. *Seminars in Orthodontics* 14: 272–89.

Moskow BS (1987) Longevity: a critical factor in evaluating the effectiveness of periodontal therapy. *Journal of Clinical Periodontology* 14: 237–44.

Moss ML (1997a) The functional matrix hypothesis revisited, 1. The role of mechanotransduction. *American Journal of Orthodontics and Dentofacial Orthopedics* 112: 8–11.

Moss ML (1997b) The functional matrix hypothesis revisited. 2. The role of an osseous connected cellular network. *American Journal of Orthodontics and Dentofacial Orthopedics* 112: 221–6.

Moss ML (1997c) The functional matrix hypothesis revisited, 3.The genomic thesis. *American Journal of Orthodontics and Dentofacial Orthopedics* 112: 338–42.

Moss ML (1997d) The functional matrix hypothesis revisited. 4. The epigenetic antithesis and the resolving synthesis. *American Journal of Orthodontics and Dentofacial Orthopedics* 112: 410–17.

Moss ML (2004) Genetics, epigenetics, and causation. *American Journal of Orthodontics and Dentofacial Orthopedics* 80: 366–75.

Mostaza YA, Tawfik KM, El-Mangoury NH (1985) Surgical-orthodontic treatment for overerupted maxillary molars. *Journal of Clinical Orthodontics* 19: 350–1.

Murphy NC (2006) In vivo tissue engineering for orthodontists: a modest first step. In: Z Davidovitch, J Mah, S Suthanarak (eds) *Biological Mechanisms of Tooth Eruption, Resorption and Movement*. Boston, MA: Harvard Society for the Advancement of Orthodontics, pp. 385–410.

Nakanishi H (1982) Experimental study on artificial tooth movement with osteotomy and corticotomy. *Journal of the Tokyo Dental College Society* 82: 219–52.

Navarov AD, Ferguson DJ, Wilcko WM, et al. (2004) Improved orthodontics retention following corticotomy using ABO objective grading system. *Journal of Dental Research* 83(Spec Iss A): abstract 2644.

Neuman D (1955) Die Bichlmayrsche keilresektion bei der kieferothopaedischen Spaetbehandlung. *Fortschrift der Kierfer-und Gesichts-Chirurgie* 1: 205–10.

Nowzari H, Yorita FK, Chang HC (2008) Periodontally accelerated osteogenic orthodontics combined with autogenous bone grafting. *Compendium of Continuing Education in Dentistry* 29: 200–6.

Oliveira K, Ferguson DJ, Wilcko WM, et al. (2006) Orthodontic stability of advanced lower incisors following selective alveolar decortications. *Journal of Dental Research* 85(Spec Iss A): abstract 0769.

Oppenheim A (1911) Tissue changes particularly in bone incident to tooth movement. *American Orthodontist* 3: 57–8.

Owen AH (2001) Accelerated Invisalign treatment. *Journal of Clinical Orthodontics* 35: 381–5.

Palomo L, Palomo JM, Bissada NF (2008) Salient periodontal issues for the modern biologic orthodontist. *Seminars in Orthodontics* 14: 229–45.

Patel SA, Sherman L, Munoz J, et al. (2008) Immunological properties of mesenchymal stem cells and clinical implications. *Archivium Immunologiae et Therapiae Experimentalis* 56: 1–8.

Rabie ABM, Chay SH, Wong AM (2000) Healing of autogenous intramembranous bone in the presence and absence of homologous demineralized intramembranous bone. *American Journal of Orthodontics and Dentofacial Orthopedics* 117: 288–97.

Rothe LE, Bollen AM, Little RM, et al. (2006) Trabecular and cortical bone as risk factors for orthodontic relapse. *American Journal of Orthodontics and Dentofacial Orthopedics* 130: 476–84.

Sanders NL (1999) Evidence-based care in orthodontics and periodontics: a review of the literature. *Journal of the American Dental Association* 130: 521–7.

Sandstedt CE (1904) Einge beitrage zur theorie der zahnregulierung, Nord. Tandl Tidsskr 5, p. 236. Cited by Gianelli AA (1969) Force-induced changes in the vascularity of the periodontal ligament. *American Journal of Orthodontics* 55: 5–11.

Schwartz AM (1932) Tissue changes incident to orthodontic tooth movement. *International Journal of Orthodontia* 18: 331–52.

Sebaoun JD, Ferguson DJ, Kantarci A, et al. (2006) Catabolic modeling of trabecular bone following selective alveolar decortication. *Journal of Dental Research* 85(Spec Iss A): abstract 0787.

Tonetti MS, D'Aiuto F, Nibali L, et al. (2007) Treatment of periodontitis and endothelial function. *New England Journal of Medicine* 356: 911–20.

Twaddle BA (2001) Dentoalveolar bone density changes following accelerated osteogenesis, Masters thesis, St. Louis University, Missouri.

Urist MR (1965) Bone: formation by autoinduction. *Science* 150: 893–9.

Waldrop TC (2008) Gummy smiles: the challenge of gingival excess: prevalence and guidelines for clinical management. *Seminars in Orthodontics* 14: 260–71.

Wilcko MT, Wilcko WM, Bissada NF (2008) An evidence-based analysis of periodontally accelerated orthodontic and osteogenic techniques: a synthesis of scientific perspective. *Seminars in Orthodontics* 14: 305–16.

Wilcko WM, Wilcko MT, Bouquot JE, et al. (2001) Rapid orthodontics with alveolar reshaping: two case reports of decrowding. *International Journal of Periodontics and Restorative Dentistry* 21: 9–19.

Wilcko WM, Ferguson DJ, Bouquot JE, et al. (2003) Rapid orthodontic decrowding with alveolar augmentation: case report. *World Journal of Orthodontics* 4: 197–205.

Williams MO, Murphy NC (2008) Beyond the ligament: a whole-bone periodontal view of dentofacial orthopedics and falsification of alveolar immutability. *Seminars in Orthodontics* 14: 246–59.

Wilson EO (1998) *Consilience, the Unity of Knowledge*, 1st edn. New York, NY: Alfred A. Knopf, Inc.

Wong RWK, Rabie ABM (1999) A quantitative assessment of the healing of intramembranous and endochondral autogenous bone grafts. *European Journal of Orthodontics* 21: 119–26.

Yokota H, Tanaka SM (2005) Osteogenic potentials with joint-loading modality. *Journal of Bone and Mineral Metabolism* 23: 302–8.

Yoshikawa Y (1987) Effect of corticotomy on maxillary retraction induced by orthopedic force. *Journal of the Matsumoto Dental College Society* 13: 292–320.

Zaky SH, Cancedda R (2009) Engineering craniofacial structures: facing the challenge. *Journal of Dental Research* 88: 1077–91.

Zhang P, Su M, Tanaka S, et al. (2006) Knee loading causes diaphyseal cortical bone formation in murine femurs. *BMC Musculoskeletal Disorders* 73: 1–12.

Zhang P, Su M, Liu Y, et al. (2007) Knee loading dynamically alters intramedullary pressure in mouse femora. *Bone* 40: 538–43.

Suggested reading

Alberts A, Johnson A, Lewis J (2007) *Molecular Biology of the Cell*, 5th edn. New York, NY: Garland Science.

Bilezikian JP, Raisz LG, Martin TJ (2008) *Principles of Bone Biology*, 3rd edn. New York, NY: Academic Press.

Clausen K, Keck D, Hiesey W (1958) Experimental studies in the nature of species, Vol 3. Environmental responses of climatic races of achillea. *Carnegie Institution of Washington Publication* 581: 1–129.

De Visser J, Hermisson J, Wagner G, et al. (1993) Perspective: evolution and detection of genetic robustness. *Evolution* 57: 1959–72.

Fisher R (1931) The evolution of dominance. *Biological Reviews* 6: 345–68.

Goss P, Peccoud J (1998) Quantitative modeling of stochastic systems in molecular biology using stochastic Petri nets. *Proceedings of the National Academy of Sciences U S A* 95: 6750–5.

Haldane JBS (1939) The theory of the evolution of dominance. *Journal of Genetics* 37: 365–74.

Lanza R (2009) *Essentials of Stem Cell Biology*, 2nd edn. New York, NY: Academic Press.

Lewontin R, Goss P (2004) Developmental canalization, stochasticity and robustness. In: E Jen (ed.) *Robust Design: A Repertoire of Biological, Ecological, and Engineering Case Studies*. New York, NY: Oxford University Press.

McAdams H, Arkin A (1997) Stochastic mechanisms in gene expression. *Proceedings of the National Academy of Sciences* USA 94: 814–19.

Rendel J (1967) *Canalization and Gene Control*. London: Academic, Logos Press.

Schmalhausen I (1949) *Factors of Evolution*. Philadelphia, PA: Blakiston.

Smith M, Sondhi K (1960) The genetics of a pattern. *Genetics* 45: 1039–50.

Waddington C (1953) Genetic assimilation of an acquired character. *Evolution* 7: 118–26.

Waddington C (1957) *The Strategy of the Genes*. London: Allen and Unwin.

22

The Application of Lasers in Orthodontics

Neal D Kravitz

Summary

As an adjunctive procedure, soft tissue laser surgery has helped many orthodontists elevate the level of patient care by increasing treatment efficacy, improving oral hygiene around fixed appliances during orthodontic treatment, and enhancing final smile esthetics. Specifically, soft tissue lasers have numerous applications in the orthodontic practice, including: gingivectomy and gingivoplasty, flattening of bulbous papillae, frenectomy, exposure of partially erupted teeth, uncovering temporary anchorage devices, operculectomy, ablation of aphthous ulcerations, and even tooth-whitening. This chapter will review the two most popular lasers used in orthodontics: the diode laser and the solid-state laser, and provide an overview of laser physics, equipment set-up, choosing an appropriate anesthetic, proper laser technique, billing and insurance codes, and laser safety.

Definition and laser physics

LASER is an acronym for 'light amplification by stimulated emission of radiation'. Fundamentally, a laser beam is a focused source of electromagnetic radiation, or light-energy. Laser light energy is defined by three properties:

- Monochromatic (of one color or wavelength)
- Directional
- Coherent.

Simply, a laser beam is a concentrated source of light energy composed of one wavelength, which travels in a specific direction, and all wavelengths of the laser light travel in phase. These properties differ from ordinary light, which is diffuse and non-coherent, allowing laser light energy to target accurately and with high intensity.

The acronym 'laser' actually describes the physics behind how a laser beam is created. A laser machine releases light-energy whenever the laser medium is stimulated. Stimulation of the laser medium causes one of its electrons to drop from a higher energy state (Q_1) to a lower energy state (Q_2), releasing light energy – a process referred to as *stimulated emission of radiation*. The energy released by the laser medium becomes amplified before exiting through a collimated tube to provide a concentrated source of light energy – the laser beam (Moritz, 2006).

Components of a laser

All lasers consist of three basic components:

- The laser medium (sometimes referred to as a gain medium)
- The pump source
- The optical cavity or optical resonator.

Laser medium

The laser medium is the 'active element' which produces the laser beam. Most elements in the periodic table can be used as media to develop a laser beam. A laser medium can be a gas, dye (in liquid), solid-state element (distributed in a solid crystal or glass matrix), or semiconductor (diode). The medium will determine the wavelength output, which primarily influences the efficacy of the laser at the target site.

Pump source

The pump source 'stimulates' the lasing medium until light-energy is emitted. Examples of pump sources include:

Integrated Clinical Orthodontics, First Edition. Edited by Vinod Krishnan, Ze'ev Davidovitch.
© 2012 Blackwell Publishing Ltd. Published 2012 by Blackwell Publishing Ltd.

electrical discharges, flash-lamps, arc-lamps, or chemical reactions. The type of pump source used depends on the type of laser medium.

Optical cavity or resonator

The laser optical cavity or resonator amplifies the light-energy. The optical cavity is a compartment of mirrors that contains the laser medium. Light-energy released from the laser medium is reflected by the mirrors back on to itself (referred to as feedback), where it may be amplified by stimulated emission before exciting the cavity. The alignment of the mirrors with respect to the laser medium will determine the exact operating wavelength of the laser system.

In summary, a laser is a special form of artificial light with specific properties. A laser beam is produced within a laser machine when the pump source stimulates the laser media, releasing light energy which amplifies as it travels through the optical cavity. The amplified light energy released from the machine is what we refer to as the laser beam. When light energy enters the target tissue, it transforms into heat – a process known as *the photothermal effect* – resulting in the vaporization of the target tissue cells.

Thermal ablation

Unlike a scalpel which slices, a laser separates tissue by *thermal ablation*. Thermal ablation is an instantaneous process of absorption, melting, and then vaporization, resulting in decomposition of the tissue. As the target cells absorb the concentrated light-energy of the laser beam, the tissue rapidly rises in temperature. The target cells instantly undergo stages of warming, welding, coagulation, protein denaturization, drying, and vaporization via a micro-explosion known as *spallation* (Sarver and Yanosky, 2005).

Thermal ablation is dependent on the amount of light energy absorbed, which is determined primarily by the wavelength of the laser. The degree of tissue absorption is influenced by:

- Laser wavelength (measured in nanometers) – a component of the laser media
- Electrical power of the surgical unit (measured in watts)
- Exposure time
- Composition and thickness of the tissues.

In summary, lasers separate tissue by thermal ablation. The type of laser media produces a specific wavelength, which among other factors, influences the degree of tissue absorption and thus the 'cutting' power of the laser.

Historical perspective

As early as 1917, American physicist Albert Einstein first proposed the theory of 'stimulated emission', the process which made lasers possible. In 1954, Charles Townes at Columbia University demonstrated a working device using ammonia gas as the active medium that produced microwave amplification and the first generation of electromagnetic radiation by stimulated emissions. This device was called the 'maser' which is an acronym for microwave amplification by stimulated emission of radiation. In 1958, Arthur Schawlow, Townes's brother-in-law, proposed the operation of optical and infrared masers, or 'lasers' – a term first coined by physicist Gordon Gould in 1957.

In 1960, the first laser to use visible light (using a ruby medium) was developed by physicist Theodor H Maiman, following the theoretical work of Einstein, Townes, and Schawlow. In 1962, Robert Hall developed the first diode or semiconductor laser. The carbon dioxide gas laser was invented by Kumar Patel in 1964, and 4 years later this laser was used to perform the first soft tissue surgery.

In 1985, Paghidiwala, tested the erbium-doped solid state laser (Er:YAG) on dental hard tissue. Nearly a decade later, in 1997, the United States Food and Drug Administration (FDA) approved the Er:YAG solid-state laser for hard tissue surgery. The following year (1998), the first diode laser was approved for soft tissue surgery. More than 25 years since Dr Paghidiwala first tested a laser on dental tissues, dental laser technology has undergone remarkable advancements in design. Contemporary dental laser machinery has become portable, compact, wireless, safer, increasingly affordable, and simpler to operate, allowing more orthodontists to incorporate soft tissue laser surgery into their practice.

Laser versus scalpel

A laser offers numerous advantages compared with conventional scalpel surgery. The most significant advantage is that a laser coagulates capillaries, seals lymphatics, and sterilizes the surgical field during ablation (Sarver and Yanosky, 2005). Separation of tissue is more precise with a laser than a scalpel (Rossman and Cobb, 1995). Additionally, minor aphthous and herpetic ulcerations – which commonly occur during the early stages of treatment as the patients get accustomed to their orthodontic appliances – can be vaporized. Laser surgery is routinely performed using only light local anesthetic or compound topical anesthetic. Furthermore, there is markedly less bleeding with laser surgery, particularly for frenal surgery, as well as minimal edema, and no need for sutures or unsightly periodontal dressing (Haytac and Ozcelik, 2006). A report suggested that laser excisions produce less scar tissue than conventional scalpel surgery (Fisher et al., 1983), although contrary evidence also exists (Buell and Schuller, 1983; Frame, 1985). Post-surgically, patients report less discomfort, fewer complications related to speaking and chewing, and require less pain medication than do patients treated with conventional scalpel surgery (Haytac and Ozcelik, 2006). The benefits of laser surgery are best summarized by Sarver and Yanosky (2005): '[soft tissue lasers] result

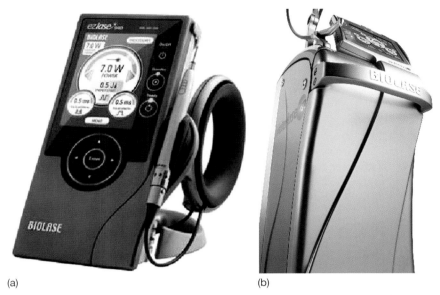

(a)   (b)

Figure 22.1 (a) Ezlase 940 diode laser and (b) Waterlase MD Turbo (Er,Cr:YSGG) erbium-doped solid-state laser (Biolase). Images are not to scale.

in shorter operative time and faster post-operative recuperation.'

The primary disadvantage of laser surgery is the operatory and upkeep expense. Some clinicians have reported additional disadvantages, such as: less tactile sensation, tissue desiccation, and poor wound healing (Baker et al., 2002). Furthermore, laser surgery is primarily excisional and performed without a flap, often resulting in no change in alveolar crest height. As such, there is a tendency for significant tissue rebounding or regrowth after laser surgery.

Diode versus solid-state lasers

The two most popular lasers used in dentistry are the *diode* and the *solid-state lasers* (Figure 22.1). Diode lasers are almost exclusively used for soft tissue surgery. Solid-state lasers, on the other hand, can be used for both soft and hard tissue surgery, such as tooth preparation, root canal debridement, and crown lengthening. The fundamental difference between a diode and a solid-state laser is the laser medium, which generates laser beams of different wavelengths. As already stated, the laser medium determines the wavelength output, which ultimately influences the efficacy of thermal ablation at the target site.

Diode (semiconductor) lasers

Diode lasers convert electrical energy into light energy. Diode lasers are known as semiconductors, as they use a media of gallium and arsenide, and occasionally indium and aluminum, whose ability to conduct electricity is between that of conductors and insulators. By doping the laser medium with impurities (dopants), stimulated emission occurs.

The wavelengths produced by diode lasers range between 810 nm and 980 nm. Light energy at these wavelengths is easily absorbed by melanin (soft tissue pigmentation) and hemoglobin, and poorly absorbed by enamel. Therefore, diode lasers are highly effective in soft tissue ablation, hemostasis, and sealing lymphatics, with low risk of damaging teeth and bone, making them ideal for soft tissue laser surgery (Kravitz and Kusnoto, 2008). Compared with other laser types, diode lasers are compact, reliable, and have a long operatory lifetime, and are packaged in portable units typically weighing less than 4.5 kg (10 lb). Connecting to the main unit is a thin, pencil-sized hand-piece containing a 200–400 μm fiberoptic tip. Newer models have handpieces that receive single-use, twist-on laser fiberoptic tips, providing a higher potential standard of cleanliness and eliminating time-consuming stripping and cleaving of the fiberoptic tip.

Priming

Before surgery with a diode laser, the fiberoptic tip must be conditioned or *primed*. All diode lasers need to have some type of pigment applied to the fiber tip in order to create a sufficient amount of energy for ablation. *Priming* is the process of concentrating heat energy at the fiberoptic tip (Tracey, 2005). Priming is performed by tapping an

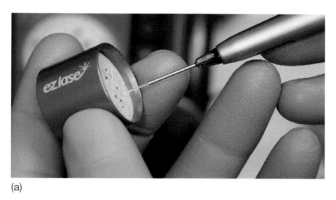
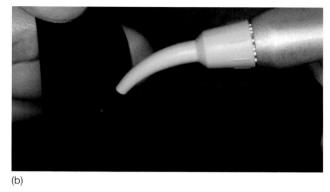

(a)   (b)

Figure 22.2 Priming a diode laser with a cork or thick, blue articulating paper. (a) EZlase 940 and (b) Odyssey Navigator (Ivoclar Vivadent).

initiated-fiberoptic tip on thick blue articulating paper (Figure 22.2), a felt tip marker, a solid color in a magazine page, or a cork. Essentially, the laser tries to ablate the pigmented region, creating a super focus of light energy. Failure to properly prime the diode laser may result in less effective tissue ablation.

During laser surgery with a diode, the fiberoptic tip should be held in *light-contact* with the tissue. For the majority of surgeries, soft tissue ablation is performed at 1.0–1.5 W, with gentle, sweeping brush strokes. All lasers are collimated; as such, the 'cutting' end is at the tip. Therefore, dragging the laser sideways tends to collect soft tissue build-up and may even damage the fiberoptic tip. During surgery with a diode laser, tissue margins may appear dark and charred. High-speed suction is critical to remove laser plume and burnt tissue smell, as well as to maintain a clear field of vision (Figure 22.3).

Solid-state lasers

Solid-state lasers use a gain medium that is a solid, rather than a liquid or gas. It should be noted that semiconductor lasers are also in the solid state, but are considered in a separate class from solid-state lasers. The active laser medium in a solid-state laser consists of a glass or crystalline matrix. Two common matrices are the yttrium aluminum garnet (YAG) and the yttrium scandium gadolinium garnet (YSGG). Comparative studies have shown little difference in efficacy between the two (Harashima et al., 2005). Atoms in the crystal are excited to produce light energy when dopants, such as erbium, chromium, and neodymium, are added to the medium (i.e. Nd:YAG, Er:YAG, or ErCr:YSGG). Erbium-doped solid state lasers are most commonly used in dentistry (Kravitz and Kusnoto, 2008).

The wavelengths produced by erbium-doped solid-state lasers range between 2780 nm and 2940 nm. Unlike diode lasers, light energy at this wavelength is easily absorbed by hydroxyapatite and surface tissue water, and therefore can

ablate both hard and soft tissues. Erbium-doped solid-state lasers are routinely used by pediatric dentists and general dentists for caries excavation, and less frequently for endodontic and periodontal procedures. When performing soft tissue laser surgery with an erbium-doped solid-state laser, the laser machine is operated at low electrical power to reduce the depth of tissue penetration (Kravitz and Kusnoto, 2008).

For most gingival surgeries, soft tissue excision may require 1.5–2.5 W depending on the tissue thickness. Coagulation with a solid-state laser requires a different setting, generally less than 1.0 W often without water spray. It should be noted that a solid-state laser will begin to ablate hard tissue at approximately 4.0–5.0 W. Solid-state lasers are packaged in larger, more complex rolling units (weighing up to 40 kg or 90 lb). The laser handpiece resembles a high-speed handpiece with removable fiberoptic tips ranging from 400 μm to 750 μm.

During surgery with an erbium-doped solid-state laser, the fiberoptic tip should be held *1 mm away* from the tissue (Hadley et al., 2000). Priming is not required as the solid-state lasing medium does not absorb pigmentation. Excision is performed with slow, short back-and-forth strokes. Coagulation is achieved under a different operatory setting, with low wattage and often no water. Tissues appear slightly reddish during excision and chalky white after coagulation. Although a solid-state later can effectively control hemorrhaging, hemostasis may be easier with a diode, particularly during more invasive soft tissue surgeries such as frenectomies.

Choosing a proper anesthetic

Soft tissue lasers both coagulate and produce a mild anesthetic effect during ablation. Accordingly, many clinicians perform soft tissue laser surgery using only light local anesthesia, strong topical anesthesia, or without any anesthesia at all. Local infiltration with 2% lidocaine, 4%

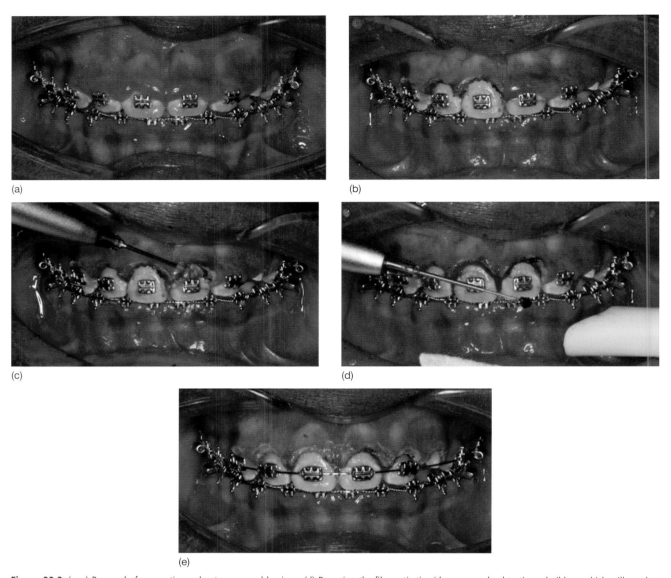

(a)

(b)

(c)

(d)

(e)

Figure 22.3 (a–e) Removal of excess tissue due to poor oral hygiene. (d) Dragging the fiberoptic tip sideways can lead to tissue build-up which will need to be removed with a 2 × 2 gauze. High-speed suction is critical to eliminate laser plume.

articaine, or occasionally 3% mepivacaine (in patients with contributory heart conditions) can be limited to the specific surgical site, i.e. interpapillary, interligamentary (the periodontal pocket), interseptal or directly into the frenum or operculum. The injection can be performed using a short or long 27 or 30 gauge needle. This method is often relatively painless, requires very little anesthesia, and is useful for anxious children who may not tolerate conventional local anesthetic technique. However, some clinicians desire a more profound anesthetic effect and prefer superior alveolar nerve blocks at the height of the mucobuccal fold.

Debate regarding compound topical anesthetics

There has been a growing interest among orthodontists and pediatric dentists in the use of strong topical compound anesthetics to be used in place of local infiltration. Compounding is the process by which the pharmacist or dentist combines, mixes, or alters pharmaceutical ingredients to create an individualized medication in accordance with a prescription (United States Pharmacopeial Convention, 2004). Essentially, compound topical anesthetics are nonregulated, custom-made, strong topical formulations.

Compound topical anesthetics are often highly viscous to prevent against run-off, include several active anesthetic agents to provide a wide spectrum of anesthetic action, and contain a vasoconstrictive agent. Specifically, common formulations include high concentrations of both amide (lidocaine and prilocaine) and ester (tetracaine) anesthetics, and small dosages of the nasal decongestant phenylephrine. Popular compound topical anesthetics, such as TAC 20% Alternate (20% lidocaine, 2% phenylephrine, 4% tetracaine) and Profound PET (10% lidocaine, 10% prilocaine, 4% tetracaine, 2% phenylephrine) are widely used by orthodontists for soft tissue laser surgery and placement of orthodontic temporary anchorage devices. These topical local anesthetics are contraindicated in elderly patients, those with hypersensitivity to ester- and amide-type local anesthetics, para-aminobenzoic acid (PABA) allergies, severe hypertension, hyperthyroidism, or heart disease. To date, compound topical anesthetics such as TAC 20% Alternate and Profound PET are neither FDA regulated nor unregulated drug products (Kravitz, 2007).

Though highly effective, concern exists regarding the safety of these anesthetics (Jeffcoat, 2004). The risks regarding use of compound topical anesthetics are the following:

- Not-regulated by the Federal Food Drug and Cosmetic Act
- Vials may be improperly mixed, measured, or labeled (Figure 22.4)
- Maximum recommended dosage (MRD) is unknown as they are intended for individual use only
- Low therapeutic index – a narrow difference between optimal dose and toxic dose
- Often contain high concentrations of ester anesthetics, which may lead to PABA anaphylaxis.

Doctors who store and repeatedly use the same compound formulation on multiple patients may be in violation of state and federal laws. To date, two deaths have been attributed to the lay use of excessive amounts of compound topical anesthetics. Clinicians who are intent on using compound topical anesthetics may consider the following protocol.

1. Review medical history to ensure no contributory health conditions.
2. Dry the mucosa with 2 × 2 gauze.
3. Apply 0.2 mL (equivalent to one cotton swab head) of topical anesthetic to the mucosa.
4. Let the topical anesthetic remain on tissue for 3–5 minutes while the doctor remains with the patient. Prolonged application can cause tissue-irritation and sloughing.
5. Suction away topical and confirm anesthesia with a periodontal probe. Anesthetic effect will last approximately 30 minutes.

Despite the risks, there is arguably a place for doctor-prescribed, doctor-applied compound topical anesthetics for use sparingly on an individualized basis. However, until these drugs become federally regulated, the large-scale pre-production of popular formulations by big pharmacies remains an end-run on manufacturing requirements, and their routine multi-patient use by either orthodontists or other dental specialists remains a questionable therapeutic practice.

Laser machine set-up

All soft tissue lasers have similar machine components and set-up steps. The main components of a dental laser machine include:

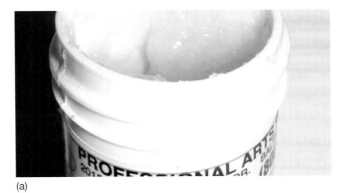
(a)

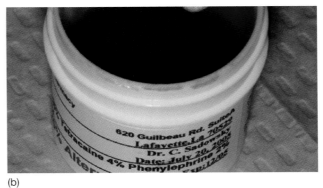
(b)

Figure 22.4 (a,b) Variability of compound topical anesthetics. Two photos of the same common-name anesthetic TAC 20% Alternate ordered from different compounding pharmacies. Note the significant difference in quality of mixture. Since compound topical anesthetics are not federally regulated, vials may be improperly labeled.

- A touch-screen control system, which incorporates factory loaded pre-sets and customizable settings such as watts, joules, and pulse repetition rates
- A handpiece with a fiberoptic tip
- Foot pedal or footswitch to initiate laser firing
- Protective goggles for the patient, the doctor, and the assistant, which blocks a range of wavelengths specific to the laser.

First, connect the power cable and footswitch, and then place a sterilized fiberoptic tip on the handpiece. Second, turn on the machine and use the touch-screen window to control the appropriate settings. Ablation of thicker tissue may require increased wattage, whereas surgeries with a likelihood of bleeding such as frenal surgery or inflamed tissue may respond better to continuous-mode laser firing rather than pulsed-mode. Erbium-doped solid-state lasers typically connect to the air-pressure valves in the chairside delivery unit and may require distilled water. Third, prepare to initiate laser firing by switching the laser from 'standby' to 'ready' mode. Finally, initiate laser firing by pressing on the footswitch. If needed, prime the laser tip at this point prior to entering the mouth. Remove foot from the pedal to cease laser initiation and move the handpiece to the mouth before initiating laser firing again (Figure 22.5).

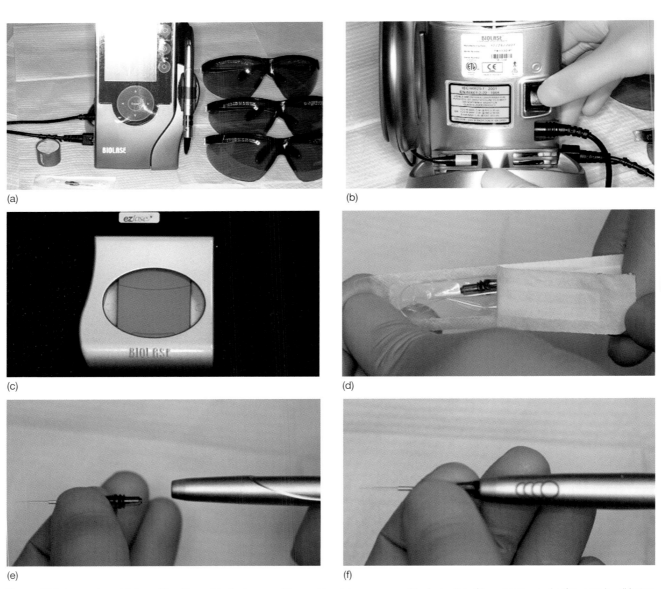

(a)

(b)

(c)

(d)

(e)

(f)

Figure 22.5 Laser set-up. (a) Laser kits will provide the laser machine and handpiece, power cable, footswitch, fiberoptic tips, and safety goggles. (b) First, connect the cables and turn on the power. (c–i) Then, twist on the fiberoptic tip. Using the touch-screen monitor, select the appropriate procedure and modify the settings as needed. When ready to initiate laser firing, touch the 'ready' button on the monitor and (j–k) step on the footswitch. (l) A red light will be visible at the end of the fiberoptic tip when the laser is initiated. Priming should begin now prior to entering the mouth.

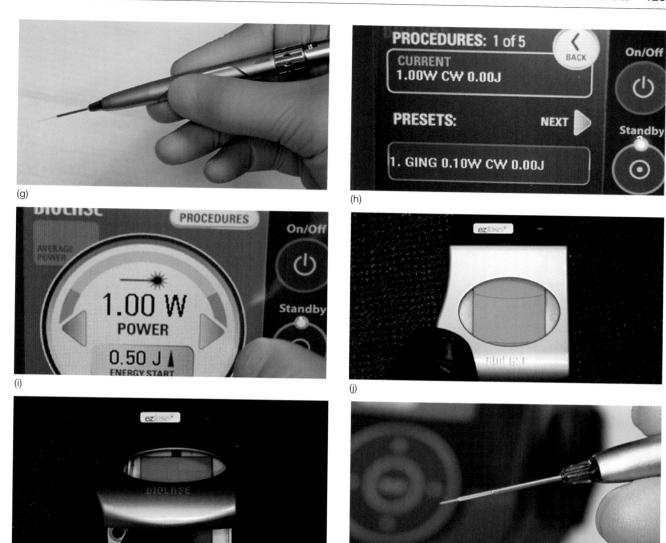

(g)

(h)

(i)

(j)

(k)

(l)

Figure 22.5 *Continued*

Procedures and surgical technique

Gingivectomy and gingivoplasty

(Recommend laser settings: diode laser: 1.0–1.5 W; erbium-doped solid-state laser: 1.5–2.5 W)

Gingivectomy is the surgical removal of a portion of gingival tissue for improved oral health, functional contour or esthetic appearance (*Glossary of Periodontal Terms*, 2001). The history of gingivectomy dates back to 1742, when Fauchard proposed a surgical procedure to remove excessive gingival tissue. In 1884, researcher and clinician Robicsek first described the semicircular excision of labial and lingual

interdental tissue prior to drilling of 'diseased' bone. In 1912, Henry Percy Pickerill's famous book, *Stomatology in General Practice*, further described the operation. By the first half of the nineteenth century, following the landmark research of Ziesel, Nodine, Orban, Kronfeld, Sischer, and Goldman, the etiology of pyorrhea or periodontal disease was no longer thought to be exclusive to bone. Nonetheless, the focus of gingivectomy surgery remained on pocket elimination and not soft tissue esthetics (Kremenak and Squier, 1997; Armitage and Robertson, 2009).

Gingivoplasty is the surgical reshaping and re-contouring of the outer surface of gingival tissue for cosmetic, physiological, or functional purposes, usually done in combination with gingivectomy. With conventional scalpel surgery, gingivoplasty corrected the thick, unnatural gingival margins left after the gingivectomy procedure. With soft tissue laser surgery, gingivectomy and gingivoplasty are almost always used simultaneously to improve gingival health and enhance smile esthetics.

Smile esthetics

Esthetic soft tissue laser surgery is aimed at producing an acceptable gingival display with proper gingival shape and contour, while incorporating the cosmetic principles of proper tooth-size and proportion.

The maxillary anterior teeth should follow two basic principles of cosmetic dentistry. First, the width of maxillary incisors should be approximately 80% the height. Second, the widths of the anterior teeth should follow the 'golden proportion'; that is, the width of the lateral incisor should be two-thirds the width of the central incisor, and the width of the mesial-half of the canine should be two-thirds the width of the lateral incisor (Sarver, 2004) (Figures 22.6, 22.7). While the need for enameloplasty is a result of tooth-shape discrepancies, the extent of incisal reduction is often guided by the amount of overbite and the length of the incisors. In patients with small incisors or large incisal fractures, enameloplasty is enhanced when working in conjunction with soft tissue laser surgery (Kravitz, 2010).

Recommended gingival shape or curvature of the gingival margin has the gingival zeniths of the maxillary lateral incisors and mandibular incisors *coinciding* with the long axes of the teeth. Alternatively, the gingival zeniths of the maxillary central incisors and canines are *distal* to their long axes (Sarver and Yanosky, 2005). In addition, the gingival height of maxillary central incisors and canines should be 0.5 mm above the maxillary lateral incisors. The maxillary lateral incisors often benefit esthetically from a 0.5 mm gingival-step as well as a 0.5 mm incisal-step (Kravitz, 2010).

Upon animated smile, the patient should reveal 1–4 mm of gingival display – the amount of exposed tissue from the gingival margins of the anterior teeth to the bottom of the upper lip (Kokich et al., 2006). Excessive gingival display may be attributed to multiple factors, such as: vertical maxillary excess, hypermobility of the upper lip, altered passive eruption, gingival hypertrophy, and hyperplasia. Gingival display will reduce slightly over lifetime as the upper lip droops with age.

Patients with severe vertical maxillary excess will benefit mostly from surgical impaction rather than soft tissue laser surgery, while patients with hypermobility of the upper lip, gingival hypertrophy (often a result of poor oral hygiene), or gingival hyperplasia (often induced by medication) respond favorably to tissue removal, as well as adjunctive plastic procedures such as collagen or botulinum toxin in the upper lip. Altered passive eruption almost always requires a surgical flap to reshape the alveolar crest and place the biologic width along the root of the tooth, rather than the crown.

Biologic width

The biologic width is the periodontal attachment located between the cementoenamel junction and the apical crest of the alveolar bone. *The distance of the biologic width is approximately 2 mm* (2.04 mm on average), composed of roughly 1 mm (0.97 mm on average) of *epithelial attachment* (otherwise known as junctional epithelium) above and 1 mm (1.07 mm on average) of *connective tissue attachment* below. Some dentists will include approximately 1 mm of sulcular depth in their definition of the biologic width, due to the challenge of restoring a tooth to the exact coronal edge of the junctional epithelium (Bargiulo et al., 1961; *Glossary of Periodontal Terms*, 2001; Camargo et al., 2007).

During gingivectomy, if the surgery extends beyond the gingival pocket and into the periodontal attachment, crestal bone will resorb, and a new biologic width will develop lower on the root surface. The biologic width tends to always remain at approximately 2 mm. Violation of the biologic width may result in the patient experiencing prolonged discomfort and gingival inflammation. Although many clinicians warn against interrupting the biologic width during gingival surgery, some crestal resorption may be needed to reduce the effects of gingival rebounding and regrowth.

Tissue rebounding

Significant tissue rebounding or marginal regeneration can occur in the weeks following gingivectomy or gingivoplasty. Experimental studies have shown that gingivectomies even extending into alveolar mucosa may regenerate as much as 50% with the formation of new attached marginal gingiva (Wennström, 1983). This can be particularly frustrating for both the clinician and patient as a second 'refinement' laser surgery may be needed to achieve optimal esthetics. Conventional scalpel surgery with apically positioned flap tends to produce less rebounding due to the crestal resorption which occurs after lifting the tissue.

Different tissue biotypes – thick or thin gingival tissue – will respond differently to inflammation, restorative trauma, parafunctional habits, and laser surgery (Fu et al., 2010). *The bone sets the tone* for gingival architecture. Dense bone with flat topography and minimal ridge atrophy is associated with thick gingival tissue; whereas, thin labial alveolar bone with ridge resorption and fenestrations is associated with thin tissue. Eighty-five percent of individuals have a thick tissue biotype. Thick gingival tissue is characterized by periodontal health, a large zone of attachment, dense fibrotic tissue, and resistance to trauma. Unfortunately, thick tissue biotypes respond poorly to laser surgery, with a high likelihood of tissue rebounding. Thin tissue biotypes are characterized by increased likelihood of

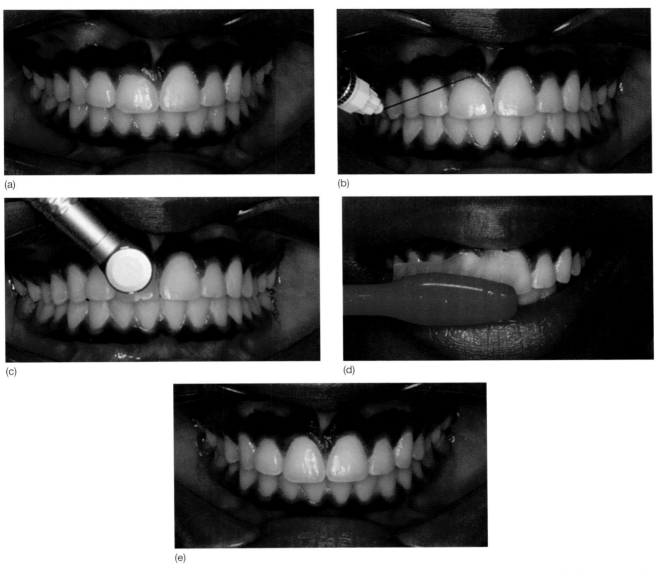

(a)

(b)

(c)

(d)

(e)

Figure 22.6 (a–c) Gingivectomy performed 1 month after debonding for improved gingival architecture esthetics using an erbium-doped solid-state laser. First, interligamentary infiltration with 4% articaine (Septocaine; 1:100 000 epinephrine) using a long 30-gauge needle. (d) After surgical excision, the patient was instructed to gently brush the gingival margins. (e) Same day final result with beautiful gingival esthetics. Note that the zeniths of the central incisors and canines are distal to their long axes and the zeniths of the laterals coincide with their long axes. Also note the 0.5 mm gingival step between the lateral and the adjacent canine and central.

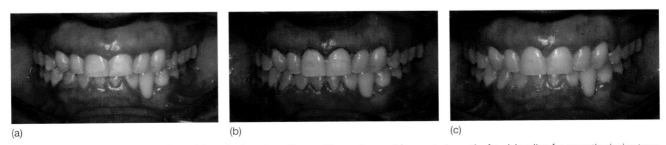

(a)

(b)

(c)

Figure 22.7 (a) Patient with missing lower left canine (wearing a flipper with a canine pontic) presents 1 month after debonding for cosmetic gingivectomy. (b) Significant improvement in gingival aesthetics immediately after surgery. (c) Moderate tissue rebounding 2 weeks after surgery.

periodontal disease, minimal zone of attachment, and friable tissue. Those with thin biotypes have a good response to laser surgery (the tissues ablate quickly) and have a low likelihood of significant rebounding.

Electrical power or wattage will influence the depth of tissue penetration and the efficacy of ablation. Routinely, gingivectomy and gingivoplasty are performed at low wattage with slow, short brush strokes. However, thicker, more fibrotic tissue may require greater electrical power and prolonged surgical exposure or slower brush strokes.

Papilla flattening

(Recommend laser settings: diode laser: 1.0–1.5 W, erbium-doped solid-state laser: 1.5–2.5 W)

Papilla flattening is the thinning, reshaping, or excision of bulbous or loose interdental papillae, often performed in conjunction with gingivectomy or gingivoplasty and limited to the anterior teeth. Ideal gingival contour or three-dimensional gingival topography is characterized by balanced, knife-edge interdental papillae. For patients with bulbous papillae, either due to poor oral hygiene, thick fibrotic tissue, or tissue bunching after space consolidation, papilla flattening can enhance gingivectomy or gingivoplasty surgery and dramatically improve gingival esthetics.

Papilla flattening is performed by operating the laser at low wattage and moving the laser tip *quickly* side to side over the selected region, as if to 'peel the layers' off the attached tissue. Loose labial or lingual interdental papilla can be excised completely (Figures 22.8–22.11).

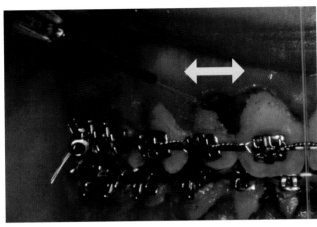

Figure 22.8 Papilla flattening performed by moving the laser side to side quickly as if to 'peel the layers' of the papilla.

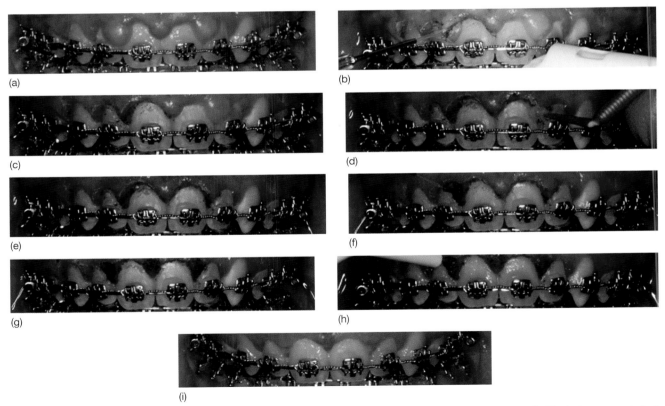

(a)

(b)

(c)

(d)

(e)

(f)

(g)

(h)

(i)

Figure 22.9 (a) Papilla flattening progression in a patient with a thick tissue biotype and bulbous papilla. (b–g) Surgery started with gingivectomy and gingivoplasty to reshape the gingival margins and papillae. A microbrush dipped in hydrogen peroxide is used to clean the gingival margins. After papilla flattening was performed, an air-water syringe was used to remove the laser char. (h) One month follow-up. Note the significant tissue rebounding; a common occurrence in patients with a thick tissue biotype.

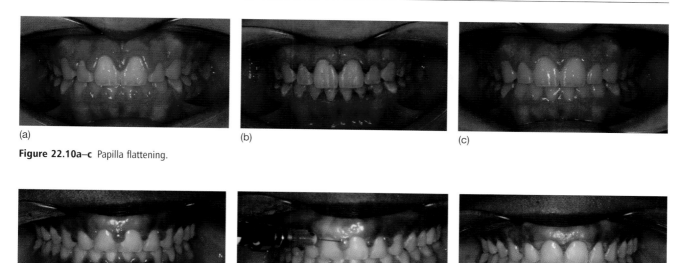

(a) (b) (c)

Figure 22.10a–c Papilla flattening.

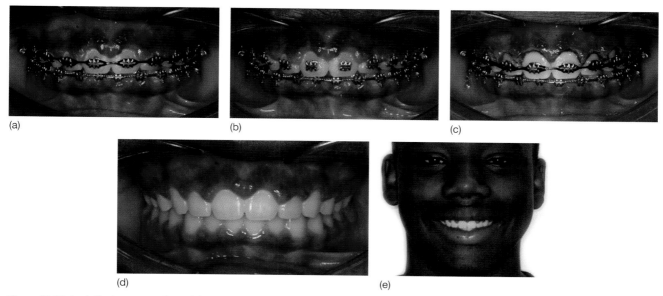

(a) (b) (c)

Figure 22.11 (a) Excision of loose papillae. (b) Infiltration with 4% articaine (Septocaine; 1:100,000 epinephrine) using a short 30-gauge needle. (c) Patient immediately following laser surgery. Note the dramatic improvement in gingival esthetics.

(a) (b) (c)

(d) (e)

Figure 22.12 (a–c) Gingivectomy performed during treatment due to poor oral hygiene. Ideally, the elastic chain and wire should be removed during gingival surgery. Note the dramatic improvement after removal of hypertrophic and edematous tissue. (d) However, even 1 month after debonding, patient still displays swollen gingival margins and signs of inadequate homecare despite having a pleasing smile (e).

Timing of surgery

The proper time to perform esthetic soft tissue laser surgery is often debated. Certainly, in patients with low clinical crown height, impacted teeth, covered temporary anchorage devices, transpositions, or poor oral hygiene resulting in gingival hypertrophy, soft tissue laser surgery *during* treatment not only aids patient homecare, but allows for better bracket repositioning and final detailing. When strictly enhancing soft tissue architecture, the clinician may consider performing laser surgery 1 month after debonding to resolve edematous tissues and allow a more accurate determination of gingival height, architecture, and pocket depth (Figures 22.12, 22.13).

Tooth and mini-implant exposure

(Recommend laser settings: diode laser: 1.0–1.5 W, erbium-doped solid-state laser: 1.5–2.5 W)

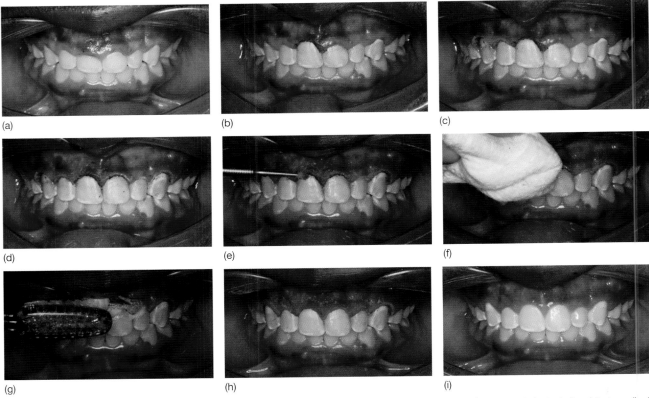

Figure 22.13 Gingivectomy for improved gingival esthetics. (a) Patient presents 1 month after debonding, with asymmetrical gingival architecture. (b–d) Beginning at the central incisor, gingival tissue reshaping was performed in one quadrant before moving to the adjacent quadrant. (e) After surgery, a microbrush was dipped in hydrogen peroxide and used to clean the gingival margins. (f,g) Remaining plume and charred tissue were cleaned with a wet gauze and toothbrush. (h) Patient immediately after surgery. (i) Patient at 1 month follow-up appointment.

Labial tooth impaction occurs in 1–2% of orthodontic patient and it is often challenging to manage (Vermette et al., 1995). Traditionally, the clinician was limited to simply waiting for the tooth to erupt, which could delay treatment for months. Uncovering an impacted canine to allow for bonding can dramatically improve treatment efficacy. The most common methods of uncovering labial impactions are excisional gingivectomy and placement of an apically positioned flap. The clinician should understand which cases need only simple window excision and which require a referral for placement of an apically positioned flap.

Excision versus apically positioned flap

Simple excision with a soft tissue laser is indicated when the canine is erupting within an adequate zone of attached tissue. The canine will be palpable and the tissue will easily blanch with finger pressure. Panoramic radiography will reveal that the crown has erupted beyond the dentoalveolus. During surgery, the clinician should make a small window within attached tissue; the excision should be small enough only to bond a bracket or button. Extrusion forces should be directed downward and under the mucogingival junction. Inadvertent forced eruption through the alveolar

mucosa may result in inadequate attachment and increase the likelihood of unsightly excessive clinical crown height (Figures 22.14–22.16).

An *apically positioned flap* is a split-thickness pedicle flap reflected from the edentulous area to expose the impacted tooth and preserve attached tissue. Apically positioned flap is indicated on labially impacted teeth erupting through alveolar mucosa or an inadequate amount of attached tissue. Surgery is performed by the periodontist or oral surgeon using the conventional scalpel technique. During the surgery, alveolar bone is removed, and the attached tissue flap is sutured apically to expose the crown. As the canine extrudes the gingiva follows with the tooth (Vanarsdall and Corn, 2004).

In addition, orthodontic temporary anchorage devices or mini-implants can become covered by soft tissue overgrowth and need surgical exposure. This is particularly true for mini-implants placed in the edentulous posterior mandibular or retromolar region due to soft tissue bunching as well as constant rubbing from the buccal mucosa and vestibular tissue. Temporary anchorage devices which become covered by inflamed gingiva have a 10% reduction in success rate.

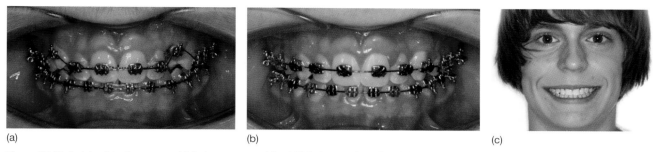

Figure 22.14 Excisional tooth exposure. (a) Patient presents with a labially impacted maxillary left canine within adequate attached tissue. A small excisional window was placed within attached tissue under the mucogingival junction. Only the minimal amount of tissue needed to bond the canine bracket was excised. The maxillary incisors were ligature-tied for anchorage. (b) After 5 months of extrusion, note the relative symmetry between the right and left clinical crown heights. (c) Final smile with optimal esthetics.

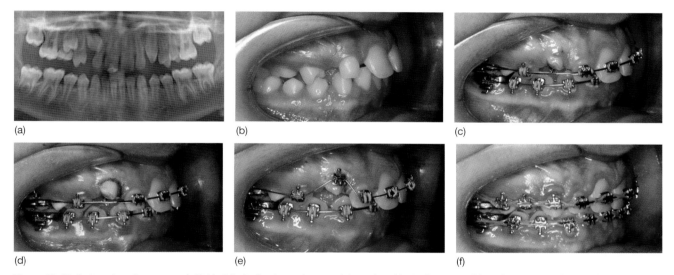

Figure 22.15 Excisonal tooth exposure. (a,b) Mesially inclined ectopic upper right canine. (c) Distalization and forced extrusion with 'piggy-back' or overlay nickel-titanium wire over the top of a heavy stainless steel archwire. (d,e) Excisional exposure within attached tissue to allow for bracket bonding and further extrusion. (f) Canine efficiently brought into proper occlusal position. Treatment continued with further finishing and detailing prior to debonding.

Typically, the mini-implant is covered by a thin layer of soft tissue or fibrino-purulent sheath. A simple slit excision around the head will quickly uncover the mini-implant. Finger pressure can be used to push the soft tissue down the body and under the gingival collar of the mini-implant. The clinician may also consider prescribing a chlorhexidine rinse, which is bactericidal and slows down further epithelialization or regrowth (Jones, 1997).

Frenectomy

(Recommend laser settings: diode laser: 1.0–1.5 W, erbium-doped solid-state laser: 1.5–2.5 W followed by coagulation at <1.0 W with no water)

A *frenectomy* or frenulectomy is the surgical removal of a small band of muscle tissue known as the frenum or frenulum from its attachment into the mucoperiosteal covering of the alveolar process. The frenum is a normal component of oral anatomy; however, a large, wide or short frenum might interfere with the normal function of the lip, cheek or tongue (*Glossary of Periodontal Terms*, 2001).

The labial frenum is the fold of muscle that attaches to the center of the upper lip and to the mucoperiosteum between the maxillary central incisors. A thick, low labial frenum in children may result in a large maxillary diastema. Interference with oral hygiene, tooth eruption, esthetics, and psychosocial concerns are contributing factors necessitating treatment of the labial frenum. When a diastema is present, treatment often includes a combination of orthodontics and soft tissue surgery (Ong and Wang, 2002). Timing of labial frenectomy is

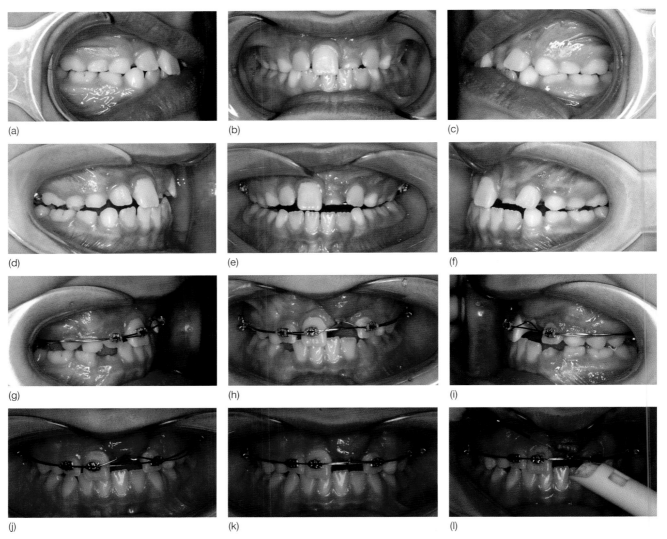

Figure 22.16 (a–f) Impacted maxillary left central incisor due to large dilacerated mesiodens. (g–k) Following maxillary palatal expansion, surgical exposure and gold chain were placed for forced eruption. 'Piggy-back' nickel-titanium wires were used to extrude the incisor. (l) Unfortunately, the incisor began erupting through the alveolar mucosa. At this point, the patient was referred to the periodontist for placement of an apically positioned flap. (m–x) Due to limited finances, the patient requested in-office surgical exposure with the full understanding that recession and excess clinical crown height were highly likely. After successful extrusion, note the discrepancy in clinical crown height between the maxillary central incisors (q). Nonetheless, acceptable smile esthetics were achieved (x) with only upper arch phase I treatment with a maxillary expander and 2 × 4 fixed appliance.

often debated; however, the popular consensus is that if orthodontic treatment is indicated, labial frenectomy should be performed only *after the diastema is consolidated as much as possible* so as to simplify the surgery and reduce the impact of scar tissue which may impede space closure (Figures 22.17, 22.18).

A short lingual frenum may result in ankyloglossia or 'tongue-tie'. Ankyloglossia is a developmental anomaly of the tongue characterized by a short, thick lingual frenum resulting in limitation of tongue movement. It occurs in 1.7–4.4% of neonates and affects four times as many boys

than girls. Ankyloglossia may result in speech defects, lingual gingival recession or even bone loss, mandibular central incisor spacing, or anterior open bite. Clinical symptoms include a classic 'heart-shape' of the tongue when raised, inability to extend the tongue past the lower lip, deviated swallow, and speech difficulties (Neville et al., 2002; Suter and Bornstein, 2009).

During surgical excision of the labial or lingual frenum, first grip the patient's lip or tongue with a 2 × 2 gauze and lift taut. The frenum should pull back and open into a rhombus-shape (Figure 22.19). The surgical procedure is

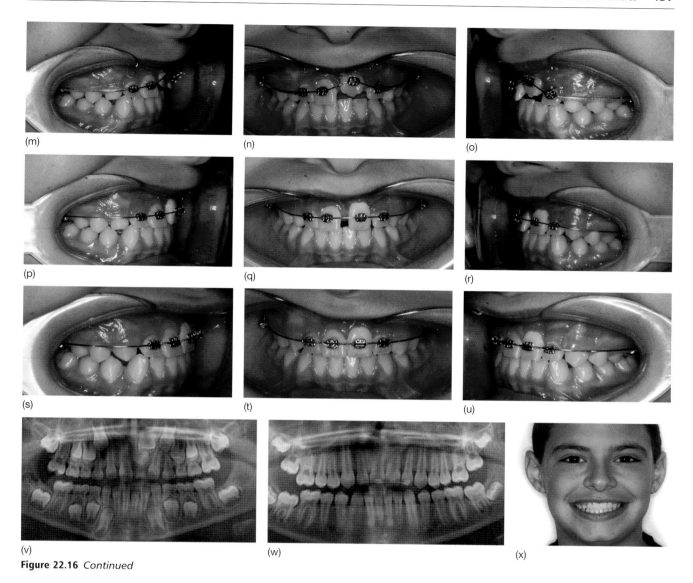

Figure 22.16 *Continued*

completed very quickly and no sutures are indicated. The patient should gain improved function immediately.

Potential complications include mild bleeding, discomfort and need for refinement surgery to excise remnants or tissue tag of the frenum on the upper lip (Figure 22.20).

Operculectomy

(Recommend laser settings: diode laser: 1.5–2.0 W, erbium-doped solid-state laser: 2.5 W)

An *operculum* is a hood of thick gingival tissue overlying the crown of an erupting tooth, typically the mandibular second or third molars. Excision of an operculum allows for banding or bonding partially erupted or impacted teeth. Occasionally, *pericoronitis* – a painful inflammatory lesion, can develop when bacteria and food debris (espe-cially popcorn seeds) are present under the operculum. As the tissue swells, the maxillary molars begin to occlude on the swollen operculum further exacerbating the condition. The patient may experience extreme pain, abscess, lymphadenopathy, and an inability to close the jaw. In the instance of pericoronitis, antibiotics should be prescribed to eliminate any infection prior to gingival surgery (Neville et al., 2002; McNutt et al., 2008).

Ablation of minor aphthous ulceration

(Recommend laser settings: diode laser: 0.5–1.0 W)

Minor aphthous ulcerations or 'canker sores' are a common occurrence in the orthodontic patient due to tissue irritation as well as stress from discomfort of tooth movement. The ulcerations are characterized by a 3–10 mm

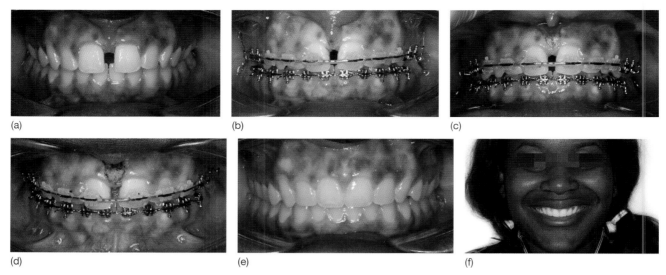

Figure 22.17 Frenectomy with an erbium-doped solid-state laser. (a) Patient with a maxillary diastema due to a thick, low frenum. (b) Consolidation with fixed appliances was performed prior to frenal surgery. (c) Holding the lip taut, the frenal fibers were excised. (c) Note that hemorrhaging was slightly harder to control with a solid-state laser. Also note the upper lip tissue-tag (the top of the frenum) that will also need to be excised. (d) After switching the laser settings to coagulation-mode (low wattage with no water), the bleeding was stopped prior to the patient leaving the office. A new elastic chain was placed to begin consolidation immediately. (e,f) Final records with beautiful gingival architecture and smile consonance.

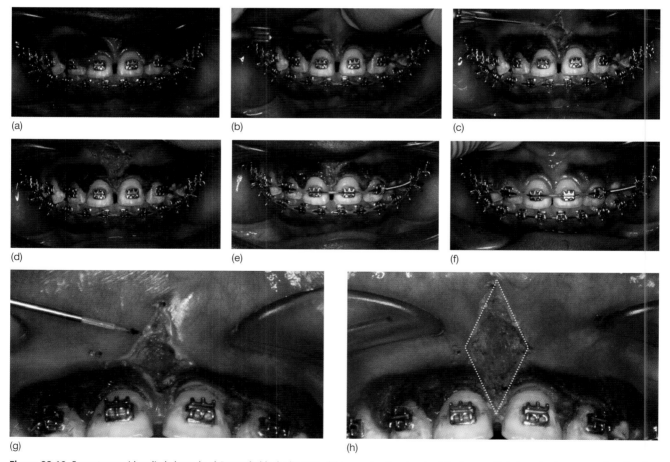

Figure 22.18 Frenectomy with a diode laser. (a–c) Doctor holds the lip taut while removing the strands of the frenum. Note how the tissue opens in a rhombus shape. (d–f) Immediately after surgery, elastic chain was placed to begin consolidation. (g) Note good tissue healing and significant space consolidation after 2 weeks. (h) Tissue opening into a rhombus-shape.

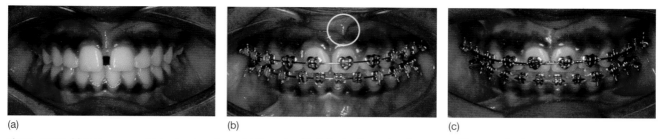

Figure 22.19 (a) Frenum opened into rhombus shape. (b) Tissue tag (circled) after incomplete frenectomy. (c) A second refinement surgery was needed to excise the remnant tissue.

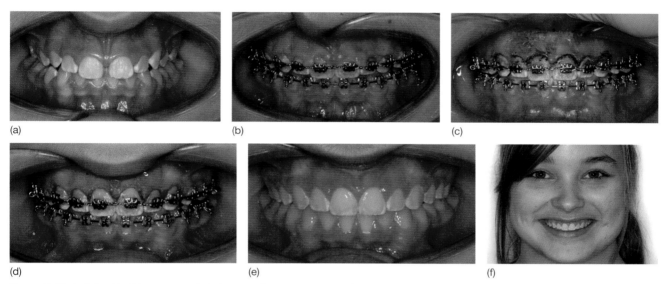

Figure 22.20 (a–f) Combined frenectomy and gingivectomy during treatment to aid consolidation and improve finishing and detailing. Space was consolidated prior to frenectomy. Gingivectomy improved crown height-to-width ratio and enabled incisal enameloplasty at the end of treatment.

diameter yellowish-white, removable fibroino-purulent membrane encircled by an erythematous halo, localized almost exclusively on nonkeratinized tissue such as the buccal mucosa, alveolar mucosa, tongue, and lips. The etiology of aphthous ulcerations includes trauma, stress, allergies (i.e. to nickel in the appliances), nutritional deficiencies, hematologic abnormalities, hormones, infectious agents, systemic conditions (i.e. immunoglobulin A deficiency, neutropenia, celiac disease), or a genetic predisposition. After relieving the etiologic agent, minor ulcerations typically heal without scarring in 7–14 days (Neville et al., 2002).

Several types of treatment are available for management of aphthous ulcerations, including: simply waiting for the mouth to heal, warm salt water rinses, hydrogen peroxide, antifungal compound medications, liquid topical anesthetics, and diode laser surgery treatment. Unlike other surgical

procedures with a diode laser, ablation of aphthous ulcerations are performed *1–2 mm away from the tissue*. The clinician should proceed with short, side-to-side brush strokes over the ulcerated area. Typically, anesthesia is not required. Postoperative management can include routine palliative treatment.

Excision of soft tissue lesions

(Recommend laser settings: diode laser: 1.0–1.5 W, erbium-doped solid-state laser: 1.5–2.5 W)

Occasionally, the orthodontic patient will present with a soft tissue lesion on the mucosa or tongue due to local irritation or trauma. In most instances, the orthodontist should refer to an oral surgeon or oral medicine specialist for evaluation and biopsy. However, in some instances, simple benign lesions, such as an irritation fibroma, pyogenic granuloma, or mucocele can be treated by the orthodontist with conservative surgical excision using a soft tissue laser.

- *Fibroma (irritation fibroma, fibrous nodule)* is a benign, asymptomatic nodular mass of dense fibrous connective tissue covered by squamous epithelium (Neville et al., 2002). A fibroma is the most common abnormal growth in the oral cavity; the most common location is the *buccal mucosa*, likely a consequence of trauma from cheek biting.
- *Pyogenic granuloma* is a non-neoplastic, smooth or lobulated erythematous mass of granulation tissue. Three-quarters of oral pyogenic granulomas are located on the *gingiva* (Neville et al., 2002). The greatest precipitating factor may be gingival inflammation from poor oral hygiene around fixed appliances.
- *Mucocele* is a dome-shaped mucosal swelling resulting from rupture of a salivary gland duct and spillage of mucin into the surrounding soft tissue (Neville et al., 2002). Over 60% of all mucoceles occur on the *lower lip*, typically resulting from local trauma such as lip-biting, bracket irritation, or inadvertent trauma from orthodontic instruments. Repeated episodes at the same location are not unusual (Figure 22.21).

When removing soft tissue lesions, the clinician should consider lifting the lesion away from the soft tissue with forceps to excise at the base. The patient may experience mild bleeding for 30 minutes following excision. *No matter how certain the diagnosis, it is important to submit all excised tissue for histological examination because malignant tumors may mimic the clinical appearance of benign growths* (Neville et al., 2002) (Figure 22.22).

Laser safety

Laser hazard classification

The major risk during laser surgery is exposure to laser radiation. Laser safety is regulated according to the American National Standards Institute's (ANSI) Z136 safety standards in the United States and the International Electrotechnical Commission (IEC) 60825 internationally. ANSI laser safety standards are the basis for Occupational Safety and Health Administration (OSHA) and state occupational safety rules. All lasers sold in the United States since 1976 are classified according to their hazard potential, power, and wavelength. Currently, there are seven laser hazard classes (Class 1, 1M, 2, 2M, 3R, 3B, and 4). Lasers used in medical or dental therapeutic use, such as soft tissue lasers, are *Class 4 products* (Kravitz and Kusnoto, 2008).

Class 4 lasers have an output power >0.5 W. At this power, eye and skin are endangered even at diffuse reflection. As such, a clinician is required to ensure the following safety precautions:

- Creation of a danger zone – typically this entails a designated surgical chair or room with a warning sign indicating that a laser is operational
- Presence of a laser safety officer (typically the orthodontist)
- Proper training of users (the orthodontist and staff)
- Consideration of potential fire hazards.

Eye and skin injury

Unquestionably, the greatest specific risk of soft tissue laser surgery is injury to the eye. The severity of injury depends

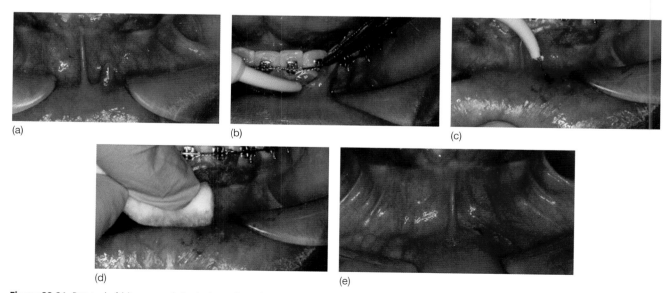

(a)   (b)   (c)

(d)   (e)

Figure 22.21 Removal of (a) a mucocele in the lower lip with a diode laser. (b,c) Holding the mucocele with Mathieu pliers to ablate at the base of the lesion. (d) After surgery, a cotton roll dipped in hydrogen peroxide was used to remove the laser char and plume. (e) Same day final results 30 minutes after surgery.

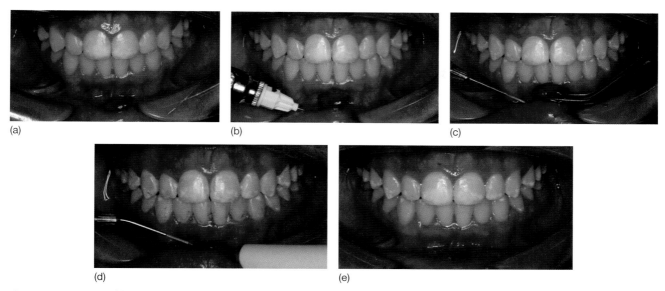

Figure 22.22 Removal of (a) an erythematous vascular lesion with a diode laser (possible diagnosis: hemorrhaging mucocele or trauma-induced hematoma). (b) Infiltration with 4% articaine (Septocaine; 1:100 000 epinephrine) at the base and the periphery of the lesion. (c) Holding the lesion taut with forceps to ablate at the base. (d) Note the high-speed suction during ablation, which is critical to remove laser plume and maintain a clear surgical field. (e) Excision and complete hemostasis 30 minutes after surgery.

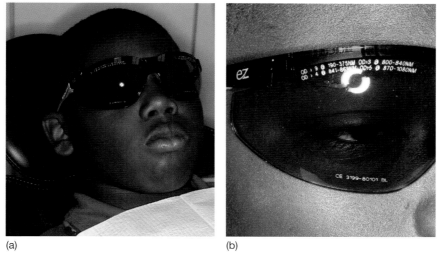

Figure 22.23 Safety goggles. (a) Proper chairside set-up with safety goggles and removal of all reflective surfaces. (b) Safety goggles protect against the wavelength generated by the laser. The specific goggles shown protect against 800–840 nm and 870–1080 nm.

on the laser wavelength, distance from the laser source, and power of the laser machine. The eye is precise at focusing light, and a split-second exposure to laser radiation may be sufficient to cause permanent injury. Retinal damage can occur at 400–1400 nm (this range is known as the retinal hazard region). The major danger is a stray laser beam reflected from a table, jewelry, or belt. Diode lasers risk retinal burns and cataract, whereas solid-state lasers risk corneal burn, aqueous flare-ups, and infrared cataract.

Skin is the largest organ of the body and poses high risk of radiation exposure, regardless of the laser used. Skin can be penetrated at wavelengths of 300–3000 nm (which includes both diodes and erbium lasers), reaching a maximum penetration at 1000 nm. The arms, hands, and head are the regions of the body most likely to be exposed to laser radiation.

Patient and operator protection
The patient and clinician should be fully covered and wavelength-specific protective goggles should be worn by the doctor, the assistant, and the patient at all times. It is imperative that the goggles block light at the appropriate wavelength and protect all possible reflective paths to the eyes (Figure 22.23). Therefore, the orange protective goggles

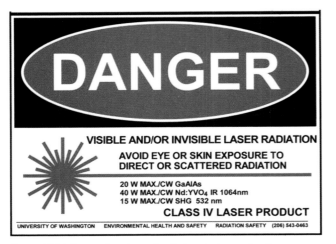

Figure 22.24 Laser safety sign to be displayed when performing surgery.

used during light curing will not suffice. Patients should remove all facial jewelry and nearby reflective surfaces should be covered or removed. Class 4 laser systems pose a fire hazard if the beam contacts flammable substances, and flame-retardant materials should be available in the office. A discernable danger zone should be created around the surgical bay with a sign reading: *Warning: Visible and Invisible Laser Radiation. Avoid Eye or Skin Exposure to Direct Scatter Radiation. Class IV laser product.* Such signs are typically provided by the laser manufacturer and are available over the internet (Kravitz and Kusnoto, 2008) (Figure 22.24).

Informed consent

Soft tissue laser surgery is currently not listed on the American Association of Orthodontics standard informed consent packet. Until then, clinicians may consider writing their own informed consent. Informed consent may vary depending on the type of laser and the procedure performed. Consent for the diode laser may include: the recommended treatment; although rare, the principal risks and complications, including postsurgical infection, swelling, bleeding, headache, temporomandibular joint (TMJ) (jaw joint) pain, tooth/gum pain, microcracks in the enamel, pulpal over-heating leading to hyperemia, shrinkage of gum tissues, muscle soreness, soft tissue numbness, postoperative discomfort, and mild bleeding; expected results and need for potential surgical refinement; and necessary follow-up care and homecare.

Postsurgical management

Immediately after the procedure, the clinician can run a microbrush or cotton roll dipped in hydrogen peroxide along the gingival margins to remove any charred tissue and laser plume. The patient should be encouraged to rinse

and gently massage the surgical area with a soft-bristle toothbrush. Bleeding and discomfort are typically minimal, with the exception of a frenal surgery, in which minor bleeding is expected for 24 hours postsurgery. Complete tissue healing will take place after 1–2 weeks, at which point the patient should be seen for a postoperative follow-up.

Billing and insurance codes

Laser surgery insurance codes provided by the American Dental Association (ADA) for common soft tissue procedures are listed under both specialties of *Periodontics (D4000–4999)* and *Oral Surgery (D7000–7999)*, and therefore will not affect the patient's orthodontic benefits. The orthodontist should stay current with annual changes in codes and definitions made to the *Current Dental Terminology* (CDT) handbook. Insurance claims often require specific information, such as quadrant, probing depths, reason for surgery, and surgical records, provided in a letter submitted along with the insurance claim (Kravitz and Kusnoto, 2008) (Table 22.1).

Conclusion

The use of soft tissue lasers offers many advantages such as improved oral hygiene, practice efficiencies, and esthetic finishing. Clinicians interested in incorporating soft tissue lasers into their practice should obtain proficiency certification, attend continuing education courses, and recognize the inherent risks associated with laser surgery. As an orthodontist committed to providing the best possible service, adjunctive procedures such as soft tissue surgery can dramatically enhance the overall treatment experience in your office.

Table 22.1 Dental codes for common soft tissue procedures

Code	Procedure
D4210	Gingivectomy/gingivoplasty – four or more contiguous teeth per quadrant
D4211	Gingivectomy/gingivoplasty – one to three contiguous teeth per quadrant
D7960	Frenectomy
D7971	Operculectomy
D7465	Aphthous ulcer
D7430	Excision of benign tumor – diameter <1.25 cm
D7430	Excision of benign tumor – diameter >1.25 cm
D7286	Biopsy of oral tissue, soft

When submitting a claim, insurance companies will ask for an accompanying letter that explains the need for surgery, the probing depths, the quadrant of surgery, and other pertinent information. Soft tissue surgical codes fall under periodontal and oral surgery insurance coverage.

References

Armitage GC, Robertson PB (2009) The biology, prevention, diagnosis and treatment of periodontal diseases: scientific advances in the United States. *Journal of the American Dental Association* 140(Suppl 1): 4S–6S.

Baker SS, Hunnewell JM, Muenzler WS, et al. (2002) Laser blepharoplasty: diamond laser scalpel compared to the free beam CO_2 laser. *Dermatology Surgery* 28: 127–31.

Bargiulo AW, Wentz FM, Orban B (1961) Dimensions and relations of the dentogingival junction in humans. *Journal of Periodontology* 32: 261–7.

Buell BR, Schuller DE (1983) Comparison of tensile strength in CO_2 laser and scalpel skin incisions. *Archives of Otolaryngology* 109: 465–7.

Camargo PM, Melnick PR, Camargo LM (2007) Clinical crown lengthening in the esthetic zone. *Journal of the California Dental Association* 35: 487–98.

Fisher SE, Frame JW, Browne RM, et al. (1983) A comparative histological study of wound healing following CO_2 laser and conventional surgical excision of canine buccal mucosa. *Archives of Oral Biology* 28: 287–91.

Frame JW (1985) Removal of oral soft tissue pathology with the CO_2 laser. *Journal of Oral and Maxillofacial Surgery* 43: 850–5.

Fu JH, Yeh CY, Chan HL, et al. (2010) Tissue biotype and its relation to the underlying bone morphology. *Journal of Periodontology* 81: 569–74.

Glossary of Periodontal Terms (2001) 4th edn. Chicago, IL: The American Academy of Periodontology.

Hadley J, Young DA, Eversole LR, et al. (2000) A laser-powered hydrdokinetic system for caries removal and cavity preparation. *Journal of the American Dental Association* 131: 777–85.

Harashima T, Kinoshita J, Kimura Y, et al. (2005) Morphological comparative study on ablation of dental hard tissue at cavity preparation by Er:YAG and Er,Cr:YSGG lasers. *Photomedicine and Laser Surgery* 23: 52–5.

Haytac MC, Ozcelik O (2006) Evaluation of patient perceptions: a comparison of carbon dioxide laser and scalpel techniques. *Journal of Periodontology* 77: 1815–19.

Jeffcoat MK (2004) Eye of newt, toe of frog: drug compounding: proceed with caution. *Journal of the American Dental Association* 135: 546–8.

Jones CG (1997) Chlorhexidine: is it still the gold standard? *Periodontology 2000* 15: 55–62.

Kokich VO, Kokich VG, Kiyak HA (2006) Perceptions of dental professionals and laypersons to altered dental esthetics: asymmetric and symmetric situations. *American Journal of Orthodontics and Dentofacial Orthopedics* 130: 141–51.

Kravitz ND (2007) The use of compound topical anesthetics: a review. *Journal of the American Dental Association* 138: 1333–9.

Kravitz ND (2010) Debanding day. *Orthodontic Products* April/May. Available at: www.orthodonticproductsonline.com/issues/articles/2010-04_08.asp (accessed 21 July 2011).

Kravitz ND, Kusnoto B (2008) Soft-tissue lasers in orthodontics: an overview. *American Journal of Orthodontics and Dentofacial Orthopedics* 133: S110–14.

Kremenak NW, Squier CA (1997) Pioneers in oral biology: the migrations of Gottlieb, Kronfeld, Orban, Weinmann, and Sicher from Vienna to America. *Critical Reviews in Oral Biology and Medicine* 8: 108–28.

McNutt M, Patrick M, Shugars DA, et al. (2008) Impact of symptomatic pericoronitis on health-related quality of life. *Journal of Oral and Maxillofacial Surgery* 66: 1482–7.

Moritz A (2006) *Oral Laser Application.* Chicago, IL: Quintessence.

Neville BW, Damm DD, Allen CM, et al. (2002) *Oral and Maxillofacial Pathology*, 2nd edn. Philadelphia, PA: WB Saunders.

Ong MA, Wang HL (2002) Periodontic and orthodontic treatment in adults. *American Journal of Orthodontics and Dentofacial Orthopedics* 122: 420–8.

Rossman JA, Cobb CM (1995) Lasers in periodontal therapy. *Periodontology 2000* 9: 150–64.

Sarver DM (2004) Principles of cosmetic dentistry in orthodontics: part 1. Shape and proportionality of anterior teeth. *American Journal of Orthodontics and Dentofacial Orthopedics* 126: 749–53.

Sarver DM, Yanosky M (2005) Principles of cosmetic dentistry in orthodontics: part 2. Soft tissue laser technology and cosmetic gingival contouring. *American Journal of Orthodontics and Dentofacial Orthopedics* 127: 85–90.

Suter VG, Bornstein MM (2009) Ankyloglossia: facts and myths in diagnosis and treatment. *Journal of Periodontology* 80: 1204–19.

Tracey S (2005) Light work. *Orthodontic Products* April/May. Available at: www.orthodonticproductsonline.com/issues/articles/2005-04_17.asp (accessed 21 July 2011).

United States Pharmacopeial Convention (2004) Good compounding practices. In: *The United States Pharmacopeia: USP 28: the National Formulary: NF 23: by Authority of the United States Pharmacopeial Convention, Inc., meeting at Washington*, April 12–16, 2000, Rockville, MD. *United States Pharmacopeial Convention* 2620: 2457.

Vanarsdall RL, Corn H (2004) Soft-tissue management of labially positioned unerupted teeth. *American Journal of Orthodontics and Dentofacial Orthopedics* 125: 284–93.

Vermette ME, Kokich VG, Kennedy DB (1995) Uncovering labially impacted teeth: apically positioned flap and closed-eruption techniques. *Angle Orthodontist* 65: 23–32; discussion 33.

Wennström J (1983) Regeneration of gingiva following surgical excision. A clinical study. *Journal of Clinical Periodontology* 10: 287–97.

23

Implant Orthodontics: An Interactive Approach to Skeletal Anchorage

Hyo-Sang Park

Summary

Many types of skeletal anchorage device have evolved in recent years, including dental implants, mini-plates, and micro- and mini-screw implants. The main advantage these devices offer is that the clinicians can move particular teeth in specific directions without causing a reciprocal movement of other dental units. The present chapter discusses the role of micro-implants and their use in interdisciplinary patient management. The ways the orthodontists interact with prosthodontists, periodontists, and oral surgeons in the placement of, as well as in the management of micro-implants are discussed and illustrated with the help of case reports. Vertical holding of molar position, intrusion and uprighting of molars, and forced eruption are discussed in detail along with the associated surgical procedures and their possible complications. The chapter emphasizes the clinician's need to be knowledgeable about the biological and mechanical principles of orthodontic tooth movement as they pertain to the use of metallic implants, in order to be able to use skeletal anchorage units in a reliable and dependable way.

Introduction

Anchorage preservation is considered to be one of the most important elements of successful orthodontic treatment. Orthodontists have always used a variety of anchorage devices, and almost all have some limitations. Extraoral appliances, which provide reliable anchorage, rely heavily on the patient's compliance, while all intraoral anchorage devices are associated with some degree of anchorage loss. The introduction of skeletal anchorage in recent decades has changed the scenario, as it provides reliable anchorage that not only does not depend on patient compliance, but also offers great precision in orthodontic tooth movement.

The usefulness of surgical screws in orthodontic anchorage was first demonstrated in a clinical trial by Creekmore and Eklund (1983), who placed a screw into the bone under the anterior nasal spine, in order to provide anchorage for intrusion of maxillary incisors. Kanomi (1997) reported intruding the lower incisors with the aid of 1.2 mm wide surgical screws placed into the mandibular symphysis. Park (1999) placed 1.2 mm wide, 5 mm long micro-screws into the interradicular bone between the maxillary second premolars and the first molars, in order to assist in the retraction of the upper anterior teeth, and demonstrated distalization of the whole maxillary dentition against the micro-screw implant. This report, demonstrating the efficacy of micro-screws as anchorage for retraction of a whole dentition finally changed the orthodontic paradigm from step-by-step tooth movement to en masse group movement (Park et al., 2001; Park and Kwon, 2004), leading to the increased proportion of non-extraction treatment, by molar distalization, in borderline cases (Park et al., 2004a, 2005). The use of skeletal anchorage to intrude the molars to achieve counterclockwise rotation of the mandible decreased the need for orthognathic surgery in the treatment of skeletal open bite (Umemori et al., 1999; Park et al., 2004b, 2006b), with similar skeletal effects.

Many types of skeletal anchorage device have evolved in recent years, including dental implants (Shapiro and Kokich, 1988), mini-plates (Umemori et al., 1999; Sherwood et al., 2002), and mini- or micro-screw implants (Creekmore and Eklund, 1983; Kanomi, 1997; Costa et al., 1998; Park,

Integrated Clinical Orthodontics, First Edition. Edited by Vinod Krishnan, Ze'ev Davidovitch.
© 2012 Blackwell Publishing Ltd. Published 2012 by Blackwell Publishing Ltd.

1999; Park et al., 2001, 2004a,b, 2005, 2006a,b; Park and Kwon, 2004). Among these devices, the mini- or micro-screw implants have gained increasing popularity because of their small size (which enables placement even in the narrow interradicular bone regions), low cost, suitability for immediate loading, and the ease of the surgical procedure involved in their placement (Park et al., 2001).

The most valuable and attractive contribution of skeletal anchorage, however, has been in pre-prosthetic orthodontic treatment. The teeth in the anchorage/reciprocal part should not be moved during pre-prosthetic orthodontic treatment, in order to avoid any alteration and/or deterioration of the occlusal interdigitation. Because of this requirement, pre-prosthetic treatment with conventional mechanics is quite difficult. To minimize adverse movement in the anchorage/reciprocal part, it has been recommended to include as many teeth as possible in this part of the orthodontic set-up, and to connect the anchor teeth to the teeth on the opposite side of the dental arch for anchorage reinforcement. However, even with all these measures, there is always a certain degree of anchorage loss. With the introduction of skeletal anchorage, it is possible now to bond brackets to a minimal number of teeth, while simultaneously eliminating the adverse reactive movements of teeth (Park, 2009). Consequently, this method is considered to be an efficient way of improving the quality of orthodontic treatment.

Interactive approaches

As mentioned above, conventional orthodontic treatment mechanics cannot provide precise control of tooth movement and reciprocal anchorage loss tends to compromise the final dental occlusion. However, the skeletal anchorage with micro-implants provides absolute anchorage that allows clinicians to move certain teeth in specific directions without much adverse effects on the rest of the dentition. In other words, the efficiency of micro-implants in controlling tooth position means orthodontists are now capable of moving teeth three-dimensionally, which is highly advantageous for subsequent prosthodontic treatment. Interactive management of pre-prosthetic cases, with close collaboration between orthodontists, prosthodontists, periodontists, and oral surgeons, is thus crucial for the successful outcome of treatment utilizing implant anchorage.

The following discussion and six case presentations demonstrate the ability to use mini-implants as a superior source of anchorage in the treatment of patients with various malocclusions.

Holding the molar vertical position

When dental implants are planned after extraction of posterior teeth, clinicians need to wait for the extraction sockets to heal or until the osseointegration of the dental implant is complete before completing the restoration. However, in the meantime, the antagonist teeth from the opposing arch may extrude. If the teeth on either side of the extracted tooth are in occlusal contact with their antagonists, the tooth with the potential to extrude can be splinted to the antagonists to minimize the extrusive movement. However, in conventional mechanics, where there are several missing or extracted teeth, holding the vertical position is usually accomplished with the help of a temporary denture. This denture might require further modification in the later stages, to remain in concordance with the dental implant placement. This concordance may have adverse effects, compromising the stability of the dental implants. However, with micro-implants, it is possible to prevent extrusion of the molars and hold their vertical position.

Case 1

A 47-year-old male patient received dental implants after extraction of the mandibular right molars. During the osseointegration period, the vertical position of maxillary right molars needed to be maintained, that is, the molars need to be prevented from extruding (Figure 23.1). The

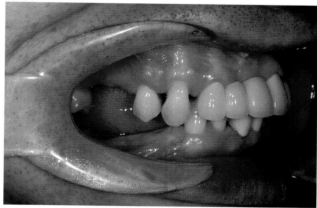

(a)

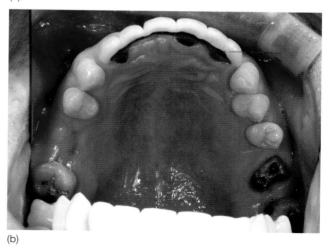

(b)

Figure 23.1 Pretreatment photograph showing missing lower right posterior teeth: (a) lateral view; (b) occlusal view.

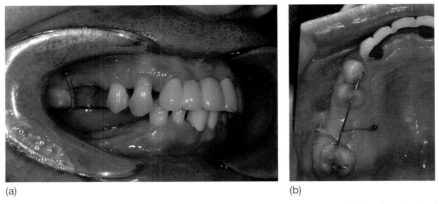

(a) (b)

Figure 23.2 A sectional wire was bonded from the premolars to the second molars and ligature wires were tied from the micro-implants to the wire: (a) lateral view; (b) occlusal view.

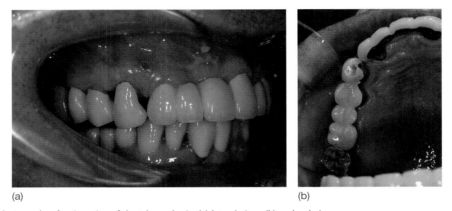

(a) (b)

Figure 23.3 Intraoral photographs after insertion of dental prosthesis: (a) lateral view; (b) occlusal view.

maxillary molar was positioned in the correct vertical plane, then requiring only maintenance of its position, with the aid of micro-implants. The maxillary right premolars and the second molars were splinted with a 0.019 × 0.025 inch stainless steel sectional wire, and a core composite resin. Two micro-implants (SH1312-08, Absoanchor, Dentos) were placed into the buccal and palatal alveolar bone and ligature wires were lightly tied from the micro-implants to the splint (Figure 23.2) to prevent extrusion of the upper molars. After completion of the implant prostheses in the lower arch, the maxillary appliance were removed (Figure 23.3).

Intrusion of molars

Intrusion of molars is one of the most frequent tooth movements in pre-prosthetic orthodontic treatment. When a molar is missing, the antagonist (molar) tooth tends to extrude and adjacent teeth tip into the extraction space. Before delivering a dental prosthesis, the extruded molar needs to be intruded and the tipped adjacent teeth have to be uprighted. Otherwise, the occlusal surface of the extruded molar will need to reduced. However, reducing occlusal surfaces can result in pulpal exposure or irritation, ending up with a root canal treatment at a later stage.

Conventional orthodontic mechanics for molar intrusion include the use of removable appliances (Alessandri Bonetti and Giunta, 1996) or a bonded lingual intruder (Chun et al., 2000); the success of treatment with removable appliances depends on patient compliance, and the appliance may be dislodged easily. A lingual intruder is bonded to the lingual surface of the teeth and has hooks for applying intrusion force. The appliance is effective, but needs to be bonded to several teeth in order to provide anchorage for the intrusion of one or two molars. In contrast, micro-implant anchorage effectively intrudes molars without any adverse movement of other teeth.

Direction of the intrusive orthodontic force

A vertical orthodontic force should pass through the center of resistance of the tooth that is to be moved to obtain pure intrusion. Otherwise, tipping of the tooth will result in the apices of the dental roots coming into contact with the buccal or lingual cortical plates of the alveolar bone, causing bone fenestrations and root resorption. These consequences appear to be minimal when the amount of intrusion is less than 1 mm.

Magnitude of the intrusive orthodontic force

Diverse opinions exist about the optimal magnitude of the intrusive force. Considering the fact that heavy forces result in root resorption, the application of a light force is desirable. Dellinger (1967) reported that 300 g of intrusion force produced more root resorption than 50 and 100 g in monkeys. Ohmae et al. (2001) reported that root resorption was observed in dogs after loading 150 g intrusion force on the molars. Costopoulos and Nanda (1996) stated that 15 g intrusion force on an anterior tooth resulted in a clinically negligible amount of root resorption in humans. Therefore, it is desirable to use a light intrusion force of about 15–20 g for an anterior tooth and of about 100 g for a molar.

Periodontal considerations

Control of periodontal as well as gingival inflammation is a prerequisite for safe application of intrusion mechanics. Melsen (1986) showed that after intrusion, the amount of marginal alveolar bone loss on the hygienic side of the dental arch was small compared with the non-hygienic side. Cardaropoli et al. (2001) demonstrated reduction in the size of infrabony pockets after intrusion of teeth, once inflammation was controlled.

Retention of teeth after intrusion

Once a prosthetic device has been made in the opposing arch, after intrusion of the extruded teeth, there appears to be no relapse in the tooth movement performed. Until this is done, the micro-implant and the orthodontic appliances should be used as retainers (Park, 2009). If there is a requirement for additional tooth movement buccolingually after intrusion of molars, criss-cross elastics can be prescribed after bonding a lingual button on the prosthesis after its insertion.

Considerations regarding the maxillary sinus

According to earlier reports, the maxillary sinus does not impose limitations on the intrusion of upper molars. One clinical case report showed bone formation around the intruded dental roots while moving a premolar into the sinus in order to develop the site for a prosthetic implant (Re et al., 2001). Similar bone formation around the protruding roots in the nasal cavity was demonstrated in dogs by Daimaruya et al. (2003). However, clinicians have to be cautious about root resorption, which can happen with the application of excessive intrusive forces.

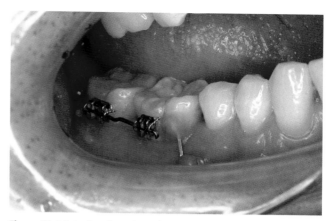

Figure 23.4 Intrusion of a molar with indirect anchorage. See text for details.

The effect of occlusion on intruded teeth

Teeth that are intruded may show slight mobility. On the other hand, the dental implant prosthesis in the opposite arch is very firm, that is, it shows no mobility. Occlusal contact of mobile, intruded teeth with the immobile antagonist may cause persistent mobility of the intruded tooth, but this can be prevented by occlusal adjustment.

Intrusion of a molar with indirect anchorage

A simple method of intruding a molar is to apply an intrusive force from the adjacent teeth, which, in turn, are connected to a micro-implant (Figure 23.4).

Position of the micro-implant

When using indirect anchorage, placement of the micro-implants perpendicular to the bone surface, rather than obliquely, is recommended because of the ease in connecting a sectional wire to a perpendicularly positioned implant. However, in certain cases, in order to prevent root resorption, it is beneficial to position the apex of the micro-implant obliquely at the level of the root apex, where the interradicular space is wider.

Micro-implants can be placed either on the buccal or the palatal side of the alveolar bone. The buccal side provides easier access for surgical placement. On the contrary, the palatal side has wider interradicular spaces and a larger amount of masticatory mucosa, which is more resistant to inflammation. However, the palatal side has poor accessibility and a palatal micro-implant causes tongue irritation.

Biomechanical considerations

When using the micro-implant as indirect anchorage for molar intrusion, the sectional wire connecting the micro-implant to the anchor tooth should be aligned as vertically

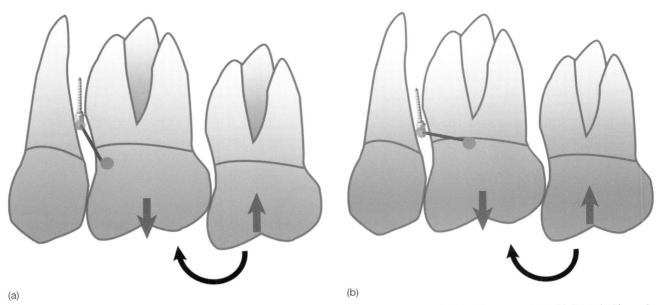

(a)   (b)

Figure 23.5 A vertically connected wire (a) from micro-implant to an anchor tooth can resist better than a horizontally connected wire (b). (Printed with permission, from Park [2009].)

as possible to be able to resist the reactive extrusive forces and moment on the anchor tooth (Figure 23.5a). If the sectional wire is horizontally aligned, the rotational moment exerted on the anchor tooth will be larger (Figure 23.5b) than when it is aligned vertically. As the micro-implants has weak resistance against torsional or rotational forces (Costa et al., 1998), the sectional wire should be connected parallel to the reaction force so that only a pushing or pulling force is loaded on the micro-implant. Thus the position of the micro-implant should be decided bearing this consideration in mind.

Case 2

A 50-year-old male patient presented with extruded maxillary second and third molars, a situation that had developed following the loss of the mandibular second molar (Figure 23.6). We decided to extract the maxillary third molar and to intrude the maxillary second molar to providing vertical space for a mandibular prosthesis. A micro-implant (SH1312-08, Absoanchor) was placed into the buccal alveolar bone between the maxillary second premolar and the first molar (Figure 23.7). A 0.016 × 0.022 inch stainless steel sectional wire was fabricated and attached with core composite (Bisfil Core, BISCO Inc.) to the second premolar, the first molar, and the head of the micro-implant (Figure 23.8). Standard 0.018 × 0.022 inch slot brackets were bonded on the buccal surfaces of the maxillary first and second molars, and to the palatal surfaces of the second premolar and molars. Sectional titanium-molybdenum (TMA) wires, 0.016 × 0.022 inch, were fabricated and ligated to apply intrusion force with an activation of 0.5 mm. Note that the application of force on both sides,

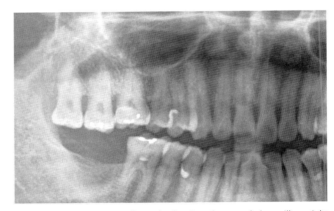

Figure 23.6 Panoramic radiograph showing the extruded maxillary right second and third molars.

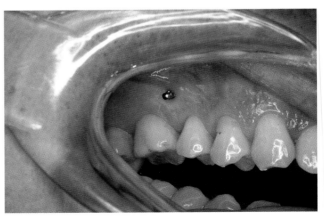

Figure 23.7 Micro-implant placed in the alveolar bone between the second premolar and first molar.

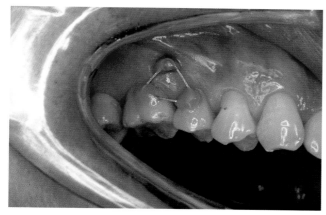

Figure 23.8 Sectional wire connected from the micro-implant to the teeth.

buccal and palatal, minimizes the tipping of the molar buccolingually (Figure 23.9). The irritation caused to the tongue by the brackets on the palatal surface can be alleviated by use of wax or silicone periodontal wound dressing (e.g. Barricaid R, Dentsply-Gendex). The appropriate intrusion was achieved after 5 months of treatment (Figures 23.10, 23.11). The same orthodontic appliance was used as a retainer while waiting for osseointegration of the lower dental implant and prosthesis. After the delivery of the dental prosthesis in the lower arch, all the appliances were removed (Figures 23.12, 23.13). As it takes 5–6 months to intrude a molar by 2–3 mm and osseointegration requires 3–6 months, to reduce the treatment time, the clinicians can perform intrusion of the upper molar

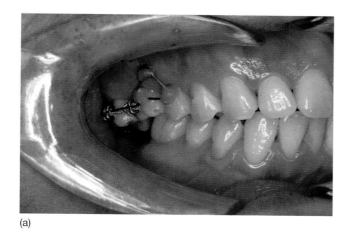

(a)

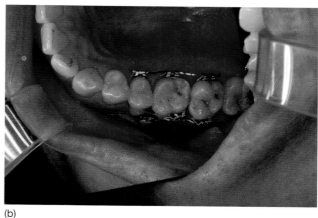

(b)

Figure 23.9 Brackets bonded on the buccal and palatal surfaces to apply intrusion force from both sides: (a) lateral view; (b) occlusal view.

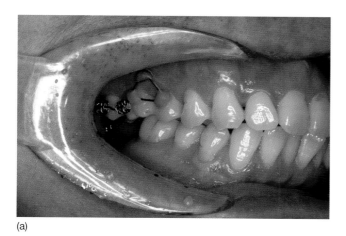

(a)

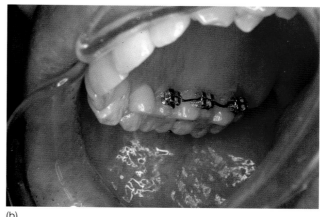

(b)

Figure 23.10 At 5 months of treatment, the second molar was intruded: (a) lateral view; (b) palatal view.

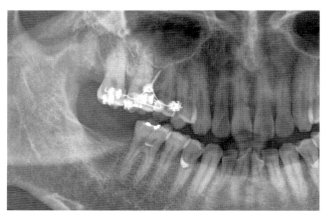

Figure 23.11 Panoramic view showing the intrusion.

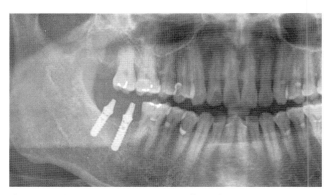

Figure 23.13 Post-treatment panoramic radiograph.

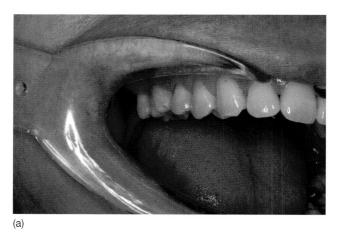

(a)

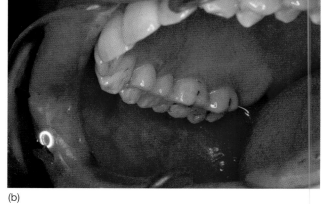

(b)

Figure 23.12 Post-treatment intraoral photographs: (a) buccal view; (b) palatal view.

and the lower dental implant placement in the same time period.

Simultaneous intrusion of two molars

One of the easy and biomechanically simple methods of intruding two molars on one side of the dental arch is to use buccal and palatal micro-implants. Tooth movement stops when the root contacts the micro-implant during intrusion. To avoid this contact, the micro-implant is placed in the apical area so that there is enough space between the micro-implant and the roots for their subsequent movement. Since the buccal interradicular space between the upper first and second molars is narrow (Park et al., 2010), micro-implants should be placed in the apical area where the space is relatively wider. Since maxillary molars have a single palatal root, there exists a wide space for the micro-implant on this side, and since the buccal root curves dis-

tally, the micro-implant needs to be inserted distal to the contact point.

In addition, to maintain the curve of Spee, the second molar should be located higher than the first molar and needs to be intruded to a greater extent. The direction of the orthodontic force depends on the position of the head of the micro-implant and the attachment on the tooth. To obtain greater intrusion of the second molar, the micro-implant should be placed distal to the contact point of the first and second molars (Figure 23.14), or occasionally, an additional micro-implant in the maxillary tuberosity can be helpful (Figure 23.15).

Owing to the weaker alveolar bone on the palatal side, which is covered by thick soft tissue, the distance from the buccopalatal midpoint of the tooth crowns to the head of the micro-implant should be greater on the palatal side than on the buccal side. The resultant horizontal

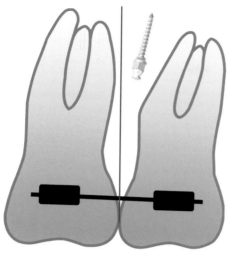

Figure 23.14 The micro-implant is placed distal to the contact point to provide a greater intrusive force for the second molar. (Printed with permission, from Park [2009].)

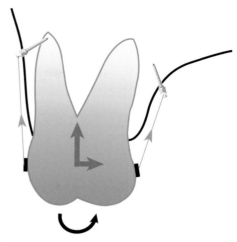

Figure 23.16 Palatal tipping of intruding molar occurs when the distance from the micro-implant to the midpoint of the teeth on palatal side is longer than on the buccal side. (Printed with permission, from Park [2009].)

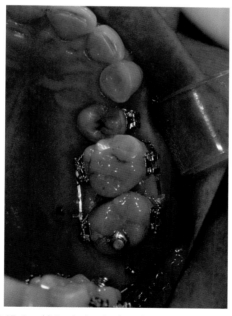

Figure 23.15 An additional micro-implant placed into the maxillary tuberosity produces a distal intrusion force to achieve greater intrusion of the second molar.

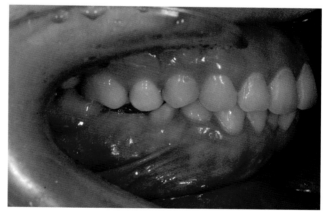

Figure 23.17 Supraerupted upper right second premolar and first molar.

component of force on the palatal side will, therefore, be stronger than on the buccal side (Figure 23.16) resulting in palatal tipping of the molar. To prevent this tipping, the buccal micro-implant should be long, and at the same time it should protrude buccally, while the palatal micro-implant should be inserted close to the gingival margin, thus reducing the horizontal component of force. The alignment of teeth can also be performed during

the intrusion by bonding brackets and adding appropriate bends to the sectional wires. Sectional wires can be bonded directly to the tooth surfaces if there is no such requirement.

Case 3

A 38-year-old female patient attended the orthodontic clinic with a supraerupted maxillary right second premolar and first molar, following the loss of the mandibular first molar (Figure 23.17). Two micro-implants (buccal: SH1312-08, palatal: SH1312-10) were placed into the buccal and palatal alveolar bone between the second premolar and the first molar (Figure 23.18). In order to provide sufficient space for intrusion, the buccal micro-implant was placed high into the vestibule. The heads of the micro-implants

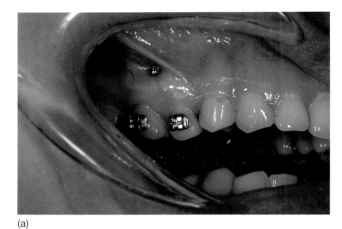

(a)

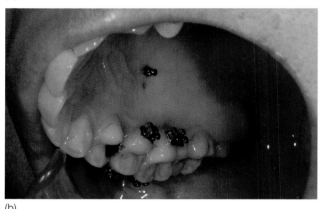

(b)

Figure 23.18 Micro-implants placed in the buccal (a) and palatal (b) alveolar bone.

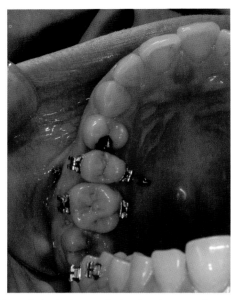

Figure 23.19 Occlusal photograph showing the same distance from the micro-implants to the midpoint of teeth on buccal and palatal sides.

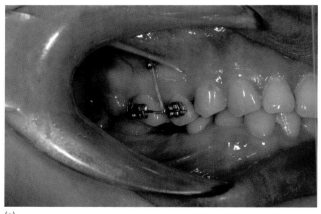

(a)

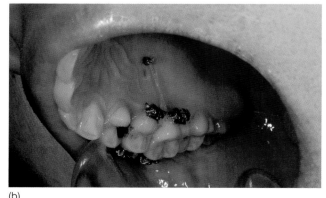

(b)

Figure 23.20 Intrusive force applied from the micro-implants to the wire: (a) buccal view; (b) palatal view.

on the buccal and palatal sides were located at the same distance from the midpoint of the crowns buccopalatally, to minimize tipping of the teeth in this plane (Figure 23.19). Standard 0.018 × 0.022 inch brackets were bonded to the buccal and palatal surfaces of the second premolar and first molar. Sectional TMA wires, 0.016 × 0.022 inch, were ligated and intrusive forces applied from the micro-implants to the wires (Figure 23.20). To reduce the treatment time, an intrusive force is usually applied immediately after insertion of the micro-implants. We prefer to use elastomeric threads such as Super thread (RMO) or Square thread (Dentos) for this purpose. These produce relatively light force, and the Square thread has the advantage of minimal food impaction. After 5 months of treatment, the second premolar and the first molar were intruded to the level of the second molar (Figure 23.21). After bonding a bracket to the second molar, further intrusion forces were applied to all three teeth. After 8 months of treatment, all three teeth showed an appropriate amount of intrusion (Figure 23.22). After attachment of the prosthesis to the

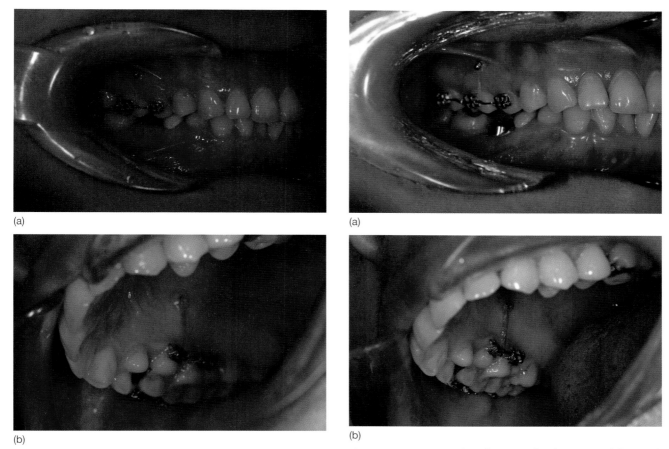

Figure 23.21 Intrusion achieved at 5 months of treatment: (a) buccal view; (b) palatal view.

Figure 23.22 Intrusion achieved at 8 months of treatment of three teeth (now including the second molar): (a) buccal view; (b) palatal view.

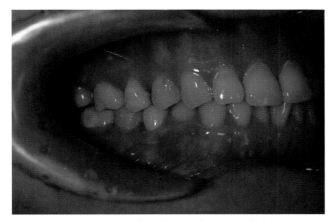

Figure 23.23 After delivery of prosthesis in the lower arch the upper appliances were removed.

lower arch, the upper appliances were removed (Figure 23.23).

Molar uprighting

It is well known that some eruption/occlusal movement of a molar occurs while the tooth is being uprighted. This eruptive/occlusal movement results from the distal tipping of the molar crown as it rotates around the tooth's center of resistance, which is located in the furcation area (Figure 23.24). Furthermore, when applying uprighting moment to the tooth with a sectional wire, an extrusive force is applied on the molar and an intrusive force on the reactive unit. Therefore, adding an intrusive force when uprighting a molar might help in minimizing traumatic occlusion later.

A mesially tipped molar can be uprighted by two types of movement, i.e. by distal movement of the crown or mesial movement of the root. Distal crown movement (Figure 23.25) is quick and easy, because only a small amount of root movement is required. However, mesial

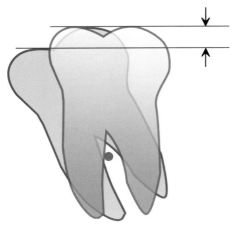

Figure 23.24 Passive eruption of a molar during uprighting. (Printed with permission, from Park [2009].)

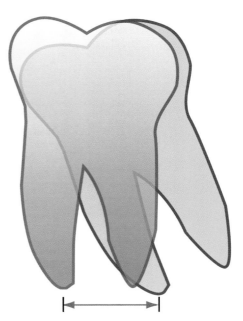

Figure 23.26 Uprighting with root mesial movement. (Printed with permission, from Park [2009].).

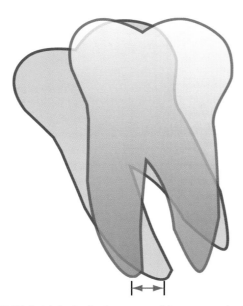

Figure 23.25 Uprighting by distal movement of the crown requires little root movement. (Printed with permission, from Park [2009].)

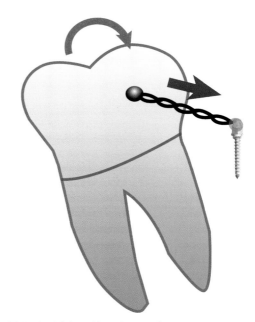

Figure 23.27 Uprighting with an intrusive force component using a micro-implant. (Printed with permission, from Park [2009].)

movement of the root (Figure 23.26) is more difficult, requiring longer treatment time, and is even more difficult in cases with a narrow alveolus.

The retromolar micro-implant: placement site and surgical procedure

When considering the position of the micro-implant, the most important issue is the final position of the micro-implant's head. This position is crucial because it determines the direction of the orthodontic force and controls the type of tooth movement. Therefore, the head of the micro-implant should be positioned at the most appropriate point both in the buccolingual and in the vertical

dimensions. In all patients, the micro-implant should be placed far enough distally to provide a sufficiently long span for distal uprighting of molars. The head of the micro-implant should be positioned lower than the attachments on the uprighting molar to generate an intrusive force during uprighting (Figure 23.27).

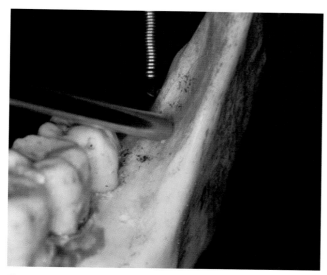

Figure 23.28 A site for retromolar area; a flat bone inner to external oblique ridge. (Printed with permission, from Park [2009].)

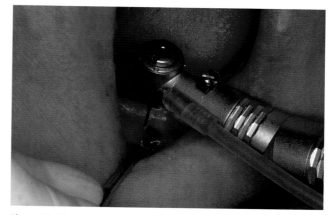

Figure 23.30 Preparation of a hole with pilot drill. (Printed with permission, from Park [2009].)

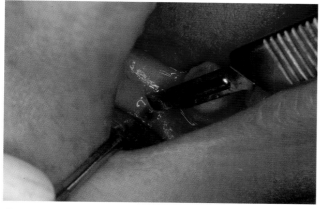

Figure 23.29 Incision for placing a micro-implant in the retro-molar area. (Printed with permission, from Park [2009].)

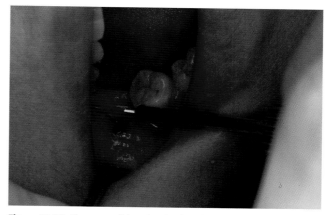

Figure 23.31 Placement of the micro-implant. (Printed with permission, from Park [2009].)

Mandibular molars tend to tip mesially and lingually when a tooth located anteriorly in the dental arch is lost. Therefore, a distobuccal force is required, in order to upright the molar. Accordingly, the head of the micro-implant should be positioned buccal and distal to the uprighting molar. The flat and triangular area inside the external oblique ridge is an appropriate site for a retromolar micro-implant (Figure 23.28). If the third molar needs to be extracted, the micro-implant can be placed at the time of the extraction.

Surgical procedure

After the administration of local anesthesia, an incision is made in the attached gingiva (Figure 23.29). Owing to the presence of thick soft tissue in this area, an incision is necessary, but it should be small, approximately 3 mm long, to minimize the need for a suture. When placing the micro-implant with the drill-free method, it should be inserted perpendicularly to the bone surface. However, as the access to the retromolar area is difficult, the micro-implants may need to inclined by 60–70° to the bone surface. In this situation, the clinician should create a hole with a pilot drill (Figure 23.30), and then insert the micro-implant (Figure 23. 31). We also have to consider the occlusion at this point because micro-implant failure often occurs due to impact from the occlusal forces generated by the maxillary second and/or third molars during chewing.

Ligature wire

The head of the micro-implant, which is exposed after surgery, often gets covered by soft tissue following healing. This necessitates the fabrication of a ligature wire extension

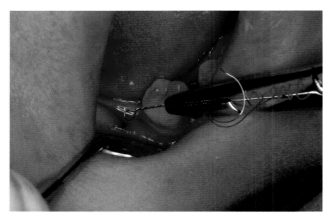

Figure 23.32 A ligature wire extension. (Printed with permission, from Park [2009].)

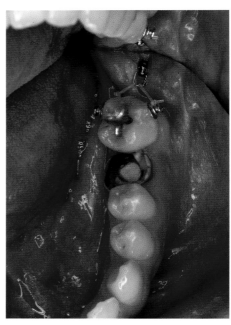

Figure 23.33 Lingual buttons on the distobuccal and distolingual line angles of the molar.

(Figure 23.32). The ligature wire should be extended in the direction of the orthodontic force. Failing to incorporate this much extension might result in trauma to the gingiva and subsequently infection.

Attachments

An elastic thread attached to a lingual button on the mesial surface of the molar can provide sufficient span for activation, but the thread might get cut by the forces of occlusion, or rotation of the uprighting molar could occur if the elastic thread slips down. Using a thread from a lingual button bonded to the distal surface of the uprighting molar will not result in the rotation of the molar. However, the span of the elastomeric thread, i.e. the distance from the micro-implant head or hook of the ligature wire extension to the distal button, is too short, and, as the molar is uprighted, the distance becomes even shorter. Bonding two lingual buttons, one on the buccal and one on the lingual surface can eliminate the tendency for rotation, while still providing an adequate span for activation of the elastomeric thread (Figure 23.33). By altering the magnitude of the force on the lingual or buccal side, the clinician can rotate the molar when required.

Considerations with regard to trauma from occlusion

The center of resistance of the molars is located at the furcation area of the roots, which means that an uprighting molar can passively erupt with the crown extruding beyond the occlusal plane (see Figure 23.24). This extrusion may cause trauma from the occlusion. For this reason, selective grinding of occlusal surface should be considered. If, however, the vertical position of the micro-implant head is located below the lingual button, the direction of orthodontic force will be backward and downward

(see Figure 23.27). In such situations, the molar is intruded and uprighted simultaneously, preventing trauma from occlusion and avoiding the need for occlusal grinding. However, in certain instances of uprighting, the distal cusp of the molar may extrude over the occlusal plane and temporary trauma from the occlusion is unavoidable. To prevent this, disclusion is necessary using an anterior bite plate or a bonded resin block on the adjacent molars.

The amount of orthodontic force

There is no need for a heavy force to upright a mesially tipped molar. Approximately 80–100 g of force should suffice. We prefer to use elastomeric threads, such as Super thread (RMO) or Square thread (Dentos), for the application of a force to the molar. Immediate loading is possible after placement of the micro-implant, because relatively weak forces are used.

Mobility

Molars that are being uprighted commonly exhibit mobility, especially in the adult patient. Because of occlusal interferences created, trauma from occlusion can result in mobility when the cusp of the lower molar extrudes beyond the occlusal plane. If the mobility is severe, the occlusal force should be reduced by increasing the intrusive component of the force or by grinding the occlusal surface selectively. After the completion of molar uprighting, a fixed retainer should be bonded for retention until the tooth is no longer mobile.

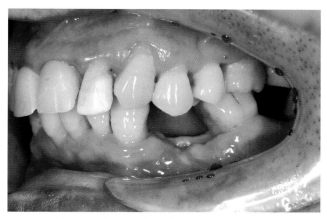

Figure 23.34 A mesially tipped lower first molar.

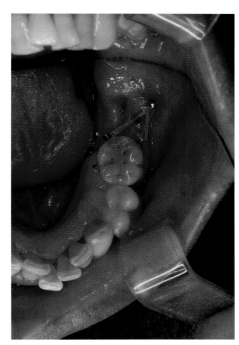

Figure 23.35 Micro-implant placed into bone distobuccal to the molar; a distal and intrusive force was applied immediately.

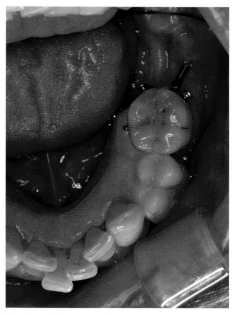

Figure 23.36 The failed micro-implant.

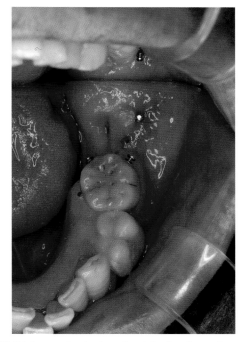

Figure 23.37 A new micro-implant placed distal to the previous one.

Case 4

A 38-year-old male patient presented with a mesially tipped lower left first molar (Figure 23.34). A micro-implant (SH1312-06, Absoanchor) was placed in the distobuccal alveolar bone (Figure 23.35). Two buttons were bonded on the distobuccal and distolingual line angles of the first molar, and a distal-driving intrusive force was applied. After 3 weeks of treatment, the micro-implant failed (Figure 23.36). Another micro-implant (SH1312-07, Absoanchor) was placed distal to the previous one at the same visit,

and a distal-driving force was continuously applied (Figure 23.37). After 3 months of treatment, the molar was mobile owing to trauma from occlusion. Occlusal adjustment was performed (Figure 23.38), and after another 3 months of treatment, the first molar was uprighted appropriately (Figure 23.39). As the patient wanted to

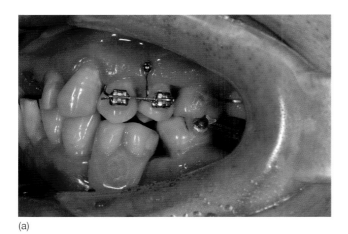

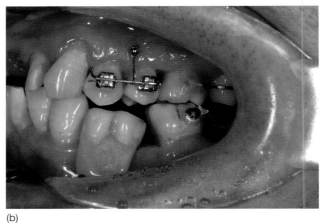

(a)   (b)

Figure 23.38 At 3 months of treatment, mobility of the molar was evident: (a) maximum intercuspation; (b) resting position.

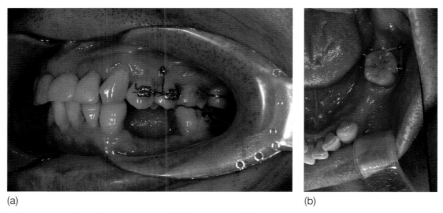

(a)   (b)

Figure 23.39 At 6 months of treatment, the molar was uprighted: (a) lateral view; (b) occlusal view.

receive a dental implant at a later date, the appliances were kept as retainers.

Molar uprighting with two joint micro-implants

By connecting two micro-implants together with a ligature wire and composite, the micro-implants become stronger and the likelihood of failure is diminished significantly. The joining of two immobile structures provides resistance to a rotational twisting force, which is the most difficult stress for one micro-implant to resist. By bonding a bracket on the head of the micro-implant, it can receive a rectangular arch wire to provide precise three-dimensional control of tooth movement. In a system using two micro-implants, it is easy to predict the course of tooth movement, because the micro-implants remain stationary, and the direction of force is altered only due to the moving teeth.

The thick and dense buccal cortical bone should be utilized for placement of the micro-implants, as the bone at the alveolar crest is thin, weak, and less dense. The implants should be inserted about 3 mm away from the alveolar crest, and 10° toward the lingual side. Micro-implants that protrude excessively toward the cheek may irritate the cheek mucosa, causing inflammation. The gap between the two micro-implants should be about 3 mm, and they should be placed parallel to each other. A space of about 1 mm should be kept between the composite material connecting the implants and the gingiva, to allow the patient to maintain oral hygiene in that area.

Case 5

A 58-year-old female patient was referred for distal uprighting of the lower right second molar. After removal of the previous dental prosthesis, a temporary crown was delivered. Mesial tipping of the tooth was not observed clinically, owing to the wrong shape of the provisional

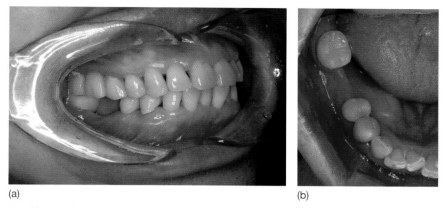

Figure 23.40 A mesially tipped lower right second molar with wrongly shaped provisional crown: (a) lateral view; (b) occlusal view.

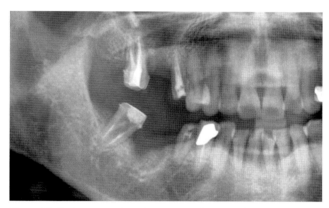

Figure 23.41 Panoramic view showing mesial tipping of the molar.

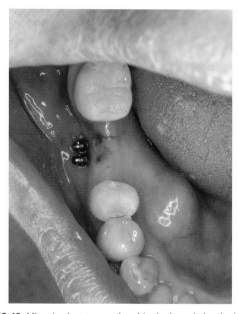

Figure 23.42 Micro-implants were placed in the buccal alveolar bone.

crown (Figure 23.40) however, it was evident on the panoramic radiograph (Figure 23.41). The provisional crown was modified to make it coincide with the direction of the roots. Two micro-implants (SH1312-08, Absoanchor) were placed in the edentulous ridge. To utilize the thick buccal cortical plate, the micro-implants were placed 3 mm buccal from the alveolar crest, inclined at an angle of 10° toward the lingual side (Figure 23.42), parallel to each other. A ligature wire was tied on the heads of the two micro-implants (Figure 23.43). Core composite was put on the heads and ligature wire (Figure 23.44), and a 0.018 × 0.022 inch slot standard edgewise bracket was bonded to the composite (Figure 23.45). A 0.016 × 0.022 inch TMA sectional wire was fabricated to apply uprighting and protraction forces to the second molar (Figure 23.46). As the second premolar also needed to be uprighted distally, it was also ligated to the TMA wire. The second molar was uprighted with mesial root movement so that the edentulous span was not increased. At 10 months of treatment, the lower second molar had uprighted and a dental prosthesis was delivered (Figure 23.47).

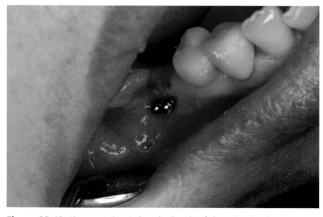

Figure 23.43 Ligature wire tied to the heads of the micro-implants.

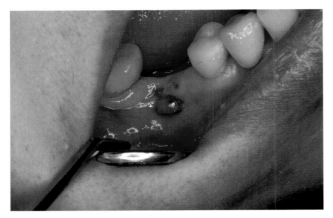

Figure 23.44 Core composite covering the heads of the micro-implants.

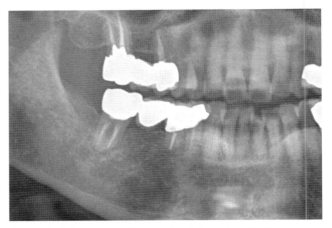

Figure 23.47 Panoramic radiograph after delivery of prosthesis.

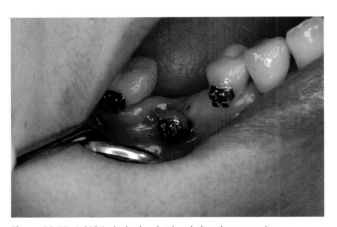

Figure 23.45 A 018 inch slot bracket bonded to the composite.

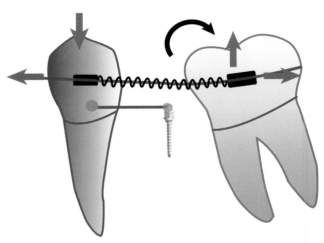

Figure 23.48 Illustration of molar uprighting with indirect anchorage. (Printed with permission, from Park [2009].)

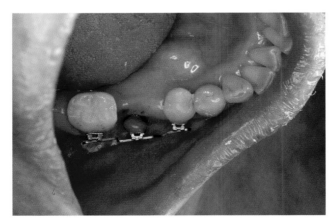

Figure 23.46 Uprighting moment applied with a 016 × 022 TMA wire.

Molar uprighting with indirect anchorage

Molar uprighting can also be performed with indirect anchorage. When the second molar is uprighted with conventional mechanics, anchorage is usually obtained from the premolars. For uprighting using indirect anchorage, in order to eliminate the movement of the anchor teeth, the tilted tooth can be connected to the micro-implants with the help of a sectional wire. The reactive force on the premolars is mesial and intrusive in nature, and the connecting wire should be aligned horizontally to resist undesirable tooth movements (Figure 23.48). For this reason, the micro-implant has to be placed near the gingival margin. The uprighting molar tends to erupt because of the extrusive force from the uprighting moment. To prevent trauma from occlusion, it is also necessary to apply an intrusive force to the uprighting molar.

Forced eruption

Forced eruption of a tooth is a necessary step in restoring a fractured or a severely decayed tooth with root involvement, which interferes with prosthetic restoration. Removable appliances can be used as anchorage, but it is difficult to precisely control tooth movement, and it is not effective in non-compliant patients. Fixed orthodontic appliances can provide better anchorage and precise control of tooth movement, but unwanted reactive movement of anchor teeth is inevitable. Furthermore, the forced eruption of a tooth without any adjacent teeth to serve as anchorage is challenging. However, treatment using micro-implant anchorage minimizes the number of teeth needed for bracket bonding; at times, it can also be more esthetic if the implant is placed in the palatal area.

Considerations regarding the alveolar bone and gingiva

The contour of the alveolar bone and gingiva often follow the extruded tooth (Koyuturk and Malkoc, 2005). This phenomenon of bone induction can be utilized while placing a dental implant at the bone defect (Mantzikos and Shamus, 1998). The dental prosthesis needs to follow the rules of biologic width (Ingber et al., 1977) to preserve periodontal support (see Chapter 22 for more details on biologic width). Therefore, coronal bone formation with forced eruption should be prevented. Periodical gingival fiberotomy can prevent coronal bone growth (Kozlovsky et al., 1988). Berglundh et al. (1991) reported that gingival fiberotomy cannot prevent coronal migration of the alveolar bone and gingiva. In our experience, it seems more practical to perform one alveolar bone resection and gingivectomy procedure than several gingival fiberotomies. The thickness of the gingiva should also be considered when performing gingivectomy. In case of thin gingiva, more gingival shrinkage is expected after gingivectomy.

Retention

Two months retention is reported to be sufficient (Felippe et al., 2003). However, relapse can occur even after 3 months of retention (Park, 2009). A fixed bonded retainer for a year might be a good retention protocol.

Orthodontic force

Excessive extrusive orthodontic forces exerted on teeth may cause root resorption and ankylosis. Determination of the appropriate extrusive forces to be applied depends on the root morphology, mainly the root diameter, length, and surface area (Ogihara and Wang, 2010). Therefore, if the tooth to be extruded is an incisor, 15 g is sufficient, whereas 60 g might be needed for a molar. For slow extrusion 30 g of force is adequate (Minsk 2000). However, if rapid extrusion is required, the force applied should be increased to 50 g (Bondemark et al., 1997).

Direction of force

The force should pass along the long axis of the tooth. Thus a hook should be fitted into the root canal, or attached to the middle of a tooth and another hook on the cantilever arm, which is attached to the implants, should be located over the middle of the erupting tooth.

Case 6

A 22-year-old female patient was referred from the department of prosthetics for extrusion of the lower right first premolar, which had severe decay and history of previous root canal treatment (Figure 23.49). It was decided that 2 mm of forced eruption would be required for the construction of a proper dental crown prosthesis. To minimize adverse reactive movement of adjacent teeth, which was expected when using adjacent teeth as anchorage, micro-implants were used for this purpose. The first step in the treatment consisted of fabricating a hook with a 0.014 inch round stainless steel wire (Figure 23.50). Note that the

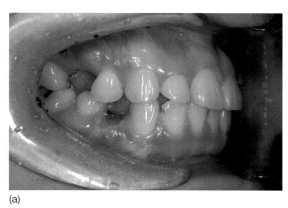
(a)

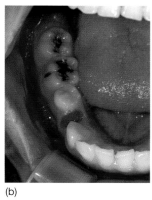
(b)

Figure 23.49 A lower right first premolar requiring forced eruption: (a) lateral view; (b) occlusal view.

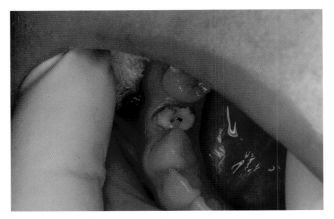

Figure 23.50 Hook cemented into the root canal.

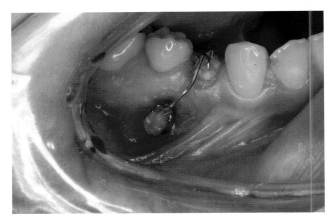

Figure 23.52 Extrusive force applied from the free end of cantilever wire to the hook on the tooth.

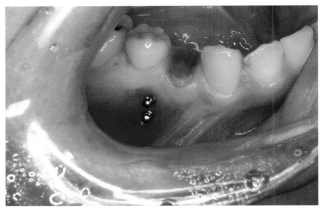

Figure 23.51 Two micro-implants placed into the alveolar bone between the first and second premolars.

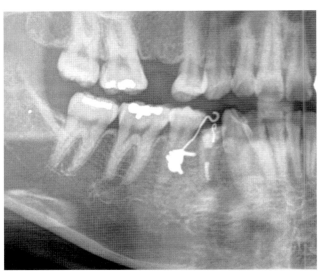

Figure 23.53 Panoramic radiograph showing appliance set-up.

hook should be as small as possible. Two micro-implants (SH1312-07, Absoanchor) were placed in the alveolar bone between the lower first and second premolars (Figure 23.51). A ligature wire was tied to the heads of the micro-implants and composite material was added to the heads. After bonding a bracket, a sectional cantilever TMA wire, 0.016 × 0.022 inch, was ligated to the bracket slot. The force was applied with a Super thread (RMO, Denver, CO, USA) (Figures 23.52, 23.53).

The hook of the cantilever sectional wire should be out of occlusal contact (Figure 23.54). As the hook determines the direction of force and resultant direction of extrusion, it should be located at the middle of the tooth (Figure 23.55). If distal movement of the tooth is required, the hook can be bent distally. After 2 months of treatment, the second premolar had erupted appropriately (Figures 23.56, 23.57). The appliances were kept *in situ* for 4 additional

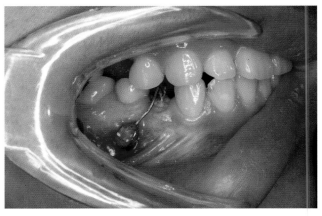

Figure 23.54 The cantilever wire should be free from occlusal contact.

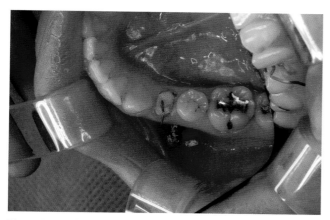

Figure 23.55 The hook of wire needs to be located at the middle of the tooth.

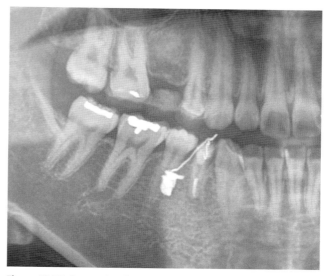

Figure 23.57 Panoramic radiograph after forced eruption.

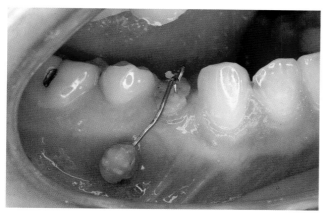

Figure 23.56 At 2 months of treatment, 2 mm of extrusion was obtained.

months for retention, after which the dental prosthesis was delivered.

Surgical placement of micro-implants

Micro-implants can be easily placed as a routine orthodontic procedure. There is a comparatively high success rate in comparison with conventional anchorage sources, but there is still a certain level of concern as they can fail. The failure rate varies according to the type of skeletal anchorage obtained, the surgical dexterity of the clinician, the placement method, the placement sites and the patient's systemic status.

The surgical procedure has a learning curve, but with the accumulation of surgical experience over a period of time, clinicians have fewer failures (Park and Kim, 1999; Park, 2003). As the literature reveals, most implant failures occur within the first 4 months of placement (Park, 2003; Moon

et al., 2010). Consequently, the first step toward success is becoming competent in the art and essence of the surgical procedure.

There are two types of surgical placement methods for micro-implants: drill method (self-tapping method) and drill-free method (self-drilling method). The drill method requires preparation of a hole with a pilot drill before placement of the micro-implant. In contrast, in the drill-free method, the micro-implants are placed without any drilling, just by twisting the micro-implant into the bone with a driver, so that it can penetrate the bone easily and is placed *in situ* firmly and precisely. As the bone thickness and density vary in different regions of the jaws (Park et al., 2008; Park and Cho, 2009) and in different individuals, the most ideal method of implant placement in patients with thick cortical bone and high density is the drill method. The drill-free method provides better initial stability in cases with bone with thin cortices and low density, as the bone is condensed during placement (Park, 2009).

Local anesthesia

To prepare the aseptic field for the selected surgical site, the site is dabbed with benzalkonium chloride ((Zephiran)-soaked gauze (Figure 23.58), although full aseptic preparation is mandatory for the whole face and mouth. Then an injection of a quarter or one-third of an ampoule of a local anesthetic is given (Figure 23.59). Mild surface anesthesia of the oral mucosa keeps the sensitivity of the nerve fibers intact in the periodontal ligament; in this way patients can alert the clinician when the pilot drill impinges or approaches the periodontal ligament. If this happens during the preparation, utmost care should be taken and the drill redirected away. Topical anesthetic

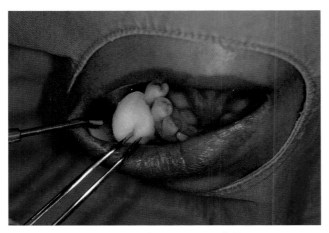

Figure 23.58 Asepsis procedure for the placement field.

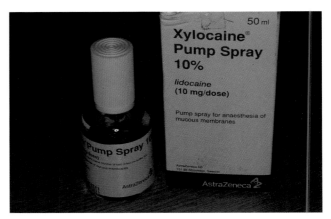

Figure 23.60 Topical anesthesia: 10% lidocaine (Xylocaine).

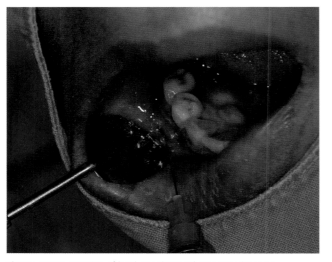

Figure 23.59 Injection of local anesthetic solution into the gingiva.

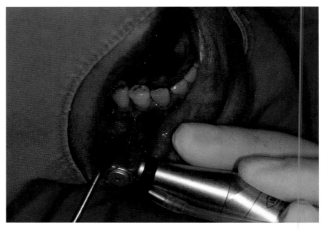

Figure 23.61 Drilling a hole with a pilot drill.

solution with 10% lidocaine (Figure. 23.60) can also be used. Ten minutes of waiting time is required so as to gain suitable depth of anesthesia. Some patients may not reach the required depth of anesthesia with topical anesthesia and may require an injection of anesthetic solution as well.

Incision

An incision is required only when the micro-implants are placed into the oral mucosa; it is not required for placement in attached gingiva or the palatal masticatory mucosa.

Drilling a hole with the pilot drill

The drill method requires making a surgical hole (Figure 23.61) before the placement of micro-implants. With due regard to the bioengineering principles governing the drill and the screw, an in-depth assessment of the mechanical procedure needs to be done. Maximum bone removal is achieved when the diameter of the drill is 85% of outer diameter of the screw, as this reduces the insertion torque (Heidemann et al., 1998). Moreover, the diameter of the drill should be smaller than the inner diameter of the screw for better contact of the latter with the bone (Oktenoglu et al., 2001). We prefer to use a 0.1–0.2 mm smaller diameter drill as compared with the inner diameter of the micro-implants used in the maxilla and 0.1 mm smaller diameter drill in the mandible. Our clinical experience with Absoanchor micro-implants SH1312 from Dentos, with specified inner diameter of 1.1 mm at the neck and 1.0 mm at the apex, endorses the statement that it is better to use

0.9 mm of pilot drill in the maxilla and 1.0 mm in the mandible for better stability.

During drilling, the site should be irrigated profusely with a coolant to reduce the heat generation. In order to minimize heat production, the drill is moved in and out from the pilot opening as the drilling proceeds into the dense cortical bone. Caution has to be observed while drilling to maintain the direction of the axis of the drill so as not to inadvertently enlarge the opening. The clinician should not apply too much pressure while drilling, because generation of heat is proportionate to the pressure applied (Tehemar, 1999). The drill hole should extend all the way through the cortical bone.

The speed of the drill, which is about 600 rpm, is far slower than the specified speed for a normal dental implant placement. This is an added advantage during the placement of orthodontic micro-implants. As a matter of fact, a drill with smaller diameter and faster speed will produce more heat, causing deleterious effects on the bone.

Placement of micro-implants

The head of the micro-implants needs to be engaged into the tip of the driver (Figure 23.62), and meticulous care should be taken to avoid touching or contaminating the threaded portion of the micro-implant. The micro-implant is inserted into the opening of the hole prepared or directly into the bone and driven into position (Figures 23.63, 23.64). The micro-implants can be placed either using a hand driver or an engine-driven driver. We prefer to use a hand driver because it allows the clinician greater tactile information regarding the density and thickness of the bone, and also detecting any root contact via proprioception transmitted through the driver into the fingers and hand. The insertion torque increases with tightening of the micro-implants and the highest insertion torque is at the last turn. If the implant is screwed in significantly beyond this point, there will be a decrease in the insertion torque. It means that the bone material interlacing with the threads of the micro-implants has been smashed and destroyed, and this is one of the causes of failure of implants.

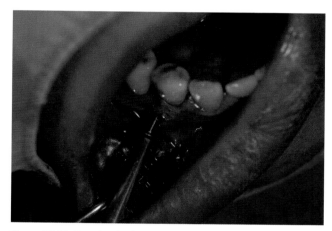

Figure 23.63 The micro-implant is introduced into the prepared hole.

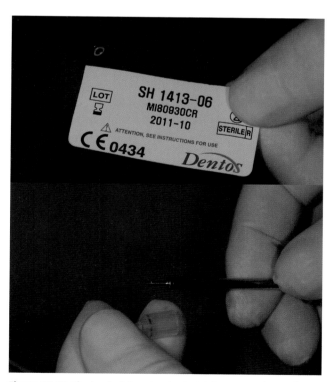

Figure 23.62 The head of the micro-implant being engaged securely into the tip of the driver.

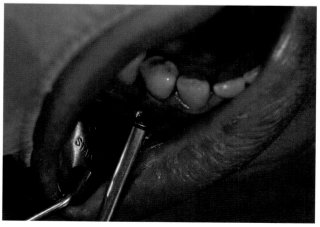

Figure 23.64 The micro-implant is tightened until the neck is flush with the bone surface.

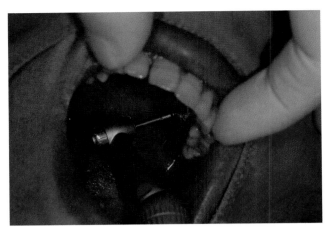

Figure 23.65 Placement of the micro-implant with an engine driver.

Therefore, the micro-implants should be tightened slowly and gently, appreciating the resistance when approaching the last turn.

Micro-implants fracture mostly at the last turn, and there is a spring-back action just before the fracture. To avoid a fracture, the clinician should stop applying tightening force at this point. Slow tightening of the micro-implants can reduce the chances of fracture. When using a low-speed drill to place micro-implants, an appropriate speed of the drill is about 25–30 rpm. Engine-driven placements are preferred in areas where there is less chance of root contacts (Figure 23.65). With the drill-free method, which requires limited instrumentation, micro-implants can be placed easily. The micro-implant itself makes the surgical opening into the bone during the screwing-in procedure.

Postoperative care

Most patients do not experience severe pain or discomfort during or after placement, or during the removal, of micro-implants. An incision followed by reflection of a flap for placing a surgical mini-plate may produce pain and postoperative swelling (Kuroda et al., 2007a). Inflammation around micro-implants occurs less frequently in the maxilla than in the mandible. Administration of antibiotics and anti-inflammatory agents for 1 day is sufficient for reducing inflammation after placement (Hossein et al., 2005). Preemptive administration of antibiotics increased the success rate of the dental implants (Laskin et al., 2000), in fact, the preoperative administration of antibiotics 2 hours prior to the surgical procedure is the most preferable approach to reduce the inflammation.

Control of oral hygiene is essential, as inflammation around the micro-implant may have a deleterious effect on its stability. We recommend educating the patient to maintain exemplary oral hygiene. A toothbrush may irritate the soft tissues around the micro-implant, hence a water flosser such as Waterpik is the best method to maintain oral hygiene. The usage of oral rinses with chlorhexidine is also recommended.

Success rate

We have studied and reported the success rate with micro-implants, which ranges from 82% to 93.3%. Our first study was conducted in 1999 and revealed 82% of success rate during the 5 months observation period (Park and Kim, 1999). The next two studies conducting in 2003 and 2006 revealed a 93% success rate (Park, 2003; Park et al., 2006a). This emphasizes the fact that with increasing experience, a higher success rate can be expected.

Success rate according to implant placement sites
The maxilla had a higher success rate than the mandible and the maxillary palatal side had 100% success rate (Park, 2003; Park et al., 2006a). The mandibular posterior teeth region has the highest rate of failure (Park, 2003; Cheng et al., 2004; Park et al., 2006a).

Timing of and factors affecting failure

Most failures occurred during the first few months of placement – in our experience, six out of 12 failures occurred within the first 2 months after placement (Park, 2003). There were three failures in the 2–6-months period and three more failures in the 7–10 months period. No failures occurred thereafter. Therefore, the surgical procedure is the most important factor in successful implant anchorage use, as is the management of the micro-implants with proper oral hygiene measures to prevent inflammatory changes.

Other factors affecting the failure of the micro-implants are very similar to those related to failure of dental implants, which can be divided into three categories: host, surgical, and management factors. The host factors include presence of systemic conditions such as diabetes, osteoporosis, and smoking, and local host factors such as the condition of the soft tissue and density of the local bone (Jaffin and Berman, 1991). These are very important in elderly patients, as they are the main population seeking prosthetic treatment and thus also pre-prosthetic orthodontic treatment. Management factors include heavy force applications, infection, and inflammation.

To be successful, micro-implants should demonstrate initial stability after placement. Occlusion with teeth in the opposite arch may cause failure (Figure 23.8). If the micro-implants contact the roots of adjacent teeth, the chances of failure increase (Kuroda et al., 2007b). However, given all these factors that can cause failure, the success rate is quite high. In order to increase the success rate, clinicians need to check for and try to eliminate every possible cause of failure with careful monitoring of the situation.

Complications

Inflammation around micro-implants

Inflammation is one of the main complications, and its presence compromises the stability of micro-implants. Micro-implants placed in the palatal vault have a higher success rate due to the presence of thicker masticatory mucosa, which is strongly resistant to inflammation when compared with the buccal side where there is thin oral mucosa (Park, 2003). According to Cheng et al. (2004), mini-screws placed in the attached gingiva have a higher success rate than those placed into the oral mucosa. They also stated that inflammation is a definite risk factor. Micro-implants placed in the oral mucosa deep in the vestibule are more prone to inflammation.

To minimize inflammation, stringent oral hygiene procedures are essential. Food debris and plaque can accumulate around the micro-implants and the nickel-titanium (NiTi) coil springs, causing inflammation. Occasionally there is calculus deposition around the micro-implants. Tooth brushing irritates the mucosa at the margins of the micro-implants and leads to unintended application of heavy forces to the micro-implants, which may dislodge Ni-Ti coil springs. A water flosser such as Waterpik or use of water spray through a three-way syringe is the best method of maintaining hygiene around micro-implants.

Swelling after surgery

Flap surgery produces postsurgical swelling after placement. In cases where there is a need for minor flap surgery, minimal swelling has been observed and in cases where no flap surgery is required, no swelling is seen (Kuroda et al., 2007a). The mandibular posterior teeth area experiences more swelling than the maxilla.

Root damage

Fabbroni et al. (2004) found that 15.9% (37 out of 232) of mini-screws placed in the maxillofacial region produced minor damage due to root contact. There were six cases of pulp necrosis resulting from root damage due to mini-screw contact (Fabbroni et al., 2004). Borah and Ashmead (1996) reported that of a total of 2300 surgical micro-screws placed in 387 patients, 13 screws had root contact (0.47%) and these occurred mostly in the mandible (ratio of 10:3 with the maxilla). However, there were no serious complications.

The consequence of root contacts can be understood in the context of the findings of studies on periodontal damage. According to Andreasen (1980), if there is less than $4\,mm^2$ of periodontal damage, the periodontal ligament will be repaired to a normal state within 8 weeks. The

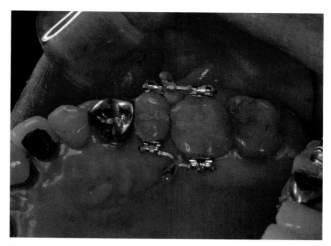

Figure 23.66 Use of bonding resin on the head reduces irritation to the tongue and cheeks.

diameter of the micro-implants ranged from 1.2 mm to 1.8 mm and they will not produce damage of more than $4\,mm^2$. Asscherickx et al. (2005) found that root damage caused by screws was repaired within 6 weeks after their removal. Root damage caused by smaller-diameter micro-implants (1.2–1.5 mm) also gets repaired faster. But bigger-diameter implants with sharp cutting edges lead to irreparable damage (Melsen, 2007). This damage may induce pulp necrosis. The drill method is better in terms of root damage, because the drill will not drive the implant into the roots as the clinician can appreciate the presence of the roots during the drilling.

Irritation to the tongue and cheek

Adult patients experience a sore tongue and cheek irritation much more than young patients. Therefore, the sharp edge at the head of the micro-implants or the edge of the Ni-Ti coil spring should be covered with bonding resin or a light-curing periodontal pack (Figure 23.66).

Conclusion

As micro-implants provide absolute anchorage and can be placed into any area of the bone, minor pre-prosthetic orthodontic treatment can be performed without adverse side effects and with minimal or no tooth anchorage requirements. To achieve their treatment goals, clinicians need to be knowledgeable about the biological and mechanical principles of orthodontic tooth movement as they pertain to the use of metallic implants, in order to be able to use skeletal anchorage units in a reliable and dependable way. They should be able and willing to communicate with appropriate specialists to provide quality care for the patient without jeopardizing the stability of micro-implants. Close collaboration with prosthodontists, oral surgeons, and periodontists will help eliminate or at least minimize complications arising from implant placement and management.

References

Alessandri Bonetti G, Giunta D (1996) Molar intrusion with a removable appliance. *Journal of Clinical Orthodontics* 30: 434–7.

Andreasen JO (1980) A time related study of periodontal healing and root resorption activity after replantation of mature permanent incisors in monkeys. *Swedish Dental Journal* 4: 101–10.

Asscherickx K, Vannet BV, Wehrbein H, et al. (2005) Root repair after injury from mini-screw. *Clinical Oral Implants Research* 16: 575–8.

Berglundh T, Marinello CP, Lindhe J, et al. (1991) Periodontal tissue reactions to orthodontic extrusion. An experimental study in the dog. *Journal of Clinical Periodontology* 18: 330–6.

Bondemark L, Kurol J, Hallonsten AL, et al. (1997) Attractive magnets for orthodontic extrusion of crown-root fractured teeth. *American Journal of Orthodontics and Dentofacial Orthopedics* 112: 187–93.

Borah GL, Ashmead D (1996) The fate of teeth transfixed by osteosynthesis screws. *Plastic and Reconstructive Surgery* 97: 726–9.

Cardaropoli D, Stefania R, Corrente G, et al. (2001) Intrusion of migrated incisors with infrabony defects in adult periodontal patients. *American Journal of Orthodontics and Dentofacial Orthopedics* 120: 671–5.

Cheng SJ, Tseng IY, Lee JJ, et al. (2004) A prospective study of the risk factors associated with failure of mini-implants used for orthodontic anchorage. *International Journal of Oral and Maxillofacial Implants* 19: 100–6.

Chun YS, Woo YJ, Row J, et al. (2000) Maxillary molar intrusion with the molar intrusion arch. *Journal of Clinical Orthodontics* 34: 90–3.

Costa A, Raffini M, Melsen B (1998) Miniscrews as orthodontic anchorage. *International Journal of Adult Orthodontics and Orthognathic Surgery* 13: 201–9.

Costopoulos G, Nanda R (1996) An evaluation of root resorption incident to orthodontic intrusion. *American Journal of Orthodontics and Dentofacial Orthopedics* 109: 543–8.

Creekmore TD, Eklund MK (1983) The possibility of skeletal anchorage. *Journal of Clinical Orthodontics* 17: 266–9.

Daimaruya T, Takahashi I, Nagasaka H, et al. (2003) Effects of maxillary molar intrusion on the nasal floor and tooth root using the skeletal anchorage system in dogs. *Angle Orthodontist* 73: 158–66.

Dellinger EL (1967) A histologic and cephalometric investigation of premolar intrusion in the Macaca speciosa monkey. *American Journal of Orthodontics* 53: 325–55.

Fabbroni G, Aabed S, Mizen K, et al. (2004) Transalveolar screws and the incidence of a dental damage: a prospective study. *International Journal of Oral and Maxillofacial Surgery* 33: 442–6.

Felippe LA, Monteiro Junior S, et al. (2003) Reestablishing biologic width with forced eruption. *Quintessence International* 34: 733–8.

Heidemann W, Gerlach KL, Grobel KH, et al. (1998) Drill free screws: a new form of osteosynthesis screw. *Journal of Craniomaxillofacial Surgery* 26: 163–8.

Hossein K, Dahlin C, Bengt A (2005) Influence of different prophylactic antibiotic regimens on implant survival rate: a retrospective clinical study. *Clinical Implant Dentistry Related Research* 7: 32–5.

Ingber JS, Rose LF, Coslet JG (1977) The 'biologic width' – a concept in periodontics and restorative dentistry. *Alpha Omegan* 70: 62–5.

Jaffin RA, Berman CL (1991) The excessive loss of Branemark fixtures in type IV bone: a 5-year analysis. *Journal of Periodontology* 62: 2–4.

Kanomi R (1997) Mini-implant for orthodontic anchorage. *Journal of Clinical Orthodontics* 31: 763–7.

Koyuturk AE, Malkoc S (2005) Orthodontic extrusion of subgingivally fractured incisor before restoration. A case report: 3-years follow-up. *Dental Traumatology* 21: 174–8.

Kozlovsky A, Tal H, Lieberman M (1988) Forced eruption combined with gingival fiberotomy. A technique for clinical crown lengthening. *Journal of Clinical Orthodontics* 15: 534–8.

Kuroda S, Sugawara Y, Deguchi T, et al. (2007a) Clinical use of miniscrew implants as orthodontic anchorage: success rates and postoperative dis-

comfort. *American Journal of Orthodontics and Dentofacial Orthopedics* 131: 9–15.

Kuroda S, Yamada K, Deguchi T, et al. (2007b) Root proximity is a major factor for screw failure in orthodontic anchorage. *American Journal of Orthodontics and Dentofacial Orthopedics* 131: 68–73.

Laskin DM, Dent CD, Morris HF, et al. (2000) The influence of preoperative antibiotics on success of endosseous implants at 36 months. *Annals of Periodontology* 5(1): 166–74.

Mantzikos T, Shamus I (1998) Case report: forced eruption and implant site development. *Angle Orthodontist* 68: 179–86.

Melsen B (1986) Tissue reaction following application of extrusive and intrusive forces to teeth in adult monkeys. *American Journal of Orthodontics* 89: 469–75.

Melsen B (2007) What influence has skeletal anchorage had on orthodontics? In: JA McNamara (ed.) *Microimplants as Temporary Orthodontic Anchorage.* Proceedings of the thirty-fourth Annual Moyers Symposium, February 24–25, Ann Arbor, Michigan. Craniofacial growth series No. 45, Needham Press, Ann Arbor, MI, pp. 1–32.

Minsk L (2000) Orthodontic tooth extrusion as an adjunct to periodontal therapy. *Compendium of Continuing Education in Dentistry* 21: 768–70.

Moon CH, Park HK, Nam JS, et al. (2010) Relationship between vertical skeletal pattern and success rate of orthodontic mini-implants. *American Journal of Orthodontics and Dentofacial Orthopedics* 138: 51–7.

Ogihara S, Wang HL (2010) Periodontal regeneration with or without limited orthodontics for the treatment of 2- or 3-wall infrabony defects. *Journal of Periodontology* 81: 1734–42.

Ohmae M, Saito S, Morohashi T, et al. (2001) A clinical and histological evaluation of titanium mini-implants as anchors for orthodontic intrusion in the beagle dog. *American Journal of Orthodontics and Dentofacial Orthopedics* 119: 489–97.

Oktenoglu BT, Ferrara LA, Andalkar N, et al. (2001) Effects of the hole preparation on screw pullout resistance and insertional torque: a biomechanical study. *Journal of Neurosurgery* 94: 91–6.

Park HS (1999) The skeletal cortical anchorage using titanium microscrew implants. *Korean Journal of Orthodontics* 29: 699–706.

Park HS (2003) Clinical study on success rate of microscrew implants for orthodontic anchorage. *Korean Journal of Orthodontics* 33: 151–6.

Park HS (2009) *Minor Tooth Movement with Microimplants for Prosthetic Treatment.* Daegu, Korea: Dentos Co Inc.

Park HS, Kim JB (1999) The use of titanium microscrew implants as orthodontic anchorage. *Keimyung Medical Journal* 18: 509–15.

Park HS, Kwon TG (2004) Sliding mechanics with microscrew implant anchorage. *Angle Orthodontist* 74: 703–10.

Park HS, Bae SM, Kyung HM, et al. (2001) Micro-implant anchorage for treatment of skeletal class I bialveolar protrusion. *Journal of Clinical Orthodontics* 35: 417–22.

Park HS, Kwon, TG, Sung JH (2004a) Nonextraction treatment with microscrew implant. *Angle Orthodontist* 74: 539–49.

Park HS, Kwon TG, Kwon OW (2004b) Treatment of openbite with microscrew implant anchorage. *American Journal of Orthodontics and Dentofacial Orthopedics* 126: 627–36.

Park HS, Lee SK, Kwon OW (2005) Group distal movement of teeth using microscrew implant anchorage. *Angle Orthodontist* 75: 602–9.

Park HS, Jeong SH, Kwon OW (2006a) Factors affecting the clinical success of screw implants used as an orthodontic anchorage. *American Journal of Orthodontics and Dentofacial Orthopedics* 130: 18–25.

Park HS, Kwon OW, Sung JH (2006b) Nonextraction treatment of an open bite with microscrew implant anchorage. *American Journal of Orthodontics and Dentofacial Orthopedics* 130: 391–402.

Park HS, Lee YJ, Jeong SH, et al. (2008) Density of the alveolar and basal bones of the maxilla and the mandible. *American Journal of Orthodontics and Dentofacial Orthopedics* 133: 30–7.

Park HS, Hwangbo ES, Kwon TG (2010) Proper mesiodistal angles for microimplant placement assessed with 3-dimensional computed tomography images. *American Journal of Orthodontics and Dentofacial Orthopedics* 137: 200–6.

Park J, Cho HJ (2009) Three-dimensional evaluation of interradicular spaces and cortical bone thickness for the placement and initial stability of microimplants in adults. *American Journal of Orthodontics and Dentofacial Orthopedics* 136: 314.e1–12.

Re S, Cardaropoli D, Corrente G, et al. (2001) Bodily tooth movement through the maxillary sinus with implant anchorage for single tooth replacement. *Clinical Orthodontics and Research* 4: 177–81.

Shapiro PA, Kokich VG (1988) Uses of implants in orthodontics. *Dental Clinics of North America* 32: 539–50.

Sherwood KH, Burch JG, Thompson WJ (2002) Closing anterior open bites by intruding molars with titanium miniplate anchorage. *American Journal of Orthodontics and Dentofacial Orthopedics* 122: 593–600.

Tehemar SH (1999) Factors affecting heat generation during implant site preparation: a review of biologic observations and future considerations. *International Journal Oral and Maxillofacial Implants* 14: 127–36.

Umemori M, Sugawara J, Mitani H, et al. (1999) Skeletal anchorage system for open bite correction. *American Journal of Orthodontics and Dentofacial Orthopedics* 115: 166–74.

24

Temporomandibular Dysfunction: Controversies and Orthodontics

Donald J Rinchuse, Sanjivan Kandasamy

Summary

Few topics in dentistry are as confusing, or given to as many controversies and dilemmas, as temporomandibular disorders (TMDs). The history of TMD is marred with debates over definition, etiology, diagnosis, and treatment. Due to the confounded nature of TMD research, as well as the ineptitude in research analysis and interpretation, a plethora of fallacious conclusions have been fostered from empirical clinical observations and research findings. The evolution of the various schools of thought and philosophies related to occlusion and TMD has certainly been fueled by the lack of understanding of the research data. Many professionals have savored the numerous self-proclaimed gurus of the day. Long-held tenets have been handed down and accepted through the generations and a certain kind of blind faith has existed regarding occlusion and TMD. Rather than relying on science and evidence, many in dentistry and orthodontics have based their beliefs on information and knowledge acquired through empiricism, authority, rationalism, and tenacity. With the promulgation of the modern day evidence-based view, more attention should be spent on objectively analyzing and evaluating the evidence rather than toward opinions, anecdotes, and empiricism. This chapter reviews the controversies and dilemmas surrounding occlusion and TMD as they relate to orthodontics. It starts with the evolution of the controversies followed by a discussion of the misconceptions pertaining to the relationship between occlusion, condyle position (centric relation), orthodontic treatment, and TMD. The orthodontist's role as well as other specialists in the management of TMD is also discussed.

Temporomandibular disorders – the evolution of controversy

The origin of the notion of the possibility of temporomandibular disorders (TMDs) dates back to the time of the ancient Egyptians (McNeill, 1997). What we refer to as TMDs today was referred to in the past by a vast array of terms such as: temporomandibular joint (TMJ) pain dysfunction syndrome, myofascial pain dysfunction syndrome, craniomandibular articulation disorders, mandibular dysfunction, TMJ disorders, and TM disorders (Rinchuse, 1987). The modern history of TMDs appears to have started in 1934. Based on the analysis of 11 cases, an otolaryngologist, Dr James Costen (1934), described a syndrome (Costen's syndrome) related to the TMJs and ears. The etiology was believed to be related to overclosure of the mandible due to loss of dental vertical dimension subsequent to tooth loss. Symptoms of Costen's syndrome include pain in and around the jaw, TMJ sounds, limited mandibular opening, and myofascial tenderness/pain, as well as ear symptoms such as dizziness, tinnitus, pain and impaired hearing. The ear/hearing effect was assumed to be due to the close anatomical proximity of the TMJ to the external auditory meatus. A decade later, a famous anatomist, Dr Harry Sicher (1948), proved Costen's syndrome as fallacious from an anatomical viewpoint. Even though Costen's proposals were disproved, it certainly initiated great interest and awareness of the TMJs among dentists. Sved (1944), Block (1947), Christensen (1970), and others, however, still supported aspects of Costen's concepts and advocated the use of bite-raising appliances to restore the vertical dimension to alleviate any TMJ/ear symptoms. Over time modifications of these appliances eventually led to the use of oral occlusal appliances or splints for TMD management, and other bite- and joint-related issues.

In 1927, McCollum founded the Gnathological Society of California, and together with colleagues Stuart and Stallard, developed and taught the principles of gnathology, which involved harmonizing occlusal and jaw relationships

Integrated Clinical Orthodontics, First Edition. Edited by Vinod Krishnan, Ze'ev Davidovitch.
© 2012 Blackwell Publishing Ltd. Published 2012 by Blackwell Publishing Ltd.

for ideal dental and TMD treatment. Originally, gnathology relied on the principles of science and much useful information was gleaned from studies involving chewing kinematics (Guttetman, 1961; Sheppard and Sheppard, 1965; Ahlgren, 1967; Gillings et al., 1973; Gibbs et al., 1977; Wickwire et al., 1981; Alexander et al., 1984) and intraoral telemetry (Graf and Zander, 1963; Pameijer et al., 1969, 1970; Glickman et al., 1970). Nonetheless, gnathology has moved away from the tenets of science to those emphasizing mechanistic, and often instrument-driven procedures.

Many well-regarded clinicians (Schuyler, 1929; Posselt, 1952; Mann and Pankey, 1963; Ramfjord and Ash, 1971) endorsed the principles of gnathology, and/or modified versions of it with their own improved instrumentation. This development undoubtedly fed the growing belief in the importance of occlusion and occlusal adjustment to the overall health of the stomatognathic system. Others such as Dawson (1974), Guichet (1979), Williamson et al. (1980) and Roth (1981a, b) popularized various techniques and recommended occlusal equilibration as an important adjunctive treatment to occlusal therapy as well as the prophylactic use of equilibration to prevent TMD.

When current evidence discredited existing notions and/or beliefs, occlusionists were quick to put new spins on old ideas. In the 1970s and early 1980s, many originally in the occlusionist camp abandoned the belief that occlusion was the primary cause of TMD. Their mantra now became that TMJ dysfunction, or craniomandibular dysfunction, was caused by eccentric (or displaced) TMJ condyles rather than discrepancies in occlusal relationships. Dentists were now orthopedists of the stomatognathic system and instead of calling the appliances used in TMJ treatments occlusal splints, they were now referred to as dental orthotics. The focus became trying to determine the most optimal condyle (or centric relation [CR]) position and working out the best method of recording it and then directing dental treatments toward it. Gelb (1977), a famous New York dentist, even went so far as to postulate that his mandibular orthopedic repositioning appliances (MORA splints)/orthotics, or any device that discluded the teeth such as an athletic mouthguard, could increase overall athletic performance. Early on, several anecdotal reports and uncontrolled and unblinded studies were used to verify this tenet. However, when blinded, controlled studies were eventually conducted, which neutralized many of the placebo/psychological effects due to subject/investigator/appliance interaction, no benefit of MORA on athletic strength/performance was found (Friedman and Weisberg, 1981; Greenberg et al., 1981; Hart et al., 1981). Nonetheless, aspects of this notion seem to resurface time and again.

In the 1970s, Jankelson (1979, 1984) refuted the gnathological ideals of the time and developed his own method of determining and recording CR or myocentric position with an instrument termed the 'Myomonitor'. The myocentric position was believed to be the optimum neuromuscular jaw relationship to serve as the basis for occlusal and TMD treatment. This myocentric position was typically found somewhere between centric relation occlusion (CRO, as per the older definition) and centric occlusion (CO). When natural dentitions did not adhere to specific myocentric or gnathological ideals, the followers of the associated philosophy would consider the dentition as not ideal and potentially pathological. Dao et al. (1988) found that the 'Myomonitor' only stimulates the distal axons of the motor neurons peripherally and not centrally, therefore only producing a simple superficial masseter muscle twitch as opposed to producing a reflex activation of the jaw closing muscles through stimulation of the motor root of the trigeminal nerve as originally purported (Jankelson et al., 1975). As a result of their findings, they questioned whether a physiological occlusal position could be established with this method.

With the development of better TMJ imaging techniques in the mid to late 1970s, Farrar and McCarty (Farrar, 1972, 1979, 1982–1983; McCarty, 1979) focused on TMJ internal derangements as the primary cause of TMJ dysfunction. Most of the TMJ internal derangements were found to be anterior-medial displacements of the TMJ disks rather than posterior disk displacements. They advocated recapturing displaced disks with the use of anterior repositioning appliances and/or TMJ surgery. Interestingly, the internal derangement camp was not able to explain the original cause of the TMJ internal derangements, although there was a focus on TMJ trauma.

The introduction of computed tomography (CT) and magnetic resonance imaging (MRI) in the mid-1980s significantly improved imaging of the TMJs. With better imaging techniques and devices, many TMJ surgical procedures were carried out during that era, with the focus on structural repair of the joint and disk and eventually replacement of the disk with autogenous or alloplastic materials. For the most part, these aggressive surgical treatments failed miserably. Around this time functional orthodontists, mostly not university trained specialists, such as Witzig and Spahl (1991), became strong advocates of advancing the mandible with the use of functional appliances with a view to encouraging mandibular growth and establishing specific occlusal and jaw relationships for the management or prevention of TMD. They also believed that 'traditional orthodontics' involving premolar extractions, headgear, and incisor retraction predisposed patients to present and future TMD.

By the 1980s there were many diverse views of TMJ dysfunction as related to cause and treatments, i.e. occlusion, condyle (CR) position, and/or TMJ internal derangements. With so many different views and controversies related to TMJ dysfunction, the American Dental Association (ADA) held a conference in June 1982. In 1983, the ADA published guidelines derived from the conference for the examination, diagnosis, and management of dysfunctions of the TMJ (Griffiths, 1983), which were now defined as temporomandibular disorders. TMDs were, and are now, considered to be a collection of musculoskeletal disorders/ dysfunctions affecting the TMJ complex and neighboring structures of the head and neck, embracing many clinical conditions with many different and diverse causes. Incidentally, the ADA then held a second conference in 1989 (McNeill et al., 1990) and the National Institutes of Health held a conference in 1996 (National Institutes of Health Technology Assessment Conference Statement, 1996) to further address the issues surrounding TMD. Much of what was determined in the first ADA TMD Conference held up well and was reinforced in the subsequent conferences. There are several TMD classifications, but for the purpose of an overview, a summarized and simplified version is provided in Box 24.1 (Griffiths, 1983; Dworkin and LeResche, 1992; Okeson, 2005).

Although the prevalence of minor disturbances of the TMJ area is common in the healthy population (popping and clicking), epidemiological studies suggest that approximately 5–12% of the population may be significantly affected by TMDs or require some form of treatment (Solberg et al., 1979; Dworkin et al., 1990). Today, TMD has moved away from the historic, mechanical, dental-based model, which primarily focused on occlusal modification or jaw repositioning (Greene and Laskin, 2000; Greene, 2001; Klasser and Greene, 2007a) to a biopsychosocial model which integrates a host of biological, clinical and behavioral factors that account for the onset, maintenance and remission of TMD (Fernandez and Turk, 1989; Dworkin and LeResche, 1992; Flor and Birbaumer, 1993; Turk et al., 1993, 1996; Dworkin and Massoth, 1994; Dworkin et al., 1994; Rudy et al., 1995; Greco et al., 1997; Mishra et al., 2000; Gardea et al., 2001; Dworkin et al., 2002a,b; Gatchel et al., 2006). Cognitive behavioral therapies (CBT) and biofeedback (BFB) are becoming recognized as the standard in the early therapy of TMD (Gardea et al., 2001; Gatchel et al., 2006). See Table 24.1 for a general summary of TMD controversies.

Recent information indicates that TMD patients exhibit greater sensitivity to experimental pain than control subjects, suggesting that nociceptive processing may be upregulated in TMD patients. The generalized hyper-excitability of their central nociceptive pathways may contribute to the development and/or maintenance of chronic TMD pain and possibly increase the likelihood of other chronic pain disorders. Further, it appears that women exhibit greater excitability of their central nociceptive neurons than men, making the female central nervous system more easily upregulated to a pathologically hyperexcitable state, contributing to the greater prevalence of various chronic pain conditions among women (Sarlani and Greenspan, 2005). Moreover, there appears to be a genetic predisposition among individuals who experience chronic pain.

In addition, it has been suggested that variations of the gene encoding for catechol-O-methyl-transferase (COMT) is associated with influencing pain regulatory mechanisms in the central nervous system. COMT is one of several enzymes that degrade catecholamines (i.e. neurotransmitters) such as dopamine, epinephrine, norepinephrine, and enkephalins. Three common COMT haplotypes have been found to account for some variability in experimental pain perception in females. These markers may in the future allow us to identify a subgroup of subjects who are at a higher risk of developing TMD (Diatchenko et al., 2005; Slade et al., 2008). These data and findings reinforce the idea that there is a paradigm shift regarding the etiology of TMD; moving away from a focus on 'chasing' occlusal contacts to 'chasing' vulnerability alleles (Stohler, 2004).

Orthodontics and TMD

It was not until the early 1970s that a serious consideration was made of a possible relationship between orthodontics

---

Box 24.1 Simplified classification system for TMD diagnosis

Masticatory muscle disorders
- Protective muscle splinting
- Masticatory muscle spasm or myospasm
- Masticatory muscle inflammation (myositis)
- Local myalgia
- Myofascial pain
- Centrally mediated myalgia

Derangements of the TMJ
- Incoordination
- Disk displacements with or without reduction

Extrinsic trauma
- Dislocation
- Fracture
- Traumatic arthritis
- Internal disk derangement
- Inflammation of the tendon(s) and/or ligament(s)

Degenerative joint diseases
- Osteoarthrosis
- Osteoarthritis

Inflammatory joint disorders with possible systemic involvement
- Rheumatoid or other autoimmune related arthritis
- Infectious arthritis
- Metabolic arthritis

Chronic mandibular hypomobility
- Ankylosis (fibrous or osseous)
- Muscle contracture
- Coronoid impedance

Growth disorders of the TMJ with skeletal and /or muscle involvement
- Congenital
- Acquired or developmental
- Neoplastic

Psychological considerations

Table 24.1 The judge and jury of temporomandibular disorder (TMD) controversies[a]

Allegation	Verdict
TMD is a single disorder with a single cause	TMD is a collection of disorders, in some of which the TMJ is not the focus
The diagnosis of TMD is based on a detailed analysis of occlusion	The 'gold standard' is based on a thorough history, clinical examination, and when indicated TMJ imaging
Dental-based model for TMD management	Medical-based model and biopsychosocial approach to TMD management
Orthodontic treatment causes TMD	Orthodontic treatment does not cause TMD
The anterior-superior-medial condyle position is the ideal	No one ideal condylar position exists and there exists a range of positions
Advocate canine protected occlusion (some tolerance for group function occlusion)	Accept all functional occlusion types, but *no interferences* (balancing and protrusive contacts tolerated, but not interferences)
Centric slides cause TMD	Large centric slides are most likely related to the result of disease rather than the cause
Favor the use of articulators in orthodontics	Use of articulators in orthodontics is not evidence based and is cost-ineffective
TMD treatments are typically based on treating the cause	TMD treatments are typically symptomatic and palliative
Believe anterior repositioning splints can recapture displaced disks	Displaced disks cannot be recaptured; retrodiskal tissues adapt to become the 'new disk'
Oral occlusal appliances work better than other TMD treatment therapies	Oral occlusal appliances are not more effective than other TMD treatment therapies

[a]The above is based on population data and may *not* apply to all clinical situations at the individual patient level.

and TMD. Arguing an orthodontic gnathological view, Roth (1973, 1976) maintained that certain functional occlusion and centric relation standards needed to be achieved in orthodontic treatments. His view was taken from the classic gnathological–prosthodontic philosophy which fostered the concepts of canine protected occlusion, retruded CR, anterior guidance, and the use of articulators in orthodontic diagnostics. Roth believed that orthodontic treatments that did not foster traditional gnathological functional goals would cause and/or predispose orthodontic patients to TMD. Purveyors of this thinking reasoned that orthodontic treatment is analogous to doing full-mouth occlusal rehabilitations, with the difference being that orthodontists did not 'cut' or modify the natural tooth structure.

Orthodontics was viewed as a cause of TMD from two perspectives. First, orthodontists who did not achieve a gnathological occlusal finish were believed to produce iatrogenic functional occlusions (i.e. functional balancing interferences) and/or eccentric condyle (or CR) positions. This then led to TMD. Second, certain orthodontic appliances or techniques (e.g. Class II or III mechanics, headgears, extractions, chin cups, certain retainers, and so on) were believed to directly cause TMD (Witzig and Spahl, 1991; Wyatt, 1987).

In 1987, a landmark US court case took place, which resulted in an unfavorable judgment against a Michigan orthodontist for purportedly causing TMD in a 16-year-old girl with a Class II Division 1 malocclusion. The orthodon-

tic treatment involved maxillary first premolar extractions and the use of a headgear. The patient filed a complaint against the orthodontist alleging that following the removal of the appliances she developed severe clicking in the TMJ with pain and crepitus. The theory was that certain orthodontic appliances and procedures could cause distal displacement of the mandible leading to TMJ internal derangements, i.e. anterior displaced TMJ disks. In this case it was alleged that the distal displacement of the mandible was due to the over-retraction and lingual inclination of the maxillary incisors. An expert witness for the plaintiff, a prominent and vocal functional orthodontist, Dr John W Witzig testified in part as follows:

In Susan's case with her type of malocclusion or her type of problem when she went to see the orthodontist, no way should headgear and retraction of the upper front teeth back toward the tongue have occurred. This left Susan with a bite that her lower jaw now bites in a displaced position, and no way should any patient be left in that condition – this is dental negligence.

JW Witzig, cited in Luecke and Johnston (1992)

Unfortunately, the jury sided with the plaintiff, awarding her US$850 000 (Pollack, 1988).

Mostly due to this famous Michigan TMD case (Brimm *v* Malloy), the debate over orthodontics causing TMD was renewed but at a more serious level. This prompted the American Association of Orthodontists (AAO) and the orthodontic community to re-examine the relationship between orthodontic treatment and TMD. Nonetheless, many subsequent investigations that were performed discredited the allegations in the Brimm case. These studies have demonstrated that orthodontic treatments performed with and without extractions and/or headgears, resulting in the retraction of maxillary incisors do *not* cause distally positioned mandibles and anterior displaced TMJ disks (Gianelly et al., 1988, 1991a,b; Gianelly, 1989a,b).

Luecke and Johnston evaluated pre- and post-treatment records of 42 'edgewise' patients with Class II Division 1 malocclusions treated in conjunction with the extraction of the upper two first premolars. About 70% of the patients showed forward displacement of the mandible and the remaining 30% exhibited distal displacement. The changes in condylar position were not correlated with incisor retraction but rather with the displacement of the buccal segments. The authors suggested that given the pronounced overjet in a Class II malocclusion, the incisors would normally go through marked retraction without touching or 'trapping' the lower incisors. It would seem that a patient's centric occlusion position is determined by the occluding cusp-fossa relationships. With combined forward growth of the midface and anchorage loss from the reciprocal closure of the maxillary extraction spaces, marked mesial movement of the buccal occlusion will occur, producing an anterior shift of the mandible rather than a distal displacement (Luecke and Johnston, 1992). Further studies by Johnston and co-workers have also shown no differences between extraction and non-extraction groups with regards to TMD (Luppanapornlap and Johnston, 1993; Beattie et al., 1994).

Chin-cup therapy in Class III malocclusions has also been implicated in causing TMD. It is believed that the applied upward and backward directed forces to the mandible will predispose patients to anterior disk displacements. However, studies on the long-term follow-up of patients and MR scans of the condyle–disk relationships in patients following chin-cup therapy have concluded that chin-cup therapy when applied with appropriate forces is not a risk factor for TMD (Gökalp et al., 2000; Arat et al., 2003).

In 1990, Reynders completed the first comprehensive literature review to evaluate whether there was a relationship between orthodontics and TMD. He reviewed all articles published from 1966 to 1988 and concluded that 'orthodontic treatment should not be considered responsible for causing TMD regardless of orthodontic technique. The data also rejects the assumption that orthodontic treatment is specific or necessary to cure signs and symptoms of TMD.' Similarly, in a review article by McNamara et al. in 1995, it was concluded that orthodontic treatment performed during adolescence generally does not increase or decrease the odds of developing TMD later in life. In addi-

tion, in 2002, Kim et al. published a meta-analysis further supporting the premise that orthodontics does not cause or predispose to TMD. A recent long-term, prospective cohort study by Macfarlene et al. (2009) conducted in South Wales, UK, initially involving over 1000 subjects, concluded that orthodontic treatment neither causes nor prevents TMD. This has been the largest longitudinal epidemiological study in orthodontics to investigate the relationship between orthodontic treatment and TMD. The study demonstrated that TMD prevalence in young adults and adolescents is the highest at age 19–20 and higher in females than in males. Female gender and TMD in adolescence were the only predictors for TMD in young adults. In addition, a large recent cross-sectional study involving randomly selected 1011 children and adolescents between the ages of 10 and 18 found that the group undergoing orthodontic treatment were not at an increased risk of TMD and bruxism (Hirsch, 2009). This author also found that the orthodontic group exhibited fewer wear facets and reported less parafunctional behavior. These studies, as well as others, over time have helped to define (and redefine) and clarify the possible relationship between orthodontics (and orthodontists) and TMD.

Centric relation controversy

CR is the position of the condyles independent of tooth contact, whereas CO is an interocclusal dental position of the maxillary teeth relative to the mandibular teeth. Other terms that have been used synonymously with CO are MI (maximum intercuspation) and ICP (intercuspal position). The definition of CR has evolved considerably over the past half-century from being a posterior position of the condyle in relation to the glenoid fossa to a posterior-superior position to eventually an anterior and superior position (Academy of Prosthodontics, 2005). Before 1968, CR was considered as the retruded most posterior condylar position. The latest edition of the Glossary of prosthodontic terms (GPT) (Academy of Prosthodontics, 2005) defines CR as 'a maxillomandibular relationship in which the condyles articulate with the thinnest avascular portion of their respective disks with the complex in the anterior-superior position against the slopes of the articular eminences.' This edition of the GPT also includes six historical definitions of CR. Unfortunately changes in the definition and concept of CR have been determined for the most part arbitrarily, and not based on science and evidence.

The current gnathological view dictates that CO should ideally be coincident with an anterior-superior CR (Klar et al., 2003; Schmitt et al., 2003; Cordray, 2006). This hypothesis was adopted despite the absence of evidentiary support. In the 1970s, Roth advocated establishing a retruded, posterior-superior 'seated' CR position when the interdigitating occlusion was in CO; that is, CR (CRO) equals CO, or CR is coincident with MI or ICP (Roth, 1973, 1976). He believed that if orthodontists failed to reach this goal of a posterior-superior seated CR position coincident with CO as part of their orthodontic treatment, patients would be prone to develop TMD symptoms. Furthermore, the attainment of a retruded, posterior-superior CR position would mitigate the development of TMD. Roth later recanted his view of retruded CR and adopted the contemporary view of antero-superior CR.

Although contemporary orthodontic gnathologists believe in attaining an anterior-superior condyle position at the same time that the teeth are in CO (CR = CO), there is little or no scientific evidence to support this view (Rinchuse, 1987). Alexander et al. (1993), using TMJ MRI, revealed that condyles are not located in the assumed positions as advocated and provided by several gnathological centric bite registrations. Several popular centric bite registrations attempting to locate retruded (posterior-superior) CR and contemporary anterior-superior CR did not correspond to the condyle positions of individuals who were TMD asymptomatic. It would appear that the attempted doctor positioning of the condyles into specific locations within the glenoid fossae through chin guidance, manipulation, and/or bite registration is essentially a blind procedure. Dentists, who believe in establishing a coincidence of CR with CO, unnecessarily subject their patients to procedures that may lead to irreversible bite alterations and increased financial costs. The location and position of the condyles in the glenoid fossa, irrespective of where that may be, has not been demonstrated to be consequential to the presence or absence of TMD symptoms (Griffiths, 1983; McNeill et al., 1990; Dixon, 1991; Mohl and Dixon, 1994).

Centric slides and TMD

Centric slides typically refer to an anterior-posterior shift, present between CO and CRO (the point of occlusal contact when the TMJs are in centric relation). In the 1960s, centric slides were believed to cause TMD (Ramfjord and Ash, 1971; Mohl, 1991). These findings, however, were based on descriptive studies that lacked control/comparison groups. Interestingly, when control/comparison groups that included subjects without TMD were included in subsequent studies, it was found that the exact same centric slides were also present and observed in subjects who did not have TMD. So the early studies possessed many false-positive findings for TMJ pain dysfunction, i.e. high sensitivity with poor specificity, which further fueled the TMD debate (Mohl, 1991).

On average and 'normally,' most centric slides are in the range of 1–2 mm. Furthermore, it has been shown that large slides (4–7 mm) are associated with degenerative changes within the TMJ. However, it appears that these large centric slides are more the result or consequence of the TMD or joint changes rather than the cause. As a result, the removal of such centric slides even in the presence of a TMJ articular disorder is not advisable (Seligman and Pullinger, 1991; McNamara et al., 1995).

Deprogramming to obtain an ideal CR

The use of 'deprogramming splints' for either the short or long term prior to taking centric bite registrations in order to obtain a more accurate record of centric relation is a controversial topic. It is believed that mandibular movements are governed by preprogrammed muscular engrams, or habitual muscular patterns. Muscle engrams are the memorized patterns of muscle activity developed from the habitual repetition of proprioceptive sensory information. Gnathologists hypothesize that these memorized patterns of the muscles of mastication may adversely change the position of the mandible in the presence of occlusal interferences. They therefore recommended the use of a deprogramming splint or other type of apparatus before obtaining centric bite registrations. It is believed that using various deprogramming splints to disclude the posterior teeth would remove any occlusal interferences or proprioceptive errors and permit the muscles of mastication to establish a more physiologic engram (Roth, 1973, 1976, 1981a, b, 1985; Roth and Rolfs, 1981; Cordray, 1996, 2006).

Orthodontic gnathologists maintain that patients need to be deprogrammed from their pre-existing occlusion prior to obtaining CR records even in patients without TMD. They contend that without the use of deprogramming splints prior to articulator mountings (especially in patients with Class II skeletal malocclusions), clinicians may miss the diagnosis of large centric sagittal slides ('Sunday bites' – greater than 2 mm) as well as slight transverse and vertical discrepancies. Finally, it is argued that the use of hand-held dental casts made from CO-generated pretreatment records (including lateral cephalograms), vis-à-vis CR records preceded by deprogramming splints, may compromise the initial orthodontic diagnosis because the true skeletal discrepancy may not be elucidated (Roth, 1973, 1976, 1981a, b; Williamson et al., 1978; Roth and Rolfs, 1981; Shildkraut et al., 1994; Cordray, 2006).

However, the evidence for using deprogrammers is equivocal and lacks a true physiologic basis. Following the use of a 'Lucia-type anterior deprogramming jig' (i.e. anterior tooth contact without posterior tooth contact) for 6 hours in TMD subjects, Karl and Foley in 1999 found small differences in before and after articulator condyle position indicator (CPI) centric recordings. Compared with traditional centric bite registrations, the differences were very minor. The most prevalent type of centric slide on average resulted in a posterior and inferior distraction of the articulator condyles from CR to CO (condyles) of 0.37 mm horizontally and 0.57 mm vertically. Conversely, Kulbersh et al. (2003a) did not find a difference in MI-CR measurements between 34 post-orthodontic subjects who wore gnathological full coverage splints for 3 weeks (24 hours/day) versus 14 post-orthodontic subjects who did not wear splints.

It would appear that the use of various deprogramming splints for either short or long periods to establish a more accurate CR are unjustified and not evidence based. It would seem that deprogramming splints simply serve to complicate and introduce more error and procedures into a gnathological treatment modality that already struggles to justify its use. Another issue is how does one know that the deprogrammed CR position is healthier or more physiological in comparison with the original position?

Articulators as a diagnostic aid in orthodontics

There is a plethora of articulator types: arcon, non-arcon, fully adjustable, semi-adjustable, polycentric hinge, and so forth. It is well established that articulators can have utility for gross fixed and removable prosthodontic and orthognathic surgical procedures to at least maintain a certain vertical dimension while preclinical laboratory procedures are performed. The issue of the use of articulators as a diagnostic aid in orthodontics has been debated since the early 1970s when Roth introduced the classic, historic philosophy of prosthodontics-gnathology to the orthodontic profession. He believed that articulator mounted dental cases would help orthodontists deduce three-dimensional CR discrepancies. Early on, Roth focused on being able to identify sagittal discrepancies such as 'Sunday bites' and later on his focus was on the orthodontic diagnoses of hidden transverse and vertical discrepancies. The orthodontic-gnathological camp argues that for a certain percentage of orthodontic patients ranging from 18.7% to 40.9% according to Utt et al. (1995) and Cordray (2006), respectively, the diagnosis of Angle's classification will be affected and different for those who have had articulator mountings. A sub-issue of the mounting debate involves whether some or all orthodontic cases need to be mounted. Not all gnathologists believe that all cases need to be mounted. Some believe that only certain ones need mounting, such as patients requiring orthognathic surgery, TMD patients, most adult patients, those with many missing permanent teeth, those with functional crossbites and midline discrepancies, and those with deviations on opening/ closing. A contemporary Roth advocate, Cordray (1996), however, believes that all cases need to be mounted based on the assertion that no practitioner can determine beforehand which patients/cases are really, or will turn out to be, the troubling ones. However, although much is written and discussed concerning articulators, the critical issue is not about the articulator mountings per se, but is and has always been about the reliability, validity, and transferability of the bite registration(s) used to 'set' or mount the casts on the articulator.

Articulators are based on the faulty concept of Posselt's 'terminal hinge axis', which dates back more than half a century (Posselt, 1950). Posselt conjectured that in the initial 20 mm or so of opening and closing, the mandible (condyles) rotates similar to a door hinge (and does not simultaneously translate). However, Posselt's hypothesis was created in the era when CR was considered a retruded, posterior position of the condyles in the glenoid fossa. During that time period, retruded CR was recorded with distal-guided pressure applied to the chin, the most apparent reason for Posselt's finding of a 'terminal hinge axis'. In 1995, Lindauer et al. demonstrated that during opening and closing, the condyles not only rotate but simultaneously translate (move downward and forward). They demonstrated that the terminal hinge axis did not exist and their findings supported an 'instantaneous center of rotation' that is different in every patient which cannot be simulated on an articulator.

Orthodontic gnathologists contend that the Roth power bite registration followed by an articulator mounting is the best way to evaluate CR (Cordray, 1996, 2006; Kulbersh et al., 2003b). However, there are a few issues with this concept. First, although the centric bite registrations are reliable, orthodontic gnathologists have not furnished any evidence (MRI data) to demonstrate that the condyles are actually in the positions they have described them to be. As discussed previously, it has been shown that on average condyles are not located in the assumed positions as advocated and produced by several gnathological centric bite registrations (Alexander et al., 1993). Second, the difference between gnathological and non-gnathological diagnostics is on average as little as 1 mm or less, and this is mostly in the vertical dimension (Kulbersh et al., 2003b). It is doubtful whether such a difference is a true health concern. Considering the errors associated with the registration and mounting process, the significance of these differences and the gnathologists' claims are further reduced. Third, in children, the TMJ condyle–glenoid fossa complex changes location with growth; the fossae on average are displaced posteriorly and inferiorly (Buschang and Santos-Pinto, 1998). Gnathologists therefore would need to perform new mountings throughout treatment in order to maintain an ideal CR. This action, however, does not occur.

In view of the above evidence, it is reasonable to conclude that the use of articulators in orthodontics is a perfunctory exercise and there is no valid evidence to support the routine mounting of dental casts to affect orthodontic diagnoses and treatment planning and eventually lead to an improvement in patients' stomatognathic health (Ellis and Benson, 2003; Rinchuse and Kandasamy, 2006). Articulator mountings are a cost-ineffective exercise and provide no additional biological information about the patient's health or disease. Diseases of the TMJ such as disk displacement and osteoarthrosis are best diagnosed with TMJ imaging (MRI) and clinical examination and not by using articulators. Interestingly, the most destructive occlusal forces of all are those produced during parafunction (bruxing and clenching) and articulators have never been used, and cannot be used, to capture and analyze these types of movements and forces.

Functional occlusion and TMD

The optimal type of functional occlusion has been debated for almost a century. There have been proponents of balanced occlusion, group function occlusion, and canine protected occlusion (CPO). Currently, the most often recommended type of functional occlusion is 'canine (mutually) protected occlusion.' The GPT (2005) defines CPO as: 'a form of mutually protected articulation in which the vertical and horizontal overlap of the canine teeth disengages the posterior teeth in the excursive movements of the mandible.' It is theoretically argued that human canine teeth are innately similar to the long dominant canine teeth present in carnivorous animals and are therefore the best teeth to protect (by disclusion) the remaining dentition from eccentric movement forces away from CR/relation occlusion (D'Amico, 1958; Okeson, 2005). Advocates further claim that CPO provides for optimal periodontal health (Goldstein, 1979) and TMD health (Roth, 1973; Roth, 1976; Roth and Rolfs, 1981; Cordray, 1996; Torsten et al., 2004; Panek et al., 2008). The basic premise of this claim involves the idea that non-working or balancing contacts (or interferences) as presented in other functional schemes (versus CPO) can produce harmful forces on lateral mandibular movements. In addition, arguments are made that CPO is the most prevalent type of functional occlusion found in the general population (D'Amico, 1958; Scaife and Holt, 1969).

Nonetheless, the evidence supporting the superiority of CPO is empirical and not scientifically based. An optimal functional occlusion is not so easily identified in nature (Ash and Ramjford, 1996). There is a plethora of evidence that supports the notion that CPO may not necessarily be better than other types of functional occlusion with no one functional occlusal scheme demonstrating any superiority in ameliorating signs and symptoms of TMD (Rinchuse and Kandasamy, 2007). It must be said, however, that there is nothing inherently 'bad' or 'wrong' with CPO, only that it may be merely one of several types of functional occlusion schemes that may harmoniously exist in humans. After a comprehensive review of the literature, Woda and others (1979) concluded that 'Pure canine protection or pure group function rarely exists and balancing contacts seem to be the general rule in populations of contemporary civilizations'. Rinchuse and Kandasamy (2007), after reviewing the literature, found that balanced occlusion was more prevalent than CPO and that this was particularly true for subjects with normal static occlusions.

A single type of functional occlusion should not be blindly recommended for all patients. This universal, dogmatic, and myopic view fails to take into consideration the significant individual variation that exists in the patient population. Parenthetically, any functional occlusal scheme which allows for and permits balancing side 'interferences' should *not* be recommended, i.e. balancing 'contacts' (which do not interfere with function or cause dysfunction or injury to any components to the masticatory system) would be permissible. If CPO is therapeutically achieved via orthodontics, it has questionable stability and longevity. One must ask the question, 'What happens to the canine teeth following attrition which inevitably occurs with age?' It would appear that CPO produced during orthodontics eventually evolves into a group function occlusion and then possibly balanced occlusion following post-treatment occlusal settling, wear, and continued facial growth and aging.

Also, achieving a CPO, while at the same time producing a 'consonant smile arc', appears to be a mutually exclusive exercise. A consonant smile arc exists when the incisal edges of the maxillary incisors and canines are parallel to and follow the curvature of the lower lip on smiling (Sarver, 2001). The unjustified deliberate extrusion or resin build-up of the maxillary canines for the sole purpose of obtaining CPO not only creates a non-consonant smile, which negatively impacts on an orthodontic patient's smile esthetics, but is possibly iatrogenic.

Today, it would seem logical to reconsider and question the validity of the age-old concept of CPO, as well as the other traditional schemes. Do subjects actually function in the side-to-side laterotrusive movement governed by the philosophical paradigm of CPO? That is, do subjects actually make direct side-to-side movements, and to the degree of a cusp-to-cusp position (3–5 mm laterally), in any type of mandibular functional movements that include mastication and/or parafunction? It may appear that the premise behind all the popular concepts of functional occlusion is essentially flawed. In the current evidence-based arena, a particular functional occlusal scheme should only be recommended for a given patient following a consideration of factors such as chewing cycle kinematics, craniofacial morphology, static occlusion type, oral health status, and parafunctional habits. At present, all these relationships are poorly understood, requiring further study and evaluation. Until these complex relationships are explored scientifically, the notion of an ideal functional occlusion will be elusive. Therefore, the routine recommendation of one type of functional occlusal scheme over any another for all patients is equivocal and unsupported by the evidence.

Asymptomatic internal derangements – need for treatment?

Internal derangements are defined as any interference with smooth joint movement. The term is used interchangeably with disk displacements in this chapter; however, it may also include disk adherences, adhesions, subluxations, and dislocations of the disk–condyle complex (de Leeuw, 2008). It appears that as many as 30% or more of TMD asymptomatic subjects have TMJ internal derangements, most commonly disk displacements (Kircos et al., 1987; Tallents et al., 1996; Larheim et al., 2001). A current debate is whether or not TMD asymptomatic subjects with TMJ internal derangements need some form(s) of dental or orthodontic treatment to mitigate the risk of developing TMDs in the future.

Although small, an associational relationship (not cause-effect) has been found between TMJ internal derangements and craniofacial morphology (Nebbe et al., 1999a,b; Flores-Mir et al., 2006). That is, reduced forward growth of the maxillary and mandibular bodies and reduced growth of the mandibular ramus (Hall, 1995; Flores-Mir et al., 2006). The assumption is that untreated (or inadequately treated) TMJ internal derangements would most likely lead to pain, degenerative joint disease, compromised mandibular growth, and other negative conditions (Hall and Nickerson, 1994; Hall, 1995). It is believed that individuals with *asymptomatic* TMJ internal derangements need treatment involving a night-time occlusal stabilizing splint initially (in the past the argument was for a repositioning splint) followed by comprehensive orthodontics. The best time to treat TMJ internal derangements is before significant disk, skeletal, and occlusal changes occur; when the individual is young and retains optimal capacity for tissue repair and growth (Hall, 1995). Further, it is assumed that the majority of the initially asymptomatic patients will become symptomatic usually after growth is complete and when the TMJs have already progressed to a non-reducing disk displacement and degenerative joint disease; a stage when any treatment rendered would be significantly less effective (Hall and Nickerson, 1994; Hall, 1995).

Nonetheless, the logical and evidence-based view is to *not* treat this group of individuals because they are essentially TMJ *asymptomatic* (Dolwick, 1995; Larheim et al., 2001). There is no scientific evidence that providing treatment will mitigate future TMD. One must respect the fact that the relationship between disk displacement and TMD is complex; the causes are multifactorial (such as trauma, genetics, stress, and pathology), and therefore cannot be simply explained by disk position (Gonzalez et al., 2008). From the perspective that it implies the need for treatment, Carlsson (2004) argues that the term 'disk displacement' is flawed. Many TMJ asymptomatic subjects who are characterized as having a 'disk displacement' merely have atypical TMJ disk locations in relation to the condyle-glenoid fossa. It has been demonstrated that, over the long term, patients with moderate to severe TMJ dysfunction with associated disk displacement without reduction will improve with minimal, or no treatment. Further, the natural course of patients with non-reducing disk displacements without treatment over time tends to be a reduction in clinical signs and symptoms with improvements in chewing movement and masticatory efficiency (de Leeuw et al., 1994; Kurita et al., 1998; Sato et al., 1998, 2002; de Leeuw, 2008). Interestingly, studies have revealed that patients with radiographic evidence of degenerative joint disease can become comfortable with progress radiographs demonstrating successful remodeling over time (Rasmussen, 1981, 1983). The retrodiskal tissue is quite adaptive and can tolerate repeated functional loading which may account for the ability of many patients to function 'off the disk' (Scapino, 1983; Blaustein and Scapino, 1986). With regard to internal derangements and growth, not all growing patients with disk displacement grow abnormally, nor do all patients with growth deficiencies have disk displacement (Dolwick, 1995; Kurita et al., 1998; Klasser and Greene, 2007a). It would seem that if disk displacements were a significant cause of mandibular growth deficiency, the signs and symptoms of disk displacement would be more common in this population than in the normal population. However, the relationship of disk displacement to pain, mandibular dysfunction, osteoarthrosis, and growth disturbances remains unclear and given the fact that each patient adapts differently to variations in disk–condyle relationships, the presence of asymptomatic internal derangements should be discussed with the patient, but in general are best left untreated.

Recapturing the TMJ disk

Although the concept was originally introduced in the 1970s by Farrar, it is still believed by some that anteriorly displaced disks, even in asymptomatic patients, need to be treated in order to avoid progression to TMD such as in degenerative disease and/or painful dysfunction (Farrar, 1972; Farrar and McCarty, 1979; Farrar, 1985). The belief is that by positioning the mandible forward with a so-called anterior positioning appliance or device, the disk would be 'recaptured' in a forward position, and then the appliance is adjusted or remade to facilitate the gradual 'walking back' of the disk–condyle relationship to a normal position. When clinicians are unsuccessful with this approach, some advocate the stabilization of this anterior position of the mandible with the help of orthodontic treatment, or prosthodontics, or orthognathic surgery. Unfortunately this practice is not based on evidence, but rather the justification for the use of repositioning splints is based on anecdotal reports, and may lead to adverse occlusal changes (Griffiths, 1983; McNeill et al., 1990; Klasser and Greene, 2007b).

Greene and Laskin (1983) wrote, 'there is no known anatomic mechanism that could account for the retraction of an anteriorly displaced disk to its normal position'. It appears that by positioning the mandible forward there is reduced activity of the muscles and the loading of the TMJs is redirected. The retrodiskal tissues are allowed to recover, facilitating adaptive and reparative changes in the retrodiskal tissues. These tissues become avascular and fibrotic, allowing the condyles to eventually move posteriorly to function 'off the disk' or articulate on the newly adapted retrodiskal tissues with no pain (Griffiths, 1983; Clark, 1986; Moloney and Howard, 1986; McNeill et al., 1990; Choi et al., 1994; Klasser and Greene, 2007b). Nonetheless, the TMJ disk(s) still remains anteriorly displaced.

Controversies regarding TMD treatments

The TMD field is no longer linked to traditional dentistry involving occlusion and jaw alignment theories but more so related to the biomedical sciences, including molecular biology. The diagnosis and clinical management of TMD patients has changed from a dental-based model to a biopsychosocial model which attempts to integrate a host of biological, clinical, and behavioral factors that may account for the onset, maintenance, and remission of TMD. Genetics (vulnerabilities related to pain), imaging of the pain-involved brain, central brain processing of thinking and emotions, endocrinology, behavioral risk-conferring factors, and psychosocial traits and states appear to be factors that are now receiving more attention and research in order to improve our understanding of TMD.

Unfortunately, many orthodontists and general dentists have still not embraced the current evidence-based developments in TMD and continue to advise TMD patients that some aspect of their occlusions is responsible for their condition. Patients end up getting complex and invasive treatments rather than the recommended evidence-based conservative care. This not only compromises the care the patient receives and the faith of the general public in the dental profession but it also fragments the dental profession with each competing group promoting its own beliefs and unsubstantiated treatment modalities.

It would appear that a significant contributing factor for the evolution of TMD management into a biomedical-based model has essentially been experimental research involving long-term follow-ups with use of placebos. The rationale behind the success of many untested TMD therapeutic procedures has been worked out based on the research design strategies of placebo studies. Greene and Laskin (2000) are credited for their series of clinical studies, and their findings were ground breaking in that, fairly high positive placebo responses were found in relation to common TMD treatments, medications, oral appliances, and occlusal equilibrations. In many instances, placebos can be as effective as or more effective than actual physical treatments. Interestingly, in a double-blind study, placebo medications given in a realistic prescription process were found to be 50% more effective than the inadvertent administration of just placebo pills (Greene and Laskin, 2000). This outcome not only reinforced the effect of the placebo on treatment effectiveness but it also revealed the importance of evaluating the various intangible factors in influencing the outcome of TMD treatments including the doctor–patient relationship and the environment in which this takes place (Greene and Laskin, 1972b).

Occlusal appliances have been used for many decades in the treatment of TMD. Generally, they have been described as relieving TMD symptoms by occlusal disengagement, relaxing jaw musculature, restoring the vertical dimension of occlusion, redirecting the loading within the joints, cognitive awareness, or by TMJ repositioning (Clark, 2008). Some proponents of occlusal splints assume that the relief they observe from their patients primarily arises from treating some aspect of a patient's occlusal or craniomandibular relationships. This effect progresses to the belief that these splint patients then need further occlusion altering procedures involving extensive and irreversible dental treatments. It was not until 1972 when Greene and Laskin found that non-occluding 'placebo' splints (simple acrylic palatal appliances) were successful in not only relieving patient symptoms (in over 40% of the patients) but also in influencing how subjects felt about their bite while they wore the splint (Greene and Laskin, 1972a).

Placebo or 'mock' equilibration carried out on TMD patients after a thorough occlusal analysis and adequate patient discussion, revealed positive placebo responses as high as 64% of the patients reporting a major or total improvement in their so-called bite relationships (Goodman et al., 1976). These placebo experiments not only highlighted the importance of the patient's beliefs or expectations but also the role of psychosocial factors in influencing the management of the TMD patient. In addition, oral occlusal appliances can change the position of the tongue and how a patient thinks about biting, positioning his or her teeth, and where they place their tongue which goes beyond a placebo effect and can generally be characterized as 'cognitive awareness'. With placebo pills, non-occluding splints, and mock occlusal adjustments being just as successful as more invasive and aggressive procedures, the understanding behind the etiology and management of TMD has gradually moved away from a mechanistic dental-centered model. Further, a common feature of all TMD treatments, including the placebos, is that they are capable of eliciting a degree of positive response in patients which has been shown to be more effective than no treatment at all.

In view of the fact that some intervention is better than none at all and some degree of success is assured even with a placebo, how can we justify putting patients through costly or cost-ineffective (both in terms of financial and quality of life) irreversible and invasive procedures to manage TMD? Realizing that TMD treatments range from irreversible dental and invasive surgical treatments to conservative physical therapies and cognitive-behavioral interventions, it would appear that a conservative biopsychosocial approach to the management of a TMD patient would be most prudent, at least in the initial treatment.

In general, TMD treatments are typically symptomatic and palliative and therefore do not usually address the cause (Greene, 2001). This situation is similar to certain chronic illnesses such as fibromyalgia in which the cause is never addressed but rather the symptoms are more or less managed. The general principle of TMD therapies is that they should be conservative and reversible (at least initially) and when at all possible have a scientific basis. TMD treatments can generally be divided into two types or phases. Type 1 is regarded as 'palliative TMD' treatment and is referred to as the initial conservative, reversible, and symptomatic treatment. Type 2 is regarded as 'definitive TMD' treatment that involves invasive and irreversible therapies that are directed at treating the cause and typically involve establishing a so-called optimal occlusion and/or correct condyle (CR) position (Greene, 2001; Turp et al., 2008). It must be noted that if a certain palliative TMD treatment 'fails', it does not necessarily mean that a more aggressive and definitive TMD treatment(s) must ensue.

Definitive TMD treatments are typically one, or a combination, of the following: orthodontics, prosthodontics, occlusal adjustments, repositioning splints, surgery and so forth (Greene, 2001). Definitive TMD treatments are rarely needed and should not be routinely performed. Invasive and irreversible TMD treatments are indicated only when a patient's symptoms persist to a point where they no longer can be managed in a conservative way; or in situations when certain diagnostic testing such as a TMJ MRI (which is still not singularly specific for a diagnosis of TMD, nor does an 'abnormal' finding axiomatically suggest the need for treatment) indicates the need for an invasive procedure. In summary, the primary responsibility of the judicious orthodontic TMD clinician is to provide TMD patients with what they most desire and need, i.e. relief from pain and a return to their normal daily activities.

Contemporary multidisciplinary, evidence-based treatment options

Orthodontists should be capable of providing scientifically based palliative, conservative and reversible TMD treatments. The majority of TMD patients can be managed (at least initially) with simple treatments such as counseling/reassurance, medications, physical therapies, and occlusal splints even though part of the therapeutic success observed may be more or less placebo and/or due to a patient's cognitive awareness (Griffiths, 1983; McNeill et al., 1990; Greene, 2001; Clark, 2008; Turp et al., 2008).

At times CBT and/or BFB may be the most appropriate initial treatment option *versus* the use of an oral occlusal appliance or splints (Gatchel et al., 2006). Nonetheless, it appears that the best available evidence suggests that occlusal splints work best initially and CBT including BFB work better later on in treatment (Turk et al., 1993, 1996; Rudy et al., 1995; Greco et al., 1997). Parenthetically, a recent systematic review based on 12 randomized controlled trials concluded that 'there is insufficient evidence for or against the use of stabilization splint therapy over other active

interventions for the treatment of temporomandibular myofascial pain' (Thurman and Huang, 2009).

There are four major categories for the treatment of muscle-generated TMD (Clark, 2008):

- Patient self-directed
- Office-based physical medicine
- Pharmacological
- Behavioral therapies.

Patient self-directed therapies are: avoidance therapies, local ice-cold therapy, stretch therapy, exercise therapy. Stretch exercises should be performed multiple times a day in order to suppress muscle tension levels (not to strengthen or condition the muscles). As a holistic approach to fitness/health including reduction of stress, more general somatic physical exercise (aerobic and anaerobic) can also be beneficial. Referral to a dietician, personal trainer, psychologist/counselor, and/or a physiotherapist may also be indicated to further supplement this aspect of management. A trained clinician can provide office-based physical medicine treatments which could include local trigger-point injection therapy, botulinum toxin injection therapy and manual physical therapy such as therapeutic massage, acupressure, acupuncture, and so forth. Pharmacological agents such as analgesic and anti-inflammatory agents (nonsteroidal anti-inflammatory drugs [NSAIDs]) are primarily aimed at axis I type TMD conditions which refer to physical factors that influence pain. Antianxiety agents, tranquilizers, and antidepressant medications would be most helpful for axis II type TMD conditions, which refer to psychological factors that influence pain. It must be mentioned that clinicians need to be well trained in this arena before embarking on the use of this type of prescription medication. We advise referring the patient to and/or working in conjunction with the patient's family medical practitioner, a clinical psychologist/psychiatrist, or oro-facial pain specialist. Behavior therapies include mind-body therapies such as autogenic training, relaxation exercises, meditation, CBT, hypnosis, guided imagery, BFB, or education on a specific disorder or that related to coping skills training (Clark, 2008). The key to the success in treating these patients is to obtain adequate diagnostic records/information, keeping thorough clinical records and involving the appropriate health professionals in the overall management of these patients. The authors cannot stress enough the importance of a multidisciplinary approach to the overall care of TMD patients, especially as the current concepts in TMD management are based around a more conservative biomedical/psychosocial model as opposed to a more occlusal-based model.

Conclusion

A possible relationship between occlusion and the TMJs was hypothesized in the 1930s and ever since dentistry has played a role in the debate on the diagnosis and management of TMD. This involvement led to many empirical causative and therapeutic hypotheses being developed based on this overemphasized relationship. The dental-based model of the past has been gradually replaced by a biomedical model based on the consideration of treatments for other chronic musculoskeletal disorders. The current biopsychosocial approach to TMD management attempts to integrate a host of biological, clinical, and behavioral factors that may account for the onset, maintenance, and remission of TMD. Genetics (vulnerabilities related to pain), imaging of the pain-involved brain, central brain processing of thinking and emotions, endocrinology, behavioral risk-conferring factors, and psychosocial traits and states appear to be factors receiving more attention and research in order to improve the understanding of TMD. Nonetheless, despite the current evidence demonstrating that the mechanistic and sometimes irreversible and invasive TMD treatment approaches of the past are no longer acceptable, some in dentistry and orthodontics are resistant to change and continue to tenaciously hold on to past unscientific beliefs to the detriment of their patients. As long as this trend continues, the quality of TMD management will be affected, negatively impacting on the comfort and well-being of TMD patients.

References

Academy of Prosthodontics (2005) Glossary of prosthodontic terms, 8th edn. *Journal of Prosthetic Dentistry* 94: 10–92.

Ahlgren J (1967) Pattern of chewing and malocclusion of teeth: A clinical study. *Acta Odontologica Scandinavia* 25(3): 3–13.

Alexander SR, Moore RN, DuBois LM (1993) Mandibular condyle position: Comparison articulator mountings and magnetic resonance imaging. *American Journal of Orthodontics and Dentofacial Orthopedics* 104: 230–9.

Alexander TA, Gibbs CH, Thompson WJ (1984) Investigation of chewing patterns in deep-bite malocclusions before and after orthodontic treatment. *American Journal of Orthodontics* 85: 21–7.

Arat ZM, Akcam MO, Gökalp H (2003) Long-term effects of chin-cup therapy on the temporomandibular joints. *European Journal of Orthodontics* 25: 471–5.

Ash MM, Ramjford S (1996) *Occlusion*, 4th edn. Philadelphia, PA: WB Saunders.

Beattie JR, Paquette DE, Johnston LE Jr (1994) The functional impact of extraction and nonextraction treatment: a long-term comparison in patients with 'borderline', equally susceptible Class II malocclusions. *American Journal of Orthodontics and Dentofacial Orthopedics* 105: 444–9.

Blaustein DI, Scapino RP (1986) Remodeling of the temporomandibular joint disk and posterior attachment in disk displacement specimen in relation to glycosaminogylcan content. *Plastic Reconstructive Surgery* 78: 756–64.

Block IS (1947) Diagnosis and treatment of disturbances of the temporomandibular joint, especially in relation to vertical dimension. *Journal of the American Dental Association* 34: 253–60.

Buschang P, Santos-Pinto A (1998) Condylar growth and glenoid fossa displacement during childhood and adolescence. *American Journal of Orthodontics and Dentofacial Orthopedics* 113: 437–42.

Carlsson G (2004) Chapter 7. Temporomandibular joint disorders. In: I Klineberg, R Jagger (eds) *Occlusion and Clinical Practice – An Evidence-Based Approach*. London: Wright, p. 68.

Choi BH, Yoo JH, Lee WY (1994) Comparison of magnetic resonance imaging before and after nonsurgical treatment of closed lock. *Oral Surgery Oral Medicine Oral Pathology* 78: 301–5.

Christensen J (1970) Effect of occlusion-raising procedures on the chewing system. *Dental Practice* 20: 233–8.

Clark GT (1986) The TMJ repositioning appliance: A technique for construction, insertion, and adjustment. *Journal of Craniomandibular Practice* 4: 37–46.

Clark GT (2008) Classification, causation and treatment of masticatory myogenous pain and dysfunction. *Oral and Maxillofacial Surgery Clinics of North America* 20: 145–57.

Cordray FE (1996) Centric relation treatment and articulator mountings in orthodontics. *Angle Orthodontist* 66: 153–8.

Cordray FE (2006) Three dimensional analysis of models articulated in the seated condylar position from a deprogrammed asymptomatic population: a prospective study. Part 1. *American Journal of Orthodontics and Dentofacial Orthopedics* 129: 619–30.

Costen JB (1934) Syndrome of ear and sinus symptoms dependent upon disturbed function of the temporomandibular joint. *Annals of Otology, Rhinology, Larygology* 43: 1–4.

D'Amico A (1958) The canine teeth: normal functional relation of the natural teeth of man. *Journal of the Southern California Dental Association* 26: 6–23.

Dao TTT, Feine JS, Lund JP (1988) Can electrical stimulation be used to establish a physiologic occlusal position? *Journal of Prosthetic Dentistry* 60: 509–14.

Dawson PE (1974) *Evaluation, Diagnosis, and Treatment of Occlusal Problems*. St Louis, MO: Mosby.

de Leeuw R (2008) Internal derangements of the temporomandibular joints. *Oral and Maxillofacial Surgery Clinics of North America* 20: 159–68.

de Leeuw R, Boering G, Stegenga B, et al. (1994) Clinical signs of TMJ osteoarthrosis and internal derangement 30 years after nonsurgical treatment. *Journal of Orofacial Pain* 8: 18–24.

Diatchenko L, Slade GD, Nackley AG, et al. (2005) Genetic basis for individual variations in pain perception and the development of a chronic pain condition. *Human Molecular Genetics* 14: 135–43.

Dixon DC (1991) Diagnostic imaging of the temporomandibular joint. *Dental Clinics of North Americ* 35: 53–74.

Dolwick LF (1995) Intra-articular disc displacement. Part I: Its questionable role in temporomandibular joint pathology. *Journal of Oral Maxillofacial Surgery* 53: 1069–72.

Dworkin SF, LeResche L (1992) Research diagnostic criteria for temporomandibular disorders: review, criteria, examinations and specifications, critique. *Journal of Cranimandibular Disorders* 6: 301–55.

Dworkin SF, Massoth DL (1994) Temporomandibular disorders and chronic pain: disease or illness? *Journal of Prosthetic Dentistry* 72: 29–38.

Dworkin SF, Huggins KH, LeResche L, et al. (1990) Epidemiology of signs and symptoms in temporomandibular disorders: clinical signs in cases and controls. *Journal of the American Dental Association* 120: 273–81.

Dworkin SF, Turner JA, Wilson L, et al. (1994) Brief group cognitive-behavioral intervention for temporomandibular disorders. *Pain* 59: 175–87.

Dworkin SF, Huggins KH, Wilson L, et al. (2002a) A randomized clinical trial using research diagnostic criteria for temporomandibular disorders-axis II to target clinic cases for tailored self-care TMD treatment program. *Journal of Orofacial Pain* 16: 48–63.

Dworkin SF, Turner JA, Mancl L, et al. (2002b) A randomized clinical trial of a tailored comprehensive care treatment program for temporomandibular disorders. *Journal of Orofacial Pain* 16: 259–76.

Ellis PE, Benson PE (2003) Does articulating study casts make a difference to treatment planning? *Journal of Orthodontics* 30: 45–9.

Farrar WB (1972) Differentiation of temporomandibular joint dysfunction to simplify treatment. *Journal of Prosthetic Dentistry* 28: 629–36.

Farrar WB (1982–1983) Craniomandibular practice: the state of the art-definition and diagnosis. *Journal of Craniomandibular Practice* 1: 4–12.

Farrar WB (1985) Disk derangement and dental occlusion: changing concepts. *International Journal of Periodontics Restorative Dentistry* 33: 713–21.

Farrar WB, McCarty WL Jr (1979) The TMJ dilemma. *Journal of the Alabama Dental Association* 63: 19–26.

Fernandez E, Turk DC (1989) The utility of cognitive coping strategies for altering pain perception: a meta-analysis. *Pain* 38: 123–35.

Flor H, Birbaumer N (1993) Comparison of the efficacy of electromyographic biofeedback, cognitive-behavioral therapy, and conservative medical interventions in the treatment of chronic musculoskeletal pain. *Journal of Consult Clinical Psychology* 61: 653–8.

Flores-Mir C, Nebbe B, Heo G, et al. (2006) Longitudinal study of temporomandibular joint disc status and craniofacial growth. *American Journal of Orthodontics and Dentofacial Orthopedics* 130: 324–30.

Friedman MH, Weisberg J (1981) Applied kinesiology-double blind pilot study. *Journal of Prosthetic Dentistry* 45: 321–3.

Gardea MA, Gatchel RJ, Mishra KD (2001) Long-term efficacy of biobehavioral treatment of temporomandibular disorders. *Journal of Behavioral Medicine* 24: 341–59.

Gatchel RJ, Stowell AW, Wildenstein L, et al. (2006) Efficacy of an early intervention for patients with acute temporomandibular disorder-related pain- a one year outcome study. *Journal of the American Dental Association* 137: 339–47.

Gelb H (1977) *Clinical Management of Head, Neck and Temporomandibular Join Pain and Dysfunction: A Multidisciplinary Approach to Diagnosis and Treatment*. Philadelphia, PA: WB Saunders.

Gianelly AA (1989a) Condylar position and class II deep bite, no overjet malocclusion. *American Journal of Orthodontics and Dentofacial Orthopedics* 96: 428–32.

Gianelly AA (1989b) Orthodontics, condylar position and TMJ status. *American Journal of Orthodontics and Dentofacial Orthopedics* 95: 521–3.

Gianelly AA, Hughes HM, Wohlgemuth P, et al. (1988) Condylar position and extraction treatment. *American Journal of Orthodontics and Dentofacial Orthopedics* 93: 201–5.

Gianelly AA, Cozzanic M, Boffa J (1991a) Condylar position and maxillary first premolar extraction. *American Journal of Orthodontics and Dentofacial Orthopedics* 99: 473–6.

Gianelly AA, Anderson CK, Boffa J (1991b) Longitudinal evaluation of condylar position in extraction and nonextraction treatment. *American Journal of Orthodontics and Dentofacial Orthopedics* 100: 416–20.

Gibbs CH, Masserman T, Reswwick JB, et al. (1977) Functional movements of the mandible. *Journal of Prosthetic Dentistry* 26: 604–20.

Gillings BRD, Graham CH, Duckmanton NA (1973) Jaw movements in young men during chewing. *Journal of Prosthetic Dentistry* 29: 616–27.

Glickman JI, Martigoni M, Haddad A, et al. (1970) Further observation on human occlusion monitored by intraoral telemetry. *International Association of Dental Research* (abstract no. 612): 201.

Glossary of Prosthodontic Terms (2005) *Journal of Prosthetic Dentistry* 94: 10–92.

Gökalp H, Arat M, Erden I (2000) The changes in temporomandibular joint disc position and configuration in early orthognathic treatment: a magnetic resonance imaging evaluation. *European Journal of Orthodontics* 22: 217–24.

Goldstein GR (1979) The relationship of canine-protected occlusion to a periodontal index. *Journal of Prosthetic Dentistry* 41: 277–83.

Gonzalez YM, Greene CS, Mohl ND (2008) Technological devices in the diagnosis of temporomandibular disorders. *Oral and Maxillofacial Surgery of North America* 20: 211–20.

Goodman P, Greene CS, Laskin DM (1976) Response of patients with myofascial pain-dysfunction syndrome to mock equilibration. *Journal of the American Dental Association* 92: 755.

Graf H, Zander HA (1963) Functional tooth contacts in lateral and centric occlusion. *Journal of Prosthetic Dentistry* 13: 1055–66.

Greco CM, Rudy TE, Turk DC, et al. (1997) Traumatic onset of temporomandibular disorders: positive effects of a standardized conservative treatment program. *Clinical Journal of Pain* 13: 337–47.

Greenberg MS, Cohen SG, Springer P, et al. (1981) Mandibular position and upper body strength: a controlled clinical trial. *Journal of the American Dental Association* 103: 576–9.

Greene CS (2001) The etiology of temporomandibular disorders: implications for treatment. *Journal of Orofacial Pain* 15: 93–105.

Greene CS, Laskin DM (1972a) Splint therapy for the myofascial pain-dysfunction (MPD) syndrome. A comparative study. *Journal of the American Dental Association* 84: 624–8.

Greene CS, Laskin DM (1972b) Influence of the doctor-patient relationship on placebo therapy for patients with myo-fascial pain-dysfunction (MPD) syndrome. *Journal of the American Dental Association* 85: 892–4.

Greene CS, Laskin DM (1974) Long-term evaluation of conservative treatment for myofascial pain-dysfunction syndrome. *Journal of the American Dental Association* 89: 1365–8.

Greene CS, Laskin DM (1983) Long-term evaluation of treatment for myofascial pain-dysfunction analysis. *Journal of the American Dental Association* 107: 235–8.

Greene CS, Laskin DM (2000) Temporomandibular disorders: moving from a dentally based to a medically based model. *Journal of Dental Research* 79: 1736–9.

Greene CS, Goddard G, Macaluso GM, et al. (2009) Topical review: placebo responses and therapeutic responses. How are they related? *Journal of Orofacial Pain* 23: 93–107.

Griffiths RH (1983) Report of the president's conference on the examination, diagnosis, and management of temporomandibular disorders. *Journal of the American Dental Association* 106: 75–7.

Guichet NF (1979) The Denar system and its application in everyday dentistry. *Dental Clinics of North America* 23: 243–57.

Gutteman AS (1961) Chop-stroke chewers. *Dental Progress* 1: 254–7.

Hall HD (1995) Intra-articular disc displacement. Part I: Its significant role to temporomandibular joint pathology. *Journal of Oral Maxillofacial Surgery* 53: 1073–9.

Hall HD, Nickerson JW (1994) Is it time to pay more attention to disc position? *Journal of Orofacial Pain* 8: 90–6.

Hart DL, Lundquist DO, Davis HC (1981) The effect of vertical dimension on muscular strength. *Journal of Orthopaedic Sports Physical Therapy* 3: 57–61.

Hirsch C (2009) No increased risk of temporomandibular disorders and bruxism in children and adolescents during orthodontic therapy. *Journal of Orofacial Orthopaedics* 70: 39–50.

Jankelson B (1979) Neuromuscular aspects of occlusion. Effects of occlusal position on the physiology and dysfunction of the mandibular musculature. *Dental Clinics of North America* 23: 157–68.

Jankelson B (1984) Three-dimensional orthodontic diagnosis and treatment. A neuromuscular approach. *Journal of Clinical Orthodontics* 18: 627–36.

Jankelson B, Sparks S, Crane PF, et al. (1975) Neural conduction of the myo-monitor stimulus: A quantitative analysis. *Journal of Prosthetic Dentistry* 34: 245–53.

Karl PJ, Foley TF (1999) The use of a deprogramming appliance to obtain centric relation. *Angle Orthodontist* 69: 117–25.

Katzberg RW, Westesson PL, Tallents RH, et al. (1996) Orthodontics and temporomandibular joint internal derangement. *American Journal of Orthodontics and Dentofacial Orthopedics* 109: 515–20.

Kircos L, Ortendahl D, Mark AS, et al. (1987) Magnetic resonance imaging of the TMJ disc in asymptomatic volunteers. *Journal of Oral Maxillofacial Surgery* 45: 852–4.

Kim MR, Graber TM, Vianna MA (2002) Orthodontics and temporomandibular disorders: a meta-analysis. *American Journal of Orthodontics and Dentofacial Orthopedics* 121: 438–46.

Klar NA, Kulbersh R, Freeland T, et al. (2003) Maximum intercuspation – centric relation disharmony in 200 consecutively finished cases in a gnathologically oriented practice. *Seminars in Orthodontics* 9: 109–16.

Klasser GD, Greene CS (2007a) Predoctoral teaching of temporomandibular disorders. *Journal of the American Dental Association* 138: 231–7.

Klasser GD, Greene CS (2007b) Role of oral appliances in the management of sleep bruxism and temporomandibular disorders. *Alpha Omegan* 100: 111–19.

Kulbersh R, Dhutia M, Navarro M, et al. (2003a) Condylar distraction effects of standard edgewise therapy versus gnathologically based edgewise therapy. *Seminars in Orthodontics* 9: 117–27.

Kulbersh R, Kaczynski R, Freeland T (2003b) Orthodontics and gnathology. *Seminars in Orthodontics* 9: 93–5.

Kurita K, Westesson PL, Yuasa H, et al. (1998) Natural course of untreated symptomatic temporomandibular joint disc displacement without reduction. *Journal of Dental Research* 77: 361–5.

Larheim TA, Westesson PL, Sano T (2001) Temporomandibular joint disk displacement: comparison in asymptomatic volunteers and patients. *Radiology* 218: 428–32.

Laskin DM (1969) Etiology of the pain-dysfunction syndrome. *Journal of the American Dental Association* 79: 147–53.

Laskin DM, Greene CS (1970) Correlation of placebo responses and psychological characteristics in myofascial pain-dysfunction patients. *International Association of Dental Research* (abstract no. 82): 119.

Lindauer SJ, Sabol G, Isaacson RJ, et al. (1995) Condylar movement and mandibular rotation during jaw opening. *American Journal of Orthodontics and Dentofacial Orthopedics* 105: 573–7.

Luecke PE, Johnston LE Jr (1992) The effect of maxillary first premolar extraction and incisor retraction on mandibular position: Testing the central dogma of 'functional orthodontics'. *American Journal of Orthodontics and Dentofacial Orthopedics* 101: 4–12.

Luppanapornlap S, Johnston LE Jr (1993) The effects of premolar-extraction: a long-term comparison of outcomes in' clear-cut' extraction and nonextraction Class II patients. *Angle Orthodontist* 63: 257–72.

Lupton DE (1969) Psychological aspects of temporomandibular joint dysfunction. *Journal of the American Dental Association* 79: 131.

Macfarlene TV, Kenealy P, Kingdon HA, et al. (2009) Twenty-year cohort study of health gain from orthodontic treatment: Temporomandibular disorders. *American Journal of Orthodontics and Dentofacial Orthopedics* 135: 692–3.

Mann AW, Pankey LD (1963) Concepts of occlusion: the PM philosophy of occlusal rehabilitation. In: GL Courtcade (ed.) *Occlusal Rehabilitation*. Philadelphia, PA: WB Saunders, pp. 621–36.

McCarty W (1979) Diagnosis and treatment of internal derangements. In: WK Solberg, GT Clark (eds) *Temporomandibular Joint Problems: Biological Diagnoses and Treatment*. Chicago, IL: Quintessence.

McCollum BB (1927) Factors that make the mouth and teeth a vital organ (articulation orthodontia). *Journal of the American Dental Association* 14: 1261–71.

McNamara JA Jr, Seligman DA, Okeson JP (1995) Occlusion, orthodontic treatment, and temporomandibular disorders: a review. *Journal of Orofacial Pain* 9: 73–89.

McNeill C (1997) History and evolution of TMD concepts. *Oral Surgery Oral Medicine Oral Pathology Oral Radiolology and Endodontics* 83: 51–60.

McNeill C, Mohl ND, Rugh JD, et al. (1990) Temporomandibular disorders: diagnosis, management, education, and research. *Journal of the American Dental Association* 120: 253–60.

Mishra KD, Gatchel RJ, Gardea MA (2000) The relative efficacy of three cognitive-behavioral treatment approaches to temporomandibular disorders. *Journal of Behavioral Medicine* 23: 293–309.

Mohl ND (1991) Temporomandibular disorders: the role of occlusion, TMJ imaging, and electronic devices- a diagnostic update. *Journal of the American College of Dentists* 58: 4–10.

Mohl ND, Dixon DC (1994) Current status of diagnostic procedures for temporomandibular disorders. *Journal of the American Dental Association* 125: 56–64.

Moloney F, Howard JA (1986) Internal derangements of the temporomandibular joint: anterior repositioning splint therapy. *Australian Dental Journal* 31: 30–9.

National Institutes of Health Technology Assessment Conference Statement (1996) Management of temporomandibular disorders. *Journal of the American Dental Association* 127: 1595–606.

Nebbe B, Major PW, Prasad NG (1999a) Female adolescent facial pattern associated with TMJ disk displacement and reduction in disk length. Part I. *American Journal of Orthodontics and Dentofacial Orthopedics* 116: 167–76.

Nebbe B, Major PW, Prasad NG (1999b) Male adolescent facial pattern associated with TMJ disk displacement and reduction in disk length. Part II. *American Journal of Orthodontics and Dentofacial Orthopedics* 116: 301–7.

Okeson JR (2005) *Management of Temporomandibular Disorders and Occlusion*, 5th edn. St Louis, MO: Mosby, pp. 121–2.

Pameijer JH, Glickman I, Roeber FW (1969) Intraoral occlusal telemetry. 3. Tooth contacts in chewing, swallowing, and bruxism. *Journal of Periodontology* 40: 253–8.

Pameijer JH, Brion M, Glickman I, et al. (1970) Intraoral occlusal telemetry. V. Effect of occlusal adjustment upon tooth contacts during chewing and swallowing. *Journal of Prosthetic Dentistry* 24: 492–7.

Panek H, Matthews-Brzozowska T, Nowakowska D, et al. (2008) Dynamic occlusions in the natural permanent dentition. *Quintessence International* 39: 337–42.

Pollack B (1988) Cases of note: Michigan jury awards \$850 000 in ortho case: A tempest in a teapot. *American Journal of Orthodontics and Dentofacial Orthopedics* 94: 358–60.

Posselt U (1950) Terminal hinge movement of the mandible. *Journal of Prosthetic Dentistry* 7: 787–9.

Posselt U (1952) Studies in the mobility of the human mandible. *Acta Odontologica Scandinavia* 10(Suppl. 10):19–160.

Ramfjord SP, Ash MM (1971) *Occlusion*, 3rd edn. Philadelphia, PA: WB Saunders.

Rasmussen OC (1981) Description of population and progress of symptoms in a longitudinal study of temporomandibular arthropathy. *Scandinavian Journal of Dental Research* 89: 196–203.

Rasmussen OC (1983) Temporomandibular arthropathy: clinical, radiographic, and therapeutic aspects, with emphasis on diagnosis. *International Journal of Oral Surgery* 12: 365–97.

Reynders R (1990) Orthodontics and temporomandibular disorders: a review of the literature (1966–1988). *American Journal of Orthodontics and Dentofacial Orthopedics* 1: 73–86.

Rinchuse DJ (1987) Counterpoint: preventing adverse effects on the temporomandibular joint through orthodontic treatment. *American Journal of Orthodontics and Dentofacial Orthopedics* 91: 500–6.

Rinchuse DJ, Kandasamy S (2006) Articulators in orthodontics: An evidence-based perspective. *American Journal of Orthodontics and Dentofacial Orthopedics* 129: 299–308.

Rinchuse DJ, Kandasamy S (2007) A contemporary and evidence-based view of canine protected occlusion. *American Journal of Orthodontics and Dentofacial Orthopedics* 132: 90–102.

Rinchuse DJ, Rinchuse DJ (1983) The impact of the American Dental Association's guidelines for the examination, diagnosis, and management of temporomandibular disorders on orthodontic practice. *American Journal of Orthodontics and Dentofacial Orthopedics* 83: 518–22.

Rinchuse DJ, Rinchuse DJ, Kandasamy S (2005) Evidence-based versus experience-based views on occlusion and TMD. *American Journal of Orthodontics and Dentofacial Orthopedics* 127: 249–54.

Roth RH (1973) Temporomandibular pain-dysfunction and occlusal relationship. *Angle Orthodontist* 43: 136–53.

Roth RH (1976) The maintenance system and occlusal dynamics. *Dental Clinics of North America* 20: 761–88.

Roth RH (1981a) Functional occlusion for the orthodontist. Part I. *Journal of Clinical Orthodontics* 15: 32–51.

Roth RH (1981b) Functional occlusion for the orthodontist. Part III. *Journal of Clinical Orthodontics* 15: 174–9, 182–98.

Roth RH (1985) Treatment mechanics for the straight-wire appliance. In: TM Graber, BF Swain (eds) *Orthodontics, Current Principles and Techniques*. St. Louis, MO: Mosby, pp. 665–716.

Roth RH, Rolfs DA (1981) Functional occlusion for the orthodontist. Part II. *Journal of Clinical Orthodontics* 25: 100–23.

Rudy TE, Turk DC, Kubinski JA, et al. (1995) Differential treatment response of TMD patients as a function of psychological characteristics. *Pain* 61: 103–12.

Sarlani E, Greenspan JD (2005) Why look to the brain for answers to temporomandibular disorder pain? *Cells Tissues Organs* 180: 69–75.

Sarver DM (2001) The importance of incisor positioning in the esthetic smile: the smile arc. *American Journal of Orthodontics and Dentofacial Orthopedics* 120: 98–111.

Sato S, Takahashi K, Kawamura H, et al. (1998) The natural course of nonreducing disk displacement of the temporomandibular joint: changes in condylar mobility and radiographic alterations at one-year follow up. *International Journal of Oral and Maxillofacial Surgery* 27: 173–7.

Sato S, Nasu F, Motegi K (2002) Natural course of nonreducing disc displacement of the temporomandibular joint: changes in chewing movement and masticatory efficiency. *Journal of Oral and Maxillofacial Surgery* 60: 867–72.

Scaife RR, Holt JE (1969) Natural occurrence of cuspid guidance. *Journal of Prosthetic Dentistry* 22: 225–9.

Scapino RP (1983) Histopathology associated with malposition of the human temporomandibular joint disc. *Oral Surgery Oral Medicine Oral Pathology* 55: 382–97.

Schmitt ME, Kulbersh R, Freeland T, et al. (2003) Reproducibility of the Roth Power Centric in determining centric relation. *Seminars in Orthodontics* 9: 102–8.

Schuyler CH (1929) Principles employed in full denture prostheses which may be applied in other fields of dentistry. *Journal of the American Dental Association* 16: 20–45.

Schwartz L (1958) Conclusions of the TMJ clinic at Columbia. *Journal of Periodontology* 29: 210–12.

Schwartz L (1959) *Disorders of the Temporomandibular Joint*. Philadelphia, PA: WB Saunders.

Seligman DA, Pullinger AG (1991) The role of functional occlusal relationships in temporomandibular disorders: a review. *Journal of Craniomandibular Facial Oral Pain* 5: 265–79.

Sheppard IM, Sheppard SM (1965) Range of condylar movement during mandibular opening. *Journal of Prosthetic Dentistry* 15: 263–71.

Shildkraut M, Wood DP, Hunter WS (1994) The CR-CO discrepancy and its effect on cephalometric measurements. *Angle Orthodontist* 64: 333–42.

Sicher H (1948) Temporomandibular articulation in mandibular overclosure. *Journal of the American Dental Association* 30: 131–9.

Slade GD, Diatchenko L, Ohrbach R, et al. (2008) Orthodontic treatment, genetic factors and risk of temporomandibular disorder. *Seminars in Orthodontics* 14: 146–56.

Solberg WK, Woo MW, Houston JB (1979) Prevalence of mandibular dysfunction in young adults. *Journal of the American Dental Association* 98: 25–34.

Stohler CS (2004) Taking stock: From chasing occlusal contacts to vulnerability alleles. *Orthodontic Craniofacial Research* 7: 157–61.

Sved A (1944) Changing the occlusal level and a new method of retention. *American Journal of Orthodontics* 5: 527–35.

Tallents RH, Katzberg RW, Murphy W, et al. (1996) Magnetic resonance imaging findings in asymptomatic volunteers and symptomatic patients with temporomandibular disorders. *Journal of Prosthetic Dentistry* 75: 529–33.

Thurman MM, Huang GJ (2009) Insufficient evidence to support the use of stabilization splint therapy over other active interventions in the treatment of temporomandibular myofascial pain. *Journal of the American Dental Association* 140: 1524–5.

Torsten J, Lundquist S, Hedegard B (2004) Group function or canine protection. *Journal of Prosthetic Dentistry* 91: 403–8.

Turk D, Zaki H, Rudy T (1993) Effects of intraoral appliance and biofeedback/stress management alone and in combination in treating pain and depression in TMD patients. *Journal of Prosthetic Dentistry* 70: 158–64.

Turk DC, Rudy TE, Kubinski JA, et al. (1996) Dysfunctional patients with temporomandibular disorders: an evaluating the efficacy of a tailored treatment protocol. *Journal of Consult Clinical Psychology* 64: 139–46.

Turp JC, Greene CS, Strub JR (2008) Dental occlusion: a critical reflection on past, present and future concepts. *Journal of Oral Rehabilitation* 35: 446–53.

Utt TW, Meyers CE Jr, Wierzba TF, et al. (1995) A three-dimensional comparison of condylar position changes between centric relation and centric occlusion using the mandibular position indicator. *American Journal of Orthodontics and Dentofacial Orthopedics* 107: 298–308.

Wickwire NA, Gibbs CH, Jacobson AP, et al. (1981) Chewing patterns in normal children. *Angle Orthodontist* 51: 48–60.

Williamson EH, Caves SA, Edenfield RJ, et al. (1978) Cephalometric analysis: comparisons between maximum intercuspation and centric relation. *American Journal of Orthodontics* 74: 672–7.

Williamson EH, Steinke RM, Murse PK, et al. (1980) Centric relation: a comparison of muscle-determined position and operator guidance. *American Journal of Orthodontics* 77: 135–45.

Witzig JW, Spahl TJ (1991) *The Clinical Management of Basic Maxillofacial Orthopedic Appliances*, Vol 3. The temporomandibular joint. Boston, MA: PSG Publishing Company.

Woda A, Vigneron P, Kay D (1979) Non-functional and functional occlusal contacts: a review of the literature. *Journal of Prosthetic Dentistry* 42: 335–41.

Wyatt WE (1987) Preventing adverse effects on the temporomandibular joint through orthodontic treatment. *American Journal of Orthodontics and Dentofacial Orthopedics* 91: 493–9.

25

Orthodontic Treatment for the Special Needs Child

Stella Chaushu, Joseph Shapira, Adrian Becker

Summary

Individuals with special needs are children or adults who are prevented by a physical or mental condition from full participation in the normal range of activities of their age groups. They usually exhibit high orthodontic treatment need, because of an increased prevalence and severity of malocclusion. Although parents may be highly motivated to improve a child's quality of life by enhancing appearance and oral function, these children are the least likely to receive orthodontic treatment. The present chapter discusses orthodontic treatment for patients with developmental disability involving behavioral problems, based on our earlier published studies and clinical experience in the treatment of this compromised minority group within the community. The chapter will discuss the major obstacles that may preclude the delivery of orthodontic treatment or are encountered during treatment and the different management modalities that may be employed to overcome the behavioral limitations in children, and will provide guidelines for the orthodontist to gain therapeutic access to these patients.

Introduction

'Special needs' is an umbrella term under which a staggering array of diagnoses may be included: from mild learning disabilities to profound mental retardation; food allergies to terminal illness; developmental delays that are transitory to those that are intractable; occasional panic attacks to serious psychiatric problems. The designation is useful for garnering needed professional help and services, setting appropriate goals, and gaining understanding for a child and his distressed family. The present chapter will focus on those children with developmental disability involving behavioral problems.

Therapeutic access

Children with behavioral issues do not respond to traditional discipline nor do they necessarily wish to be subjected to the various procedures they may need to undergo. Their intellectual level is also not adequate for them to understand the need for compliance in the intricacies of a standard biomechanical apparatus. They require specialized and, often, simplified strategies that are tailored to their specific abilities and disabilities. If these important steps are not considered by the operator, therapeutic access may be impossible to obtain. The clinician needs to be understanding, flexible, and creative.

There are several specific areas in which the special needs patient will unintentionally obstruct the delivery of treatment (Becker and Shapira, 1996) and this is because he or she typically has shortcomings not usually seen in the normal child, such as (Shapira et al., 1999):

- Increased apprehension, reduced understanding, limited tolerance and short attention span
- Exaggerated gag reflex (which seems to be a consequence of fear)
- Inability to remain still for any appreciable time; uncontrolled body movements
- Reduced level of cooperation
- Drooling.

Under these conditions simple exercises such as the taking of radiographs or dental impressions become tasks of major proportions. In order to achieve these normally modest and simple aims, behavior modification techniques may need to be employed, with or without specific

---

Integrated Clinical Orthodontics, First Edition. Edited by Vinod Krishnan, Ze'ev Davidovitch.
© 2012 Blackwell Publishing Ltd. Published 2012 by Blackwell Publishing Ltd.

pharmacological aids and/or through conscious and deep sedation or with general anesthesia.

Over the past 20 years or so, both the absolute number and proportion of special needs children in society has increased (Waldman et al., 2000), in spite of prenatal diagnostic techniques and the improvement in prenatal identification of congenital anomalies. The main reasons are first, sophisticated medical care, both perinatal and adult, that has increased the survival rate of the newborn and their overall life expectancy. Second, given the enlightened attitude of society today, changing social policies and legislation, many more special needs children are seen as an integral part of their family, within adoptive families, or in sheltered housing and are thus far more visible in general, while three decades ago they were largely housed in institutions. This gradual but palpable process of 'mainstreaming' has brought about a greater awareness and appreciation on the part of the general public.

With their higher public profile, the present-day affluent society of the Western world has created a general improvement in quality of life for these children that, in turn, expresses itself in an increased demand for esthetics and normal function. The aim is acceptance into society, including the opportunity for employment towards self-sufficiency. As the direct result, the concern for facial appearance has become an item for discussion among their parents and this has generated a demand for orthodontic treatment (Becker and Shapira, 1996).

In general, the main goals of orthodontics are to improve the alignment and occlusion of the teeth and thus, to contribute to one of the more important factors involved in improvement of the facial appearance (Shaw et al., 1980). However, its efficacy is limited and cannot provide a satisfactory answer for every situation. Individual benefits that are principally associated with the patient's own concept of him/herself might have been gained by the patient and these are often strongly influenced by those around him (Sticker, 1970).

Studies of the effects that dental appearance has on individuals and their surroundings have found this to be extremely important in overall facial esthetics (Lew, 1993). In adverse conditions, it is a principal focus for teasing among school children (Shaw et al., 1980), has a significant emotional impact on the individual, and is a factor used in social acceptability and personality judgment by others (Shaw, 1981).

In their everyday life, special needs children comprise a group of individuals who depend heavily on their families and others for their needs and welfare. From earlier observations (Oreland et al., 1987), we learn that they have malocclusion, which is more frequent, more severe, and more skeletally based than in the general population. Several conditions, such as cerebral palsy, Down syndrome, and mental retardation, exhibit increased prevalence of specific dental features (Cohen and Winer, 1965; Franklin

et al., 1996), which can adversely affect function (Proffit et al., 2007). Yet, these patients are those least likely to receive orthodontic treatment.

Beneficial but not essential

The pediatric dentist must treat a patient to eliminate dental disease and to relieve pain, regardless of whether the child is cooperative in the dental chair and diligent in his routine homecare. At the same time, the dentist is duty-bound to encourage behavior alteration in both these areas. By contrast, orthodontics performed under these adverse conditions is contraindicated since a successful outcome is doubtful and iatrogenic damage, in the form of caries and gingival inflammation, is likely. Thus, while treatment need is often high and its object beneficial, orthodontics must still be considered to be an elective item. The order must therefore be reversed, with a sustained level of oral hygiene being first achieved, and this is the point where parental involvement will usually be essential.

Motivation and expectation

The motivation for treatment in most of these cases comes from the parents of the disabled child, rather than from other medical or dental professionals (Becker et al., 2000). A majority of these children live at home, receiving daily one-on-one attention from highly motivated parents and siblings, who are often prepared to sacrifice much to improve the child's wellbeing (Becker et al., 2000). Certainly many of the children will be sufficiently aware to believe that treatment is desirable, but there is a deep abyss between their 'in principal' agreement and the compliance that will be needed when the first clinical steps need to be taken.

The wearing of a simple orthodontic appliance, together with maintaining adequate oral hygiene either alone or permitting the parents to do it, may represent the first challenge of accepting responsibility on the part of the child. The special needs child is usually positively influenced by praise and compliments from the practitioner, the parent and those around him/her, when certain functions and stages are completed successfully and this all combines to form an environment that encourages compliance. A marred facial appearance is the principal factor motivating the request for orthodontic treatment among normal children but, in the present context, recognition of poor oral health and function and their improvement are parallel aims (Becker et al., 2000).

Patient management

Special needs patients need much more time and understanding for progress to be made in treatment and this requirement may exceed the patience of many otherwise highly productive providers, since it is difficult to rise to the challenge and yet blend it with the smooth running efficiency of a regular orthodontic office (Waldman et al., 2000;

Becker et al., 2001). Sedation or general anesthesia sessions are sometimes needed and it makes sense to include other specialists to perform any required endodontic, oral surgery, and restorative procedures, taking advantage of the potential that these modalities provide (Chaushu and Becker, 2000). An orthodontic environment that can accommodate all these specialists and provide a trained anesthetist close at hand is unlikely outside a hospital-type setting, which limits the capability of the purely orthodontic practice for the duration of the only the simplest of cases of this type.

Pretreatment visits and patient assessment

Although true for every orthodontic case, there are four specific aims which have special relevance here, with the exception that in the present context they invariably demand more than a single visit to evaluate them. Morbidity due to medical conditions that feature hypotony and myopathy is high among this group, which means that food is not cleared from the mouth efficiently in normal function, manual dexterity is poor and most subjects practice no oral hygiene whatsoever. Pre-treatment visits are therefore essential and are used for four specific purposes:

- To allay the patient's anxiety and raise confidence level in the dental chair
- To evaluate the existing level of homecare, to point out to both child and parent where it may be lacking
- Demonstrate how improvement can and must be achieved always with parental supervision, often with their active participation, as a precondition to acceptance for treatment
- To assess the level of actual compliance and whether this can be maintained through treatment.

At the first visit, the child and parent are shown the debris surrounding the teeth, the collections of food in the palatal vault, in the cheek area and elsewhere, together with the accompanying gingival inflammation, and are taught to recognize this situation. In order for the child to reach a level of oral hygiene consistent with the pursuit of orthodontic treatment, it is inevitable that the parent must be the dominant tooth brusher, with the child 'finishing off' the exercise to include him or her in accepting responsibility that will take them through later life. The act of tooth brushing carried out by a parent on a daily basis is itself a potentially helpful exercise, since it familiarizes the child with the insertion of foreign items into the oral cavity in a non-threatening environment, which helps to overcome apprehension and gagging (Becker and Shapira, 1996). Perhaps the most reliable sign of a good and potentially compliant patient is seen at the visit after oral hygiene instruction has been given and its importance stressed. The patient and parent arrive with an optimistic disposition, having put into practice what they have learned. However, the acid test is not merely to see clean teeth, but to check for the resolution of the gingival inflammation.

It has to be recognized that most visits for later orthodontic treatment will usually require using behavior management techniques and that sedation and general anesthesia will only be used for lengthy and involved procedures – perhaps two or three sessions for the duration of the treatment. For this reason, time spent in pretreatment preparation and evaluation is usually well spent (Chaushu and Becker, 2000). If the patient is unable to achieve a healthy mouth, the orthodontist should refuse to treat at that time and suggest follow-up at a later date.

Drawing up a tentative treatment plan

Treatment plans are usually the product of the gathering and collation of information contributed from a clinical examination, from photographic and radiographic records, a cephalometric analysis, plaster casts, and other aids to diagnosis and, under normal conditions, these records are simply and routinely acquired. In the present circumstances, these same diagnostic aids become a major undertaking which can frighten the child for months or years to come, if badly managed.

The answer may often be to formulate a general direction of treatment based on a clinical examination only and delay the needed diagnostic records for the first sedation session. This initial and tentative treatment plan may then be confirmed or adjusted in accordance with the new information. In this way, the first sedation session may be used for alginate impressions (to be rapidly cast), intraoral radiographs and photographs (to be quickly processed and viewed), a full treatment plan devised on the spot and, perhaps a further impression to make an initial simple removable plate. Other activities that may be usefully brought into this single session include scaling, fissure sealants, and minor restorations or even root treatments for traumatized central incisors, which is a common occurrence in these patients. At the conclusion of this important visit, the new records are studied and a reasoned working treatment plan established. This level of patient management requires a high degree of diagnostic and clinical skill on the part of the lead orthodontist.

Control of adverse behavior during treatment

Orthodontics involves many visits for a variety of different treatment activities and functions and it must be clear from the outset that negative behavior cannot be controlled with general anesthesia at every visit. Certainly for the more anxious special needs patient, the difficult, the exacting, and the protracted visits and those in which more meticulous biomechanics is needed, pharmacological assistance will be needed, but these need to be properly planned and kept to a minimum. This means that the use of the 'tell-show-do' behavior modification techniques, with positive and negative reinforcement, needs to become the modus operandi for the most part of any treatment program, leaving a decision to be made regarding the supplementary modalities needed for those procedures that are poorly tolerated (Becker and Shapira, 1996).

A conscious and highly anxious patient can be brought to a relaxed state by pharmacological agents through several routes, including inhalation (nitrous oxide and oxygen), transmucosally (midazolam via nasal drops), orally (chloral hydrate, valium, midazolam), or intravenously (propofol). Through the use of these agents, the patient's compliance may be assured for the duration of the treatment, increasing the range of procedures that may be performed on the unwilling and apprehensive patient, even permitting the orthodontist to provide treatment formerly considered impossible. Combinations of these drugs, such as midazolam (anxiolytic, sedative and amnestic) with nitrous oxide (analgesic and relaxing effects) can produce conscious sedation with virtually no side effects and may be used inexpensively for relatively short procedures (Malamed, 1995). General anesthetic carries with it the accompanying need for short term hospitalization, specialized operating theatre, and preoperative and postoperative care. Nevertheless, until recently it was considered the only answer for the more involved and lengthy procedures, such as the placement of a fully bracketed fixed appliance, possibly combined with the extraction of teeth in appropriate cases, despite the attendant morbidity and much higher cost (Jackson, 1967; Chadwick and Asher-McDade, 1997).

Several years ago, we introduced intravenous deep sedation as an alternative to general anesthesia and this has permitted us to increase the uptake of greater numbers of very difficult patients (Chaushu et al., 2002b) without the need for an operating room. The orthodontic clinic is the ideal environment to carry out orthodontic procedures, but it is required to be properly equipped for sedation with the availability of the services of an anesthetist, if sedation is to be performed. The sedation agent used is intravenous propofol, which induces a safe level of sedation very rapidly and is relatively free of side effects. Risk of aspiration and other emergencies is very low and the patient's vital reflexes are maintained for the duration of the sedation. Intubation is not usually necessary and recovery is very fast. This modality permits medium duration procedures to be undertaken, including collaboration with oral surgery and endodontic specialists in the comprehensive treatment of the patient. Intravenous sedation has greatly improved our ability to achieve therapeutic access in these patients and has facilitated the smooth pursuit of treatment on an outpatient basis (Chaushu et al., 2002b).

Adapting orthodontics to the special needs child

Modifications to orthodontic treatment and the manner in which it is delivered are needed, if success is to be achieved with these patients.

- Pragmatic treatment aims: Ideal results are not always achievable because various adverse factors may be present in the particular individual, which dictate aiming for more limited goals.
- Record taking: We have already mentioned the problems involved in taking impressions and how these may be circumvented. Intraoral radiographs are often just as difficult to take in these cases, when the child is fully conscious, and these may need to be taken under sedation. On the other hand, extraoral films, such as panoramic radiographs and cephalograms are usually better tolerated. However, holding the head of a frightened child in a cephalostat, or having him/her sit still in a particular posture for several seconds while the X-ray tube circles the head, may not be possible and sedation may not be an asset in this situation. Accordingly, diagnosis may have to be made with fewer diagnostic aids, placing greater emphasis on the clinical examination.
- Modular treatment: A problem list should be drawn up and its various components prioritized into modules, beginning with the simpler tasks and progressing to the next, while being prepared to make adaptive alterations that may be needed at each stage.
- Simplified treatment methods:
  - Placement of removable appliances is very simple, is easily learned, and well tolerated (Becker et al., 2001). Adjustment and activation are made outside the mouth, which means that the patient's mouth is not disturbed by the operator's hands and by the insertion and manipulation of dental instruments. Oral hygiene is considerably easier than with fixed appliances, both for parent and child. It is recommended to continue their use to achieve as much as possible before moving on to the fixed appliance stage or, possibly, even to be in the position to occasionally eliminate it. Care should be taken in the design and construction of the removable appliance to include several retention clasps, so that even the more rebellious child with limited dexterity will have difficulty in removing it, until quickly becoming accustomed to its presence.
  - Appliances with a long range of action should be preferred, to increase the time between visits. The use of a removable plate with a headgear cured into the acrylic and worn full time has been found to be very acceptable (Becker and Shapira, 1996; Becker et al., 2001) to these patients and the corrective influence of this *en bloc* appliance on a severe Class II relationship may be dramatic (Thurow, 1975). It is simple to use, requires few visits for adjustments, and, above all, is extremely safe since, with no detachable parts, it contrasts very favorably with a headgear that slots into molar tubes. With its use, fewer premolar extractions are needed and, therefore, there are fewer corrective root movements to deal with later.

— When extractions are nevertheless necessary, the Class II relation is more efficiently corrected with this removable integral headgear appliance than with Class II elastics, with which both child and parent are often highly dexterity challenged. This means that space closure will need to be completed with intra-arch mechanics, which are far more reliable, since they are placed by the operator.

— With the Class II corrected to a Class I relationship, the remainder of the treatment is best carried out with a fixed appliance which offers minimum frictional resistance to sliding mechanics, such as the Tip-Edge Plus or the self-ligating bracket systems. Breakages may occasionally occur, although experience has shown that this is less of a problem than in a healthy patient, possibly due to the hypotonic facial and masticatory musculature.

— Mechanics may often be simplified by non-routine extractions and this should certainly be considered in this subgroup of the population, if not among healthy individuals.

Special considerations with orthodontics under sedation

Certain precautions are necessary when treating the sedated patient and the most important concern relates to aspiration because of partial or total loss of the patient's protective reflexes. It is essential to prevent the leakage of water, saliva, blood, debris, or loose orthodontic brackets into the airway, to avoid laryngospasm or tracheal or bronchial infection. Children with cerebral palsy and muscular dystrophy may have an impaired cough reflex due to their condition and thus are at greater risk. The best way to significantly reduce this palpable danger is to use a rubber dam under these circumstances (Chaushu et al., 2000b). When this is impossible, as with impression taking, band fitting and the cementation of soldered lingual/palatal arches, an oropharyngeal pack is mandatory. Indirect bonding has also been used in these situations and has much to recommend it (Thomas, 1979).

Molar band placement is more difficult when the patient cannot bite on a band-seating instrument or bite stick and it is difficult to apply manual pressure, particularly in the mandible, when the anesthetist is trying to hold the jaw forward to increase the size of the airway. However, band cementation requires less critical and less stringent conditions of saliva control than bracket bonding and, wherever possible, should be performed in a separate visit, before the sedation session. If the special needs individual has been taken patiently through the stages outlined above, this is usually possible to achieve and, if so, is of considerable advantage.

Bracket bonding must be as accurate and as perfect as possible, to reduce the chances of bond failure later on, as a rebond will be much more difficult. The operator should use the method and materials that they are most comfortable with and have proved to be the most reliable. Aluminum oxide sandblasting is recommended, provided suitable precautions regarding aspiration are in place. Anti-sialogog drugs should be used if needed.

Relapse and retention

Teeth move throughout life, whether or not orthodontic treatment had been performed. Accordingly, when a beautiful result has been achieved with any patient, it needs to be maintained with a suitable retainer for a long period of time. For some, the degree of change/relapse that will occur post-retention is hardly noticeable. For others it may be very marked, due to an untreated or unaccounted for underlying etiologic factor. Special needs individuals have a very high prevalence of abnormal soft tissue behavior, including tongue thrusting and abnormal anterior oral seal, which are not often amenable to treatment. Retention, therefore, is more important than for the healthy child population.

'Active' retention, with high-pull headgear, twin-blocks, and the like is sometimes needed against the recurrence of some of the more severe skeletal Class II and open bite cases. Some of these may be surgical cases from the outset, but because of their poor health or other reasons, a conservative approach had been advised.

Failures

Most of the failures that we see are due to noncompliance with the retaining devices and, inevitably, re-treatment may be necessary, although not before parent and child accept that more disciplined retention will be assured in the end. As noted above, some medical conditions may generate the adverse changes. Myopathies and cerebral palsy tend to cause further vertical growth and only some of this can be controlled with 'active' retention, even with good cooperation.

Post-treatment parental evaluation

There can be no question that those parents who request treatment for their special needs child are highly motivated and most appreciative of the efforts made in the delivery of treatment in these difficult circumstances. But they are not a random sample of parents with special needs children. Nevertheless, when polled in a survey, they expressed considerable satisfaction at the results achieved (Becker et al., 2000). From their subjective view of their child, they pointed to improvement in oral function, swallowing and drooling, speech and in their chewing movements, in addition to improvement in their facial and dental appearance. Among those children who were sufficiently aware of improvement, the parents reported greater self-confidence and a pride in their appearance (Becker et al., 2001).

Case descriptions

As noted in the introduction to this chapter, the list of medical and psychological diagnoses that may place a child in the realm of 'special needs' is inordinately long and it is beyond the scope of this chapter to describe the orthodontic management in all of them. Accordingly, a case description of the two most commonly seen conditions among special needs children in which orthodontic treatment is likely to be highly beneficial, and in which special attention needs to be given to compliance and management issues, will be presented here.

Cerebral palsy

Cerebral palsy affects 2/1000 live-born children (Longo and Hankins, 2009). It refers to a group of chronic conditions affecting body movements and muscle coordination, caused by brain damage occurring during fetal development or infancy. Cerebral palsy patients can be classified by the type of movement problem into three subgroups:

- Spastic – inability of a muscle to relax
- Athetoid – inability to control muscle movement
- Ataxic – impaired balance and coordination.

Alternatively, they may be grouped by the body parts involved, such as hemiplegia (one arm and one leg), diplegia (both legs), and quadriplegia (all the limbs, trunk, and neck). There are several associated neurological features including epilepsy, mental retardation, learning disabilities, and attention deficit-hyperactivity disorder (Blair and Watson, 2006).

The skeletal features include Class II jaw relationship, increased lower facial height, backward mandibular rotation, broad mandible and anterior open bite. The oral characteristics are uncontrolled head and tongue movements, forward tongue posture, hypotonic orofacial musculature, grossly incompetent lips, and drooling (Strodel, 1987; Rodrigues dos Santos et al., 2003). The following dental features are commonly seen: Class II Division 1 malocclusion, an anterior open bite, a posterior crossbite due to the wide mandibular dental arch, gingival inflammation and traumatized upper incisors (Franklin et al., 1996; Carmagnani et al., 2007).

Treatment need is very high (Oreland et al., 1987; Vittek et al., 1994) (Patient 1: Figures 25.1, 25.2), but these patients present a plethora of justifiable reasons why treatment is likely to be denied. Typically, they exhibit exaggerated apprehension and reduced understanding. This, together with their physical impairment and involuntary movements, undermines their ability to cooperate. In addition they have drooling (Harris and Purdy, 1987), a highly sensitive gag reflex, and poor oral hygiene (Guare Rde and Ciamponi, 2003), with food accumulation and stagnation which is largely due to poor muscle function.

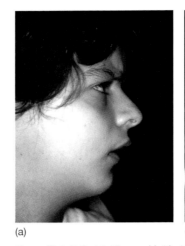 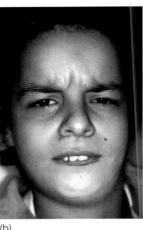

(a)   (b)

Figure 25.1 Patient 1: 10-year-old girl with ataxic cerebral palsy. Pretreatment facial photographs showing the convex profile due to marked retrusion of the mandible: (a) profile, (b) frontal.

In the case of normal children, some recent evidence is not supportive of two-phase orthodontic treatment and demonstrates that in spite of temporary skeletal change that may occur in the younger patient, early treatment does not provide patients with any advantage over those treated at a later age, in regard to the long-term outcome in Class II patients (Dolce et al., 2007; Harrison et al., 2007). It is critical to be aware that children with cerebral palsy often experience falls and, without the ability to protect themselves with their hands, traumatic injury to the maxillary incisors is more frequently seen than in normal children. It is for this reason that prevention of trauma and its consequences is mandatory and a short course of early treatment to reduce an increased overjet is to be encouraged (Patient 1: Figure 25.3). This treatment should be initiated as early as possible after eruption of the maxillary incisors, at 8–10 years of age and it should also be aimed at improving a skeletal discrepancy, by restraining the forward and downward growth of the maxilla or by encouraging forward growth of the mandible. Completion of phase 1 should see a reduction of the Class II dental relationship to allow better lip cover and thus protect these teeth from incidental trauma (Patient 1: Figure 25.4). The second justification for a phase 1 treatment is the orthodontic reduction of displaced anterior teeth following trauma, especially in cases of accidental intrusion or bucco/lingual displacement.

Following traumatic intrusion, the long-term survival of the injured tooth hangs in the balance. In the absence of timely treatment, pulp necrosis, inflammatory root resorption, ankylosis, replacement resorption and loss of marginal bone support are likely to occur (Andreasen and

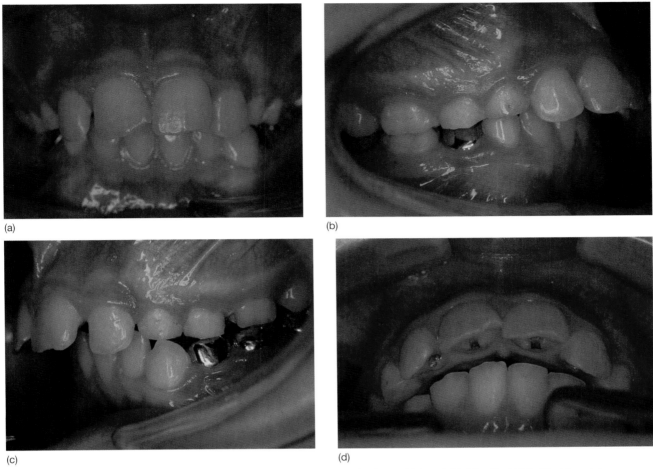

Figure 25.2 Patient 1: pretreatment intraoral views showing a Class II Division 1 malocclusion: (a) frontal, (b) right side, (c) left side, (d) overjet.

Andreasen, 1994). It should be clearly understood and appreciated that the alternative to extraction and prosthodontic replacement in the special needs population subgroup is not an option to be countenanced lightly. Three options are available for reduction and realignment of dislodged teeth (Chaushu et al., 2004):

- Observation alone, in the optimistic expectation of spontaneous re-eruption
- Immediate surgical repositioning into their presumed previous locations
- Early orthodontic repositioning, which is largely a valid procedure to be initiated during a period of up to 3 months' post-trauma.

Observation in anticipation of spontaneous re-eruption of a traumatically intruded tooth is highly unreliable, but isolated successes have been reported (Shapira et al., 1986). Nevertheless, in the more severely intruded teeth, access for

root canal therapy may then only be provided after extensive gingivectomy (Tronstad et al., 1986).

Surgical repositioning has been advocated to immediately relocate moderately or severely intruded teeth and to provide early access for root canal treatment in order to prevent infection pursuant to pulpal necrosis. However, this operation has also been reported as actually increasing the incidence of ankylosis, pulp necrosis, and loss of marginal bone (Chaushu et al., 2004; Andreasen et al., 2006).

Orthodontic repositioning of traumatically displaced teeth has been shown to be superior to the other alternatives, in terms of tooth loss during the follow-up period (Chaushu et al., 2004; Andreasen et al., 2006). Regardless of treatment approach, external inflammatory root resorption and marginal bone loss are frequent complications, and the incidence of root resorption appears to be similar between the three treatment approaches (about 40%). Marginal bone loss was higher in those teeth treated by observation

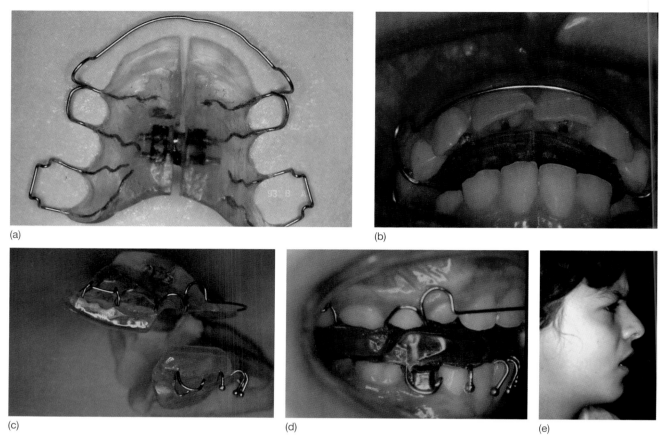

Figure 25.3 Patient 1: phase I treatment was initiated with the aim of preventing trauma by reducing the increased overjet. (a) The simple acrylic 'trainer' removable expansion appliance with anterior bite plane. (b) Removable appliance in mouth. (c) Twin-block appliance to encourage mandibular growth. (d) Twin-block appliance in mouth. (e) Profile view with twin block appliance in situ.

only than in those repositioned either in a one-step surgical approach or over time by orthodontic traction (Chaushu et al., 2004). Thus, it seems that if the tooth remains in its embedded position in the bone, there is the strong likelihood of bone loss, while if the tooth is relocated in its original position, and the normal relationship between the tooth and the bone is re-established, marginal bone loss is minimized.

The aims of phase 2 treatment are to align the teeth, to relieve crowding and to close down open bites, while maintaining the achieved skeletal sagittal interarch relationship (Patient 1: Figure 25.5). This goal is usually achieved with the use of fixed multibracketed appliances, with headgear or extraction support, in the full permanent dentition (Patient 1: Figures 25.6, 25.7).

In the presence of an abnormal growth direction, deleterious hypotonic muscle behavior and poor function, maintenance of the achieved result becomes the major concern. A regimen of active retention is sometimes needed to main-

tain the treated outcome by restraining maxillary growth, with the aid of a high-pull extraoral removable en bloc appliance (Thurow, 1975), or preventing clockwise mandibular rotation using a chincap. Despite these precautions, subsequent changes in late adolescence/early adulthood may still occur and dictate the need for a phase 3 intervention involving orthognathic surgery, although this option must only be recommended with due consideration and careful assessment of the individual patient in this subgroup of the population.

Down syndrome

Down syndrome is an autosomal genetic disorder, caused by an extra chromosome 21, with an incidence of 1/800–1000 live births. The patient has a short stature, mental retardation, and phenotypic abnormalities including oral, cardiovascular, hematopoietic, musculoskeletal, nervous, and behavioral anomalies (Hawli et al., 2009). Down syndrome individuals are prone to the development of

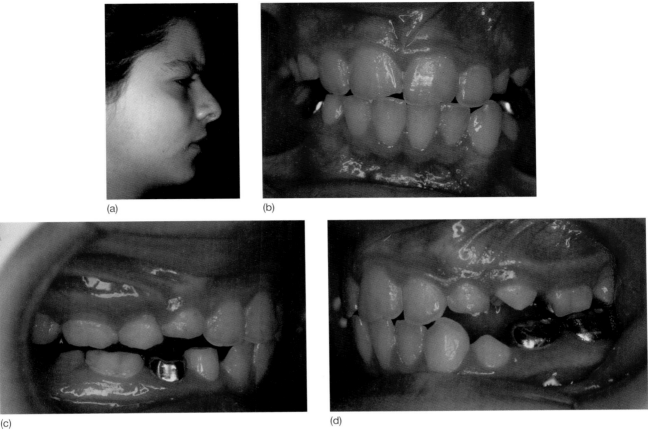

Figure 25.4 Patient 1: interim photographs at the end of phase I, showing the improvement in the appearance due to correction of the skeletal Class II skeletal relationship and the overcorrection of dental relationships. (a) Profile, (b) frontal, (c) right, and (d) left views.

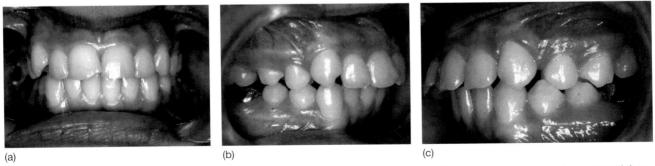

Figure 25.5 Patient 1: intraoral views before the beginning of phase II treatment with fixed appliances. The upper first left molar has been extracted due to caries with compensatory extraction of the upper second right premolar. (a) Frontal view, (b) right side, and (c) left side.

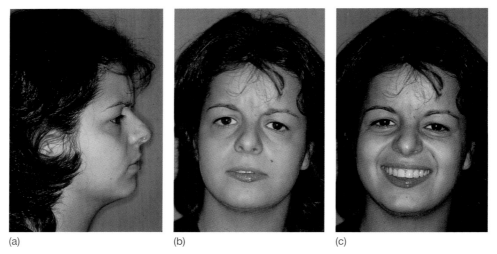

(a)   (b)   (c)

Figure 25.6 Patient 1: post-treatment facial photographs showing the marked improvement in the esthetics of the face and profile. (a) Profile, (b) frontal, and (c) smile.

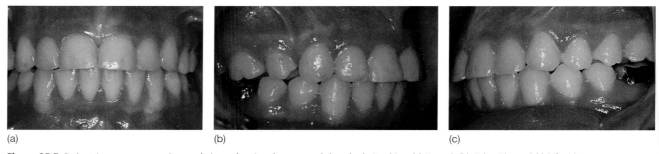

(a)   (b)   (c)

Figure 25.7 Patient 1: post-treatment intraoral views showing the corrected dental relationships. (a) Frontal, (b) right side, and (c) left side.

infectious, malignant, and autoimmune diseases (Desai, 1997). There is also a high incidence of hypothyroidism (Fort et al., 1984; Goday-Arno et al., 2009) and delayed motor function (Vicari, 2006).

Down syndrome patients are characterized by many skeletal and dental anomalies, which have been widely reported in the literature. A skeletal Class III pattern is usually present due to an underdeveloped midface. The maxilla is deficient in all three planes of space: it is retruded in the sagittal plane, narrow in the coronal plane and short in the vertical plane. The palate is V-shaped and high (Limbrock et al., 1991; Desai and Flanagan, 1999). The mandible is usually of normal size (Reuland-Bosma and Dibbets, 1991) but, because of the decreased lower facial height, there is overclosure of the mandible, resulting in a relative mandibular prognathism (Patient 2: Figures 25.8–25.10).

Down syndrome patients are characterized by many dental anomalies, including Class III dental relationship with anterior and posterior crossbites, which have been reported in the literature (Oliveira et al., 2008). Dental abnormalities in the number (fewer), size (smaller) and morphology (peg-shaped and other morphological deficiencies) (Cohen and Winer, 1965; Townsend, 1983; Peretz et al., 1996), and the timing of their development (late dentition) (Garn et al., 1970) are constant features of this syndrome. There is an increased incidence of canine/premolar transpositions and of impacted canines (Roger, 1994; Shapira et al., 2000). The tongue is large and is postured forward at rest and during function (Glatz-Noll and Berg, 1991). There is often an open mouth posture and mouth breathing, in part due to the hypotonic musculature (Morris et al., 1982; Merrick et al., 2000), and recurrent chronic upper respiratory infections (Shott, 2006). Salivary output

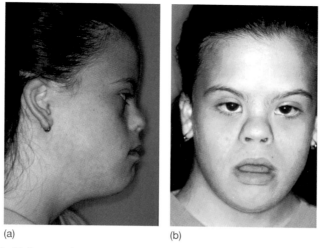

(a)   (b)

Figure 25.8 Patient 2: 13-year-old child with Down syndrome. Pretreatment facial photographs: (a) profile, (b) frontal.

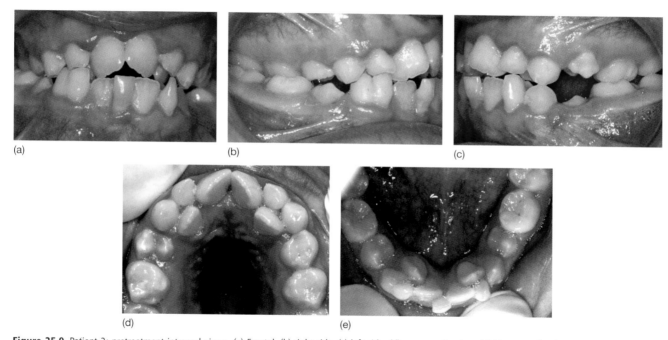

(a)   (b)   (c)

(d)   (e)

Figure 25.9 Patient 2: pretreatment intraoral views. (a) Frontal, (b) right side, (c) left side, (d) upper occlusal, and (e) lower occlusal.

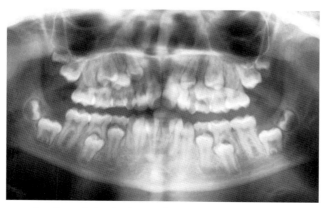

Figure 25.10 Patient 2: pretreatment panoramic radiograph showing impacted maxillary canines and a missing lower incisor.

is reduced and this is reflected as dry lips and oral mucosa, with frequent ulceration (Chaushu et al., 2002a,c, 2007). The salivary immune system is impaired – a characteristic which itself is a potential etiologic factor of the recurrent upper respiratory infection (Chaushu et al., 2002a,c). Bruxism is a common finding.

Several previous studies have shown that Down syndrome individuals have an increased prevalence of periodontal disease compared with normal, age-matched control groups and other mentally disabled patients of similar age distribution (Orner, 1976; Reuland-Bosma and van Dijk, 1986). The prevalence of periodontitis under the age of 30 is close to 100% and is in sharp contrast with the low incidence of caries (Orner, 1976). The progression and severity, as well as the clinical characteristics of the periodontal destruction reported in Down syndrome individuals, are consistent with the early-onset/aggressive periodontitis disease pattern (Shaw and Saxby, 1986; Cichon et al., 1998).

Because of the high prevalence and severity of skeletal and dental abnormalities, Down syndrome patients present high orthodontic treatment need (Oreland et al., 1987; Desai, 1997). From the skeletal point of view, they commonly need maxillary expansion and protraction, to correct/improve the skeletal Class III jaw relationship and the profile esthetics (Patient 2: Figures 25.11, 25.12). Dentally, they generally need alignment of their teeth, opening/closing spaces of congenitally missing teeth and resolution of impactions and transpositions. However, the clinician encounters many obstacles in pursuing successful orthodontic treatment. Their behavior is often problematic because of reduced understanding and increased apprehen-

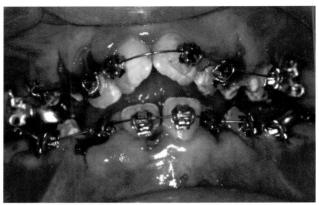

(a)

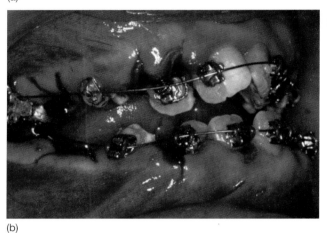

(b)

Figure 25.11 Patient 2: views at the conclusion of intravenous sedation. (a) Frontal and (b) right side.

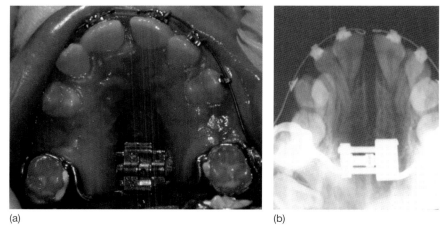

(a)   (b)

Figure 25.12 Patient 2: expansion of the upper arch. (a) Clinical view and (b) radiographic occlusal view.

sion, short attention span and limited tolerance. Although our experience shows that most of these patients can be treated at the chairside using the regular behavior management techniques, some need sedation or general anesthesia for the more extensive procedures and potentially painful appointments, such as bonding/debonding of brackets or extractions of deciduous teeth (Chaushu and Becker, 2000; Chaushu et al., 2002b). Other impediments are the increased incidence of macroglossia and open mouth posture. These, together with the hypotonic musculature that might impede closing of an anterior open bite, cause relapse of a successfully achieved result. In addition, these patients require close monitoring from the periodontal aspect because of the highly increased risk for periodontal disease. Early-onset periodontitis is an aggressive disease which should be diagnosed and treated with due attention and speed. Sometimes, the orthodontic appliances have to be removed and treatment halted during the period of periodontal treatment only to be restarted after improvement in the periodontal status has been achieved.

Dividing the orthodontic treatment into two phases is indicated in cases of significant skeletal discrepancy. In these cases, phase I treatment is performed at an age of 8–10 years and its main aim is to treat the posterior and anterior crossbite by maxillary expansion and protraction. The best way to achieve this goal is to use a banded or bonded rapid palatal expansion appliance with hooks for the simultaneous maxillary protraction with a face mask. We usually recommend the use of a custom-made facemask, which can be constructed on a plaster impression of the face. This kind of facemask fits the patient's face, can be made with clear acrylic chin and forehead pads, and is less obvious to those around. This is better accepted by the patient in comparison to those seen in an orthodontic catalog.

Phase II treatment is usually initiated at an age of 12–15 years, depending on the delay in dental age. It is aimed at aligning the teeth, closing or opening spaces of congenitally missing teeth, treating impactions and tooth transpositions (Patient 2: Figures 25.13–25.16). This treatment is performed with fixed appliances which can usually be placed at the chairside, unless multiple procedures are needed, in which case a sedation session may be planned to accommodate all of these at a single session.

In cases of severe jaw discrepancies in patients after cessation of growth, orthognathic surgery may be planned for maxillary expansion and a down-sliding advancement (Janson et al., 2009).

Conclusion

Special needs patients suffer to a greater extent and from more grotesque malocclusions than healthy patients; anxiety and apprehension levels are far greater than among their peers and they have a much reduced threshold

of understanding, tolerance, and compliance. It follows, therefore, that in order for the orthodontist to achieve therapeutic access, a structured approach to their treatment is required. This includes the need for considerably more chairside time, the exploitation of the full range of behavior management modalities and a breakdown of the treatment into individual self-contained tasks, in a modular approach. Above all, there is the essential requirement for a caring, patient, and persevering attitude on the part of the treatment delivery team, which includes the orthodontist, the chairside assistant and the parent, together with the occasional services of several other specialists, chief among them being the anesthetist.

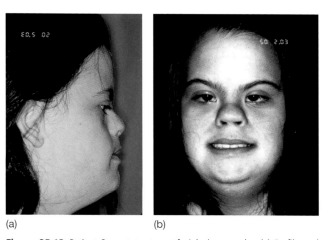

(a)   (b)

Figure 25.13 Patient 2: post-treatment facial photographs. (a) Profile and (b) frontal views.

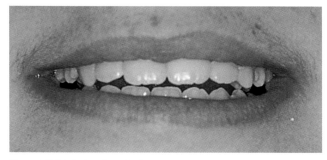

Figure 25.14 Patient 2: smile line.

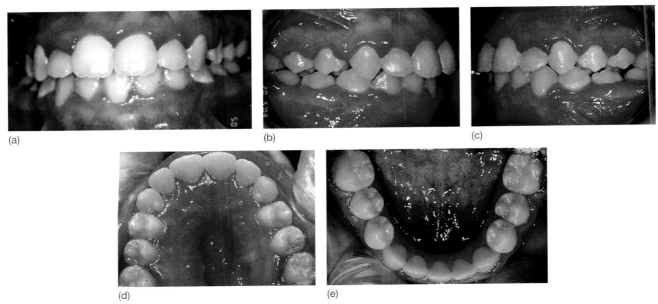

(a) (b) (c)

(d) (e)

Figure 25.15 Patient 2: post-treatment intraoral views: (a) frontal, (b) right side, (c) left side, (d) upper, and (e) lower views.

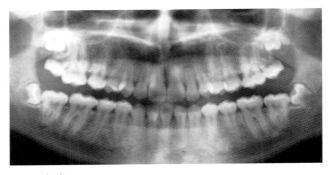

Figure 25.16 Patient 2: post-treatment panoramic view.

References

Andreasen J, Andreasen FM (1994) *Textbook and Color Atlas of Traumatic Injures to the Teeth*. Copenhagen: Munksgaard.

Andreasen JO, Bakland LK, Andreasen FM (2006) Traumatic intrusion of permanent teeth. Part A clinical study of the effect of treatment variables such as treatment delay, method of repositioning, type of splint, length of splinting and antibiotics on 140 teeth. *Dental Traumatology* 22: 99–111.

Becker A, Shapira J (1996) Orthodontics for the handicapped child. *European Journal of Orthodontics* 18: 55–67.

Becker A, Shapira J, Chaushu S (2000) Orthodontic treatment for disabled children: motivation, expectation, and satisfaction. *European Journal of Orthodontics* 22: 151–8.

Becker A, Shapira J, Chaushu S (2001) Orthodontic treatment for disabled children – a survey of patient and appliance management. *Journal of Orthodontics* 28: 39–44.

Blair E, Watson L (2006) Epidemiology of cerebral palsy. *Seminars in Fetal Neonatology and Medicine* 11: 117–25.

Carmagnani FG, Goncalves GK, Correa MS, et al. (2007) Occlusal characteristics in cerebral palsy patients. *Journal of Dentistry for Children* 74: 41–5.

Chadwick SM, Asher-McDade C (1997) The orthodontic management of patients with profound learning disability. *British Journal of Orthodontics* 24: 117–25.

Chaushu S, Becker A (2000) Behaviour management needs for the orthodontic treatment of children with disabilities. *European Journal of Orthodontics* 22: 143–9.

Chaushu S, Zeltser R, Becker A (2000) Safe orthodontic bonding for children with disabilities during general anaesthesia. *European Journal of Orthodontics* 22: 225–8.

Chaushu S, Becker A, Chaushu G, et al. (2002a) Stimulated parotid salivary flow rate in patients with Down syndrome. *Special Care Dentist* 22: 41–4.

Chaushu S, Gozal D, Becker A (2002b) Intravenous sedation: an adjunct to enable orthodontic treatment for children with disabilities. *European Journal of Orthodontics* 24: 81–9.

Chaushu S, Yefenof E, Becker A, et al. (2002c) A link between parotid salivary Ig level and recurrent respiratory infections in young Down's syndrome patients. *Oral Microbiology and Immunology* 17: 172–6.

Chaushu S, Shapira J, Heling I, et al. (2004) Emergency orthodontic treatment after the traumatic intrusive luxation of maxillary incisors. *American Journal of Orthodontics and Dentofacial Orthopedics* 126: 162–72.

Chaushu S, Chaushu G, Zigmond M, et al. (2007) Age-dependent deficiency in saliva and salivary antibodies secretion in Down's syndrome. *Archives of Oral Biology* 52: 1088–96.

Cichon P, Crawford L, Grimm WD (1998) Early-onset periodontitis associated with Down's syndrome–clinical interventional study. *Annals of Periodontology* 3: 370–80.

Cohen MM, Winer RA (1965) Dental and facial characteristics in Down's syndrome (mongolism). *Journal of Dental Research* 44(Suppl): 197–208.

Desai SS (1997) Down syndrome: a review of the literature. *Oral Surgery Oral Medicine Oral Pathology Oral Radiology and Endodontics* 84: 279–85.

Desai SS, Flanagan TJ (1999) Orthodontic considerations in individuals with Down syndrome: a case report. *Angle Orthodontist* 69: 85–8.

Dolce C, McGorray SP, Brazeau L, et al. (2007) Timing of Class II treatment: skeletal changes comparing 1-phase and 2-phase treatment. *American Journal of Orthodontics and Dentofacial Orthopedics* 132: 481–9.

Fort P, Lifshitz F, Bellisario R, et al. (1984) Abnormalities of thyroid function in infants with Down syndrome. *Journal of Pediatrics* 104: 545–9.

Franklin DL, Luther F, Curzon ME (1996) The prevalence of malocclusion in children with cerebral palsy. *European Journal of Orthodontics* 18: 637–43.

Garn SM, Stimson CW, Lewis AB (1970) Magnitude of dental delay in trisomy G. *Journal of Dental Research* 49: 640.

Glatz-Noll E, Berg R (1991) Oral dysfunction in children with Down's syndrome: an evaluation of treatment effects by means of video registration. *European Journal of Orthodontics* 13: 446–51.

Goday-Arno A, Cerda-Esteva M, Flores-Le-Roux JA, et al. (2009) Hyperthyroidism in a population with Down syndrome (DS). *Clinical Endocrinology* 71: 110–14.

Guare Rde O, Ciamponi AL (2003) Dental caries prevalence in the primary dentition of cerebral-palsied children. *Journal of Clinical Pediatric Dentistry* 27: 287–92.

Harris SR, Purdy AH (1987) Drooling and its management in cerebral palsy. *Developmental Medicine and Child Neurology* 29: 807–11.

Harrison JE, O'Brien KD, Worthington HV (2007) Orthodontic treatment for prominent upper front teeth in children. *Cochrane Database Systematic Reviews* 3: CD003452.

Hawli Y, Nasrallah M, El-Hajj Fuleihan G (2009) Endocrine and musculoskeletal abnormalities in patients with Down syndrome. *Nature Reviews Endocrinology* 5: 327–34.

Jackson EF (1967) Orthodontics and the retarded child. *American Journal of Orthodontics* 53: 596–605.

Janson M, Janson G, Sant'Ana E, et al. (2009) Orthognathic treatment for a patient with Class III malocclusion and surgically restricted mandible. *American Journal of Orthodontics and Dentofacial Orthopedics* 136: 290–8.

Lew KK (1993) Attitudes and perceptions of adults towards orthodontic treatment in an Asian community. *Community Dentistry and Oral Epidemiology* 21: 31–5.

Limbrock GJ, Fischer-Brandies H, Avalle C (1991) Castillo-Morales' orofacial therapy: treatment of 67 children with Down syndrome. *Developmental Medicine and Child Neurology* 33: 296–303.

Longo M, Hankins GD (2009) Defining cerebral palsy: pathogenesis, pathophysiology and new intervention. *Minerva Ginecologica* 61: 421–9.

Malamed S (1995) *Sedation: A Guide to Patient Management*. St. Louis, MO: Mosby.

Merrick J, Ezra E, Josef B, et al. (2000) Musculoskeletal problems in Down Syndrome European Paediatric Orthopaedic Society Survey: the Israeli sample. *Journal of Pediatric Orthopedics Part B* 9: 185–92.

Morris AF, Vaughan SE, Vaccaro P (1982) Measurements of neuromuscular tone and strength in Down's syndrome children. *Journal of Mental Deficiency Research* 26: 41–6.

Oliveira AC, Paiva SM, Campos MR, et al. (2008) Factors associated with malocclusions in children and adolescents with Down syndrome. *American Journal of Orthodontics and Dentofacial Orthopedics* 133: 489. e1–8.

Oreland A, Heijbel J, Jagell S (1987). Malocclusions in physically and/or mentally handicapped children. *Swedish Dental Journal* 11: 103–19.

Orner G (1976) Periodontal disease among children with Down's syndrome and their siblings. *Journal of Dental Research* 55: 778–82.

Peretz B, Shapira J, Farbstein H, et al. (1996) Modification of tooth size and shape in Down's syndrome. *Journal of Anatomy* 188(Pt 1): 167–72.

Proffit W, Fields HW, Sarver DM (2007) *Contemporary Orthodontics*. Elsevier, St Louis, MO.

Reuland-Bosma W, Dibbets JM (1991) Mandibular and dental development subsequent to thyroid therapy in a boy with Down syndrome: report of case. *ASDC Journal of Dentistry for Children* 58: 64–8.

Reuland-Bosma W, van Dijk J (1986) Periodontal disease in Down's syndrome: a review. *Journal of Clinical Periodontology* 13: 64–73.

Rodrigues dos Santos MT, Masiero D, Novo NF, et al. (2003) Oral conditions in children with cerebral palsy. *Journal of Dentistry for Children* 70: 40–6.

Roger K (1994) Facial dysmorphism and syndrome diagnosis. In: K Roger (ed.) *Pediatric Orofacial Medicine and Pathology*. London: Chapman and Hall Medical Co., pp. 42–74.

Shapira J, Regev L, Liebfeld H (1986) Re-eruption of completely intruded immature permanent incisors. *Endodontics and Dental Traumatology* 2: 113–16.

Shapira J, Becker A, Moskovitz M (1999) The management of drooling problems in children with neurological dysfunction: a review and case report. *Special Care Dentist* 19: 181–5.

Shapira J, Chaushu S, Becker A (2000) Prevalence of tooth transposition, third molar agenesis, and maxillary canine impaction in individuals with Down syndrome. *Angle Orthodontist* 70: 290–6.

Shaw L, Saxby MS (1986) Periodontal destruction in Down's syndrome and in juvenile periodontitis. How close a similarity? *Journal of Periodontology* 57: 709–15.

Shaw WC (1981) The influence of children's dentofacial appearance on their social attractiveness as judged by peers and lay adults. *American Journal of Orthodontics* 79: 399–415.

Shaw WC, Addy M, Ray C (1980) Dental and social effects of malocclusion and effectiveness of orthodontic treatment: a review. *Community Dentistry and Oral Epidemiology* 8: 36–45.

Shott SR (2006) Down syndrome: common otolaryngologic manifestations. *American Journal of Medical Genetics Part C Seminars in Medical Genetics* 142C: 131–40.

Sticker G (1970) Psychological issues pertaining to malocclusion. *American Journal of Orthodontics* 58: 276–83.

Strodel BJ (1987) The effects of spastic cerebral palsy on occlusion. *ASDC Journal of Dentistry for Children* 54: 255–60.

Thomas RG (1979) Indirect bonding: simplicity in action. *Journal of Clinical Orthodontics* 13: 93–106.

Thurow RC (1975) Craniomaxillary orthopedic correction with en masse dental control. *American Journal of Orthodontics* 68: 601–24.

Townsend GC (1983) Tooth size in children and young adults with trisomy 21 (Down) syndrome. *Archives of Oral Biology* 28: 159–66.

Tronstad L, Trope M, Bank M, et al. (1986) Surgical access for endodontic treatment of intruded teeth. *Endodontics and Dental Traumatology* 2: 75–8.

Vicari S (2006) Motor development and neuropsychological patterns in persons with Down syndrome. *Behaviour Genetics* 36: 355–64.

Vittek J, Winik S, Winik A, et al. (1994) Analysis of orthodontic anomalies in mentally retarded developmentally disabled (MRDD) persons. *Special Care Dentist* 14: 198–202.

Waldman HB, Perlman SP, Swerdloff M (2000) Orthodontics and the population with special needs. *American Journal of Orthodontics and Dentofacial Orthopedics* 118: 14–17.

Index

Aarskog syndrome 114, 120
abfraction 60
abrasion of teeth 60
  see also enamel demineralization and
    erosion
acetylsalicylic acid 48
achondroplasia 42, 105–6, 114, 148–9
acromegaly 43–4, 183, 184
actinomycosis 244, 248–9
activator appliance 220
acute necrotizing ulcerative gingivitis
    (ANUG) 244, 245
acute suppurative parotitis (ASP) 246–7
Addison's disease 50, 192
adenoid cystic carcinomas 327–30
adenoidectomies 201–3
adenoids 196–7
  anomalies 197–201
  investigations 222–7
  removal 201–3
adhesives, biomimetic 375–6
adolescence 77
  diet and food choices 89
adrenal disorders, general 192
adrenal insufficiency 183, 192
aerobic infections, affecting oral cavity
    243–5
agenesis see dental agenesis
airway imaging 198–9, 222
airway obstruction
  ENT referrals 197–201
  impact on facial length 199–201
  measurement and evaluation 198–9
  otolaryngology 201–3
  see also obstructive sleep apnea (OSA)
alcohol use 6
  see also fetal alcohol syndrome
allergens 47, 373
allergic disorders 47
allografts 389, 403–18
  see also alveolar bone grafts
alopecia totalis 9, 11
alveolar bone grafts 162–3, 401–2
  contraindications 415–16
  future research needs 418
  harvesting methods 406–8
  post-surgery evaluations 411–12
  surgical protocols 408–11
  transmucal penetration and cell
    rejuvenation 412–15
  use of stem cell technologies 401–18

alveolar bone modelling 169–70, 171,
    394–6
  with stem cell technologies 401–18
alveolar cleft closures 162–3
alveolar drift 169–70
amelo-onchohypohydrotic dysplasia 113
amelogenesis imperfecta 60–2, 109, 112,
    114
American Board of Clinical Geneticists
    (ABMG) 110–11
anemia
  hemolytic 47
  sickle cell 47–8
angiomas, facial 39
Angle, Edward Hartley 2, 380
ankylosis of teeth 303–5
anorexia nervosa 60, 89
  impact on orthodontic treatment 88
antidepressants 87
antipsychotics 87
antiviral agents 47
ANUG see acute necrotizing ulcerative
    gingivitis (ANUG)
anxieties over treatment, underlying causes
    70
Apert syndrome 42, 113–14, 143–8
apexification techniques 293–5
apnea 214
  see also obstructive sleep apnea
appearance concerns 69–70
appliances (general considerations)
  cariogenic problems 286
  pulpal reactions 286–8
  see also biomedical engineering;
    individual named appliances;
    materials science
application service provider (ASP) solutions
    17
appointment scheduling, IT software 16
archwires
  coatings 371–2
  mechanical properties 369–72
  nonmetallic 368–9
  surface properties 366–8
archwire-bracket friction studies 366–8
asthma 46
attention deficit hyperactivity disorder
    (ADHD) 77
attractiveness 72–3
  ethno-cultural differences 75–6
  perceptual basis 73–4

physical basis 73
  quantitative analysis 74–5
audiological tests 206–7
autoimmune diseases 6–7, 39–40, 49, 114,
    254–5
autoimmune polyendocrinopathy 114
autotransplantation 300–3
azotemia 47

bacterial infections 241–8
  management principles 397–8
  within oral cavity 243–5, 397–400
basal cell carcinoma (nevoid) 42, 112,
    113–14, 123
Binder syndrome see maxillonasal
    dysplasia
bio-Oss 389
bioglass materials 389
biological status of patient 5–9
biomaterials 383–4
  design requirements 383
  see also tissue engineering
biomedical engineering
  background and past research
    366–73
    archwire-bracket friction 366–8
    fabrication of nonmetallic archwires
      368–9
    force measurements 372
    mechanical properties of archwires
      369–72
    use of finite element analysis
      372–3
  current studies and potential applications
    373–7
    biomimetic adhesives 375–6
    brackets with force measurement
      centres 375
    self-cleaning materials 376–7
    self-healing materials 374–5
    shape memory polymers 373–4
  see also tissue engineering
biomedical engineers 366
bisphosphonate treatment, jaw necrosis
    174
blastomycosis 259
bleeding disorders 49, 50
bleeding index 398
Bloch-Sulzberger syndrome see
    incontinentia pigmenti
blood transfusions 49

Integrated Clinical Orthodontics, First Edition. Edited by Vinod Krishnan, Ze'ev Davidovitch.
© 2012 Blackwell Publishing Ltd. Published 2012 by Blackwell Publishing Ltd.